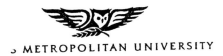

1996 UPDATE

Core Concepts in Health

Brief Seventh Edition

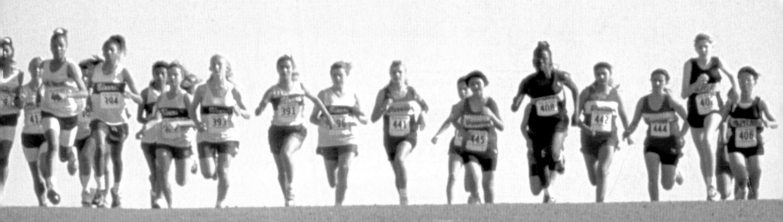

Paul M. Insel • Walton T. Roth
Stanford University

L. McKay Rollins • Ray A. Petersen
Brigham Young University

Mayfield Publishing Company
Mountain View, California
London • Toronto

Library of Congress Cataloging-in-Publication Data
Core concepts in health / Paul M. Insel . . . [et al.]. -- Brief 7th ed.
    p.   cm.
    "1996 update"
    Includes bibliographical references and index.
    ISBN 1–55934–540–3
    1. Health. I. Insel, Paul M.
RA776.C83 1994b
613—dc20
                         93–19012
                             CIP

Manufactured in the United States of America
10 9 8 7 6 5 4 3 2 1

Mayfield Publishing Company
1280 Villa Street
Mountain View, California 94041

Sponsoring editor, Serina Beauparlant; *developmental editors,* Kirstan Price and Kathleen Engelberg; *production editors,* Lynn Rabin Bauer and Carol Zafiropoulos; *manuscript editor,* Joan Pendleton; *art director and cover designer,* Jeanne M. Schreiber; *text designer,* Detta Penna; *illustrators,* Dale Glasgow, Robin Mouat, Kevin Somerville, Pamela Drury Wattenmaker; *photo researcher,* Melissa Kreischer; *cover photographer,* © Tony Stone Images/Don Lowe; *proofreader,* Carol Carter; *manufacturing manager,* Randy Hurst. This text was set in 10.5/12 Berkeley Book by Graphic Typesetting Services and printed on 45# Chromatone LG by Banta Company.

Text and photo credits

Sources

Page 86, "What's Lurking in Your Family Tree" Copyright 1992 by Consumers Union of U.S., Inc., Yonkers, NY 10703-1057. Reprinted by permission from Consumer Reports on Health, September 1992.

Page 221, Reprinted from June 1994 *Mayo Clinic Health Letter* with permission of Mayo Foundation for Medical Education and Research, Rochester, MN 55905. For subscription information, call 1-800-333-9037.

Photo Credits

Chapter 1, pg. 1, © David Madison 1990; pg. 5, © Anthony Edgeworth/The Stock Market; pg. 11, © Bob Daemmrich/The Image Works; pg. 14, © Sam Forencich

Chapter 2, pg.19, © David Young-Wolff/PhotoEdit; pg. 21, © Tony Savino/The Image Works; pg. 27, © Tony Freeman/PhotoEdit; pg. 30, © Jeff Zaruba/The Stock Market

Chapter 3, pg. 36, © Jonathan A. Meyers/JAM Photography; pg. 39, © Suzanne Arms; pg. 40, © Elizabeth Crews; pg. 48, © 1992 B. Kramer/Custom Medical Stock Photo

Chapter 4, pg. 52, © Dorothy Littell Greco 1992/Stock Boston; pg. 54, © Frank Siteman/Stock Boston; pg. 60, © Suzanne Arms; pg. 66, © Phil Borden/PhotoEdit

Chapter 5, pg. 70, © Suzanne Arms; pg. 75, © Bob Daemmrich/The Image Works; pg. 81, © Joel Gordon 1992; pg. 91, © Alexander Tsiaras/Stock Boston; pg. 98, © Suzanne Arms

Chapter 6, pg. 102, © Joel Gordon; pg. 104, © Joel Gordon 1991; pg. 105, © Jonathan A. Meyers/JAM Photography; pg. 106, © Joel Gordon 1991; pg. 109, © Joel Gordon 1988; pg. 111, © Joel Gordon; pg. 120, © Joel Gordon 1988 (left); pg. 120, © Joel Gordon 1992 (right)

Chapter 7, pg. 127, © Bob Daemmrich/The Image Works; pg. 130, © Mary Kate Denny/PhotoEdit; pg. 135, © Edrington/The Image Works; pg. 146 © Stacy Pick/Stock Boston

Chapter 8, pg. 155, © G. Azar/The Image Works; pg. 164, © Owen Franken/Stock Boston; pg. 173, © Mugshots 1989/Gabe Palmer/ The Stock Market

Chapter 9, pg. 178, © Mark Antman/The Image Works; pg. 181, © Bob Daemmrich/Stock Boston; pg. 186, © L. Dardelet/Explorer/ Photo Researchers; pg. 193, © Charles Gupton/Stock Boston

Chapter 10, pg. 205, © David Madison 1989; pg. 206, © Bob Daemmrich/Stock Boston; pg. 212, © David Madison 1992; pg. 220, © Jonathan A. Meyers/JAM Photography 1993

Chapter 11, pg. 229, © David Madison 1992; pg. 231, © Jon Feingersh/The Stock Market; pg. 233, © 1988 David H. Wells/The Image Works; pg. 241, © David Madison 1991

Chapter 12, pg. 249, © J. Griffin/The Image Works; pg. 254, © Joel Gordon 1991; pg. 270, © David Austen/Stock Boston; pg. 275, © 1987 Blair Seitz/Photo Researchers

Chapter 13, pg. 284, © Omikron/Photo Researchers; pg. 289, © 1991 Aaron Haupt/Stock Boston; pg. 298, © Joel Gordon 1991; pg. 306, © Joseph Gianetti/Stock Boston

Chapter 14, pg. 311, © Matthew McVay/Stock Boston; pg. 316, © Joel Gordon 1991; pg. 323, © Lynne Ann DeSpelder 1989; pg. 330, © Bob Daemmrich/The Image Works

Chapter 15, pg. 335, © James R. Fisher 1982/Photo Researchers; pg. 336, © Frank Siteman 1992/Stock Boston; pg. 337, © Rafael Macia/Photo Researchers; pg. 342, © 1995 David Toy

Preface to the Brief Seventh Edition

Now in its seventh edition, *Core Concepts in Health* has maintained its leadership in the field of health education for nearly 20 years. Since we pioneered the concept of self-responsibility for personal health in 1976, hundreds of thousands of students have used our book to become active, informed participants in their own health care. Each edition of *Core Concepts* has brought improvements and refinements, but the principles underlying the book have remained the same. Our commitment to these principles has never been stronger than it is today, and it is reflected as fully in this Brief Edition as in the Seventh Edition of *Core Concepts* on which this edition is based. We have prepared the Brief Edition to accommodate instructors whose courses—sometimes carrying only one hour of credit—afford too little time for the complete range of topics and the level of detail of the larger edition.

OUR GOALS

Our goals in writing this book can be stated simply:

- To present scientifically based, accurate, up-to-date information in an accessible format
- To involve students in taking responsibility for their health and well-being
- To instill a sense of competence and personal power in students

The first of these goals means making expert knowledge about health and health care available to the individual. *Core Concepts* brings scientifically based, accurate, up-to-date information to students about topics and issues that concern them—exercise, stress, nutrition, weight management, contraception, intimate relationships, HIV infection, drugs, alcohol, and a multitude of others. Current, complete, and straightforward coverage is balanced with "user-friendly" features designed to make the text appealing. Written in an engaging, easy-to-read style and presented in a colorful, open format, *Core Concepts* invites the student to read, learn, and remember. Boxes, tables, artwork, photographs, and many other features highlight areas of special interest throughout the book.

The second of our goals is to involve students in taking responsibility for their health. *Core Concepts* uses innovative pedagogy and unique interactive features to get students thinking about how the material they're reading relates to their own lives. We invite them to examine their emotions about the issues under discussion, to consider their personal values and beliefs, and to analyze their health-related behaviors. Beyond this, for students who want to change behaviors that detract from a healthy lifestyle, we offer guidelines and tools, ranging from samples of health journals and personal contracts to detailed assessments and behavior change strategies.

Perhaps our third goal in writing *Core Concepts in Health* is the most important: to instill a sense of competence and personal power in the students who read the book. Everyone has the ability to monitor, understand, and affect his or her own health. Although the medical and health professions possess impressive skills and have access to a huge body of knowledge that benefits everyone in our society, people can help to minimize the amount of professional care they actually require in their lifetime by taking care of their health—taking charge of their health—from an early age. Our hope is that *Core Concepts* will continue to help young people make this exciting discovery—that they have the power to shape their own futures.

CONTENT OF THE BRIEF EDITION

The Brief Seventh Edition of *Core Concepts* focuses on the health issues and concerns of greatest importance to students. The content of this edition remains essentially the same as the Brief Sixth Edition, with coverage of stress, mental health, intimate relationships, sexuality, substance use and abuse, nutrition, weight management, exercise, cardiovascular disease, cancer, sexually transmissible diseases, and aging. Because of the growing recognition of the close connection between humans and their environment, we have included a new chapter on environmental health (Chapter 15) in this edition.

For this edition, all chapters were carefully reviewed, revised, and updated. The latest information from scientific and health-related research is incorporated in the text, and newly emerging topics and issues are discussed. The following list gives a sample of some of the current concerns addressed in the seventh edition:

- The changing profile of the epidemic of HIV infection and the latest approaches to treatment
- The new food labels and the Food Guide Pyramid
- The newest contraceptive methods, including the female condom, contraceptive implants, and Depo-Provera injections

- Effects of environmental tobacco smoke on nonsmokers
- Physician-assisted suicide
- Family violence
- The links between people's feelings and states of mind and their physical health
- Destruction of the ozone layer
- Hostility and heart disease
- Alzheimer's disease

Of course, the health field is dynamic, with new discoveries, advances, trends, and theories reported every week. Ongoing research—on the role of a high-fat diet in certain cancers, for example, or on the genetic links in Alzheimer's disease—continually changes our understanding of the human body and how it works. For this reason, no health book can claim to have the final word on every topic. Yet within these limits, *Core Concepts* does present the latest available information and scientific thinking on innumerable topics.

A NEW LOOK

One thing that will be immediately apparent to past users of *Core Concepts* is that the book has a fresh and exciting new look. *Core Concepts* has always set the standard in the field for innovative graphics and illustrations, and this edition is no exception. A major part of this new look is the illustration program, which includes new renderings of the best art from the sixth edition and many new illustrations. Much of the anatomical art has been prepared by a medical illustrator in a dramatic new style that is both visually appealing and highly informative. These illustrations help students understand such important information as how blood flows through the heart; how the digestive system works; how stress affects the body; and how to use a diaphragm. Many graphs, charts, and other illustrations have also been rendered in a dynamic, colorful, and appealing new style. These lively and abundant illustrations will particularly benefit those students who learn best from visual images.

The overall design of the book itself is also new—more dynamic, more colorful, and better able to catch and hold students' attention. A compelling photographic image appears at the opening of each chapter, suggesting an important theme of that chapter; the photos within the chapters are all in color and most are new. All the chapter elements have been designed and coordinated to make each page both visually appealing and easy for students to read and follow.

Taken together, these visual elements—new design, new illustrations, new photos—provide powerful pedagogical tools and create a colorful and inviting look.

FEATURES OF THE BRIEF SEVENTH EDITION

As a concise version of the Seventh Edition of *Core Concepts in Health*, this Brief Edition builds on the features that attracted and held our readers' interest in the previous six editions. One of the most popular features has always been the **boxes**, which allow us to explore a wide range of current topics in greater detail than is possible in the text itself. Over half the boxes are new to the seventh edition, and many others have been significantly revised or updated. A major change to the box program in this edition is the division of the boxes into five categories, each marked with a unique icon and label.

 Dimensions of Diversity boxes are part of our commitment to reflect and respond to the diversity of the student population. These boxes give students the opportunity to identify any special health risks that affect them because of who they are, as individuals or as members of a group. They also broaden students' perspectives by exposing them to a wide variety of viewpoints on health-related issues. The different dimensions reflected include gender, socioeconomic status, race or ethnicity, and age. The principles embodied by these boxes are described in the first box in the series, "Health Issues for Diverse Populations," which appears in Chapter 1. Topics covered in later chapters include special risks for women who smoke, variations in alcohol metabolism, and attitudes toward aging and the elderly.

In addition, some of the Dimensions of Diversity boxes highlight health issues and practices in other parts of the world, allowing students to see what Americans share with people in other societies and how they differ. Students have the opportunity to learn about laws and attitudes toward contraception in other countries, the pattern of HIV infection around the world, and other topics of interest.

 Sound Mind, Sound Body boxes explore the close connection between mind and body. Drawn from studies in psychoneuroimmunology, these boxes focus on total wellness by examining the links between people's feelings and states of mind and their physical health. By looking at these boxes, students can learn how stress affects the immune system, for example; the health benefits of intimate relationships; the links between hostility and cardiovascular disease; how exercise affects mood; and so on.

 A Closer Look boxes highlight current health topics of particular interest to students. Topics include the common cold, family violence, condoms, preventive medicine for healthy adults, and physician-assisted suicide.

Tactics and Tips boxes distill from each chapter the practical advice students need in order to apply information to their own lives. By referring to these boxes, students can easily find ways to reduce the amount of fat in their diets, to support their immune systems, to protect themselves from drunk drivers, to improve communication in their relationships, to use medications safely and effectively, and so on.

Vital Statistics boxes, figures, and tables highlight important facts and figures in a memorable format that often reveals surprising contrasts and connections. From boxes, tables, and figures marked with the Vital Statistics label, students can learn about drinking among college students, world population growth, the average American diet, cancer incidence, and a wealth of other information. For students who grasp a subject best when it is displayed graphically, numerically, or in a list or table, the Vital Statistics feature provides an alternative way of approaching and understanding the text.

In addition to the new box program, the most popular and useful features of *Core Concepts* have been retained and revised for this edition. **Personal Insight** is a revised and broadened version of Exploring Your Emotions, a feature that appeared in previous editions of *Core Concepts*. Each Personal Insight asks open-ended questions designed to encourage self-examination and heighten students' awareness of their feelings, values, beliefs, thought processes, and past experiences. These questions have been formulated in a nonjudgmental way to foster honest self-analysis, and they appear at appropriate points throughout the chapter.

Take Action, appearing at the end of every chapter, suggests hands-on exercises and projects that students can undertake to extend and deepen their grasp of the material. Suggested projects include interviews, investigations of campus or community resources, and experimentation with some of the behavior change techniques suggested in the text. Special care has been taken to ensure that the projects are both feasible and worthwhile.

New to the seventh edition is **Journal Entry**, a feature which also appears at the end of each chapter. These entries suggest ways for students to use their Health Journal (which we recommend they keep while using *Core Concepts*) to think about topics and issues, explore their own views, and express their thoughts in written form. They are designed to help students deepen their awareness and understanding of their own health-related behaviors.

Making wise choices about health requires students to sort through and evaluate health information. To help students become skilled evaluators, each chapter contains at least one **Critical Thinking** Journal Entry. These entries help students develop their critical thinking skills, including finding relevant information, separating fact from opinion, recognizing faulty reasoning, evaluating information, and assessing the credibility of sources. Critical Thinking Journal Entry questions do not have right or wrong answers; rather, they ask students to analyze, evaluate, or take a stand on a particular issue.

The **Behavior Change Strategies** that conclude many chapters offer specific behavior management/modification plans relating to the chapter's topic. Based on the principles of behavior management that are carefully explained in Chapter 1, these strategies will help students change unhealthy or counterproductive behaviors. Included are strategies for dealing with test anxiety, quitting smoking, planning a personal exercise program, phasing in a healthier diet, and many other practical plans for change.

An innovative **Built-In Study Guide** is included in the back of the book. Printed on perforated pages for easy removal, the study guide provides sample test questions to help students prepare for examinations, plus additional opportunities for self-assessment in the form of Wellness Worksheets.

New and revised tables also add interest to the text. From the tables students can quickly learn about such topics as the effects of smoking, the fat content of foods, and guidelines for cholesterol and blood pressure levels.

Also designed for quick reference is the **appendix,** "The Facts About Fast Food," following Chapter 9 (Nutrition Facts and Fallacies). It provides students with a handy guide to the nutritional content of the most commonly ordered menu items at seven popular fast food restaurants. Especially useful is the information about the fat and sodium content of each item and its proportion of fat calories to total calories. A "Red Cross First Aid Chart" appears inside the back cover of the text, providing information that can save lives. These guides offer students the kind of information they can keep and use for years to come.

LEARNING AIDS

Although all the features of *Core Concepts in Health* are designed to facilitate learning, several specific learning aids have also been incorporated into the text. **Chapter outlines** provide an overview of the contents of the following pages, orienting students at the outset of each new subject area. Important terms appear in boldface type in the text and are defined in a **running glossary,** helping students handle a large and complex new vocabulary.

Chapter summaries offer students a concise review and a way to make sure they have grasped the most important concepts in the chapter. Also found at the end of every chapter are **selected bibliographies** and annotated **recommended readings,** which have been expanded and carefully updated for this edition. Students can use these lists to extend and broaden their knowledge of particular topics or pursue subjects of interest to them. A complete **index** at the end of the book includes references to glossary terms in boldface type.

TEACHING TOOLS

Available to qualified adopters of the Brief Edition of *Core Concepts in Health* is a comprehensive package of supplementary materials that enhance teaching and learning. Included in the package are the following items:

- Instructor's Resource Guide
- Wellness Worksheets
- Transparency acetates
- Videotapes
- Health Risk Appraisal software
- Nutrition Analysis software
- Brownstone Academic Management System

The **Instructor's Resource Guide** for the Brief Edition contains a variety of teaching aids, all revised and updated for the seventh edition: learning objectives for each chapter; extended chapter outlines; suggestions for student activities; listings of additional resources, including films, books, and periodicals; and health crossword puzzles. The guide includes a complete set of examination questions that provides instructors with a large bank of questions to choose from when creating tests. The multiple choice and true/false questions have been carefully reviewed, and the answer keys list the page number in the text where the answer is found. The Instructor's Resource Guide also includes more than 60 transparency masters, providing additional lecture resources for instructors.

A set of 80 **Wellness Worksheets** helps students become more involved in their own health and be better prepared to implement successful behavior change programs. Most of the worksheets provide assessment tools that help students learn more about their health-related attitudes and behaviors. Some are strictly knowledge-based and help increase students' comprehension of key concepts. Seventeen of the Wellness Worksheets are included in the built-in study guide located at the end of the Brief Edition; the complete set of 80 worksheets is available in an easy-to-use pad for students.

The set of **transparency acetates,** many in full color, provides material suitable for lecture and discussion purposes. These acetates do not duplicate the transparency masters in the Instructor's Resource Guide, and many of them are from sources other than the text.

Our exciting **videotapes** give instructors the opportunity to illustrate and extend coverage of the most current and compelling health-related topics treated in the text. For information about the videos, instructors should contact their Mayfield representative or call 1-800-433-1279.

The computerized **Health Risk Appraisal software** package provides students with a self-assessment tool that alerts them to their personal risk areas and advises them on how to improve their risk profile. Designed for IBM-compatible computers, the program provides a detailed two-page report for each user.

The completely new **Nutrition Analysis software** package allows students to assess their current daily diet, evaluate menus, and compare their diets to current nutrition guidelines. Students receive a printout that includes an easy-to-understand scoring system and suggestions for improving food choices.

The **Brownstone Academic Management System** gives instructors a powerful, easy-to-use method of handling time-consuming tasks such as creating tests and calculating and entering grades. It is available for IBM-compatible and Apple computers. The Microtest program from the Chariot Software Group is available for Macintosh computer users.

A NOTE OF THANKS

The efforts of innumerable people have gone into producing this Brief Edition of *Core Concepts in Health.* The book has benefited immensely from their thoughtful commentaries, expert knowledge and opinions, and many helpful suggestions. We are deeply grateful for their participation in the project.

Academic Contributors

Roger Baxter, M.D., Internist and Infectious Disease Specialist, Kaiser Permanente Medical Center, Oakland, California
Immunity and Infection

Virginia Brooke, Ph.D., University of Texas at Galveston
The Challenge of Aging

Boyce Burge, Ph.D., *Healthline*
Cardiovascular Disease and Cancer

Thomas Fahey, Ed.D., California State University, Chico
Exercise for Health and Fitness

Paul Insel, Ph.D., Stanford University
Taking Charge of Your Health; Stress: The Constant Challenge; Tobacco and Alcohol; The Use and Abuse of Psychoactive Drugs; Cardiovascular Disease and Cancer

Bea Mandel, R.N., M.P.H., Executive Director, PRIDE, College of Health and Human Development, Pennsylvania State University
Immunity and Infection

Joyce D. Nash, Ph.D., Pacific Graduate School of Psychology
Weight Management

David Quadagno, Ph.D., Florida State University
Sexuality, Pregnancy, and Childbirth

Walton T. Roth, M.D., Stanford University School of Medicine
Mental Health

James H. Rothenberger, M.P.H., University of Minnesota
Environmental Health

Albert Lee Strickland and Lynne Ann Despelder, Cabrillo College
The Challenge of Aging

Bryan Strong, Ph.D., University of California at Santa Cruz, and Christine DeVault
Intimate Relationships; Sexuality, Pregnancy, and Childbirth

Jared R. Tinklenberg, M.D., Palo Alto Veterans Administration Medical Center and Stanford University
Tobacco and Alcohol

Mae V. Tinklenberg, R.N., N.P., M.S., Fair Oaks Family Health Center
Contraception and Abortion: Current Issues

Gordon Wardlaw, Ph.D., R.D., Ohio State University
Nutrition Facts and Fallacies

Academic Advisers and Reviewers

Carolyn M. Allred, Central Piedmont Community College
Dianne Bartley, Middle Tennessee State University
Lori J. Bechtel, Pennsylvania State University, Altoona Campus
Michael S. Davidson, Montclair State University
Thomas M. Davis, University of Northern Iowa
Jan Dodson, Middle Tennessee State University
David F. Duncan, Brown University
R. Daniel Duquette, University of Wisconsin at La Crosse
Cheryl Ellis, Middle Tennessee State University
Mary E. Etherington, California State University, Northridge
Marilyn Green, Middle Tennessee State University
Jo Hill, New Mexico State University
Roberta B. Hollander, Howard University
Catherine E. King, Floyd College
Mark J. Kittleson, Southern Illinois University
Becky Kennedy Koch, Ohio State University
Loretta Liptak, Youngstown State University
Beverly Saxton Mahoney, Pennsylvania State University
Anne Nadakavukaren, Illinois State University
Sandra Neal, Middle Tennessee State University
James V. Noto, San Diego State University
Judy Oaks, Director, Center for Personal Recovery
Anne O'Donnell, Santa Rosa Junior College
Andrea Port Jacobs, Howard Community College
Bruce M. Ragon, Indiana University
Kerry J. Redican, Virginia Polytechnic Institute and State University
Janet Reis, University of Illinois at Urbana-Champaign
Mary Rose-Colley, Lock Haven University

James Rothenberger, University of Minnesota
John P. Sciacca, Northern Arizona University
Melinda Joy Seid, California State University, Sacramento
Philip A. Sienna, Mission College
David A. Sleet, San Diego State University
Thea Siria Spatz, University of Arkansas at Little Rock
Molly H. Whaley, Middle Tennessee State University
Carol A. Wilson, University of Nevada, Las Vegas
Richard W. Wilson, Western Kentucky University

A special note of thanks is due to Bryan Strong and Christine DeVault, authors of Mayfield's new text, *Human Sexuality*, available for adoption as of January 1994.

Finally, the book could not have been published without the efforts of the staff at Mayfield Publishing Company and the *Core Concepts* book team: Erin Mulligan, Sponsoring Editor; Kirstan Price and Kate Engelberg, Developmental Editors; Linda Toy, Production Director; Carol Zafiropoulos, Production Editor; Jeanne M. Schreiber, Art Director; Pam Trainer, Permissions Editor; Melissa Kreischer, Photo Researcher; Martha Branch, Manufacturing Manager; Julie Wildhaber, Editorial Assistant; Larisa North, Production Assistant. To all, we express our deep appreciation.

Paul M. Insel
Walton T. Roth
L. McKay Rollins
Ray A. Petersen

About the 1996 Update

Because changes in health-related information occur so rapidly, and because we are committed to providing comprehensive, accurate information on the most pressing current issues, we have prepared this updated version of the Brief Seventh Edition of *Core Concepts in Health*. The overall content, organization, and features of the seventh edition remain in place, but within this framework, key topics and issues have been updated with the most recent information available.

CONTENT AND ORGANIZATION

Coverage has been updated in two general ways:

- Wherever more recent statistics have become available, we have replaced older figures with newer ones. For example, we have been able to update statistics on the incidence of various diseases, including AIDS, cancers, and CVD; on rates of use of tobacco, alcohol, and other drugs; and on leading causes of death among Americans.

- Where important new issues or topics have arisen, or where new information has become available in key areas, we have incorporated this information in text or boxes. Examples include binge drinking on college campuses; the growing use of inhalants; new vaccines, including one for chicken pox; the use of AZT to lessen prenatal transmission of HIV; and recent federal actions related to smoking.

FEATURES AND LEARNING AIDS

All the student-oriented features and learning aids of the Seventh Edition have been retained: boxes, Personal Insights, Take Action, Journal Entry, Critical Thinking Journal Entry, Behavior Change Strategies, running glossary, and chapter outlines and summaries. The appendix has been updated, including fast food facts on Taco Bell's new low-fat entrees. The selected bibliographies and recommended readings have also been updated.

Recent research findings and new statistics have been incorporated in a number of boxes, and four new boxes have been added to highlight key current issues:

Listening to Prozac

Domestic Abuse and Violence: A Question of Control

Sexual Behavior in the 1990s

Sexual Decision Making: Is Abstinence the Right Choice for You?

TEACHING TOOLS

The Instructor's Resource Guide, the Wellness Worksheets, the examination questions, and the transparency acetates have been updated to match the text. Approximately 25 percent of the examination questions are new with this updated version of *Core Concepts*. A new set of videotapes is also available. For the 1996 Update, all line art from the text is available on CD-ROM and all transparency masters are available on electronic presentation software. For more information about the teaching tools, contact your Mayfield representative or call 1-800-433-1279.

ACKNOWLEDGMENTS

The material on sexually transmissible diseases in Chapter 13, "Infection and Immunity," was updated by Fred Kroger, Centers for Disease Control and Prevention.

The examination questions were updated by Phyllis Murray, Eastern Kentucky University.

David Quadagno would like to thank Jennifer Neal for her assistance in updating the material on sexuality in Chapter 5, "Sexuality, Pregnancy, and Childbirth."

We would also like to thank the academic advisors and reviewers for the 1996 Update:

Patricia M. Alt, Towson State University
Lori J. Bechtel, Pennsylvania State University, Altoona
David A. Birch, Indiana University
Sandra Bonneau, Golden West College
Michael S. Davidson, Montclair State University
Lori Dewald, Shippensburg University
Dalen Duitsman, Iowa State University
R. Dan Duquette, University of Wisconsin, La Crosse
Sylvia Burnett Elbaz, Kingsborough Community College, City University of New York
Sandra J. Gourley, Lake Land College
B. Lee Green, University of Alabama
Steven B. Hafen, Catonsville Community College
Jo Hill, New Mexico State University
Donna Quimby Jackson, University of Arkansas at Little Rock

Richard A. Kaye, Kingsborough Community College, City University of New York

Randy Kirkpatrick, Arkansas Tech University

Kiyoka Koizumi, Brooklyn College, City University of New York

Carolyn G. Matthews, Auburn University

Phyllis Murray, Eastern Kentucky University

Judith G. Nelson, Burlington County College

Larry W. North, Arizona State University

Kerry J. Redican, Virginia Polytechnic Institute and State University

Janet S. Reis, University of Illinois

Carol J. Teske, Kutztown University

Beverly Triana-Tremain, Collin County Community College

Chris M. Tuten, Western Carolina University

Carol A. Wilson, University of Nevada, Las Vegas

Richard W. Wilson, Western Kentucky University

Finally, we would like to thank the staff at Mayfield Publishing Company, particularly the members of the *Core Concepts* book team: Serina Beauparlant, Sponsoring Editor; Kirstan Price and Kate Engelberg, Developmental Editors; Linda Toy, Production Director; Lynn Rabin Bauer and Carol Zafiropoulos, Production Editors; Jeanne M. Schreiber, Art Director; Pam Trainer, Permissions Editor; Melissa Kreisher and Brian Pecko, Photo Researchers; Randy Hurst, Manufacturing Manager; Julie Wildhaber, Editorial Assistant; Larisa North, Production Assistant; Danilo Purlia, Promotions Director; Marshall Sanderford, Marketing Manager; Jonathan Silvers, Marketing Product Manager. To all, we express our deep appreciation.

Paul M. Insel
Walton T. Roth
L. McKay Rollins
Ray A. Petersen

Brief Contents

Contents

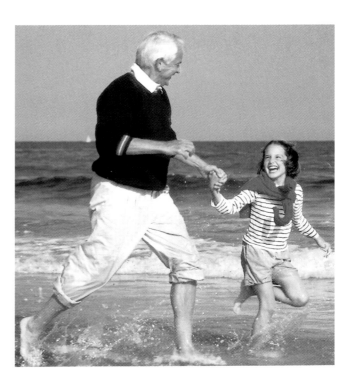

CHAPTER 4
INTIMATE RELATIONSHIPS   52

CHAPTER 5
SEXUALITY, PREGNANCY, AND CHILDBIRTH   70

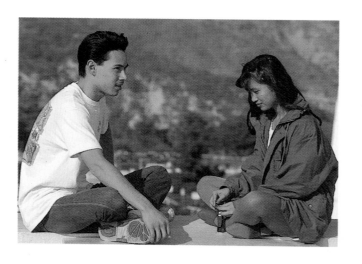

CHAPTER 6
CONTRACEPTION AND ABORTION: CURRENT ISSUES   102

CHAPTER 7
TOBACCO AND ALCOHOL   127

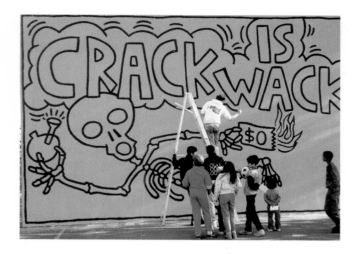

CHAPTER 11
EXERCISE FOR HEALTH AND FITNESS 229

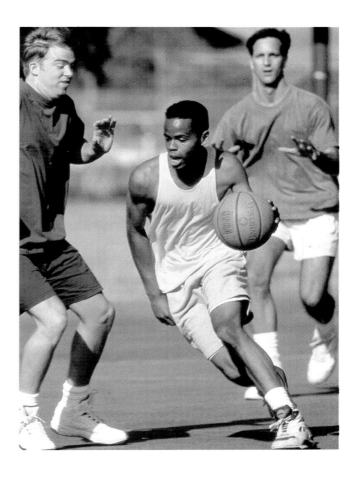

CHAPTER 12
CARDIOVASCULAR DISEASE AND CANCER 249

CHAPTER 15
ENVIRONMENTAL HEALTH 335

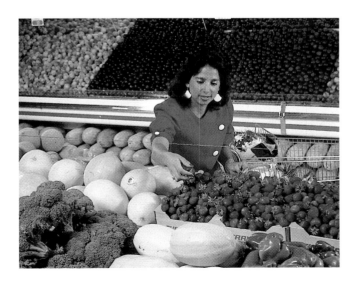

BOXES

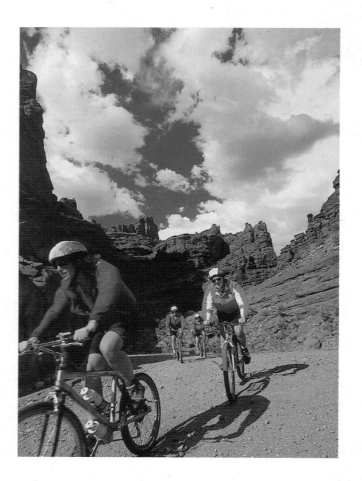

1

Taking Charge of Your Health

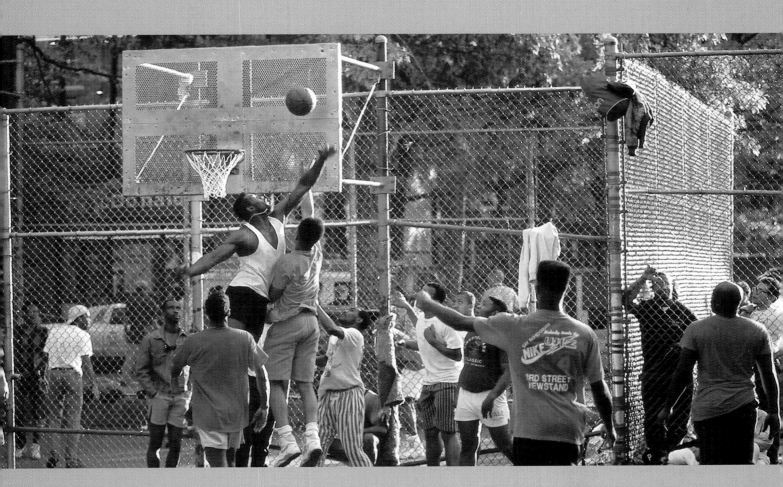

CONTENTS

Today, many people are striving for optimal health. A century ago, such a goal was unknown—people counted themselves lucky just to survive. A child born in 1890, for example, could expect to live only about 40 years. Killers such as polio, smallpox, diphtheria, measles, and mumps took the lives of a tragic number of infants and children in the days before vaccinations. Youngsters who escaped those threats still risked death from infectious diseases such as tuberculosis, typhus, or dysentery. In 1918 alone, 20 million people died in a flu epidemic. Millions of others lost their lives to common bacterial infections in the era before antibiotics. Environmental conditions—unrefrigerated food, poor sanitation, and air polluted by coal-burning furnaces and factories—contributed to the spread and the deadliness of these diseases.

The picture today is quite different. Over the past 100 years, life spans have nearly doubled. A sense of empowerment over our health has replaced the fatalism that prevailed in the last century. Today, our most serious health threats are chronic illnesses such as heart disease and cancer—diseases that we have the power to help prevent. Medical research has given us guidelines we can use to prolong our lives. Beyond that, it has provided us with information we can use to enjoy a quality of life unimagined by our grandparents.

The message of this book is that optimal health is something everyone can have. Achieving it requires knowledge, self-awareness, motivation, and effort; but the benefits last a lifetime. Optimal health comes mostly from a healthy lifestyle—patterns of behavior that promote and support your health now and as you get older. In the pages that follow, you'll find current information and suggestions about topics in health that you can use to build a better lifestyle.

WHAT IS HEALTH?

What exactly is meant by the term *health?* The definition is influenced by how people lead their lives, and today's ideas about health are very different from those held in 1890. Let's look briefly at how the concept of health has evolved over a century.

Health as the Absence of Illness

In the past, a person who was free from pain, disability, and symptoms of disease was considered healthy. From the earliest times, epidemics of infectious diseases have periodically swept around the world, ravaging whole populations. The worst outbreak of bubonic plague took more than 25 million lives in Europe in the fourteenth century, but it was only one of more than 100 major outbreaks dating back to biblical times. Entire tribes of Native Americans were wiped out by infectious diseases brought to this country by European colonizers. No age

was immune from the terrors of epidemic, whether of malaria, measles, syphilis, cholera, or some other contagious disease. No wonder health was defined as simply the absence of illness. Throughout history, this was the best one could hope for. When medical science began to unravel the mystery of these diseases and bring them under control, life expectancies rose and death rates fell.

Health as Longevity: Is Longer Better?

Once antibiotics were introduced for widespread use in the 1940s, people speculated that all diseases might soon be conquered by modern medicine. An age of medical miracles seemed just around the corner. Health began to be defined in terms of longevity—how long people could expect to live.

But as communicable disease yielded to antibiotics, vaccines, and public health campaigns, a different set of diseases emerged as a major health threat. A new pattern of death took shape. By the 1950s, degenerative diseases such as coronary heart disease, cancer, stroke, diabetes, atherosclerosis, and cirrhosis had replaced pneumonia and influenza as the leading causes of death in the United States.

Degenerative diseases spawned new treatments—open heart surgery, chemotherapy and radiation, organ transplants, and others—but they were less successful than earlier innovations had been. They were also enormously expensive and raised a new set of social and ethical questions. Many people began to question the value of some of the most advanced procedures, such as heart-lung transplants, which seem to lead to incapacitating strokes, and life-support systems, which sometimes are used to keep people alive in a permanent vegetative state. Merely being alive—with minimal physical and mental functions, supported by machines or in a coma—was now seen as a kind of living death.

It became apparent that quantity of life without quality of life is no blessing (Figure 1-1). It also became clear that the best treatment for the new killers is prevention—people taking care of their own bodies. A number of habits and behaviors were identified as culprits in the development of disease; others seemed to promote health. Many of these factors—diet, work, play, sexual and reproductive choices, and the environment in which we live—turned out to be things that individuals can themselves control. Health cannot be prescribed; physicians and the health establishment can do little more than provide information, advice, and encouragement—the rest is up to each individual.

Wellness: The New Health Goal

No longer do we consider health to be simply the absence of disease. Today we view it also as the presence of **vitality**—the ability to function with vigor and live actively, energetically, and fully. Vitality comes from **wellness**, a

Ages of Health Advancement

A study of death rates over the last century illustrates the dramatic changes that have taken place in the nature of health problems and the solutions to these problems. The figure below shows overall death rates in the United States (age-adjusted) from 1885 to the present, with the times at which major medical innovations became available.

- Over 70 percent of the decline in death rate between 1885 and the present occurred *before* the most significant medical innovations were introduced, during a period dominated by improvements in the environment and in our public health policies.

- The discovery of antibiotics in the 1930s accelerated the decline in U.S. death rates for a period of about 20 years.

- The decline slid to a stop in the early 1950s as problems still responsive to antibiotics began to disappear. Over

the next 20 years (early 1950s to early 1970s), there was almost no reduction in death rate or increase in life expectancy. Ironically, this is the period when many of our most expensive medical innovations were introduced.

- Death rates again began to decline in the early 1970s and continued to fall into the 1990s. Although the death rate for AIDS rose, mortality rates for heart disease, cancer, stroke, lung disease, injuries, and pneumonia and influenza all declined. This decline coincided with reduced rates of smoking, lower-fat diets, and increased attention to disease and injury prevention.

Adapted from Centers for Disease Control and Prevention. 1994. *Monthly Vital Statistics Report*, vol. 43, no. 6, supplement, December 8; and D. M. Vickery. 1978. *Life Plan for Your Health* (Reading, Mass.: Addison-Wesley), pp. 17–18.

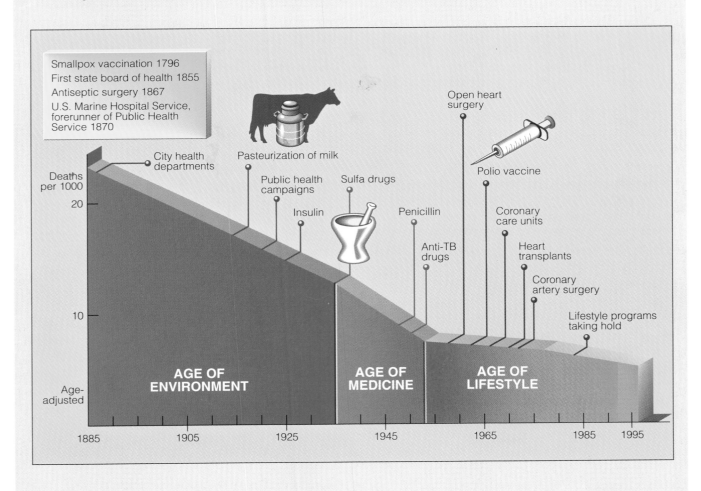

Smallpox vaccination 1796
First state board of health 1855
Antiseptic surgery 1867
U.S. Marine Hospital Service, forerunner of Public Health Service 1870

Deaths per 1000

City health departments

Pasteurization of milk

Public health campaigns

Insulin

Sulfa drugs

Penicillin

Anti-TB drugs

Open heart surgery

Polio vaccine

Coronary care units

Heart transplants

Coronary artery surgery

Lifestyle programs taking hold

AGE OF ENVIRONMENT

AGE OF MEDICINE

AGE OF LIFESTYLE

Age-adjusted

1885   1905   1925   1945   1965   1985   1995

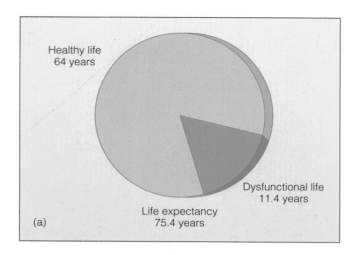

(a)

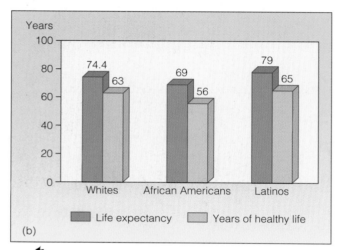

(b)

VITAL STATISTICS

Figure 1-1 *Quantity of life vs. quality of life.*
(a) Years of healthy life as a proportion of life expectancy, U.S. population. (b) Years of healthy life vs. life expectancy for whites, African Americans, and Latinos in the United States. Adapted from National Center for Health Statistics. 1994. *Healthy People 2000 Review, 1993.* Hyattsville, Md.: Public Health Service. Publication No. (PHS) 94-1232-1.

state of optimal physical, emotional, intellectual, spiritual, interpersonal, social, environmental, and even planetary well-being. At all ages and at all levels of physical and mental ability, people can increase their vitality and wellness.

Physical Health   Optimal physical health requires eating well, exercising, avoiding harmful habits, making responsible decisions about sex, learning and watching for the symptoms of disease, getting regular medical and dental check-ups, and taking steps to prevent injuries at home, on the road, and on the job. The habits you develop and the decisions you make today will determine to a great extent not only how many years you will live but also the quality of life you will enjoy during those years.

Emotional Health   Optimism, trust, self-esteem, self-acceptance, self-confidence, self-control, satisfying relationships, and an ability to share feelings are just some of the qualities and aspects of emotional wellness. Emotional health is a dynamic state that fluctuates with your physical, intellectual, spiritual, and interpersonal health. Maintaining emotional wellness requires monitoring and exploring your thoughts and feelings, identifying obstacles to emotional well-being, and finding solutions to emotional problems, with the help of a therapist if necessary.

Intellectual Health   The hallmarks of intellectual wellness include an openness to new ideas, a capacity to question and think critically, and the motivation to master new skills. A sense of humor, creativity, and curiosity are others. An active mind is essential to overall wellness, for it is your mind that learns, evaluates, and stores health information. Your mind detects problems, finds solutions, and directs behavior. People who enjoy intellectual wellness never stop learning. They relish new experiences and challenges and actively seek them out.

Spiritual Health   To enjoy spiritual health is to possess the capacity for love, compassion, forgiveness, altruism, joy, peace, and fulfillment. Spiritual wellness is a state of harmony and balance between oneself and others and between inner needs and the demands of the world. It is an antidote to cynicism, anger, bitterness, fear, anxiety, and pessimism. Organized religions help many people develop spiritual health. Many other people find meaning and purpose in their lives on their own, through nature, art, meditation, political action, or good works.

Interpersonal and Social Health   Satisfying relationships are basic to both physical and emotional health. We need loving, supportive people in our lives. And we need to be needed by them. Developing interpersonal health means learning good communication skills, developing the capacity for intimacy, and cultivating a support network of caring friends or family members. Social health means participating in and contributing to your community, country, and world.

Environmental or Planetary Health   Increasingly, personal health depends on the health of the planet. Wellness requires learning about and protecting yourself from environmental hazards—and doing what you can to reduce or eliminate them.

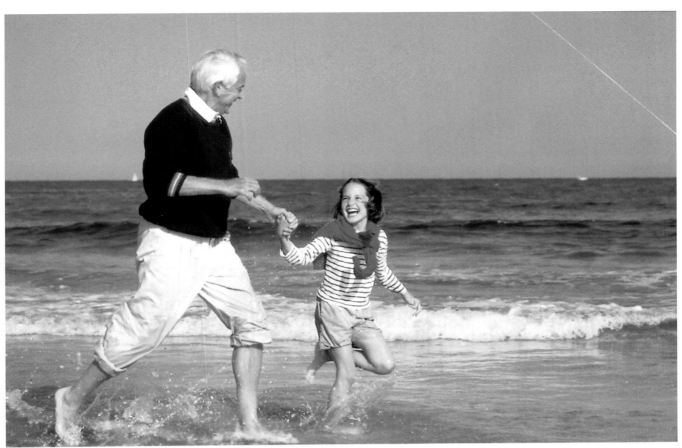

With wellness comes vitality, exuberance, a capacity for joy—and for fun. What makes you feel vital?

CHOOSING WELLNESS

This wellness model of health has a far-reaching effect on how we view ourselves and live our lives. We now have greater control over our health than human beings have ever had before—and greater responsibility for it as well.

Factors That Influence Wellness

Scientific research is continually revealing new connections between our habits and emotions and the level of health we enjoy. For example, heart disease, the nation's number one killer, is associated with cigarette smoking, high levels of stress, habitually hostile and suspicious attitudes toward the world and the people in it, a high-fat diet, and a sedentary way of life (Table 1-1). Other habits are beneficial. Regular exercise, for example, can help to prevent heart disease, high blood pressure, diabetes, osteoporosis, and depression and may reduce the risk of colon cancer, stroke, and back injury. As we learn more about how our actions affect our bodies and minds, we can make informed choices for a healthier life.

Of course, our behavior isn't the only factor involved in health. Our heredity, the environment we live in, and whether we have access to adequate health care are other important influences. These factors, which vary both for individuals and for groups, can interact in ways that produce either health or disease. For example, a sedentary lifestyle combined with a genetic predisposition to diabetes can greatly increase an individual's risk of developing diabetes. If this person also lacks adequate health care, he or she is much more likely to suffer dangerous complications from diabetes and have a lower quality of life.

But in many cases, behavior can tip the balance toward health even where inheritance or environment are negative factors. For example, breast cancer can run in families, but it also may be associated with being overweight and inactive. A woman with a family history of breast can-

Vitality The ability of an organism to function with vigor.
Wellness Optimal health and vitality, encompassing physical, emotional, intellectual, spiritual, interpersonal, social, and environmental well-being.

TERMS

Health Issues for Diverse Populations

We Americans are a diverse people. Our ancestry is European, African, Asian, Pacific Islander, Latin American, and Native American. We live in cities, suburbs, and rural areas, working at every imaginable occupation, in luxury, comfort, and poverty. In no other country in the world do so many diverse people live and work together every day. And in no other country is the understanding and tolerance of differences so much a part of the political and cultural ideal. We are at heart a nation of diversity, and, though we often fall short of our goal, we strive for justice and equality among all people.

When it comes to health, most differences among people are insignificant—the majority of health issues concern us all equally. We all need to eat well, exercise, manage stress, and cultivate satisfying personal relationships. We need to know how to protect ourselves from heart disease, cancer, sexually transmitted diseases, and injuries. We need to know what to do when we're sick and how to use the health care system.

But some of our differences—differences among us both as individuals and as members of groups—do have important implications for health. Some of us, for example, have inherited predispositions to develop certain health problems, such as high cholesterol or osteoporosis. Some of us have grown up eating foods that raise our risk of heart disease or obesity. Some of us live in environments that increase the chances that we'll smoke cigarettes or abuse alcohol. These health-related differences among individuals and groups can be biological—determined genetically—or cultural—acquired as patterns of behavior through daily interactions with our families, communities, and society. Many health conditions are a function of biology and culture combined. A person can have a genetic predisposition to a disease, for example, but won't actually develop the disease itself unless certain lifestyle factors are present, such as stress or a poor diet.

When we talk about health issues for diverse populations, we face two related dangers. The first is the danger of stereotyping, of talking about people as groups rather than as individuals. It's certainly true that every person is an individual with his or her own unique genetic endowment as well as unique experiences in life. But many of these influences are shared with others of similar genetic and cultural background. Statements about these group similarities can be useful; for example, they can alert people to areas that may be of special concern for them and their families.

The second danger is that of overgeneralizing, of ignoring the extensive biological and cultural diversity that exists among peoples who are grouped together. Groups labeled Latino or Hispanic, for example, include Mexican Americans, Puerto Ricans, Cuban Americans, people from South and Central America, and other Spanish-speaking peoples. Similarly, the population labeled Native American includes hundreds of recognized tribal nations, each with its own genetic and cultural heritage. It's important to keep these considerations in mind whenever you read about different populations.

Health-related differences among groups can be identified and described along several different dimensions, including the following:

Gender. Men and women have different life expectancies, different reproductive concerns, and different incidences of many diseases, including heart disease, cancer, stroke, cirrhosis of the liver, and osteoporosis. Men are more likely to develop heart disease in middle age. Women are more affected by issues involving contraception and reproductive choices. They live longer than men. They have lower suicide rates. They are more likely to be poor.

Socioeconomic status. Many health differences in our society are related to income level. People with low income have higher rates of infant mortality, of traumatic injury and violent death, and of many diseases, including cancer, heart disease, tuberculosis, and HIV infection. They are more likely to eat poorly, be overweight, smoke, drink, and use drugs. They have less access to health care services and medical insurance. Poverty is a far more important predictor of poor health than is any factor of race or ethnicity. However, it is often mixed with other factors in a way that makes it difficult to distinguish what causes what. A factor that may be even more closely associated with health status is level of educational attainment.

Race/ethnicity. Some genetic diseases are concentrated in certain gene pools, the result of each ethnic group's relatively distinct history. Sickle-cell anemia occurs almost exclusively among people of African ancestry. Tay-Sachs disease afflicts people of Eastern European Jewish heritage. Cystic fibrosis is more common among Northern Europeans. In addition to biological differences, many cultural differences occur along ethnic lines. Ethnic groups may vary in their traditional diets; their patterns of family and interpersonal relationships; their attitudes toward tobacco, alcohol, and other drugs; and their health beliefs and practices, to name just a few differences.

Four broad racial/ethnic minority groups are usually distinguished in American society—African Americans or blacks; Latinos; Asian and Pacific Islander Americans; and Native Americans. Each has some special health concerns.

- African Americans are the largest minority group, making up more than 12 percent of the American population. Although African Americans are represented in every socioeconomic group, one-third live below the poverty line. For a poorly understood variety of economic, genetic, and lifestyle reasons, the health status of African Americans lags behind that of the total population in several areas, including life expectancy and incidence of chronic and infectious disease.

The leading causes of death among African Americans are the same as for the overall population: heart disease, cancer, and stroke. But African Americans have higher rates of death due to homicide and infant mortality, and lower rates of death due to suicide. Among African Americans between the ages of 25 and 44, AIDS is now the leading cause of death. African American men die from strokes at almost twice the rate of men in the total population. Strokes are related to high blood pressure, which is twice as common among blacks as among the total population. Also contributing to cardiorespiratory problems is sickle-cell anemia.

Cancer is another special concern. African American men have a higher risk of cancer than do nonblack men, with a 25 percent higher risk for all cancers and a 45 percent higher risk for lung cancer. African American men face a 40 percent greater risk for prostate cancer than do whites, giving them the highest prostate cancer risk of any population group in the world.

African Americans also face increased risk for developing glaucoma and of becoming blind from glaucoma. Diabetes is a special concern for black women, especially those who are overweight.

- Latinos are the second largest and fastest growing minority group in the United States, making up about 10 percent of the total population. About two-thirds of the Latino population are of Mexican descent; 13 percent are of South or Central American background; 10 percent are Puerto Rican; and almost 5 percent are Cuban American. There are many cultural and biological differences among the various Latino populations, but they are frequently grouped together, often under the umbrella term *Hispanic*. This label is somewhat misleading, since many Latinos are of mixed Spanish and American Indian descent, or of mixed Spanish, Indian, and African American descent. Nevertheless, *Hispanic* is the term most commonly used in studies and statistics to identify Latino populations.

Overall, the leading causes of death for Latinos are the same as those for the general population—heart disease and cancer—but Latinos tend to have lower rates of death from heart disease, stroke, and cancer than do non-Hispanic whites and African Americans. Latinos have higher rates of death from homicide and infant mortality than do non-Hispanic whites, but they have lower rates of death from suicide and lung diseases. They also have lower incidence of high cholesterol, high blood pressure, and osteoporosis. Some special concerns are diabetes, gallbladder disease, and overweight, all probably related to American Indian descent. The birth rate among Latinos is higher than that of the total population, and the use of contraceptives is relatively low.

- Asian and Pacific Islander Americans, like Latinos, are characterized by diversity. They represent about 3.5 percent of the total population. The two oldest and largest groups are Japanese Americans and Chinese Americans. Other groups include Vietnamese, Laotians, Cambodians, Koreans, Filipinos, Asian Indians, Native Hawaiians, and other Pacific Islanders. Numbering over 9 million people, they speak more than 30 different languages and represent a similar number of distinct cultures.

Health differences also exist among these groups. For example, Southeast Asian men have higher rates of lung cancer and liver cancer than does the rest of the population, and Hawaiian women have higher than average rates of breast cancer. Diabetes is a concern among Asian Americans; its appearance may be triggered by the American diet. Among recent immigrants from Southeast Asia, tuberculosis and hepatitis B are serious health problems. Tobacco use is another concern; among some Southeast Asians, over 90 percent of the men smoke.

- Native Americans, also called American Indians and Alaska Natives, number about 2.2 million people. Most Native Americans embrace a tribal identity, such as Sioux, Navaho, or Hopi, rather than the identity of Native American.

Native Americans have lower rates of death from heart disease, strokes, and cancer than does the overall population, but they also have high rates of early death. For those under 45, causes of death include unintentional injuries (accidents), homicide, suicide, and cirrhosis; many of these problems are linked to alcohol abuse. Diabetes is very prevalent, occurring in over 20 percent of all adults in some tribes. Many Native Americans have limited access to health care services.

These are just some of the "dimensions of diversity"—differences among people and groups that are associated with different health concerns and problems. Other factors too, such as age or disability, are associated with particular health concerns. In this book, topics and issues in health that affect different American populations are given special consideration. Look for these discussions in boxes labeled "Dimensions of Diversity." Also discussed in these boxes are health issues and practices in other parts of the world. These explorations beyond the borders of the United States broaden our view, showing us both what we share with people in other societies and how we differ—our common concerns and our divergent solutions. All of these discussions are designed to deepen our understanding of the core concepts of health, vitality, and wellness in the context of ever-growing diversity.

Rank	Cause of Death	Number	Percent of Total Deaths	Lifestyle Factors
1	Heart disease	717,706	33.0	D I S
2	Cancers	520,578	23.9	D I S A
3	Strokes	143,769	6.6	D I S
4	Accidents	127,759	5.9	S A
	(Motor vehicle)	(40,982)	(1.9)	
	(All others)	(86,777)	(4.0)	
5	Chronic obstructive lung diseases	91,938	4.3	S
6	Pneumonia and influenza	75,719	3.5	S
7	Diabetes mellitus	50,067	2.3	D I
8	AIDS	33,566	1.5	
9	Suicide	30,484	1.4	A
10	Homicide	25,488	1.2	A
	All causes	2,175,613	100.0	

Key:

D Cause of death in which diet plays a part.
I Cause of death in which an inactive lifestyle plays a part.
S Cause of death in which smoking plays a part.
A Cause of death in which excessive alcohol consumption plays a part.

Source: Centers for Disease Control. 1994. Advance Report of Final Mortality Statistics, 1992. *Monthly Vital Statistics Report*, December 8, 1994, Vol. 43(6), p. 68.

cer is less likely to develop and die from the disease if she controls her weight, exercises regularly, does breast self-exams, and has regular mammograms taken.

Similarly, a young man with a family history of obesity can maintain a normal weight by being careful to balance calorie intake against activities that burn calories. If your life is highly stressful, you can lessen the chances of heart disease and stroke by learning ways to manage and cope with stress. If you live in an area with severe air pollution, you can reduce the risk of lung disease by not smoking. You can also take an active role in improving your environment. Behaviors like these allow you to make a difference in how great an impact heredity and environment will have on your health.

A Wellness Profile

What does it mean to be healthy today? A basic list of important behaviors and habits includes the following:

- Having a sense of responsibility for your own health and taking an active rather than passive stance toward your life
- Learning to manage stress in effective ways
- Maintaining high self-esteem and mentally healthy ways of interacting with other people
- Understanding your sexuality and having satisfying intimate relationships

- Avoiding tobacco and other drugs; using alcohol wisely, if at all
- Eating well, exercising, and maintaining normal weight
- Knowing when to treat your illnesses yourself and when to seek help
- Understanding the health care system and using it intelligently
- Knowing the facts about cardiovascular disease, cancer, infections, sexually transmitted diseases, and injuries and using your knowledge to protect yourself against them
- Understanding the natural processes of aging and dying and accepting the limits of human existence
- Understanding how the environment affects your health and taking appropriate action to improve it

This may seem like a tall order, and in a sense it *is* the work of a lifetime. But the habits that you establish now are crucial: They tend to set lifelong patterns. Some behaviors do more than set up patterns—they produce permanent changes in your health. If you become addicted to drugs or alcohol at age 20, for example, you may be able to kick the habit, but you will never again be a non-addict; you will always face the struggle of a recovered addict. If you contract gonorrhea, you may discover later that your reproductive organs were damaged without your realizing it, making you infertile or sterile. If you ruin your knees doing the wrong exercises or hurt your back in an automobile crash, you won't have them to count on when you're older. Some things just can't be undone.

Personal Insight What sorts of health habits did your parents and other family members have when you were growing up? Were they active or sedentary? Did they smoke? What kind of foods did they eat? How have your own health habits been influenced by those of your family members?

GETTING DOWN TO BASICS: HOW DO YOU REACH WELLNESS?

Your life may not resemble that described by the Wellness Profile at all. You probably have a number of healthy habits and some others that place your health at risk. Taking steps to reduce these risks will be a challenge at first, but as you make progress toward wellness, it will get easier. At first you'll be rewarded with a greater sense of control over your life, a feeling of empowerment, higher self-esteem, and more joy in life. These benefits will encourage you to make further improvements. Over time, you'll come to know what wellness feels like—more energy; greater vitality; deeper feelings of curiosity, interest, and enjoyment; and a higher quality of life.

Taking Charge of Your Health: Knowledge, Motivation, Commitment, and Sense of Control

What makes you act the way you do? Countless factors come into play in determining your behaviors, both internal and external, both rational and irrational—knowledge, emotions, values, ideals, habit, circumstances, beliefs, and perceptions about yourself and the world.

To make good decisions, you need facts and information about topics and issues in health. To put those behavior changes into action, you also need knowledge about yourself—where you fit into the health picture and what strengths you can draw on to change your behavior and improve your health.

Motivation is another prerequisite for change. Although some people are motivated by long-term goals, such as avoiding disease that may hit them in 20 or 30 years, most are more likely to be provoked to action by shorter-term, more personal goals. Looking better, being more popular with the opposite sex, doing better in school, getting a good job, improving at a sport, and gaining higher self-esteem are common sources of motivation.

Motivation has to be built on commitment, the resolve to stick with a plan no matter what temptations you encounter. Commitment provides a turning point when you bring the full force of your resolve to change a particular situation. With deeply rooted habits, it often takes a while to build up to the level of commitment you need to conquer a habit. Many smokers, for example, don't succeed in quitting until their third or fourth try.

Whether you succeed in changing behaviors is rooted in how strongly you believe you will succeed, what you unconsciously intend, and the kind of support you can draw from family and friends. Perhaps the most crucial factor is how active or passive you want to be about your life. Who is controlling your life? Is it your parents, your friends, your school, circumstances, the stars? Or is it you? When you succeed in making changes, it is because *you* have taken charge of your life. You have come to see that what you do is within your control.

A Plan for Action: Behavior Self-Management

Most of your behaviors are habits you've learned. They may be deeply ingrained, long-standing habits; but they're still habits, and you can unlearn them the same way you learned them. The key is to approach them in a systematic way. The approach recommended in this book is based on principles of behavioral self-management that have proven effective in helping people make changes in their lives. As you read about different areas of health in the chapters that follow, you can apply the self-management model to your own behavior to help you plan and carry out changes in your life.

The first time you use this approach to behavioral self-management you should have two goals in mind. You should want to change a specific behavior, but more importantly, you should also want to learn how to use this approach. Once you have learned this eight-step plan, you can use it in many situations throughout your life.

Your key to success is to be consistent and to persist. Don't skip steps or rush through the plan. You may think you know everything there is to know about your target behavior, but people are almost always surprised by patterns that emerge from carefully recorded daily accounts of their thoughts and actions. Intervening in the chain of events that occur before and after a behavior is the basis of behavior self-management. This approach provides surprisingly powerful tools that you can use to make the changes that you want in your life. Let's consider now the actual steps involved in putting together a behavior management program.

Step 1: Select a Behavior The heart of the behavior self-management model is isolating a **target behavior** that you wish to change and identifying the circumstances that trigger it and the consequences that follow. Once you know these, you can intervene in this chain of events to change your behavior.

Date _____ November 5 _____   Day   M (TU) W   TH   F   SA   SU

Time of day	M/S	Food eaten	Cals.	H	Where did you eat?	What else were you doing?	How did someone else influence you?	What made you want to eat what you did?	Emotions and feelings?	Thoughts and concerns?
7:30	M	1 C Crispix cereal 1/2 C skim milk coffee, black 1 C orange juice	110 40 — 120	3	dorm cafeteria	reading newspaper	eating w/ friends, but I ate what I usually eat	I always eat cereal in the morning	a little keyed up & worried	thinking about quiz in class today
10:30	S	1 apple	90	1	library	studying	alone	felt tired & wanted to wake up	tired	worried about next class
12:30	M	1 C chili 1 roll 1 pat butter 1 orange 2 oatmeal cookies 1 soda	290 120 35 60 120 150	2	cafeteria terrace	talking	eating w/ friends; we decided to eat at the cafeteria	wanted to be part of group	excited and happy	interested in hearing everyone's plans for the weekend
3:00	S	candy bar	250	1	hallway	waiting for next class	alone	wanted a break	bored	thinking about next class
6:30	M	4 oz roast chicken 3/4 C mashed potatoes 3/4 C peas 1/2 C ice cream 1 soda	205 150 90 125 150	3	student union	talking w/ friends	we all got ice cream for dessert	best thing available for dinner	relaxing w/friends	thinking about paper to write this evening
10:30	S	hot chocolate 1 C plain popcorn	100 25	1	living room	watch TV w/roommates	just went along with the group	it was already fixed	tired of studying; wanted a break	nothing in particular
		TOTAL FOR DAY	2230							

M/S = Meal or snack   H = Hunger rating (0-3)

Figure 1-2 *Sample health journal.*

The first time you use this self-management model it may be wise to select a behavior that is fairly simple. Once you have learned the steps, you can take on more complex behaviors. The first target behavior you choose should be something you really want to change so that you will be motivated and thus more apt to succeed. The behavior can be either something you want to stop doing or something you want to start doing. The behavior should be something that occurs fairly consistently or routinely in your life rather than something you do only occasionally. The behavior should also be something that is observable and can be counted and recorded. The behavior may be related to physical, emotional, intellectual, spiritual, or social health. It may be wise to consider several behaviors you want to change and then select one that meets the criteria listed in this paragraph.

Step 2: Monitor Your Behavior and Gather Data Begin your project by keeping a careful record of the behavior you wish to change (your target behavior) and the cir-

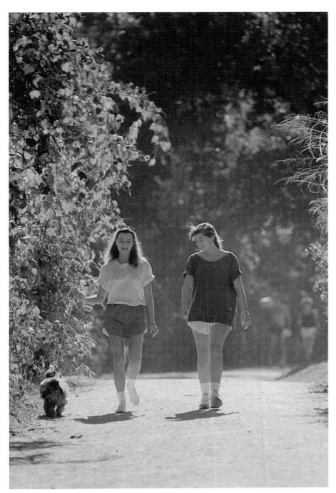

A beautiful day, a spectacular setting, a friendly companion—all conspire to make exercise a satisfying and pleasurable experience for these people. Choosing the right activity and doing it the right way are important elements in a successful health behavior management plan.

cumstances surrounding it. You want to know what your behavior was like before you started the project so you can accurately evaluate your progress. You can keep these records in a health journal. Write the details of your behavior along with observations and comments. Note exactly what the activity was, when and where it happened, what you were doing, and what your feelings were at the time (see the sample journal in Figure 1-2). Keep your journal for about a week or two to get solid information about the behavior you want to change.

Try to determine what external or internal stimuli are associated with the behavior you want to change. **External stimuli** are events or sensations in the environment that trigger a behavior. **Internal stimuli** are thoughts and feelings that trigger an action. Try to identify the "payoffs" or consequences that reinforce the behavior. **Positive reinforcers** encourage you to repeat a behavior by adding something positive that makes you feel good. **Negative reinforcers** encourage behavior by covering up or removing something that is unpleasant. Both types of reinforcers help a behavior remain a habit, one by adding something and increasing pleasure, the other by removing something and decreasing discomfort. Sometimes a behavior is supported by both positive and negative reinforcers. You will be more apt to succeed in changing your behavior if you understand and are prepared to deal with these factors.

Step 3: Analyze the Data and Identify Patterns After you have collected data on the behavior, analyze it to identify patterns in stimuli and responses. Be sure to note the connection between your feelings and such external stimuli as time of day, location, situations, and actions of others around you.

Step 4: Set Specific goals Whatever your ultimate goal, it's a good idea to break it down into a few steps, or "chunks." This is sometimes called shaping. Your plan will seem less overwhelming and more manageable, increasing the chance you'll stick to it. You'll also build in more opportunities to reward yourself (as discussed in Step 6) as well as more milestones you can use to measure your progress. It's also a good idea to prioritize your specific goals. Take the easier steps first and then work up to the harder ones. If you think through your goals carefully, you will probably succeed.

Step 5: Plan to Track Your Progress Create a plan for recording your progress. You may want to keep several different types of records. One may be used to track your daily activities and any relevant details related to specific goals. You can also use your journal to record the feelings that accompany your success or lack of progress. Plan to chart your progress on a graph that can be posted in a prominent place. This has proven to be a very effective motivator or reminder for many people. Plan to analyze your progress regularly so that you can revise your plan if necessary.

TERMS

Target behavior An isolated behavior selected as the object of a behavior change program.

External stimuli (cues) Factors from outside the person that arouse activity.

Internal stimuli Factors from within the person that arouse activity.

Positive reinforcers Something added to the environment following a behavior that results in an increase in the frequency of the behavior.

Negative reinforcer Something removed from the environment following a behavior that results in an increase in the frequency of the behavior.

It takes motivation to change. But how do you get motivated? The following strategies may help:

- Write down potential benefits of the change. If you want to lose weight, your list might include increased ease of movement, energy, and self-confidence.

- Now write down the costs of not changing.

- Frequently visualize yourself achieving your goal and enjoying its benefits. If you want to manage time more effectively, picture yourself as a confident, organized person who systematically tackles important tasks and sets aside time each day for relaxation, exercise, and friends.

- Discount obstacles to change. Counter thoughts such as "I'll never have time to shop for and prepare healthy foods" with thoughts such as these: "Lots of other people have done it and so can I."

- Bombard yourself with propaganda. Subscribe to a self-improvement magazine. Take a class dealing with the change you want to make. Read books and watch talk shows on the subject. Post motivational phrases or pictures on your refrigerator or over your desk. Listen to motivational tapes in the car. Talk to people who have already made the change.

- Build up your confidence. Remind yourself of other goals you've achieved. At the end of each day, mentally review your good decisions and actions. See yourself as a capable person, one who is in charge of his or her health.

Step 6: Devise a Plan of Action That Includes Appropriate Strategies   The following strategies have proven to be effective in helping to change certain types of behavior in particular situations. You might think of them as ammunition to be used against any obstacles you encounter.

- *Plan alternatives.* It may help to be prepared to change your environment, including people, places, and things. For example, if certain people are likely to make it difficult for you to follow your plan, it may be best to not spend time with those people, at least for a while. If you are tempted by something, such as a vending machine, along your usual route, it may be wise to devise another route.

- *Reward yourself.* Another very powerful way to affect your target behavior is by setting up a reward system that will reinforce your efforts. Carefully plan your rewards—what they will be and when they will be given. Giving yourself instant, real rewards for good behavior along the way will help you stick with your plan. Most people find it difficult to change long-standing habits for rewards they can't see right away. Plan your rewards so they can be given when you meet specific goals. Rewards should be special, inexpensive, and consistent with your goals. Don't reward yourself for sticking to your diet for a week by eating a big meal.

- *Use a role model.* Find someone who has reached the goal you are striving for. Once you start looking, you may be surprised at the number of people you will find. Talk to them about how they did it. Find out what strategies worked for them and what you can borrow from their experience. When the going gets rough, it may help to hold your model in your mind.

- *Rehearse success.* Think about situations where your target behavior is usually triggered. Plan what you will say or what you will do in these situations. Be prepared for various contingencies. This strategy is also called imagery. The more vivid or close to reality the rehearsal is, the more effective it will be.

- *Find a buddy.* Look around and you will likely find people who want to make the same changes you do. Recruit someone to join your program or join a group that is working toward similar goals. Having social support makes it easier to stick with your program. Not wanting to let your buddy down may keep you on track.

- *Use a witness.* A witness does not participate in your program as a buddy does, but he or she is interested in your success and can observe your efforts. Witnesses can be part of your personal contract (see Step 7), help you in some activities, and act as an umpire to verify your success when a subjective judgment is needed.

Step 7: Make a Personal Contract   Once you have set your goals and developed a plan of action, turn your plan into a personal contract. A serious personal contract states your objective and your commitment to reach it. Your contract should include information about your plan, such as when you will start, the steps you will use along the way, how you will measure your progress, and the date you expect to reach your final goal. It is often helpful to have someone witness the contract.

A Personal Contract for Change

All of us are familiar with the power of signed contracts. Documentation that commits our word, money, and/or property carries a strong impact and results in a higher chance of follow-through than do casual, offhand promises. Contracts can be used to try to change a health behavior if they include the time, date, and details of the behavior change program. Some target behaviors, such as quitting smoking or giving up candy snacks, lend themselves to contracts with very specific goals. Often a witness is also asked to sign the contract; this helps to set in motion the support and encouragement of a social network. Contracts help prevent procrastination by specifying the dates and other details of the behavioral tasks and goals. They also act as reminders of a personal commitment to change.

Let's take the example of Michael, who wants to break a long-standing habit of eating candy and chips every afternoon and evening. Setting up a formal contract and program for giving up these snacks will help him succeed in changing his behavior.

Michael begins by keeping track of his snacking in a journal. He discovers that he always buys candy or a bag of chips at the snack bar on campus between two of his afternoon classes. In the evenings, he eats several candy bars or a large bag of chips while he studies at home.

Next, Michael sets specific goals for his program. He sets a start date for his program and decides to break it into two parts. He will begin by cutting out his afternoon snack of candy or chips. Once he successfully reaches this goal, he'll concentrate on his evening snacking. He decides to allow himself three weeks for each half of his behavior change program.

To help increase his chances of success, Michael decides to make several changes in his behavior to help control his urges to buy and eat candy and chips. He plans to bring a healthy snack, such as an apple or orange, to eat between his afternoon classes. He decides to avoid going near the snack bar; instead, he'll spend his between-class break taking a 15-minute walk around campus or reading in the student union. To help break his evening habit, he decides to try studying at the library instead of at home; when he's at home, he'll try studying in a different room. He also plans to stock the refrigerator with healthy snacks that he can have when he feels the urge to snack on candy or chips.

Finally, Michael decides on some rewards he'll give himself when he meets his goals, choosing things he likes that aren't too expensive. Now he's ready to create and sign a behavior change contract. He decides to enlist one of his housemates as a witness to his contract; he also asks his housemate to check on his progress and offer encouragement. (Contracts can be completed without a witness, but many people find that having another person involved in their program provides a motivational boost.)

Once Michael has signed his contract, he's ready to begin. He can increase his chances of success by continuing to monitor his behavior and his snacking urges in his health journal.

My Personal Contract for Giving Up Snacking on Candy and Chips

I agree to stop snacking on candy and chips twice every day. I will begin my program on _10/4_ and plan to reach my final goal by _11/15_. I have divided my program into two parts, with two separate goals. For each step in my program, I will give myself the reward listed.

1. I will stop having candy or chips for an afternoon snack on _10/4_.
(Reward: _new CD_)

2. I will stop having candy or chips for an evening snack on _10/25_.
(Reward: _Concert_)

My plan for stopping my snacking includes the following strategies:
1. _Avoid snack bar by taking a walk or reading at student union._
2. _Eating healthy snacks instead of candy and chips._
3. _Studying at the library instead of at home._

I understand that it is important for me to make a strong personal effort to make this change in my behavior. I sign this contract as an indication of my personal commitment to reach my goal.

Witness: _Michael Cook_ _9/28_
Katie Lim _9/28_

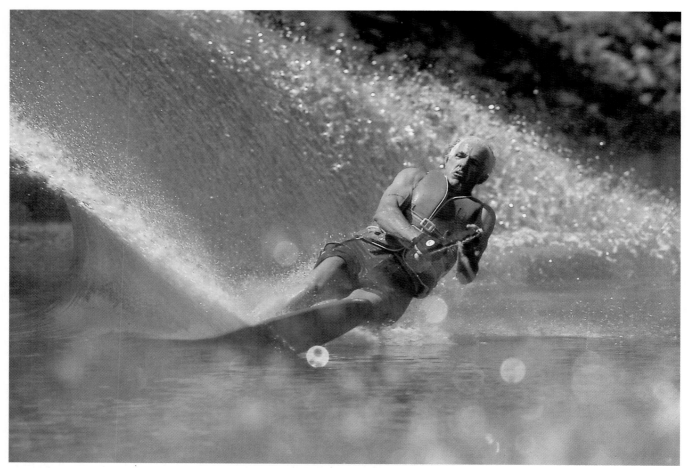

A 60-year-old man who water-skis like a 30-year-old gets his strength from years of vigorous activity. If you want to enjoy vigor and health in *your* middle and old age, begin now to make the choices that will give you lifelong vitality.

Step 8: DO IT After the seven preparatory steps, it's time to start on the program. Realize that lasting change takes time. Be prepared for obstacles and disappointments. The more important the change the more difficult it may be. Be persistent. Evaluate your progress at regular intervals and don't be afraid to revise your program if necessary. When you slip, be easy on yourself. Feeling guilty and blaming yourself work against you. Remember that the first time you use this eight-step program, the primary goal is to learn how to make the program work. As soon as you have successfully completed one behavior change program, you can start again on another target behavior.

Personal Insight How do you feel about the idea of putting together and carrying out a plan for changing some part of your behavior? Have you ever taken this kind of deliberate action before? Do you feel uneasy about the idea? Is it exciting?

BEING HEALTHY FOR LIFE

Your first few behavior management projects may never go beyond the project stage. Those that do may not all succeed. But as you taste success and begin to see progress and changes, you'll start to experience new and surprising positive feelings about yourself. You'll probably find that you're less likely to buckle under stress. You may begin opening doors to different types of people and to a new world of enjoyable physical and social events. You may accomplish things you never thought possible—winning a race, climbing a mountain, breaking a nicotine habit, having a lean, muscular body. Being healthy takes extra effort, but the paybacks in energy and vitality are priceless.

Once you've started, don't stop. Assume health improvement is forever. Tackle one area at a time, but make a careful inventory of your health strengths and weaknesses and lay out a long-range plan. Take on the easier problems first and then use what you learned to attack

We usually think of health and wellness as personal matters, things we deal with on our own—by exercising and managing stress, for example—or in conjunction with our physicians when we get sick. But did you know that the U.S. government has a vital interest in the health of all Americans? A healthy population is the nation's greatest resource, the source of its vigor and wealth. Poor health, in contrast, drains the nation's resources and raises national health care costs. As the embodiment of our society's values, the federal government also has a humane interest in people's health.

In 1990 the U.S. Department of Health and Human Services published a report entitled *Healthy People 2000: National Health Promotion and Disease Prevention Objectives*. The work of thousands of health professionals, this 700-page document, updated annually, sets forth health goals for the United States to be achieved by the year 2000. It also provides a framework within which individuals, communities, health care professionals, and government can work toward those goals. The broad national goals proposed by *Healthy People 2000* are the following:

- *To increase the span of healthy life for all Americans.* This means not only adding years to the life span but also enhancing the quality of life. Although the average American life span is almost 76 years, a person may have a disabling stroke at 60, followed by 16 years of impaired life. The national goal is to increase years of healthy life for all Americans from 64 (the figure in 1991) to 65.

- *To reduce health disparities among Americans.* Many health problems disproportionately affect certain populations in the United States, including some age groups, people with low income, certain racial and ethnic minorities, and people with disabilities. For example, life expectancy for whites at birth has been gradually increasing for many years, but African American males experienced an unprecedented decline in life expectancy every year from 1984 to 1989. Although life expectancy for black males began edging up again beginning in 1990, it remains about eight years shorter than that of white men. White females also have a longer life expectancy than black females, although the disparity is smaller. *Healthy People 2000* calls for reducing, and finally eliminating, these disparities among groups, most of whom have historically been disadvantaged economically, educationally, and politically.

- *To secure access to preventive health services for all Americans.* Preventive services, such as prenatal care,

nutritional counseling, and cancer screening, are the key to long-term improvements in national health. Because these services are usually offered in the course of regular, basic care, this third goal means increasing the number of people who have a primary source of health care and adequate health insurance coverage.

These three goals—healthy lives for more Americans, elimination of disparities among groups, and access to necessary preventive services for everyone—are the broad aspirations of *Healthy People 2000* for American society. Giving substance to these broad goals are hundreds of specific objectives in many different "priority areas." These objectives are in the form of measurable targets for the year 2000—for example, to increase to at least 30 percent the proportion of people who engage in moderate daily physical activity, up from 22 percent in 1985.

The report groups these priority areas into three broad categories—Health Promotion, Health Protection, and Preventive Services. The first category, Health Promotion, encompasses areas involving individual actions and behaviors. Examples of these areas include physical fitness, nutrition, tobacco, alcohol and other drugs, family planning, and mental health. In these areas, health improvements will be made by educating people about healthy lifestyle choices and encouraging them to make those choices. The second category, Health Protection, encompasses areas involving environmental improvements—areas in which people's health needs to be protected on a wide scale, including food and drug safety, protection from unintentional injuries (accidents) and environmental health. The third category, Preventive Services, encompasses areas involving clinical services, such as prenatal care and childhood immunizations.

Healthy People 2000 takes special notice of a changing attitude among Americans that supports its aspirations—an emerging sense of personal responsibility as the key to good health. This new perspective is seen in the concern Americans have about smoking and drug abuse, for example; in our emphasis on physical and emotional fitness; in our interest in good nutrition; and in our concern about the environment. As you have seen in this chapter, personal responsibility—taking charge of your health—is the perspective upon which *Core Concepts in Health* is built. As you move on to other chapters, you will also see that the priority concerns of *Healthy People 2000* are the principal topics covered in this book. In many ways, personal health goals are not different from national aspirations.

---

more difficult areas. Look over your shoulder to make sure you don't fall into old habits. Keep informed about the latest health news and trends; research is constantly providing new information that directly affects daily choices and habits.

Making Changes in Your World

You can't completely control every aspect of your health. At least three other factors—heredity, health care, and environment—play important roles in your well-being. After you quit smoking, for example, you may still be inhaling smoke from other people's cigarettes. Your resolve to eat better foods may suffer a setback when you can't find any healthy choices in vending machines.

But you can make a difference—you can help create an environment around you that supports a healthy lifestyle. You can help support nonsmoking areas in public places. You can speak up in favor of more nutritious foods and better physical fitness facilities. You can include nonalcoholic drinks at your parties. You can vote for measures that improve access to health care for all people and support politicians who sponsor them.

You can also work on the larger environmental challenges facing us: air and water pollution, traffic congestion, overcrowding and overpopulation, depletion of the ozone layer of the atmosphere, toxic and nuclear waste disposal, and many others. These difficult issues need the attention and energy of people who are informed and who care about health. On every level, from personal to planetary, individuals can take an active role in shaping their environment.

What Does the Future Hold?

Sweeping changes in lifestyle have resulted in healthier Americans in recent years and could have even greater effects in the years to come. Heart disease deaths, although still high, have dropped by more than half since 1950. Stroke rates dropped nearly 30 percent between 1982 and 1992. Average blood pressure and cholesterol levels have declined by small but significant amounts. Problems remain, of course—psychological, emotional, and learning disorders, along with hearing and speech impairments, are on the rise among children; access to health care is a critical problem; unacceptable disparities in health risks exist between races and ethnic groups; and **HIV infection** looms as an immense challenge for all of us. But all these problems can be addressed at least in part by individuals taking charge of their health and working to improve the health of the nation and the world.

In your lifetime, you can choose an active role in the movement toward increased awareness, greater individual responsibility and control, healthier lifestyles, and a healthier planet. Your choices and actions will have a tremendous impact on your present and future health. You have the opportunity to reach levels of wellness that your ancestors could only imagine. The door is open, and the time is now—you simply have to begin.

TERMS

HIV Infection   A chronic, progressive disease that damages the immune system; caused by the human immunodeficiency virus (HIV). Its most severe form, AIDS, is characterized by severe suppression of the immune system, leading eventually to death.

SUMMARY

- A healthy lifestyle promotes optimal health. Through knowledge, self-awareness, motivation, and effort, everyone can achieve optimal health.

What Is Health?

- Ideas about health have changed over the years. Whereas once it was considered to be the absence of disease and disability, advances in medical science in the twentieth century led people to start thinking of health in terms of longevity.

- As chronic diseases such as coronary heart disease and cancer became the leading causes of death in the United States, people recognized that merely being alive is not the same as health.

- Today, health is perceived as a matter of *wellness*— having a sense of vitality and overall well-being in life. Health is dynamic and multidimensional; it incorporates physical, emotional, intellectual, spiritual, interpersonal, societal, and environmental factors.

Choosing Wellness

- People today have greater control over their health than ever before. Being responsible for one's health means making choices and adopting habits and behaviors that will ensure wellness.

- Scientific research regularly makes connections between wellness or disease and certain lifestyles or behaviors. Although heredity, environment, and health care all play roles in wellness and disease, behavior can mitigate their effects.

- Behaviors and habits that reinforce wellness include (1) taking an active, responsible role in one's health, (2) managing stress, (3) maintaining self-esteem and good interpersonal relationships, (4) understanding sexuality and having satisfying intimate relationships, (5) avoiding tobacco and other drugs and restricting alcohol intake, (6) eating well, exercising, and maintaining normal weight, (7) knowing about illnesses and how to treat them, (8) understanding and wisely using the health system, (9) knowing about diseases and accidents and protecting yourself against them, (10) understanding the processes of aging and dying, and (11) understanding the environment and its effects on your health and working to improve it.

Getting Down to Basics: How Do You Reach Wellness?

- Knowledge about topics in health and about oneself is necessary to achieve wellness.

- Motivation is one of the most important factors in

behavior change. Most people are motivated most strongly by short-term, personal goals rather than long-term goals such as avoiding disease later in life.

- Commitment is a third necessary factor in behavior change. It involves the full force of the resolve to change.

- The fourth and perhaps most important factor in behavior change is taking control of one's life, taking an active role in living and maintaining health. With motivation and commitment, habits that have been learned can be unlearned through behavioral self-management.

- The best way to begin a behavior self-management program is to choose one target behavior and follow a systematic eight-step program to change. Consistency and persistence are highly important.

- The eight steps to behavior management are (1) select a behavior, (2) monitor the behavior and gather data, (3) analyze the data and identify patterns, (4) set specific goals, (5) plan to track your progress, (6) devise a plan of action, (7) make a personal contract, and (8) start on the program.

- Strategies for success include planning alternatives, rewarding yourself, using a role model, rehearsing success, finding a buddy, and using witnesses.

Being Healthy for Life

- Each small success in a behavior-management program leads to increased self-esteem and increased motivation to continue.

- Although people can't control every aspect of their health, individuals can make a difference in improving the environment—from insisting on nonsmoking areas in local restaurants to working on planetary issues like nuclear waste disposal and depletion of the ozone layer.

TAKE ACTION

1. Ask some older members of your family (parents and grandparents) what they recall about patterns of health and disease when they were young. Do they remember any large outbreaks of infectious disease? Did any of their friends or relatives die while very young or die of a disease that can now be treated? How have health concerns changed during their lifetime?

2. Choose a person you consider a role model and interview him or her. What do you admire about this person? What can you borrow from his or her experiences and strategies for success?

JOURNAL ENTRY

1. Purchase a small notebook to use as your health journal throughout this course. At the end of each chapter, we include suggestions for journal entries—opportunities to think about topics and issues, explore and formulate your own views, and express your thoughts in written form. These exercises are intended to help you deepen your understanding of health topics and your own behaviors in relation to them. For your first journal entry, make a list of the positive behaviors that enhance your health (such as jogging and getting enough sleep). Consider what additions you can make to the list or how you can strengthen or reinforce these behaviors. (Don't forget to congratulate yourself for these positive aspects of your life.) Next, list the behaviors that detract from wellness (such as smoking and eating a lot of candy). Consider which of these behaviors you might be able to change. Use these lists as the basis for self-evaluation as you proceed through this book.

2. *Critical Thinking:* Making smart choices about your health requires critical thinking. You have to sort through and evaluate the information you receive and then make intelligent decisions on the basis of what you've heard or read. Critical thinking involves knowing where and how to find relevant information, how to separate fact from opinion, how to recognize faulty reasoning, how to evaluate information, and how to assess the credibility of sources. Consider, for example, the typical newspaper story describing new scientific findings about cholesterol, caffeine, or AIDS treatment. As a health consumer, you have to read the article critically to understand its implications. In evaluating such an article, remember that a single scientific study isn't sufficient to "prove" anything; results have to be repeated in other studies in order to be valid. Remember, too, that in their eagerness for news, the media often distort the meaning of studies. Wait and see how findings are interpreted by a number of experts. And don't forget to look askance at any findings cited in advertising; the motive, of course, is to persuade you to buy something.

   In this book, a number of Journal Entry items are designed to help you sharpen your critical thinking skills. For your first Critical Thinking Journal Entry, write a short essay describing your sources of health information. Do you rely on newspaper or magazine articles? On television? On friends and family members? What criteria do you use to evaluate this information, to assess its credibility, and to make health decisions?

3. Think about what troubled you most during the past week. In your health journal, write down the names of three or four people who might be able to help you with whatever troubled you. If the problem persists, consider starting at the top of your list and talking to this person about it.

4. Think of the last time you did something you knew to be unhealthy primarily because those around you were doing it. How could you have restructured the situation or changed the environmental cues so that you could have avoided the behavior? In your health journal, describe several possible actions that will help you avoid the behavior the next time you're in a similar situation.

5. Make a list in your health journal of rewards that are meaningful to you. Add to the list as you think of new things to use. Refer to this list of rewards when you're developing plans for behavior change.

SELECTED BIBLIOGRAPHY

American Cancer Society. 1995. *Cancer Facts and Figures—1995*. Atlanta: American Cancer Society.

Barsky, A. J. 1988. *Worried Sick: Our Troubled Quest for Wellness*. Boston: Little, Brown.

Fries, James F. 1994. *Living Well*. New York: Addison-Wesley.

Fries, J. F., and L. M. Crapo. 1981. *Vitality and Aging*. New York: W. H. Freeman.

Hiatt, H. H. 1987. *America's Health in the Balance: Choice or Chance?* New York: Harper and Row.

Justice, B. 1988. *Who Gets Sick: How Beliefs, Moods, and Thoughts Affect Your Health*. Los Angeles: Jeremy P. Tarcher.

National Center for Health Statistics. 1994. *Healthy People 2000 Review, 1993*. Hyattsville, Md.: Public Health Service. DHHS Pub. (PHS) 94-1232-1.

———. 1992. *Monthly Vital Statistics Report*, 40(13), 30 September.

National Institutes of Health. 1994. *Vision Research, A National Plan 1994–1998*. A Report of the National Advisory Eye Council. National Eye Institute.

Reader's Digest. 1988. *The Complete Manual of Fitness and Well-Being: A Lifetime Guide to Self-Improvement*. Pleasantville, N.Y.: Reader's Digest.

Samuels, M., and N. Samuels. 1988. *The Well Adult*. New York: Summit Books.

Travis, J., and R. S. Ryan. 1988. *Wellness Workbook*. Berkeley: Ten Speed Press.

U.S. Bureau of the Census. 1993. *The Hispanic Population in the U.S.*

U.S. Bureau of the Census. 1994. *Resident Population Estimates by Race, Sex, and Age*. October.

U.S. Department of Health and Human Services. 1994. Advance report of final mortality statistics, 1992. *Monthly Vital Statistics Report* 43(6) (Supplement, 8 December).

———. 1990. *Healthy People 2000: National Health Promotion and Disease Prevention Objectives*. Washington, D.C.: U.S. Government Printing Office, DHHS Pub. (PHS) 91-50213.

RECOMMENDED READINGS

The following are highly readable monthly or bimonthly newsletters and magazines filled with the latest research and thinking on health-related topics.

Consumer Reports on Health (101 Truman Avenue, Yonkers, NY 10703-1057)

Harvard Health Letter (Palm Coast Data, P.O. Box 420285, Agency Dept., Palm Coast, FL 32142)

Health (formerly *Hippocrates* and *In Health*) (Hippocrates Partners, P.O. Box 56863, Boulder, CO 80322-6863)

Healthline (830 Menlo Ave., Suite 100, Menlo Park, CA 94025)

Mayo Clinic Health Letter (Mayo Foundation for Medical Education and Research, Neodata, P.O. Box 2606, Boulder, CO 80322)

Mental Medicine Update: The Mind/Body Health Newsletter (P.O. Box 381065, Boston, MA 02238-1065)

University of California at Berkeley Wellness Letter (P.O. Box 420148, Palm Coast, FL 32142)

Stress: The Constant Challenge

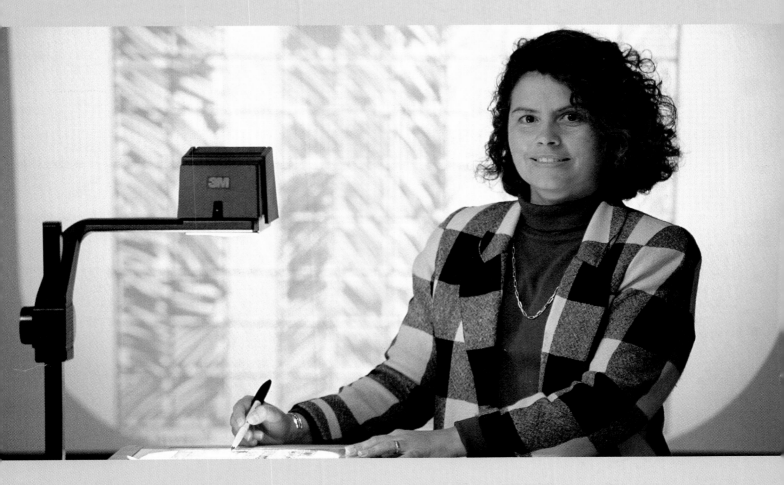

CONTENTS

Everybody talks about **stress**. People say they're "over-stressed" or "stressed out." They may blame stress for headaches or ulcers, and they may try to combat stress with aerobics classes—or drugs. But what is stress? And why is it important to manage it wisely?

Most people associate stress with negative events: the death of a close relative or friend, financial problems, or other unpleasant life changes that create nervous tension. But stress isn't merely nervous tension. And it isn't something to be avoided at all costs. In fact, complete freedom from stress is death. Before we explore more fully what stress is, consider this list of common stressful situations or events:

> Interviewing for a job
> Running in a race
> Being accepted to college
> Going out on a date
> Watching a basketball game
> Getting a promotion

Obviously, stress doesn't arise just from unpleasant situations. Stress can also be associated with physical challenges and the achievement of personal goals. Physical and psychological stress-producing factors can be either pleasant or unpleasant. What's crucial is how the individual responds, whether in positive, life-enhancing ways or in negative, counterproductive ways.

As a college student, you may be in one of the most stressful periods of your life. You may be on your own for the first time, or you may be juggling the demands of college with the responsibilities of a job, a family, or both. Financial pressures may be intense. Housing and transportation may be sources of additional hassles. You're also meeting new people, engaging in new activities, learning new information and skills, and setting a new course for your life. Good and bad, all of these changes and challenges are likely to have a powerful effect on you, both physically and psychologically. Respond ineffectively to stress, and eventually it will take a toll on your sense of well-being and overall health. Learn effective responses, however, and you will enhance your health and gain a feeling of control over your life.

WHAT IS STRESS?

Just what is stress, if such vastly different situations can cause it? No one has explored the biochemical and environmental aspects of stress more thoroughly than Hans Selye, an endocrinologist and biologist. Selye defines stress as "the nonspecific response of the body to any demand." What is a "nonspecific response"? It's the body's total biological response, from sweating palms to a pounding heart to a stress-producing situation. What is "nonspecific" about this response? No matter what the specific stressful situation that provokes it—a date, a final exam, or a flat tire—the physical response is the same. This response can vary in intensity—sometimes your heart races faster and your palms sweat more—but it is always limited to the same basic set of physical reactions.

In common usage, the word *stress* is used to refer to two different things: situations that trigger physical and emotional reactions and the reactions themselves. In this text, we'll use the more precise terms **stressor** to refer to situations that trigger physical and emotional reactions and the term **stress response** to refer to those reactions. A date and a final exam, then, are stressors; sweaty palms and a pounding heart are symptoms of the stress response. We'll use the term *stress* to describe the general physical and emotional state that accompanies the stress response. A person on a date or taking a final exam experiences stress.

Each individual's experience of stress depends on many factors, including the nature of the stressor. Stress triggered by a pleasant stressor, such as a date or a party, is called **eustress**. On the other hand, **distress** stems from an unpleasant stressor, such as a flat tire or a bad grade.

Physical Responses to Stressors: General Adaptation Syndrome

The light turns green and you step off the curb. Almost before you see it, you feel a car speeding toward you. With just a fraction of a second to spare, you leap safely out of harm's way. In that split second of danger, and in the moments following it, you have experienced a predictable series of physical reactions. Hans Selye termed this predictable pattern the **general adaptation syndrome (GAS)**. Selye divided GAS into three distinct stages: alarm, resistance, and exhaustion.

TERMS

Stress   The sum of the physical and emotional reactions to any stimulus that disturbs the organism's homeostasis.

Stressor   Any physical or psychological event or condition that produces stress.

Stress response   The physiological changes associated with stress.

Eustress   Stress resulting from pleasant stressors.

Distress   Stress resulting from unpleasant stressors.

General adaptation syndrome (GAS)   A pattern of stress responses described by Hans Selye as having three stages: alarm, resistance, and exhaustion.

Sympathetic nervous system   A division of the autonomic system that reacts to danger or other challenges by almost instantly putting the body processes in high gear.

Autonomic nervous system   The branch of the peripheral nervous system that, largely without conscious thought, controls basic body processes; subdivided into the sympathetic and parasympathetic systems.

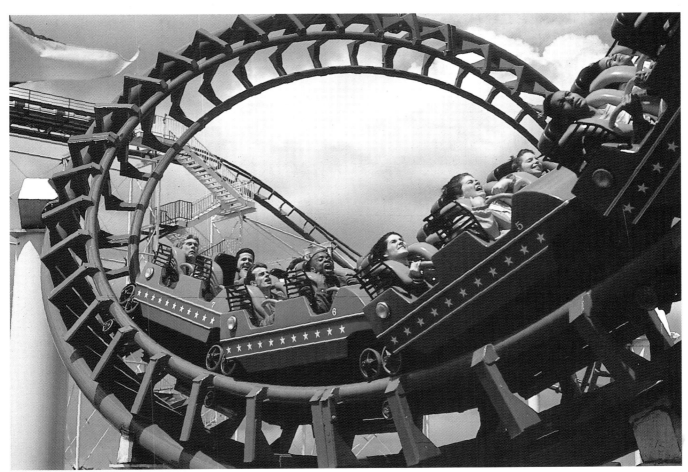

The experience of stress depends on many factors, including the nature of the stressor. Exciting experiences like this amusement park ride can produce a stimulating kind of stress known as eustress.

GAS: Alarm The instant you sense the oncoming car, an internal alarm sounds and the **sympathetic** branch of your **autonomic nervous system** takes command. For the most part, this part of your nervous system operates independently of conscious thought. It controls your heart rate, breathing, blood pressure, digestion, and hundreds of other functions you usually take for granted. It is also responsible for mobilizing your body for physical action in response to a stressor.

As the car travels toward you, you feel only fear. Your sympathetic nervous system, however, knows exactly what to do—and does it with breathtaking speed and efficiency. Its control center in the brain, the **hypothalamus**, orders the **pituitary gland** to release a chemical messenger called **adrenocorticotropic hormone (ACTH)** into the bloodstream. When ACTH reaches the **adrenal glands**, located just above the kidneys, it stimulates them to release **cortisol** and other key **hormones** into the bloodstream. Simultaneously, sympathetic nerves instruct your adrenal glands to release the hormones **epinephrine**, or adrenaline, and **norepinephrine**, which in turn trigger a series of profound changes as they circulate

TERMS

Hypothalamus A part of the brain that activates, controls, and integrates the autonomic mechanisms, endocrine activities, and many body functions.

Pituitary gland The "master gland," closely linked with the hypothalamus, that controls other endocrine glands and secretes hormones that regulate growth, maturation, and reproduction.

Adrenocorticotropic hormone (ACTH) A hormone, formed in the pituitary gland, that stimulates the outer layer of the adrenal gland to secrete its hormones.

Adrenal glands Two glands, one lying atop each kidney, their outer layer (cortex) producing steroid hormones such as cortisol, and their inner core (medulla) producing the hormones epinephrine and norepinephrine.

Cortisol A steroid hormone secreted by the cortex (outer layer) of the adrenal gland; also called *hydrocortisone*.

Hormones Chemical messengers produced in the body and transported by the bloodstream to target cells or organs for specific regulation of their activities.

Epinephrine A hormone secreted by the medulla (inner core) of the adrenal gland; also called *adrenaline,* the "fear hormone."

Norepinephrine A hormone secreted by the medulla (inner core) of the adrenal gland; also called *noradrenaline,* the "anger hormone."

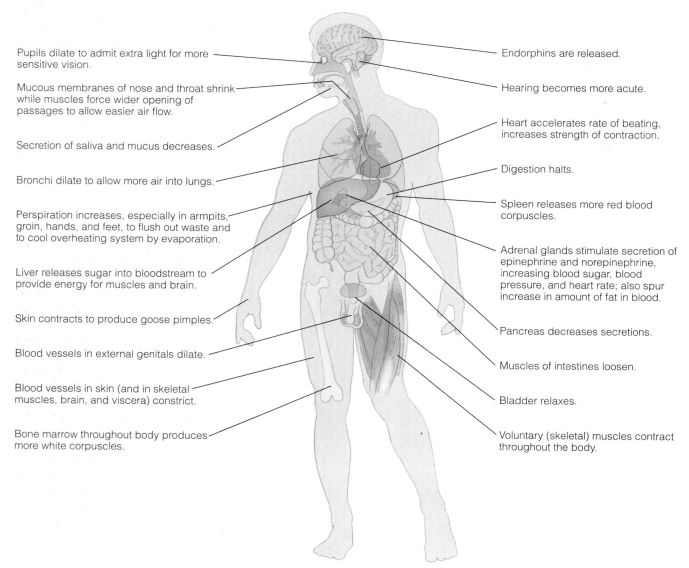

Pupils dilate to admit extra light for more sensitive vision.

Mucous membranes of nose and throat shrink while muscles force wider opening of passages to allow easier air flow.

Secretion of saliva and mucus decreases.

Bronchi dilate to allow more air into lungs.

Perspiration increases, especially in armpits, groin, hands, and feet, to flush out waste and to cool overheating system by evaporation.

Liver releases sugar into bloodstream to provide energy for muscles and brain.

Skin contracts to produce goose pimples.

Blood vessels in external genitals dilate.

Blood vessels in skin (and in skeletal muscles, brain, and viscera) constrict.

Bone marrow throughout body produces more white corpuscles.

Endorphins are released.

Hearing becomes more acute.

Heart accelerates rate of beating, increases strength of contraction.

Digestion halts.

Spleen releases more red blood corpuscles.

Adrenal glands stimulate secretion of epinephrine and norepinephrine, increasing blood sugar, blood pressure, and heart rate; also spur increase in amount of fat in blood.

Pancreas decreases secretions.

Muscles of intestines loosen.

Bladder relaxes.

Voluntary (skeletal) muscles contract throughout the body.

Figure 2-1 *The alarm reaction.*

throughout your body (Figure 2-1). Your hearing and vision become more acute. Bronchi dilate to allow more air into your lungs. Your heart rate accelerates to pump more oxygen through your body. Your liver releases extra sugar into your bloodstream to provide an energy boost for your muscles and brain. Your digestion halts. You perspire more to cool your skin. **Endorphins** are released to relieve pain in case of injury. Blood cell production increases. These almost instantaneous changes give you the heightened reflexes and strength you need to dodge the car.

The alarm response, or **fight-or-flight reaction,** is a part of our biological heritage. It's a survival mechanism that has served humankind well. In modern life, however, the alarm response is often absurdly inappropriate. It can be triggered by a party invitation, stumbling over a doorstep, or being insulted, as well as by physical threats like an out-of-control car. The alarm response prepares your body for physical action, regardless of whether physical action is a necessary or appropriate response to a particular stressor.

GAS: Resistance   Your body resists dramatic changes. Whenever normal functioning is disrupted, such as during the alarm reaction, your body strives for **homeostasis,** a state in which blood pressure, heart rate, hormone levels, and other vital functions are maintained within a narrow range of normal. Once a stressful situation ends, the **parasympathetic** branch of your autonomic nervous system takes command and halts the alarm reaction. It initiates the **adaptive reactions,** or adjustments, necessary to restore homeostasis. Your parasympathetic ner-

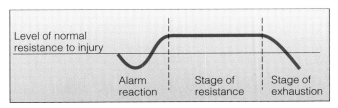

Figure 2-2 *General Adaptation Syndrome.*
In Selye's experiments, rats subjected to cold at first exhibited the hormonal changes typical of the alarm reaction but then adapted to life at lower temperatures. After several months, however, they lost their acquired resistance, and exhaustion set in.

vous system calms your body down, slowing rapid heartbeat, drying sweaty palms, and returning breathing to normal. Gradually, your body resumes its day-to-day "housekeeping" functions, such as digestion and temperature regulation. Damage that may have been sustained during the alarm reaction is repaired. The day after you narrowly dodge the car, you wake up feeling fine. The resistance phase of the GAS has enabled you to get on with your everyday life.

GAS: Exhaustion   What if, instead of getting on with your everyday life, you found yourself confronted with a string of severe stressors? Your financial aid is cut, and you are forced to work more hours each week at your part-time job. Your bicycle is stolen. You do poorly in several courses and are placed on academic probation. You break up with the person you've been dating for the last six months. Your father suffers a heart attack. This group of events would cause your body to respond over and over with an alarm reaction. Some people in extreme circumstances—men and women who serve on the front lines in battle, hostages, prisoners of war, and victims of chronic domestic or neighborhood violence—are forced to confront life-and-death emergencies every day.

As you might imagine, both the mobilization of forces during the alarm reaction and the restoration of homeostasis during the resistance stage require a considerable amount of energy. If a stressor persists, or if a series of stressors occur in succession, readily available stores of energy can be depleted. Worse, reserves of **adaptive energy** can be drained as well. When these adaptive energy reserves are used up, general exhaustion results. This is not the sort of exhaustion people complain of after a long, busy day. It's a life-threatening type of physiological exhaustion characterized by such symptoms as distorted perceptions and disorganized thinking.

In laboratory experiments, Selye subjected rats to conditions that put them under extreme stress. He found that the rats responded with an alarm reaction when they first encountered a stressor. Over time, though, their nervous systems learned to view the stressor as normal and estab-

lished a new homeostasis. However, the rats were able to sustain this resistance to the stressor for only a limited time. If the stressor continued, exhaustion eventually set in (Figure 2-2).

The Stress Response in Everyday Modern Life   Few of us will suffer a string of disasters or endure combat in our homes or on a battlefield. But modern life, even when it's going well, consists of countless stressors. Some of them—noise, overcrowding, overwork, discrimination, competition, and economic pressures, for instance—go on not just for a few minutes but for days, weeks, months, or a lifetime.

Everyday stressors don't often lead to terminal exhaustion. But there is evidence that over the long term they can kill us just the same. Selye argues that cardiovascular disease, the leading cause of death in this country, is a "disease of adaptation"—a disease that results when the body is subjected too often to the drastic demands of the stress response. Selye also considers ulcers, some mental disorders, and possibly cancer as diseases of adaptation. These and other stress-linked diseases are discussed more fully later in the chapter.

GAS is a survival mechanism meant to mobilize us for fight or flight in rare life-and-death emergencies. Our bodies aren't designed to withstand its heavy demands on an ongoing basis. Ironically, the strains and hassles of life in a civilized world have transformed this life-saving mechanism into a potentially life-threatening one. How do you know if you're overstressed? Symptoms of stress can be physical, emotional, or behavioral; they include stiff neck, headache, skin problems, allergy or asthma attacks, frequent colds or low-grade infections, gastrointestinal problems, emotional instability, depression, inability to concentrate, fatigue, sleep disturbances, changes in eating habits, and increased use of alcohol, tobacco, or other drugs. Of course, you don't have to experience them all to realize you're encountering too many stressors too frequently. And some of the signals may be

Endorphins   Brain secretions that have pain-inhibiting effects.

Fight-or-flight reaction   A defense reaction that prepares the organism for conflict or escape by triggering hormonal, cardiovascular, metabolic, and other changes.

Homeostasis   A state of stability and consistency in the physiological functioning of an organism.

Parasympathetic nervous system   A division of the autonomic system that tones down the excitatory effect of the sympathetic system, slowing metabolism and restoring energy supplies.

Adaptive reaction   The organism's attempt to readjust its activities and restore homeostasis when the demands of stress have disturbed the body's equilibrium.

Adaptive energy   Limited body reserves that are activated when the body feels exhausted.

TERMS

symptoms of a medical problem unrelated to stress. In general, though, such signals are distinct warnings about a problem that requires your attention. Ignoring or worrying about such symptoms will only add to the problem. If your body is trying to tell you something, it's important to listen.

Emotional and Behavioral Responses to Stressors: Individual Variation

Physically, everyone responds to stressors in basically the same, predictable way. Emotionally and behaviorally, though, individuals may respond in very different ways. You may feel relaxed and confident about taking exams but be nervous about talking to members of the opposite sex, while your roommate may love challenging social situations but be very nervous about taking tests. A poor grade on a group project may prompt you to go for a 10-mile jog, while other members of your project team respond by eating chocolate or getting drunk. What accounts for these differences? Emotional and behavioral responses to stressors depend on a complex set of factors that includes temperament, health, life experiences, beliefs and ideas, and coping skills.

Common emotional responses to stressors include anxiety, depression, and fear. Although we often can moderate or learn to control them, emotional responses are determined in part by inborn personality or temperament. Some people seem to be born nervous and irritable, and others are innately calm and even-tempered.

Our behavioral responses to stressors are controlled by the **somatic nervous system,** which manages our conscious actions. This means we can *choose* how we behave in response to the stressors in our lives. Depending on the stressor involved, effective behavioral responses may include crying, talking, or hugging; exercising, meditating, or laughing; or learning time management skills, finding a more compatible roommate, or looking for a different job. Inappropriate behavioral responses include overeating and using tobacco, alcohol, or other drugs. Effective behavioral responses promote mental and physical health and allow us to function at our best. Ineffective behavioral responses to stressors can harm our mental and physical health and can even become stressors themselves.

Let's consider the different emotional and behavioral responses of two students, Amelia and David, to a common stressor—the first exam of the semester. Both students feel anxious as the exam is passed out. Amelia relaxes her muscles and then starts by writing the answers she knows. On a second pass through the exam, she concentrates carefully on the wording of each question. Some material comes back to her, and she makes educated guesses on the remaining items. She spends the whole hour writing as much as she can and checking her answers. She leaves the room feeling calm, relaxed, and confident that she has done well on the exam.

David responds to his initial anxiety with more anxiety. He finds that he doesn't know some of the answers, and he becomes more worried. The more upset he gets, the less he can remember; and the more he blanks out, the more anxious he gets. He begins to imagine the consequences of failing the course and berates himself for not having studied more. David turns in his paper before the hour is up, without checking his answers or going back to the questions he skipped. He leaves feeling depressed and angry at himself.

Why are their responses so different? David may respond anxiously to many situations in life. He may be less confident of his academic abilities than Amelia. He might have blanked out during an exam in the past and so was worried that it would happen again. He may also have poor study and time management skills. Amelia may have a calmer temperament. She may have more confidence in her academic abilities, stemming from a long record of success in school. She may be able to focus her attention and study effectively despite distractions.

Behavioral, emotional, and physical responses are intimately interrelated. The more intense the physical response, the stronger the emotional response, and vice versa. Effective behavioral responses can break this cycle; ineffective ones only worsen it. Sometimes people have such intense emotional responses and such ineffective or counterproductive behavioral responses to stressors that they need professional assistance to learn to cope. More often, however, people can learn to handle stressors on their own.

Personal Insight   How do you respond when you're in a frustrating situation such as a traffic jam? Do you find that such situations really bother you at some times but not at others? What else is going on in your life when you stay calm? When you fly off the handle? Do you find that your relationships with others suffer when you're under stress?

STRESS AND DISEASE

The role of stress in disease is complex. Much depends on the individual and the situation. What is clear is that people who have too many stressors in their lives or who handle stressors poorly are at risk for a wide range of problems. In the short term, the problem might just be a cold, a stiff neck, or a stomach ache. In the long term, the problems can be more severe—cardiovascular disease, high blood pressure, or impairment of the immune system. As researchers learn more about the connections between mind and body, the list of illnesses linked to stress grows.

Most of us have wondered at one time or another about the connections between mind and body. Can states of mind affect our health? Can negative feelings like fear and anger make us sick? Can positive feelings like hope and a "will to live" help make us well? How can our elusive, intangible minds have an effect on our solid, flesh-and-blood bodies? Recently, medical research has begun to provide some scientific answers to these questions.

One of the most fruitful areas of mind-body research has been **psychoneuroimmunology** (PNI for short)—the study of the connections among the brain, the **endocrine system,** and the immune system. Advances in technology in the past decade or two have allowed researchers to begin to explore the biochemistry of these connections. Chief among their discoveries is the finding that a complex and busy electrochemical communication system links the brain and the rest of the body. The brain secretes dozens of hormones and hormonelike substances that carry information and messages throughout the body. Some of these substances, such as endorphins, function as painkillers. Others, such as interferons, trigger immune defenses against cancer.

Researchers have also found that other hormonelike substances called neuropeptides serve to coordinate the functions of the brain, glands, and immune system. Neuropeptides have been referred to as "the biochemicals of the emotions"—substances that translate emotions into bodily events. Neuropeptides are produced and received by both brain and immune cells, so that the brain and the immune system share a biochemical "language," which also happens to be the language of the emotions. Surprisingly enough, the entire lining of the intestines is also equipped with neuropeptide receptors, perhaps accounting for our tendency to experience emotions as "gut feelings."

Other mind-body investigations have focused on such areas as the effect of emotions and attitudes on the cardiovascular system and the effect of exercise on mood. These and innumerable other discoveries have persuaded many medical scientists that the mind and body are best seen not as separate entities but as parts of a fully integrated system—the living, breathing human being. What enters the mind finds its way into the body. Thoughts, feelings, attitudes, moods, psychological states may all be mirrored in the functioning of the body. Numerous studies have shown that the negative feelings of fear and anger—the hallmarks of the stress response—as well as depression, frustration, despair, and helplessness produce negative changes in the body's chemistry, dampening the immune response. Studies also suggest that the positive emotions—love, hope, joy, confidence, determination—might provide a buffer against the effects of stress.

The scientific study of mind-body connections is still in its infancy. Some of its findings have been distorted by the popular press with extravagant and unscientific claims about the "healing powers of the mind." Such claims do a disservice to the research they supposedly represent, creating false expectations—and guilt—in people with life-threatening diseases. Scientists point out that although mind-body connections are real, more research is needed before we fully understand their nature and their extent.

The realization that mind and body are intimately connected gives new meaning to the notion of "a sound mind in a sound body." The implication is that we can't cultivate mental and physical health separately and independently; instead, we need to understand that the two work together. There is no such thing as a purely psychological event or a purely physical event; the two are inseparable in the living organism.

Cardiovascular Disease

The most serious long-term effect of stress on the body is probably high blood pressure. In the alarm phase of the stress response, heart rate increases and blood vessels constrict, causing blood pressure to rise. Chronic high blood pressure is a major cause of **atherosclerosis,** a disease in which the lining of the blood vessels becomes damaged and caked with fatty deposits. These deposits can block arteries, causing heart attacks and strokes. Atherosclerosis is a leading cause of disability and death from cardiovascular disease.

Recent research suggests that certain types of emotional responses increase an individual's risk of cardiovascular disease. People who tend to react to situations with anger and hostility, or who are cynical and mistrustful, are more likely to have heart attacks than are people with less explosive, more trusting personalities.

TERMS

Somatic nervous system The branch of the peripheral nervous system that governs motor functions and sensory information; largely under our conscious control.

Atherosclerosis The buildup of hard yellow plaques of fatty material in the lining of arteries that have become damaged due to advancing age or high blood pressure; a leading cause of heart disease and stroke.

Psychoneuroimmunology The study of the interactions among the brain, the endocrine system, and the immune system.

Endocrine system The system of glands that secrete hormones into the blood to influence metabolism and other body processes.

Impairment of the Immune System

Sometimes you seem to get sick when you can least afford it—during exam week, or when you're going on vacation, or when you have a big job interview. A growing body of evidence suggests that this is more than mere coincidence. It appears that stressors can have a direct bearing on the body's ability to fight off viruses and other disease agents. Studies have shown that anxiety, depression, anger, overexertion, and sleep deprivation are all associated with a temporary decline in immune function. In one study, British investigators administered nose drops spiked with cold viruses to 394 healthy men and women. The test subjects who experienced the most stressors in the previous year were the most likely to catch colds.

Other Health Problems

Other diseases and conditions that may be triggered or aggravated by stress include injuries, allergies, asthma, backaches, cancer, eczema, HIV infection, hives, impotence, insomnia, irritable bowel syndrome, menstrual irregularities, migraines, panic attacks, psoriasis, and ulcers. Stress can also contribute to such psychological problems as depression, anxiety, and post-traumatic stress disorder. Repetitive-stress injury (RSI) is a recent addition to the list of conditions linked to stress. A 1992 study conducted by the National Institute for Occupational Safety and Health found that RSI occurred most frequently in those workers who experienced the greatest job insecurity, productivity demands, surges in workload, and lack of control over work methods. RSI causes mild to severe pain or numbness in the wrist, hand, fingers, elbow, neck, or shoulder. Typists, keyboard operators, cashiers, meat-cutters, and others who use their hands in repetitive motions are vulnerable to this painful and potentially crippling ailment.

TECHNIQUES FOR MANAGING STRESS

Stress surrounds us; it is an inevitable part of life. We face environmental stressors, social stressors, and stressors originating in our mind. What can you do about all this stress? A great deal. By shoring up your social support systems, developing and maintaining healthy exercise and eating habits, and mastering simple techniques to identify and moderate individual stressors, you can learn to control the stress in your life, instead of allowing it to control you. The effort is well worth the time: People who manage stress effectively not only are healthier, but they also have more time to enjoy life and accomplish goals.

Social Support

People need people. One study of 173 college students living in overcrowded apartments, for example, found those with strong social support systems were less dis-

tressed by their cramped quarters. Allow yourself time to nourish and maintain a network of people at home, at work, at school, or in your community on whom you can count for emotional support, feedback, and nurturance. When you share your fears, frustrations, and joys with others, your problems seem easier to face and your pleasures seem richer.

If yours is one of the many families that doesn't function very well as a support system for its members, create a second "family" of people with whom you have built meaningful ties. Support groups or religious organizations are valuable for some people: One study found stress levels decreased as religious attendance increased—even when subjects did nothing else to manage stress.

Exercise

One recent study from the National Academy of Sciences found that taking a long walk can be effective in reducing anxiety and blood pressure. Another study found that just a brisk 10-minute walk leaves people feeling more relaxed and energetic for up to 2 hours. Regular exercise has even more benefits. Researchers have found that people who exercise regularly react with milder physical stress responses before, during, and after exposure to stressors. People who took three brisk 45-minute walks a week for 3 months reported that they perceived fewer daily hassles. Their sense of general well-being also increased.

It's not hard to incorporate light to moderate exercise into your day. Walk to class or bike to the store instead of driving. Use the stairs instead of the elevator. Take a walk with a friend instead of getting a cup of coffee. Go bowling, play tennis, or roller-skate instead of seeing a movie. Make a habit of taking a brisk after-dinner stroll. Plan hikes and easy bike outings for the weekends. Play softball or Ping-Pong. Take a tai chi or yoga class. Garden. Once you begin to make sensible exercise a daily part of your life, you may find it hard to live without.

Nutrition

A healthy diet will give you an energy bank to draw on whenever stress strikes. Eating wisely also will enhance your feelings of self-control and self-esteem. Learning the principles of sound nutrition is easy, and sensible eating habits rapidly become second nature when practiced regularly.

Avoiding or limiting caffeine is also important in stress management. Although one to two cups of coffee a day probably won't hurt you, caffeine is a mildly addictive stimulant that leaves some people jittery, irritable, and unable to sleep. Tea, cola, and some other soft drinks, chocolate, and more than a thousand over-the-counter drugs, including cold remedies and weight-loss preparations, also contain caffeine, sometimes in fairly high doses.

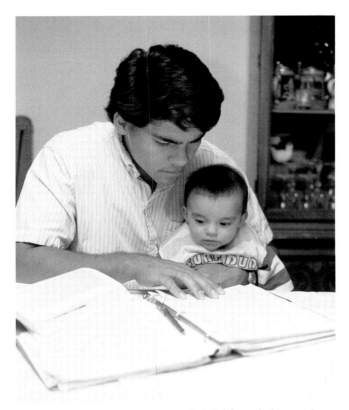

Managing the many commitments of adult life, including work, school, and parenthood, can sometimes feel overwhelming and produce a great deal of stress. Time management skills, including careful scheduling and prioritizing, help this father cope with busy days.

It's also a good idea to stay away from high-potency vitamin formulations and amino acid supplements that are sometimes touted as remedies for stress. So-called stress vitamins usually contain vitamins C, E, and B-complex. These capsules or tablets are worthless for reducing tension or anxiety, and they could add to your stress. Some supplements contain up to 80 times the U.S. Recommended Dietary Allowance (RDA) for B vitamins and 16 times the RDA for vitamin C. Megadoses can cause stomach irritation and other potentially unpleasant side effects. Amino acid supplements can be even more risky. Some popular authors and health food aficionados recommend amino acid supplements for people who want to manage stress, improve concentration, or alter their mood. There is no evidence that such use of these supplements is effective, but there is tragic evidence it can be unsafe. A number of deaths in the late 1980s and early 1990s due to a rare blood disorder have been attributed to a still-unidentified contaminant of the amino acid L-tryptophan, which is touted as a cure for premenstrual syndrome, depression, insomnia, and anxiety.

Time Management

A surprising number of the stressors in most people's lives relate to time. Many people never seem to have enough time, and they continually feel overwhelmed by the pace of their lives; others seem to have too much time on their hands and are often bored. Learning to manage your time successfully is crucial to coping with the stressors you face every day.

Procrastination is probably the single biggest time management problem for most of us. It can sabotage personal relationships, college life, and careers. Reasons for procrastination are as numerous as the excuses people invent for it (such as "I'll wait until I'm inspired" or "What difference will this make in the planetary scheme of things?"). In general, procrastination camouflages self-doubt, an unreasonable desire for perfection, or a reluctance to make changes. The best solution? Stop thinking or talking about what you're going to do, and "just do it." Here, in abridged form, are tips from two psychologists who are reformed procrastinators: "Visualize your progress. Optimize your chances. Stick to a time limit. Don't wait until you feel like it. Watch out for your excuses. Focus on one step at a time. Get beyond the first obstacle. Reward yourself after you've made some progress. Be flexible about your goal. It doesn't have to be perfect."

Even if you never procrastinate, time pressures can create stress. Try one, or all, of the following steps to manage your time more productively and creatively:

- Set priorities. Divide your tasks into three groups: essential, important, and trivial. Focus on the first two. Ignore the third.

- Schedule tasks for peak efficiency. You've undoubtedly noticed you're most productive at certain times of the day (or night). Schedule as many of your tasks for those hours as you can.

- Set realistic goals. Attainable goals spur you on. Impossible goals, by definition, generate frustration and failure.

- Write down your goals. Make sure they're realistic and attainable. Then fully commit yourself to achieving them.

- Budget enough time. For each project you undertake, calculate how long it will take to complete. Then tack on another 10 or 15 percent—or even 25 percent—as a buffer against mistakes or unanticipated problems.

- Break up long-term goals into short-term ones. Instead of waiting for or relying on large blocks of time, use short snatches of time to start a project or keep it moving. Say you have a 50-page report due and are about to panic. Divide the assignment into three tasks: research, outlining, and writing. Now budget enough half-hour or hour-long time slots to complete each task. Your steady progress will make you feel so much better that you'll be encouraged to plow on.

- Visualize the achievement of your goals. By mentally rehearsing your performance of a task, you can reach your goal quite smoothly because, after all, you'll have traveled that road before.

- Sleep on it. Before going to sleep, take five minutes to write down in order of priority the problems you expect to encounter tomorrow. Then ignore them. While you're asleep, your unconscious mind will be hard at work tackling those problems. When you deal with them by rank the next day, you may be surprised at how easily you'll be able to work them out.

- Delegate responsibility. Asking for help when you have too much to do is no cop-out; it's good time management. Just don't delegate to others the jobs you know you should do yourself, such as researching a paper.

- Say no when necessary. If the demands made on you don't seem reasonable, say no—tactfully, but without guilt or apology.

- Give yourself a break. Allow time for play—free, unstructured time when you ignore the clock. Don't consider this a waste of time. Play renews you and allows you to work more efficiently.

Relaxation Techniques

According to Herbert Benson of Harvard Medical School, relaxation techniques can trigger the relaxation response—a physiological state characterized by a feeling of warmth and quiet mental alertness. This is the opposite of the fight-or-flight response. When the relaxation response is triggered, heart rate, breathing, and metabolism slow down. Blood pressure and oxygen consumption decrease. At the same time, blood flow to the brain and skin increases, and brain waves shift from an alert, beta rhythm to a relaxed, alpha rhythm. Practiced regularly, relaxation techniques can counteract the debilitating effects of stress. When an Oregon nursing professor taught relaxation techniques to 38 nursing students in one recent study, she found they scored 7 points lower on scales of anxiety and depression after only 3 weeks. A matched group of students who received no training gained 2 points over the same time period.

Progressive relaxation, imagery, and meditation are three relaxation techniques that are among the most popular and easiest to learn. They require a minimal amount of time to learn and perform, and each can be done individually. Other techniques, such as massage, self-hypnosis, and biofeedback, require a partner or professional training or assistance.

If you decide to try one of these techniques, practice it daily until it becomes natural to you, and then use it whenever you feel the need. You may feel calmer and more refreshed after each session. If one technique doesn't seem to work well enough for you after you've given it a good try, have a go at another one. You'll know you've mastered a deep relaxation technique when you start to see subtle changes in other areas of your life: You may notice you've been encountering fewer hassles, working more efficiently, or enjoying more free time.

Progressive Relaxation Unlike most of the others, this simple method requires no imagination, willpower, or self-suggestion. You simply tense, and then relax, the muscles in your body, one by one. The technique, also known as deep muscle relaxation, helps you to become aware of the muscle tension that occurs when you're under stress. When you consciously relax those muscles, other systems of the body get the message and ease up on the stress response.

Here's what you do: Start, for example, with your right fist. Inhale as you tense it. Exhale as you relax it. Repeat. Next, contract and relax your right biceps. Repeat. Do the same with your left arm. Then, beginning at your forehead and ending at your feet, contract and relax your other muscles. Repeat each contraction at least once, breathing in as you tense, breathing out as you relax. To speed up the process, tense and relax more muscles at one time—both arms simultaneously, for instance. With practice, you'll be able to relax very quickly and effectively by clenching and releasing only your fists.

Imagery Imagery, or visualization, allows you to daydream without guilt. Elite athletes have found that the technique enhances sports performance, and visualization is even part of the curriculum at training camps for U.S. Olympic athletes. You can use the technique to help you relax, change your habits, or perform well, whether on an exam, a stage, or a playing field.

The next time you feel stressed, close your eyes. Imagine yourself floating on a cloud, sitting on a mountaintop, or lying in a meadow. What do you see and hear? Is it cold? Or damp? What do you smell? What do you taste? Involve all your senses. Your body will respond as if your imagery were real. An alternative: Close your eyes and imagine a deep purple light filling your body. Now change the color into a soothing gold. As the color lightens, so should your distress. Imagery also can enhance performance. If you're worried about doing well at a task, visualize yourself performing it flawlessly.

Meditation Meditation is a way of politely telling the mind to shut up for a while. The need to periodically stop the incessant mental chatter is so great that, from ancient times, hundreds of forms of meditation have developed in cultures all over the world. Because meditation has been at the core of many Eastern religions and philosophies, it has acquired an "Eastern" mystique that has caused some people to shy away from it. Yet meditation requires no

Several years ago, Herbert Benson developed a simple, practical technique for eliciting the relaxation response. Here's the basic procedure he recommends:

1. Pick a word, phrase, or object to focus on. If you like, you can choose a word or phrase that has a deep meaning for you, but any word or phrase will work. In Zen meditation, the word *mu* (literally, "absolutely nothing") is often used. Some meditators prefer to focus on their breathing.

2. Take a comfortable position in a quiet environment, and close your eyes if you're not focusing on an object.

3. Relax your muscles.

4. Breathe slowly and naturally. If you're using a focus word or phrase, silently repeat it each time you exhale. If you're using an object, focus on it as you breathe.

5. Keep your attitude passive. Disregard thoughts that drift in.

6. Continue for 10 to 20 minutes, once or twice a day.

7. After you've finished, sit quietly for a few minutes with your eyes first closed and then open. Then get to your feet.

Suggestions

Allow relaxation to occur at its own pace; don't try to force it. Don't be surprised if you can't tune your mind out for more than a few seconds at a time. It's nothing to get angry about. The more you ignore the intrusions, the easier doing so will get.

If you want to time your session, peek at a watch or clock occasionally, but don't set a jarring alarm.

The technique works best on an empty stomach—before a meal or about two hours after eating. Avoid times of day when you're tired—unless you want to fall asleep.

Although you'll feel refreshed even after the first session, it may take a month or more to get noticeable results. Be patient. Eventually the relaxation response will become so natural that it will occur spontaneously, or on demand, when you sit quietly for a few moments.

---

special knowledge or background. We all know how to meditate; we need only discover that we do and then put our knowledge to use. Whatever philosophical, religious, or emotional reasons may be given for meditation, its power derives from its ability to elicit the relaxation response.

Meditation helps you to tune out the world temporarily, relieving you from both inner and outer stresses. It allows you to transcend past conditioning, fixed expectations, and the trivial pursuits of the psyche; it clears out the mental smog. The "thinker" takes time out to become the "observer"—calmly attentive, without analyzing, judging, comparing, or rationalizing. Regular practice of this quiet awareness will subtly carry over into your daily life, encouraging physical and emotional balance no matter what confronts you.

Cognitive Techniques

Some stressors arise in our own minds. Ideas, beliefs, perceptions, and patterns of thinking can add to our emotional and physical stress responses and get in the way of effective behavioral responses. Each of the techniques described below can help you change unhealthy thought patterns to ones that will help you cope with stress. As with any skill, mastering these techniques takes practice and patience.

Worry Constructively Worrying, someone once said, is like shoveling smoke. Think back to the worries you

had last week. How many of them were needless? Worry only about things you can control. Try to stand aside from the problem, consider the positive steps you can take to solve it, and then carry them out. You've done what you can; you can quit worrying.

Moderate Expectations Expectations are exhausting and restricting. The fewer expectations you have, the more you can live spontaneously and joyfully. The more you expect from others, the more often you will feel let down. Trying to meet the expectations others have of you is often futile as well. In fact, the surest road to failure is to try to please everyone around you. That's a road you can choose to bypass. As therapist Fritz Perls put it, "I don't exist to fulfill your expectations, and you don't exist to fulfill mine."

Monitor Self-Talk If you catch your mind beating up on you—"Late for class again! You can't even cope with college! How do you expect to ever hold down a professional job?"—change your inner dialogue. Talk to yourself as you would to a child you love: "You're a smart, capable person. You've solved other problems; you'll handle this one. Tomorrow you'll simply schedule things so you get to class with a few minutes to spare."

Weed Out Trivia You can burden your memory with too much information. A major source of stress is trying to "store" too much data. Forget unimportant details

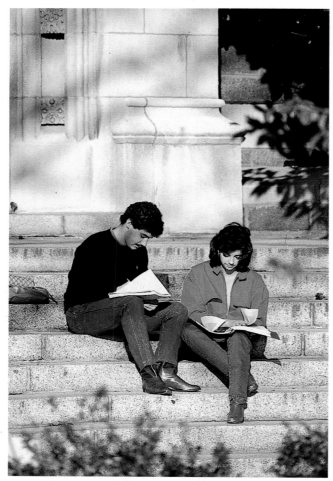

These students have found an effective strategy for dealing with the anxiety of an upcoming exam. By focusing directly on preparing for the test, they avoid self-defeating thoughts and needless worrying, give each other needed emotional support, and maximize their chances of success.

blood pressure dip below normal. You are relaxed. Ridicule, cynicism, and sarcasm don't have the same effects, however. Neither does gruesome or offensive humor, which is an unconscious means of dealing with fears and anxieties. Therapeutic humor, in contrast, reflects a healthy appreciation of life's absurdities and paradoxes. Therapeutic humor gives you a break, even if a short one, from the hassles of daily life. It detaches you from both your situation and yourself. Cultivate the ability to laugh at yourself, and you'll have a handy and instantly effective stress reliever.

Go with the Flow Remember that the branch that bends in the storm doesn't break. Try to flow with your life, accepting the things you can't change. Be forgiving of faults, your own and others'. Instead of anticipating happiness at some indefinite point in the future, realize that pleasure is integral to being alive. You can create it every day of your life. View challenges as an opportunity to learn and grow. Be flexible. In this way you can make stress work for you rather than against you, enhancing your overall health.

Personal Insight How did people in your family cope with stress when you were growing up? Were their methods successful? Do you use the same methods (or nonmethods) they did? Are there people around you who use different methods that you could try?

CREATING A PERSONAL PLAN FOR MANAGING STRESS

What are the most important sources of stress in your life? Are you coping successfully with these stressors? There is no single strategy or program for managing stress that will work for everyone. The most important starting point for a successful stress management program is to learn to listen to your body. When you learn to recognize the stress response and the emotions and thoughts that accompany it, you'll be in a position to take charge of that crucial moment and handle it in a healthy way.

Identifying Stressors

Before you can learn to manage the stressors in your life, you have to identify them. A strategy many experts recommend is to keep a stress journal for a week or two. Each time you feel or display a stress reaction, record the time and the circumstances in your journal. Note what you were doing at the time, what you were thinking or feeling, and the outcome of your response.

After keeping your dairy for a few weeks, you should

(they will usually be self-evident). Keep your memory free for essential ones.

Live in the Present Do you clog your mind by reliving past events? Clinging to experiences and emotions, particularly unpleasant ones, can be a deadly business. Clear your mind of the old debris; let it go. Free yourself to enjoy what's happening now.

Cultivate Your Sense of Humor When it comes to stress, laughter may be the best medicine. Even a fleeting smile produces changes in your autonomic nervous system that can lift your spirits. And a few minutes of belly laughing can be as invigorating as brisk exercise. Hearty laughter elevates your heart rate, aids digestion, eases pain, and triggers the release of endorphins and other pleasurable and stimulating chemicals in the brain. After a good laugh, your muscles go slack; your pulse and

Like "planned spontaneity" or "intentional accident," "learned laughter" may sound like a contradiction. But according to William F. Fry, Jr., an emeritus professor of psychiatry at Stanford University and an authority on the physiology of mirth, you can teach yourself to laugh more. Fry, who calls himself a gelotologist (from the Greek root *gelos,* meaning laughter), says laughter defuses anger, lifts depression, increases alertness, enhances learning, promotes creativity and cooperation, fosters mental health, and may help prevent disease. It's also one of the most enjoyable ways to cope with stress.

Next time you're down or anxious, rent a Laurel and Hardy video or leaf through a book of *Far Side* cartoons. In his book *The Healing Power of Humor,* author Allen Klein also recommends these smile-inducing strategies:

- Collect silly props: clown noses, bubbles, "arrow" headbands. Put on the clown nose the next time you feel yourself getting anxious about an exam. Try blowing bubbles after an argument with your roommate.

- Have a punch line ready. When life deals you a blow— a bad grade, for example—try one of these widely applicable lines: "Oh, what an opportunity for growth and learning," "Take it back, it's not what I ordered," or "Beam me up, Scotty."

- Exaggerate to the point of absurdity. If you're having a bad day, pretend you're in the I-had-the-worst-day-in-the-world Olympics.

- Keep a photo of yourself laughing in a place where you can see it often.

- Smile when you feel down or tense. Sometimes mood follows facial expression.

- Identify traits you don't like in yourself and poke a little bit of fun at one of them at least once a day. Klein, who is bald, collects baldness jokes.

- Learn to view setbacks and annoyances as tests of your sense of humor.

For more information about the power of laughter, contact the Humor Project at 110 Spring Street, Saratoga Springs, NY 12866 (518-587-8770).

---

be able to spot some patterns. You may notice, for example, that mornings are usually the most stressful part of your day. Or you may discover that when you're angry at your roommate, you're apt to respond with behaviors that only make matters worse. Once you've outlined the general pattern of stress in your life, you may want to focus in on a particularly problematic stressor or on an inappropriate behavioral response you've identified. Keep a stress log for another week or two that focuses just on the early morning hours, for example, or just on your arguments with your roommate. The more information you gather, the easier it will be to develop effective strategies for coping with the stressors in your life.

Designing Your Program

Earlier in this chapter, you learned about many different techniques for combating stress. Now that you've identified the key stressors in your life, it's time to choose the techniques that will work best for you and create an action plan for change. Finding a buddy to work on stress management with you can make the process more fun and increase your chances of success. Some experts recommend drawing up a formal contract with yourself like the one shown in Figure 2-3.

Whether or not you complete a contract, it's important to design rewards into your plan. You might treat yourself to breakfast in a favorite restaurant on the weekend if you eat a nutritious breakfast every weekday morning. If you practice your relaxation technique faithfully, you might reward yourself with a long bath or an hour of pleasure reading at the end of the day. It's also important to evaluate your plan regularly and redesign it as your needs change. Under times of increased stress, for example, you might want to focus on good eating, exercise, and relaxation habits. Over time, your new stress management skills will become almost automatic. You'll feel better, accomplish more, and reduce your risk of disease.

Getting Help

If the techniques discussed so far don't provide you with enough relief from the stress in your life, you might want to consult a peer counselor, join a support group, or participate in a few psychotherapy sessions. Your student health center or student affairs office can tell you whether your campus has a peer counseling program. Such programs are usually staffed by volunteer students who have received special training that emphasizes the preservation of confidentiality. Peer counselors can steer you to other campus or community resources, or simply provide you with an understanding ear.

Support groups are typically organized around a particular issue or problem. In your area, you might find a support group for first-year students; for reentering students; for single parents; for students of your race, ethnic group, religion, or national origin; for people with eating disorders; or for rape survivors. The number of such

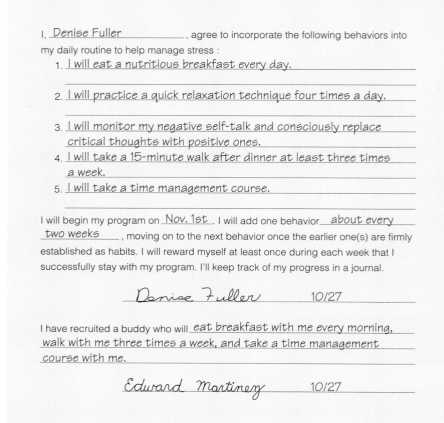

I, <u>Denise Fuller</u>, agree to incorporate the following behaviors into my daily routine to help manage stress :

1. <u>I will eat a nutritious breakfast every day.</u>

2. <u>I will practice a quick relaxation technique four times a day.</u>

3. <u>I will monitor my negative self-talk and consciously replace critical thoughts with positive ones.</u>

4. <u>I will take a 15-minute walk after dinner at least three times a week.</u>

5. <u>I will take a time management course.</u>

I will begin my program on <u>Nov. 1st</u>. I will add one behavior <u>about every two weeks</u>, moving on to the next behavior once the earlier one(s) are firmly established as habits. I will reward myself at least once during each week that I successfully stay with my program. I'll keep track of my progress in a journal.

Denise Fuller   10/27

I have recruited a buddy who will <u>eat breakfast with me every morning, walk with me three times a week, and take a time management course with me.</u>

Edward Martinez   10/27

Figure 2-3 *Sample contract for a stress management program.*

groups has increased in recent years, as more and more people discover how therapeutic it can be to talk with others who share the same situation.

Short-term psychotherapy can also be tremendously helpful in dealing with stress-related problems. Your student health center may offer psychotherapy on a sliding-fee scale; the county mental health center in your area may do the same. If you belong to any type of religious organization, check to see whether pastoral counseling is available. Your physician can refer you to psychotherapists in your community. Not all therapists are right for all people, so be prepared to have initial sessions with several. Choose the one you feel most comfortable with.

SUMMARY

- Stress-creating situations can be physical or psychological, pleasant or unpleasant. How people respond to stress helps determine their sense of well-being and their feeling of control over their health and their lives.

What Is Stress?

- In Hans Selye's terms, stress is "the body's total biological response to any demand." Physically, everyone responds to stressors in generally the same way.

- The body's response to stress, or general adaptation syndrome (GAS), has three stages: alarm, resistance, and exhaustion. GAS is controlled by the autonomic nervous system.

- The alarm stage of GAS is the fight-or-flight reaction. The sympathetic nervous system stimulates the release of chemical messengers that trigger changes in the body that mobilize it for action.

- The resistance stage of GAS, controlled by the parasympathetic nervous system, allows the body to readjust; body systems are regulated, and any damage sustained is repaired. Both the alarm and the resistance stages require considerable energy.

- The exhaustion stage occurs only if the body's reserves of energy (including adaptive energy) are depleted in a stress response; the results are distorted perceptions, disorganized thinking, and—in extreme cases—death.

- Most stresses of modern life can't be handled with a physical response; moreover, many of them continue indefinitely. A person whose body is constantly mobilized against these stresses may become a victim of "diseases of adaptation."
- Emotional and behavioral responses to stressors vary among individuals based on factors such as temperament, past experiences, beliefs, and coping skills. Emotional responses can be moderated; behavioral responses can be controlled.

Stress and Disease

- The relationships between stress and disease is complex. Too many stressors or lack of coping skills can increase a person's risk of illness or disease.
- Stress can contribute to high blood pressure and atherosclerosis. People who tend to respond to stressors with anger and hostility are at increased risk for cardiovascular disease.
- Both emotional and physical stressors lead to a decline in the body's immune response; stress, therefore, affects our ability to fight infection.
- Stress can trigger or aggravate many other health problems, from asthma to post-traumatic stress disorder.

Techniques for Managing Stress

- Stressors from a variety of sources are an inevitable part of life. Appropriate responses to stressors offer protection against the damaging effects of stress.
- Emotional and social support systems help buffer people from the effects of stress and make illness and disease less likely.
- Exercise is a coping technique that reduces anxiety and increases energy.
- Good nutrition helps the body build an energy bank necessary for coping with stress.
- Time management is an effective coping technique for those who tend to procrastinate.
- The relaxation response is the opposite of the fight-or-flight response; techniques that trigger it counteract the physiological effects of chronic stress.
- Progressive relaxation involves tensing and then relaxing parts of the body; practice leads to the ability to quickly relax. The use of imagery or visualization is a form of daydreaming or imagining; it aids not only in relaxing, but also in healing, changing habits, and improving performance. Through meditation, the world with all its stresses can be tuned out.

- There are many cognitive strategies that can help an individual cope with stress; these include worrying constructively, monitoring self-talk, and cultivating a sense of humor.

Creating a Personal Plan for Managing Stress

- People can create successful individualized programs for coping with stress. Stressors and inappropriate behavioral responses can be identified and studied with a stress journal or log. Completing a contract and recruiting a buddy can help a program succeed.
- Additional help in dealing with stress is available from peer counseling, support groups, and psychotherapy.

TAKE ACTION

1. Choose a friend or family member who seems to deal particularly well with stress. Interview that person about his or her methods of managing stress. What strategies does he or she employ? What can you learn from that person that can be applied to your own life?

2. Investigate the services available in your community to help people deal with stress, such as peer counseling, support groups, and time management classes. If possible, visit or gather information on one or more of them. Write a description and evaluation of their services, including your personal reactions.

3. Read through the stress management techniques described in the chapter and choose one to try for a week. If possible, select a behavior or strategy, such as regular exercise or systematic time management, that you've never tried before. After a trial period, evaluate the effectiveness of the strategy you chose. Did your stress level decrease during the week? Were you better able to deal with daily hassles and any more severe stressors that you encountered?

JOURNAL ENTRY

1. Watch for the physical changes of the stress response when you're in stressful situations. In your health journal, keep a stress log in which you note how many times in a day you experience the stress reaction to some degree. Also include a brief description of the circumstances surrounding your stress reaction. Is your life more or less stressful than you expected?

2. *Critical Thinking:* Some techniques for stress reduction, including meditation, imagery, and hypnosis, are considered strange or unscientific by

some people. Find out more about one such stress reduction technique through library research. What evidence can you find to support or oppose the idea that the techniques can help people manage stress? Based on your research, write a brief essay in your health journal that gives your opinion on the stress management technique you've chosen. As you consider the evidence, be sure to look closely at your sources of information.

3. Think about all the different environments in which you function, including your classrooms, the student union, the dorm, your house. Are some more stressful than others? Make a list of the environments ordered from the most stressful to the least stressful. Indicate next to each environment the reasons you think it is stressful or nonstressful. Now start at the top of your list and record three or more ways to reduce the stressful impact these environments have on you.

4. Make a list of daily hassles that you commonly encounter, such as being awakened early by loud neighbors, standing in long lines for lunch, or repeatedly misplacing your keys. Divide your list into two groups: those stressors you may be able to avoid and those that are inevitable. For each stressor that is potentially avoidable, describe a strategy for eliminating it from your life. For stressors that are inevitable, make a list of effective coping mechanisms.

BEHAVIOR CHANGE STRATEGY

DEALING WITH TEST ANXIETY

Are you a person who doesn't perform as well as you should on tests? Do you find that anxiety interferes with your ability to study effectively before the test and to think clearly in the test situation? If so, you may be experiencing test anxiety. People suffering from test anxiety often see tests as threatening, feel inadequate to cope with them, concentrate on the negative consequences of doing poorly, and anticipate failure, which becomes a self-fulfilling prophecy. They often feel so helpless that they can't mobilize their resources to deal with the problem.

If test anxiety is a problem for you, try some of the following strategies:

- Before the test, find out everything you can about it— its format, the material to be covered, the criteria used to grade essay answers. Ask the instructor for practice materials.

- Devise a study plan. This might include forming a study group with one or more classmates or outlining what you will study, when, where, and for how long.

- Once in the test situation, sit away from possible distractions, listen carefully to instructions, and ask for clarification if you don't understand a direction.

- During the test, answer the easiest questions first. If you don't know an answer and there is no penalty for incorrect answers, guess. If there are several questions you have difficulty answering, review the ones you have already handled. Figure out approximately how much time you have to cover each question or part of the test.

- For math problems, try to estimate the answer before doing the precise calculations.

- For true-false questions, look for qualifiers such as *always* and *never.* Such questions are likely to be false.

- For essay questions, look for key words in the question that indicate what the instructor is looking for in the answer. Develop a brief outline of your answer, sketching out roughly what you will cover. Stick to your outline and keep track of the time you're spending on your answer. Don't let yourself get caught with unanswered questions when the time is up.

- Remain calm and focused throughout the test. Don't let negative thoughts rattle you. If you start to become nervous, take some deep breaths and relax your muscles completely for a minute or so.

The best way to counter test anxiety is with successful test-taking experiences. The more times you succeed, the more your test anxiety will recede. If you find that these strategies aren't sufficient to get your anxiety under control, you may want to seek professional help with the problem. But whatever approach you use, it's wise to take action as early as possible to keep test anxiety from significantly interfering with your education plans and career goals.

SELECTED BIBLIOGRAPHY

American College of Sports Medicine. 1990. *The Recommended Quantity and Quality of Exercise for Developing and Maintaining Cardiorespiratory and Muscular Fitness in Healthy Adults.* Indianapolis: American College of Sports Medicine.

Back, E. E., and others. 1993. Risk factors for developing eosinophilia myalgia syndrome among L-tryptophan users in New York. *Journal of Rheumatology* 20(4): 666–72.

Benson, H., with W. Proctor. 1987. *Your Maximum Mind.* New York: Random House.

Birmaher, B., and others. 1994. Cellular immunity in depressed, conduct disorder, and normal adolescents: Role of adverse life events. *Journal of the American Academy of Child and Adolescent Psychiatry* 33(5): 671–78.

Brosschot, J. F., and others. 1994. Influence of light stress on immunological reactivity to mild psychological stress. *Psychosomatic Medicine* 56(3): 216–24.

Burka, J. B. 1990. *Procrastination: Why You Do It, What to Do About It.* Reading, Mass.: Addison-Wesley.

Cohen, S., and others. 1991. Psychological stress and susceptibility to the common cold. *New England Journal of Medicine* 325(9): 606–612.

Flach, J., and L. Seachrist. 1994. Mind-body meld may boost immunity. *Journal of the National Cancer Institute* 86(4): 256–58.

Glaser, R., and others. 1993. Stress and the memory T-cell response to the Epstein-Barr virus in healthy medical students. *Health Psychology* 12(6): 435–42.

How to beat insomnia. 1994. *Consumer Reports on Health*, March.

Johansson, N. 1991. Effectiveness of a stress management program in reducing anxiety and depression in nursing students. *College Health* 40:125–129.

Karasek, R., and T. Theorell. 1990. *Healthy Work: Stress, Productivity, and the Reconstruction of Working Life.* New York: Basic Books.

Klein, A. 1989. *The Healing Power of Humor.* Los Angeles: Jeremy P. Tarcher.

Lepore, S., and others. 1991. Dynamic role of social support in the link between chronic stress and psychological distress. *Journal of Personality and Social Psychology* 61(6): 899–909.

Lutgendorf, S. K., and others. 1994. Changes in cognitive coping strategies predict EBV-antibody titre change following a stressor disclosure induction. *Journal of Psychosomatic Research* 38(1): 63–78.

Ornstein, R., and D. Sobel. 1989. *Healthy Pleasures.* Reading, Mass.: Addison-Wesley.

Peterson, M. L., and others. 1991. Stress and pathogenesis of infectious disease. *Reviews of Infectious Diseases* 13:710–20.

Selye, H. 1976. *The Stress of Life*, rev. ed. New York: McGraw-Hill.

———. 1979. Stress: The basis of illness. In *Inner Balance: The Power of Holistic Health*, ed. E. M. Goldwag. Englewood Cliffs, N.J.: Prentice-Hall.

Sleep: Are you getting enough? 1994. *Harvard Women's Health Watch*, March.

Farquhar, J. W. 1987. *The American Way of Life Need Not Be Hazardous to Your Health.* Reading, Mass.: Addison-Wesley. *Based on the research from the Stanford Heart Disease Prevention Program; describes effective stress management and encourages habits that will reduce the incidence of premature strokes and heart attacks.*

Hanson, P. G. 1986. *The Joy of Stress.* Kansas City: Andrews, McMeel and Parker. *Engagingly presented, compact, well-tested advice from a Canadian doctor who shows how to turn stress into an ally rather than an enemy.*

Kabat-Zinn, J. 1990. *Full Catastrophe Living (Using the Wisdom of Your Body and Mind to Face Stress, Pain, and Illness).* New York: Dell. *Describes the program of the Stress Reduction Clinic at the University of Massachusetts Medical Center, which teaches the application of meditation to counteract the deleterious effects on health of stress from physical and emotional pain, work, other people, time pressure, and other sources.*

Lazarus, R. 1991. *Emotions and Adaptation.* New York: Oxford University Press. *Written by one of the foremost authorities on stress and adaptation, this book provides a theory of emotional processes that explains how different emotions are elicited and expressed and how the emotional range of an individual develops over his or her lifetime.*

Matheny, K. B., and R. J. Riordan. 1992. *Stress and Strategies for Lifestyle Management.* Atlanta: Georgia State University Business Press. *Includes practical and realistic insights into managing stress and changing maladaptive lifestyles. It contains separate chapters on stress inoculation and creating stress-free relationships.*

Schafer, W. 1992. *Stress Management for Wellness*, 2nd ed. Fort Worth: Harcourt Brace Jovanovich. *Presents basic information on stress and wellness and many different stress-management techniques; contains a separate chapter on college stress.*

Spiegel, D. 1993. *Living Beyond Limits.* New York: Random House. *Written by the pioneering Stanford University School of Medicine researcher, this book describes how he showed that support groups can help breast cancer patients live longer, higher quality lives.*

RECOMMENDED READINGS

Achterberg, J., and others. 1994. *Rituals of Healing.* New York: Bantam. *Describes clinically validated mind-body techniques that may facilitate healing and increase health and well-being.*

Adler, N., and K. Matthews. 1994. Health psychology: Why do some people get sick and some stay well? *Annual Review of Psychology* 45:229–259. *Summarizes current understanding of the effects of stress, lifestyles, and coping styles on health.*

Antonovsky, A. 1990. *Learned Resourcefulness.* New York: Springer-Verlag. *Presents a variety of strategies for managing and coping with stress and increasing self-control and adaptive behavior.*

Cousins, N. 1989. *Head First: The Biology of Hope.* New York: E. P. Dutton. *An entertaining account of some of the scientific evidence for the view that positive emotions can help combat serious illness, drawn from the author's own experience of illness and his exchanges with many patients.*

Dement, W. C. 1992. *The Sleepwatchers.* Stanford, Calif.: Stanford Alumni Association. *An entertaining discussion of sleep and dreams by one of the world's foremost authorities on sleep.*

3

Mental Health

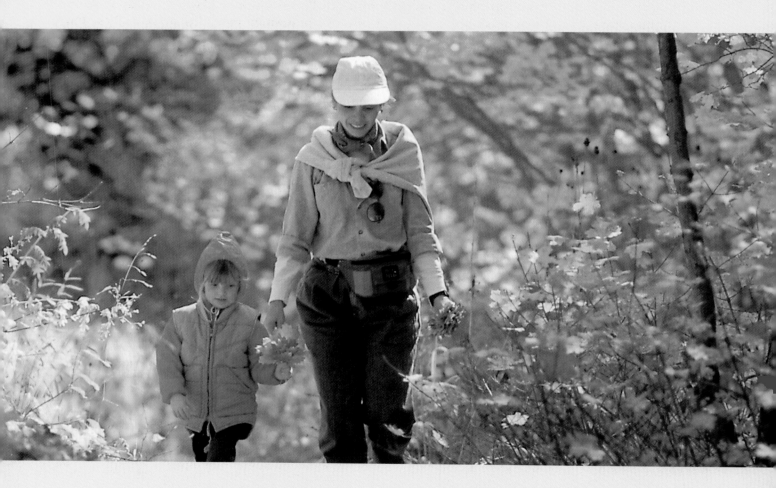

CONTENTS

What is *mental* health? We see this question become the focus of battles in legislatures and courts, where expert witnesses contradict each other on whether defendants were mentally healthy enough to have been responsible for their acts or whether people are so mentally ill that they should be treated with medicine or hospitalized involuntarily. When the perpetrator of an especially heinous crime is found "mentally incompetent to stand trial" or "not guilty by reason of insanity," it's not unusual to hear mental illness declared a "myth" promoted by the mental health "establishment."

Is mental health a myth? We don't think so. We think there is such a thing as mental health just as there is physical health (and the two are intertwined). Just as your body can work well or poorly, giving you feelings of pleasure or pain, your mind can also work well or poorly, giving you happiness or unhappiness.

WHAT MENTAL HEALTH IS NOT

Mental health is not the same as mental **normality.** Being mentally normal simply means being close to average. You can define your normal body temperature because a few degrees above or below this temperature always means physical sickness. But your ideas and attitudes can vary tremendously without your losing efficiency or feeling emotional distress. And psychological diversity is valuable; living in a society of people with varied ideas and lifestyles makes life interesting. Such a society can respond creatively to unexpected challenges.

Conforming to social demands is not necessarily a mark of mental health. If you don't question what's going on around you, you're not fulfilling your potential as a thinking, questioning human being. Never seeking help for personal problems also does not mean that you are mentally healthy, any more than seeking help proves that you are mentally ill. Unhappy people may not want to seek professional help because they don't want to reveal their problems to others, may fear what their friends might think, or may not know whom to ask for help. People who are severely disturbed mentally may not even realize they need help, or they may become so suspicious of other people that they can be treated only against their will.

And we cannot say people are "mentally ill" or "mentally healthy" on the basis of symptoms alone. Life constantly presents problems. Time and life inevitably change the environment and change our minds and bodies, and changes present problems. The symptom of anxiety, for example, can help us face a problem and solve it before it gets too big. Someone who shows no anxiety may be refusing to recognize problems or refusing to do anything about them. A person who is anxious for good reason is likely to be judged more mentally healthy in the long run than someone who is inappropriately calm.

Finally, we cannot judge mental health from the way people look. All too often a person who seems to be OK and even happy suddenly takes his or her own life. Usually such people lack close friends who might have known of their desperation.

WHAT MENTAL HEALTH IS

Mental health can be defined either negatively as the absence of sickness or positively as the presence of wellness. Abraham Maslow, an American psychology professor, eloquently described an ideal of mental health in his book *Toward a Psychology of Being.* He was convinced that psychologists were too preoccupied with people who had failed in some way. He also did not like the way psychologists tried to reduce human striving to physiological needs or drives. According to Maslow, there is a *hierarchy of needs*, listed here in order of decreasing urgency: physiological needs, safety, being loved, maintaining self-esteem, and self-actualization (Figure 3-1). When urgent needs like the need for food are satisfied, less urgent needs take priority. Most of us are well fed and feel reasonably safe, so we are driven by higher motives. Maslow's conclusions were based on his study of a group of visibly successful people who seemed to be living at their fullest. He called these people **self-actualized**; he thought they had fulfilled a good measure of their human potential and suggested that such people all share certain qualities.

Realism

Self-actualized people are able to deal with the world as it is and not demand that it be otherwise. If you are realistic, you know the difference between what is and what you want. You also know what you can change and what you cannot. Unrealistic people often spend a great deal of energy trying to force the world and other people into their ideal picture. Realistic people accept evidence that contradicts what they want to believe, and if it is important evidence, they modify their beliefs.

Acceptance

Mentally healthy people are able to largely accept themselves and others. Self-acceptance means that they have a positive **self-concept** or self-image, or appropriately high

Normality The mental characteristics attributed to the majority of people in a population at a given time.

Self-actualized Describes a person who has achieved the highest level of growth in Maslow's hierarchy.

Self-concept The ideas, feelings, and perceptions one has about oneself.

TERMS

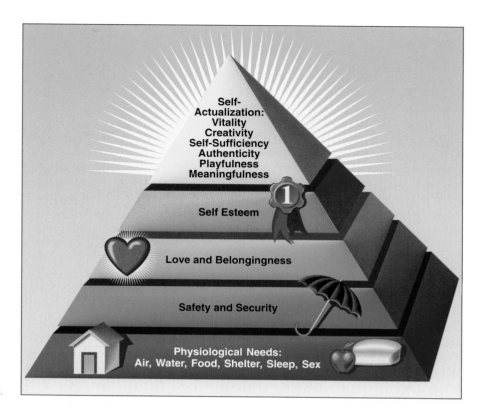

Figure 3-1 *Maslow's hierarchy of needs.* *Source:* A. Maslow. 1970. *Motivation and Personality,* 2nd ed. (New York: Harper and Row).

self-esteem. They have positive but realistic mental images of themselves and have positive feelings about who they are, what they are capable of, and what roles they play. People who feel good about themselves are likely to live up to their positive self-image and enjoy successes that in turn reinforce these good feelings. A good self-concept is based on a realistic view of personal worth—it does not mean being egocentric or "stuck on yourself."

Autonomy

Mentally healthy people are able to direct themselves, acting independently of their social environment. Autonomy is more than freedom from physical control by something or someone outside the self. Many people, for example, shrink from being themselves and from expressing their own feelings because they fear disapproval and rejection. They are unable to act freely and respond only to what they feel as outside pressure. Such behavior is **other-directed.** In contrast, **inner-directed** people find guidance from within, from their own values and feelings. They are not afraid to be themselves. Mentally free people act because they choose to, not because they are driven or pressured.

Being free can give healthy people certain childlike qualities. Very small children have a quality of being "real." They respond in a genuine, spontaneous way to whatever happens. Someone who is genuine needs no pretenses. Being free and genuine means not having to plan words or actions to get approval or to make an im-

pression. It means being aware of feelings and being willing to express them; in other words, being unselfconsciously oneself, here and now. This quality is sometimes called **authenticity;** such people are *authentic,* the "real thing."

Capacity for Intimacy

Healthy people are capable of physical and emotional intimacy. They can expose their feelings and thoughts to other people. They are open to the pleasure of intimate physical contact and to the risks and satisfactions of being close to others in a caring, sensitive way.

Creativity

Mentally healthy people are creative and have a continuing fresh appreciation for what goes on around them. They are not necessarily great poets, scientists, or musicians, but they do live their everyday lives in creative ways: "A first-rate soup is more creative than a second-rate painting." Creative people seem to see more and to be open to new experiences; they don't fear the unknown. And they don't need to reduce uncertainty or to avoid it, but actually find it an attractive and stimulating part of their lives.

How did Maslow's group achieve their exemplary mental health, and (more importantly) how can *we* attain it? Maslow himself did not answer that question, but we have a few suggestions. Undoubtedly it helps to have

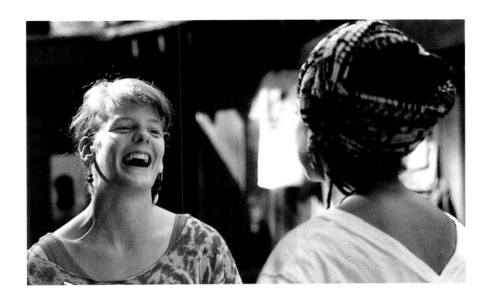

Self-actualized people respond in a genuine, spontaneous way to what happens around them.

been treated with respect, love, and understanding as a child, to have experienced stability and to have been given a sense of mastery. As adults, since we cannot redo the past, we must concentrate on meeting current psychological challenges in ways that will lead to long-term mental wellness.

MEETING LIFE'S CHALLENGES

Life is full of challenges—large and small. Everyone, regardless of how fortunate in having the right genes and the right family, must learn to cope successfully with new situations and new people. To develop mental wellness, each of us must continue to grow psychologically, developing new and more sophisticated coping mechanisms to suit our current lives. We must develop an adult identity that enhances our self-esteem and autonomy. To interact with others in a positive and meaningful way, we must also learn to communicate honestly and to avoid being defensive.

Growing Up Psychologically

Along the path from birth to old age, we are confronted with a series of challenges. How we respond to these challenges influences the development of personality and identity. A primary task beginning in adolescence is the development of an adult identity. A personal identity is a unified sense of self characterized by attitudes, beliefs, and ways of acting that are genuinely one's own. People who have developed identities know who they are, what they are capable of, what roles they play, and what their place is among their peers. They have a sense of their own uniqueness but also appreciate what they have in common with others. They view themselves realistically and

can assess their own strong and weak points without relying on the opinions of others. Achieving an identity also means that one can form intimate relationships with others while maintaining a strong sense of self.

Our identities evolve as we interact with the world and make choices about what we'd like to do and whom we'd like to model ourselves after. Early identities are often modeled after parents—or the opposite of parents, in rebellion from what they represent. Later, peers, rock stars, movie and sports heroes, and religious figures are added to the list of possible models. In high school and college, young people often join cliques that assert a certain identity—the "jocks," the "brains," the "stoners," or the "in-crowd." Although much of an identity is internal—a way of viewing oneself and the world—it can include things such as styles of talking and dressing, ornaments like earrings, and particular hairstyles. Early identities are rarely permanent, however, and at some point most of us adopt a more stable, individually tailored identity that ties together the experiences of childhood and the expectations and aspirations of adulthood.

Developing an identity is an important part of mental wellness. Without an identity, we begin to feel confused about who we are. Until we have "found ourselves," we cannot have much self-esteem because a self is not firmly in place.

Self-esteem   Satisfaction and confidence in oneself; the valuing of oneself as a person.

Other-directed   Guided in behavior by the values and expectations of others.

Inner-directed   Guided in behavior by an inner set of rules and values.

Authenticity   Genuineness.

TERMS

Achieving Realistic Self-Esteem

Positive self-esteem means regarding your self, which includes all aspects of your identity, as good, competent, and worthy of love. Ideally, a positive self-concept begins in childhood, based on experiences within the family and outside it. Children need to develop a sense of being loved and being able to give love and to accomplish their goals. If they feel rejected or neglected by their parents, they may fail to develop feelings of self-worth. They may grow to have a negative concept of themselves.

Another quality of the self-concept is its integration. An integrated self-concept is one that a person has made his or her own—it doesn't feel like someone else's mask or costume that doesn't quite fit. Important building blocks for the self-concept are personality characteristics and mannerisms of the parents, which children can take in uncritically without knowing they have done so. Later, they are surprised when they catch themselves acting like one of their parents, especially if they always objected to such behavior in that parent. Eventually, such building blocks should be reshaped and integrated into a new individual personality.

A further quality of the self-concept is its stability. Stability depends on the integration of the self and its freedom from contradictions. People who have received mixed messages about themselves from parents and friends may have contradictory self-images, which defy integration and which make them open to startling shifts of self-esteem. At times they regard themselves as entirely good, capable, and lovable—an ideal self—and at other times they see themselves as entirely bad, incompetent, and unworthy of love. While at the first pole, they may develop such an inflated ego that they totally ignore other people's needs and see others only as instruments for fulfilling their own desires. At the other pole, they may feel so small and weak that they run for protection to someone who seems powerful and caring. At neither extreme do such people see themselves or others realistically, and their personal relationships with other people are filled with misunderstandings and ultimately with conflict.

As an adult, you sometimes run into situations that challenge your self-concept: Your attempts to accomplish a goal may end in failure. You can react to such challenges in several ways. The best approach is to acknowledge that something has gone wrong and try again, adjusting your goals to your abilities without radically revising your self-concept. A less useful reaction is to deny that anything

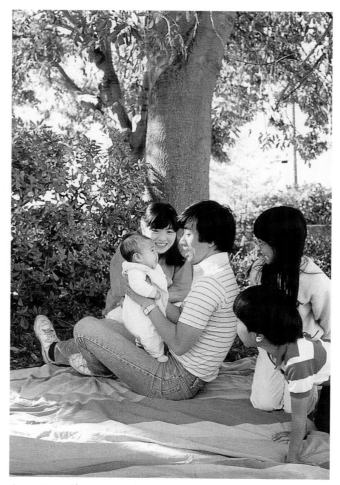

A positive self-concept begins in infancy. Knowing that she's loved and valued by her family gives this 3-month-old a solid basis for lifelong mental health.

went wrong or to blame someone else. These attitudes preserve a good self-concept temporarily, but in the long run they keep you from mastering the challenge. The worst reaction is to develop a lasting negative self-concept in which you feel bad, unloved, and ineffective—in other words, become demoralized. Instead of coping, the demoralized person gives up, reinforcing the negative self-concept and setting in motion a vicious circle of bad self-concept and failure.

One method for fighting demoralization is to recognize and test your negative thoughts and assumptions about yourself and others. The first step is to note exactly when an unpleasant emotion—feeling worthless, wanting to give up, feeling depressed—occurs or gets worse, to identify the events or daydreams that trigger that emotion, and to observe whatever thoughts come into your head just before or during the emotion. It is helpful to keep a systematic daily record of such events, which you can examine to develop more rational responses. It may be hard

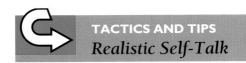
Do your patterns of thinking make events worse than they truly are? Do negative beliefs about yourself become self-fulfilling prophecies? Substituting realistic self-talk for negative self-talk can help you build and maintain self-esteem and cope better with the challenges in your life. Here are some examples of common types of distorted negative self-talk, along with suggestions for more accurate and rational responses.

Negative Self-Talk	Realistic Self-Talk
Focusing on negatives	
School is so discouraging—nothing but one hassle after another.	School is pretty challenging and has its difficulties, but there certainly are rewards. It's really a mixture of good and bad.
Expecting the worst	
Why would my boss want to meet with me this afternoon if not to fire me?	I wonder why my boss wants to meet with me. I guess I'll just have to wait and see.
Overgeneralizing	
(After getting a poor grade on a paper) Just as I thought—I'm incompetent at everything.	I'll start working on the next paper earlier. That way, if I run into problems, I'll have time to consult with the TA.
Minimizing	
I won the speech contest, but none of the other speakers was very good. I wouldn't have done so well against stiffer competition.	It may not have been the best speech I'll ever give, but it was good enough to win the contest. I'm really improving as a speaker.
Blaming others	
I wouldn't feel so lousy today if I hadn't had so much to drink at the party last night. Someone should have stopped me.	I overdid it last night. Next time I'll make different choices.
Expecting perfection	
I should have got 100 percent on this test. I can't believe I missed that one problem through a careless mistake.	Too bad I missed one problem through carelessness, but overall I did very well on this test. Next time I'll be more careful.
Believing you're the cause of everything	
Sarah seems so depressed today. I wish I hadn't had that argument with her yesterday; it must have really upset her.	I wish I had handled the argument better, and in the future I'll try to. But I don't know if Sarah's behavior is related to what I said, or even if she's depressed. In any event, I'm not responsible for how Sarah feels or acts—only she can take responsibility for that.
Thinking in black and white	
I've got to score 10 points in the game today. Otherwise, I don't belong on the team.	I'm a good player or else I wouldn't be on the team. I'll play my best—that's all I can do.
Magnifying events	
They went to a movie without me. I thought we were friends, but I guess I was wrong.	I'm disappointed they didn't ask me to the movie, but it doesn't mean our friendship is over. It's not that big a deal.

Adapted from W. Schafer. 1992. *Stress Management for Wellness,* 2nd ed. (Fort Worth: Harcourt Brace Jovanovich), pp. 227–31.

to figure out a rational response until hours or days after the event that upsets you, but once you get used to the way your mind works, you may be able to catch yourself thinking negatively and change the thought process before it goes too far.

Being Less Defensive

Sometimes our wishes come into conflict with people around us or with our conscience, and we become frustrated and anxious. If we cannot resolve the conflict by changing the external situation, we try to resolve the conflict internally by rearranging our thoughts and feelings. These mental **defense mechanisms** allow us to protect ourselves against unacceptable thoughts or comfort ourselves when under pressure. Common defense mechanisms include projection, repression, denial, rationalization, daydreaming, sublimation, and humor. The drawback of many of these mechanisms is that although they succeed temporarily, they are dead ends that make finding ultimate solutions much harder. Repression or denial, for example, in which a person removes an unpleasant feeling or memory from awareness or refuses to acknowledge it, may banish a problem in the short term, but ultimately the problem needs to be dealt with or it will return. Rationalization—giving a false, acceptable reason when the real reason is unacceptable—can keep people from developing a realistic view of themselves and identifying ways to change their lives for the better. Some of these mechanisms, such as humor and sublimation (transforming aggressive or sexual impulses into socially approved forms), can be very useful for coping as long as they do not keep us from being what we want to be.

Recognizing your favorite mechanisms can be difficult, because they probably have become automatic habits, occurring outside of your conscious awareness. But lack of awareness is never complete—we each have some inkling about how our mind operates. Try to look at yourself as an objective, outside observer would and analyze your thoughts and behavior in a concrete psychologically stressful situation from the past. Having insight into what defenses you typically use can lead to new, less defensive and more effective ways of coping in the future.

Maintaining Honest Communication

Another important area of psychological functioning is relating to others and communicating honestly with them. It can be very frustrating for us and for people around us if we cannot communicate what we want and feel. Others can hardly respond to our needs if they don't know what those needs are. The first step is for us to realize what we want to communicate and then to express it clearly. For example, how do you feel about going to the party instead of to the movie? Do you care if your roommate types a paper late into the night? Some people know what they want others to do, but don't state it clearly because they are afraid that the request or they themselves will be rejected. Such people might benefit from **assertiveness** training. They need to learn to insist on their rights, to bargain for what they want, and to say no or yes depending on the situation.

PSYCHOLOGICAL DISORDERS

All of us have felt anxious, and in dealing with the anxiety have thought less rationally than when we were calm. Al-most all of us have had periods of feeling down. Such feelings are normal responses to the ordinary challenges of life. But when emotions or irrational thoughts are strong enough to interfere with daily living, they can be regarded as symptoms of a psychological disorder.

Anxiety Disorders

Fear is a basic and useful emotion. It provides motivation for self-protection and learning to cope with new or potentially dangerous situations. Only when fear is out of proportion to real danger can it be considered a problem. Anxiety is another word for fear, referring especially to a feeling of fear that is not directed toward any definite threat. Only when anxiety is experienced almost daily or in life situations that recur and cannot be avoided, does it qualify anyone for a diagnosis of anxiety disorder.

The broad concept of anxiety disorders covers a variety of human problems. Here are the main types:

- *Simple phobia* is probably the most common and most understandable anxiety disorder, since many of us have a few specific fears—for example, fears of animals such as snakes or certain locations such as high or closed places. Sometimes these fears originate in bad experiences with the feared objects, but often there is no such explanation.

- *Social phobias* are similar to simple phobias, but they occur in interpersonal contexts. People with social phobias fear humiliation or embarrassment while being watched by others. Fear of speaking in public is perhaps the most common social phobia. Extremely shy people can have social fears that extend to almost all social situations.

- *Panic disorder* is characterized by sudden unexpected surges in anxiety, accompanied by symptoms such as rapid and strong heartbeats, shortness of breath, loss of physical equilibrium, and a feeling of losing mental control. Such attacks—the hallmark of **panic disorder**—usually begin in the early twenties.

- *Obsessive-compulsive disorder* applies to people with obsessions or compulsions or both. **Obsessions** are recurrent, unwanted thoughts or impulses. For example, a person may brood over whether he or she contracted HIV infection during a handshake; or a person may persistently wonder if he or she has done something unacceptable, such as having hit a pedestrian while driving. **Compulsions** are repetitive, difficult-to-resist actions associated with obsessions. A common compulsion is hand washing, associated with an obsessive fear of contamination by dirt.

- *Post-traumatic stress disorder* is a reaction to severely traumatic events (events that produce a sense of terror and helplessness) such as physical violence to oneself or loved ones. Such traumas occur in personal assaults like rape or military combat, natural disasters

Shyness is a form of social anxiety, a fear of what others will think of our behavior or appearance. Most people experience shyness in certain situations and are familiar with the telltale physical signs: pounding, rapid heartbeat; blushing; increased perspiration and clammy hands; butterflies in the stomach; trembling hands and legs; and a dry mouth. The accompanying feelings of self-consciousness, embarrassment, and unworthiness can be overwhelming. In order to escape these unpleasant feelings, a shy person may avoid volunteering or speaking up in public, refrain from making eye contact, and shun social gatherings and interpersonal interaction whenever possible.

Being shy is not the same thing as being introverted. Introverts prefer solitude to society, while shy people often long to be more outgoing. But it's often their own thoughts and beliefs that prevent shy people from enjoying the social interaction they crave. They dread being evaluated negatively by others, and, in anticipation of negative feedback, they become excessively self-conscious and self-critical. They resist positive feedback and tend to blame themselves for everything.

What causes people to become shy? Recent research indicates that the trait is at least partly inherited. Studies conducted by Harvard psychologist Jerome Kagan on children as young as 4 months showed that when faced with unfamiliar people or situations, shy infants and toddlers are frightened and upset and often withdraw. About 20 percent of children exhibit this type of response. At the other end of the spectrum, about 25 to 30 percent of children are consistently fearless, responding with calm or even delight to unfamiliar stimuli. These two temperaments remain fairly steady over time: Kagan's studies indicate that about half of the timid toddlers and 90 percent of the fearless ones will exhibit the same tendencies at age 7. Studies of identical twins also point to a genetic component in the development of shyness.

But for shyness as for many health concerns, biology is not destiny. About half of all shy children outgrow their shyness, just as others acquire it later in life. A variety of factors may be involved in the development of shyness in people who were not shy as infants. Possible culprits include stressors in the family environment, lack of support or emotional expressiveness in the family, or parental overemphasis on correct behavior. People may become shy as a result of one or more particularly negative social encounters or if they learn early to be uncertain about their intelligence or their appearance. Shyness can also occur if a person believes that he or she lacks the social skills needed for rewarding social interaction.

Approximately 30 to 40 percent of Americans think of themselves as shy, and about three-quarters of this group wish they weren't shy. For some, shyness is a serious problem, causing loneliness and depression. Because they have difficulty speaking up and believing in themselves, shy people are more likely to be underemployed. However, many shy people learn to work around their shyness. Some do better in structured rather than spontaneous settings and are able to experience positive social interaction through careful planning. About 20 percent of shy people are "shy extroverts"—people who, perhaps because of their shyness, have mastered ways to tell jokes or "work a crowd." Shyness may also have its upside: Shy people tend to be gentle, supportive, kind, and sensitive.

For people concerned about their own shyness or shyness in their children, several programs and strategies are available. Parents can help their shy children by accepting them as they are and by nurturing their self-esteem and sense of belonging. For shy adults, shyness classes, assertiveness training groups, and public speaking clinics offer training in social and cognitive skills, assertiveness, and changing negative self-perceptions. These programs are described in greater detail in the Behavior Change Strategy at the end of the chapter.

If you're worried about being shy, try to remember that shyness is widespread and that there are worse fates. The poet William Blake was so shy he could scarcely utter a sentence in public, so he made his pronouncements on paper. And they turned out just fine.

---

like floods or earthquakes, and accidental disasters like fires and airplane and automobile crashes. Symptoms include reexperiencing the trauma in dreams and intrusive memories, trying to avoid anything associated with the trauma, and numbing of feelings. Sleep disturbances and other symptoms of anxiety and depression may also be present.

Therapies for anxiety disorders range from medication to psychological interventions that concentrate on a person's thoughts or behavior. As we discuss later, different

TERMS

Defense mechanisms   Mental mechanisms for controlling anxiety.

Assertiveness   Expressing wishes forcefully, but not necessarily hostilely.

Panic disorder   A syndrome of severe anxiety attacks accompanied by physical symptoms.

Obsession   Recurrent irrational, unwanted thoughts.

Compulsion   Irrational, repetitive, forced action, usually associated with an obsession.

Many popular statements made about suicide are false or true only in some cases. These statements may be false generalizations from a few atypical cases, wishful thinking, or just ignorance. People often conceal details about suicides, which promotes false assumptions such as the following:

Myth   People who really intend to kill themselves do not let anyone know about it.

Fact   This belief is a convenient excuse for doing nothing when someone says he or she might commit suicide. In fact, most people who eventually commit suicide *have* talked about doing it.

Myth   People who made a suicide attempt but survived did not really intend to die.

Fact   This may be true for certain people, but people who seriously want to end their life may fail because they misjudge what it takes. Even a pharmacist may misjudge the lethal dose of a drug.

Myth   People who succeed in suicide really wanted to die.

Fact   We cannot be sure of that either. Some people were trying only to make a dramatic gesture or plea for help but miscalculated.

Myth   People who really want to kill themselves will do it regardless of any attempts to prevent them.

Fact   Few people are single-minded about suicide even at the moment of attempting it. People who are quite determined to take their lives today may change their minds completely tomorrow.

Myth   Suicide is proof of mental illness.

Fact   Many suicides are committed by people who do not meet ordinary criteria for mental illness, although people with depression, schizophrenia, and other mental illnesses have a much higher than average suicide rate.

Myth   Certain groups of the population are immune to suicide: alcoholics because they have alcohol as a crutch, elderly men because they have achieved a stable life adjustment, and black teenagers because they are not achievement-oriented.

Fact   Certain groups do have low suicide rates, but not these—the first two groups mentioned have much higher than average suicide rates, and the suicide rate for black 15- to 24-year-olds is about the same as for whites of the same age.

Myth   People inherit suicidal tendencies.

Fact   Certain kinds of depression that lead to suicide can be inherited. But many examples of suicide running in a family can be explained by factors such as psychologically identifying with a family member who committed suicide, often a parent.

Myth   All suicides are irrational.

Fact   Maybe by some standards all suicides are "irrational." But many people find it at least understandable that someone might want to commit suicide, for example, when approaching the end of a terminal illness or when facing a long prison term.

---

models of human nature lead to different ideas of causes and appropriate treatments.

Mood Disorders

Depression is the most common expression of a mood disorder. Depression comes in many kinds and degrees. Demoralization is usually part of any depression, but it's not the whole story. The following description of severe depression shows what it can include:

- A feeling of sadness and hopelessness
- Loss of pleasure in doing usual activities
- Poor appetite and weight loss
- Insomnia, especially early morning awakening
- Restlessness or, alternatively, lethargy
- Thoughts of worthlessness and guilt
- Inability to concentrate
- Thoughts of suicide

Not all these features are present in every depressive episode. Sometimes instead of poor appetite and insomnia, the opposite occurs—eating too much and sleeping too long. Amazingly, people can suffer the majority of symptoms of depression without feeling sad or hopeless or in a depressed mood, although they usually do experience a loss of interest or pleasure in things. In some cases, depression is a clear-cut reaction to specific events, such as the loss of a loved one or failing in school or work, while in other cases no trigger event is obvious.

One of the principal dangers of severe depression is suicide. Although suicide can happen unpredictably and even in the absence of depression, the chances of its happening are greater if the symptoms are numerous and severe. Additional danger signals include the following:

- Expressing the wish to be dead, or revealing contemplated methods
- Increasing social withdrawal and isolation
- A sudden, inexplicable lightening of mood (which

No drug has captured the attention of the public in the last few years like fluoxetine, which goes by the trade name Prozac. This compound was the first of a new class of psychotherapeutic drugs called selective serotonin reuptake inhibitors (SSRIs). Serotonin is an important neurotransmitter in the brain, so pharmaceutical chemists thought that drugs that modify its action were likely to have important psychological effects. They were right. Prozac is an effective antidepressant in a little over half of people with moderate to severe depression. In addition, Prozac does not have the nasty side effects of tricyclic antidepressants, the type that had previously been most commonly prescribed. Patients hated the dry mouth, blurred vision, constipation, and weight gain that tricyclics caused. Prozac's fewer side effects has made nonpsychiatric physicians willing to prescribe it and patients willing to take it.

The first news reports on Prozac were negative—a husband blamed it for his wife's suicide and a woman said it made her kill her mother. Then Peter Kramer, a psychiatrist in private practice, focused public attention on the more positive aspects of Prozac with his best-selling book, *Listening to Prozac*. In it, he claimed that the drug could change unwanted personality traits in people who were not suffering from depression or another mental illness. Shy or pessimistic people could become more outgoing and optimistic; insecure people could begin to feel more able to cope. Kramer based his conclusions not on a research study in the usual sense, but on observations of patients he was treating and "listening to" in his practice. If Kramer is right, a revolution could take place in how psychoactive drugs are used.

Instead of drugs being taken for a "mental illness" and "symptoms," they could be taken to alter unwanted personality traits. But there are grounds for suspicion. Our society has had much experience with drugs for making ordinary unhappiness go away—alcohol and heroin are two examples—and that experience can only be called disastrous. In the end, such substances have led to abuse, dependence, and physical sickness.

Is Prozac dangerous too? Not in the sense that physical dependence is likely. Prozac does not have the immediate calming or mood-elevating effects that are characteristic of most drugs that have the potential for abuse. In fact, it takes weeks for its effects to appear. And users have virtually no withdrawal symptoms when they stop taking the drug (withdrawal symptoms are a hallmark of physical dependence on a drug). But every drug has side effects, some of which are immediate and others of which may show up only after long usage. One of the most common and annoying side effects of Prozac is a decrease in sexual pleasure for both men and women. Prozac also tends to decrease appetite for food sometimes to the point of nausea, which leads to weight loss.

It is uncertain whether Prozac or any other drug can alter personality traits in a positive way in people who are already psychologically well, and such uses have sparked ethical debate. However, there is no doubt that Prozac is useful for treating significant depression or anxiety. Because of Prozac's success, four new SSRIs have been approved by the FDA—Zoloft (sertraline), Paxil (paroxetine), Effexor (venlafaxine), and Luvox (fluvoxamine). It remains to be seen whether they differ significantly from Prozac in any way.

---

can mean the person has finally decided to commit suicide)

Certain risk factors also increase the likelihood of suicide:

- A history of previous attempts
- A suicide by a family member or friend
- Readily available means, such as guns or pills
- Addiction to alcohol or drugs
- Serious medical problems

If you are severely depressed or know someone who is, expert help from a mental health professional is essential. Don't try to do it all yourself. If you suspect one of your friends is suicidally depressed, try to get him or her to see a professional.

Don't be afraid to discuss the possibility of suicide with people you fear are suicidal. You won't give them an idea they haven't already thought of. And asking direct questions is the best way to determine if someone seriously intends to commit suicide. Encourage your friend to talk

and to take positive steps to improve his or her situation. If you feel there is an immediate danger of suicide, ensure that the person is not left alone, especially when he or she is emotionally upset and more likely to act impulsively. If you must leave your friend alone, have your friend promise not to do anything to harm himself or herself without first calling you. Get qualified help as soon as possible.

If your friend refuses help, you might try to contact your friend's relatives and tell them that you are worried. If the depressed person is a college student, you may need to let someone in your health service or college administration know your concerns. Finally, most communities have emergency help available, often in the form of a hotline telephone counseling service run by a suicide prevention agency (check the yellow pages).

Treatment for depression depends on its severity and on whether the depressed person is suicidal. The basic treatment is usually some kind of psychotherapy, which may be combined with drug therapy. "Uppers" such as amphetamines are not good antidepressants. More effective are special drugs that work over a period of two or more weeks. Therefore, when suicidal impulses are too strong, hospitalization for a week or so may be necessary. Electroconvulsive treatment is an effective therapy for severe depression when other approaches have failed.

Mania is a less common feature of mood disorder. People who are manic are restless, have a lot of energy, need little sleep, and often talk nonstop. They may devote themselves to fantastic projects and spend more money than they can afford. Many manic people swing between manic and depressive states, a syndrome called bipolar disorder because of the two opposite poles of mood. Tranquilizers are used to treat individual manic episodes, while special drugs like the salt *lithium carbonate* taken daily can prevent future mood swings.

Schizophrenia

Schizophrenia can be severe and debilitating or quite mild and hardly noticeable. Although people are capable of diagnosing their own depression, they usually don't diagnose their own schizophrenia, because schizophrenics often can't see that anything is wrong. This disorder is not rare; in fact, 1 out of 100 people has a schizophrenic episode sometime in his or her lifetime, most commonly starting in adolescence. Some general characteristics of schizophrenia include the following:

- *Disorganized thoughts.* Thoughts may be expressed in a vague or confusing way that is difficult to follow.

- *Inappropriate emotions.* Sometimes all emotion seems to be absent, and at other times emotions are strong but inappropriate.

- *Delusions.* People with delusions—firmly held false beliefs—may think that their minds are controlled by outside forces, that people can read their minds, that they are a great personage like Jesus Christ, or that they are being persecuted by a group like the CIA.

- *Auditory hallucinations.* Schizophrenics may hear people talking about them and to them when no one is present.

- *Deteriorating social and work functioning.* Social withdrawal and increasingly poor performance at school or work may be gradual at first.

A schizophrenic person needs help from a mental health professional. Suicide is a risk in schizophrenia, and expert treatment can reduce that risk and minimize the social consequences of the illness by shortening the period when symptoms are active. The keystone of treatment is regular medication. Sometimes hospitalization is needed temporarily to relieve family and friends from responsibility for restraining erratic behavior.

Personal Insight When you see people talking to themselves or acting strangely on the street, how do you feel? What do you do? Do you wonder what's going on in their mind? Do you label them as "sick"? What do you think causes them to act so strangely?

GETTING HELP

Knowing when self-help or professional help is required for mental health problems is usually not as difficult as knowing how to start or which professional to choose.

Self-Help

If you have a personal problem that you would like to solve, an intelligent way to begin is to find out what you can do on your own. Some problems are specifically addressed in this book. Behavioral and some cognitive approaches are especially useful for helping yourself. All of these involve becoming more aware of self-defeating actions and ideas and combating them in some way: being more assertive when you find yourself backing down; taking the risk of communicating honestly; improving your self-esteem by counteracting thoughts, people, and actions that undermine it; and confronting things you're afraid of rather than avoiding what you fear. Get more information about solving personal problems by seeing what books are available in the psychology or self-help sections of the library or bookstore. Be selective, however—avoid self-help books that make fantastic claims that deviate from mainstream psychological thought.

Expressing your feelings is important too. Just being able to share what's troubling you with an accepting, empathetic person can bring relief. Comparing notes with people who have problems similar to yours can give you new ideas about coping. Many self-help groups work on the principle of bringing together people with similar problems to share their experiences and support each other. Some support groups are for the families of people with problems; Al-Anon, for the families of alcoholics, is an example.

For some people, religious belief and practice may promote psychological health. Religious organizations provide a social network and a supportive community, and religious practices, such as prayer and meditation, offer a path for personal change and transformation of the self.

TERMS

Schizophrenia A mental disorder that involves a disturbance in thinking and in perceiving reality.

Express Your Feelings

Is it true that expressing your feelings is better for your health than keeping a stiff upper lip? Apparently it is. Numerous studies have suggested that people who hold in their feelings are more prone to illness. Now, researchers have reviewed a dozen experiments and concluded that expressing your emotions can help keep you healthy.

In the typical study design, half the subjects were randomly assigned to spend 15 to 20 minutes a day for several days reliving a traumatic experience, either by talking into a tape recorder or writing about it. The other subjects talked or wrote about more mundane subjects, such as their plans for the rest of the day.

After several weeks or months, the subjects who grappled with painful experiences reported fewer illnesses, had fewer visits to physicians, or had better immune function, in all but one of the studies. Why might expressing bottled-up emotions improve health? Researchers suggest that holding back emotions requires physical work that puts a chronic strain on the body.

As the studies illustrate, it doesn't take much talking or writing to have a beneficial effect. Nor do you have to reveal your deepest secrets to others—a notebook or tape recorder is audience enough.

Source: "Mind/Body Update," Consumer Reports on Health, August 1992.

Professional Help

Sometimes self-help or talking to nonprofessionals is not enough. More objective, more expert, or more discreet help is needed. Many people have trouble accepting the need for professional help to handle personal problems, and often the people who most need help are the most unwilling to get it. You may find yourself someday having to overcome your own reluctance toward seeking help or the reluctance of a friend for whom you want to get help.

In some cases, professional help is optional. Some people are interested in improving their mental health in a general way by going into individual or group therapy to learn more about themselves and how to interact with others. Certain therapies teach people how to adjust the effect of what they say and do on people around them. Clearly, seeking professional help for these reasons is a matter of individual choice. Interpersonal friction among family members or between partners often falls in the middle between necessary and optional. Successful help with such problems can mean the difference between painful divorce and a satisfying relationship.

Sometimes it is difficult to determine whether someone needs professional help, but it is important to be aware of behaviors that may indicate a serious problem. The following are some strong indications that you or someone else needs professional help:

- If depression, anxiety, or other emotional problems begin to interfere seriously with performance at school, work, or in getting along with other people

- If suicide is attempted or is seriously considered (refer to the danger signals listed in this chapter)

- If symptoms such as hallucinations, delusions, incoherent speech, or loss of memory occur

- If alcohol or drugs are used to the extent that they impair normal functioning during much of the week, if finding or taking drugs occupies much of the week, or if reducing their dose leads to psychological or physiological withdrawal symptoms

Mental health workers belong to several professions. *Psychiatrists* are medical doctors with five years of medical training after college, followed by three years of training in psychiatry. *Clinical psychologists* have usually completed a Ph.D. degree requiring at least four years of graduate work after college. *Social workers* typically have master's degrees requiring at least two years of graduate study. The requirements for licensed *counselors* varies from state to state. Some clergymen have special training in *pastoral counseling* in addition to their religious studies.

These professional groups differ somewhat in their roles. Psychiatrists are experts in deciding whether a medical disease lies behind psychological symptoms. Psychiatrists are usually involved if medication or hospitalization is required. All mental health professionals are trained to practice some kind of psychological therapy, but most restrict themselves to only one or two of the approaches described in this chapter. Psychologists have been important in developing behavioral and cognitive therapies and are often expert in these therapies or in psychoanalytically inspired therapies. Social workers have much experience in finding community support for the seriously ill. In hospitals and clinics, various mental health professionals join together in treatment teams. Psychiatric nurses often are important members of these teams.

Where do you actually find these professionals when you need them? College students are usually in a good position to find inexpensive mental health care. Larger colleges have both health services that employ psychia-

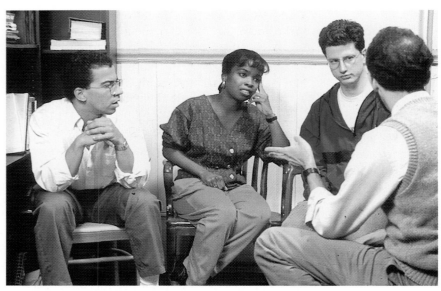

Group therapy is just one of many different approaches to psychological counseling. If you have concerns you would like to discuss with a mental health professional, shop around to find the approach that works for you.

trists and psychologists and counseling centers staffed by professionals and students (peer counselors). For less severe problems, psychology and education departments may offer student counselors. Student newspapers sometimes list self-awareness groups sponsored by student organizations. Remember, though, that peer counselors are not professionals, and for problems of the kind listed earlier in this section it is better to go to someone with more training and experience. Self-awareness groups are also not really suitable for people who are in a crisis or not functioning.

Community mental health resources may include a school of medicine or teaching hospital with outpatient psychiatric clinics that offer psychological testing, diagnostic screening, and the ongoing services of psychiatrists, psychologists, and social workers. Psychologists, counselors, or psychiatrists working in the community are listed in the local telephone book. Rather than choosing a name at random, get recommendations from a family physician, clergy, friends who have been in therapy, or community agencies.

Financial considerations are important. Be sure to check what kind of mental health benefits your personal health insurance or prepaid medical plan provides. At the time of this writing treatment by a psychiatrist in a private practice setting could cost $130 or more for a 45-minute session. Therapists in private practice charge more than those affiliated with centers or large institutions, and psychiatrists usually charge more than psychologists, who charge more than social workers or counselors. Group therapy is generally cheaper than individual therapy. Some therapists have a sliding-fee scale based on the client's income. If you are not adequately covered by a health plan, don't let that stop you from getting help; investigate low-cost alternatives. City, county, and state governments often support mental health clinics for those who can afford to pay little or nothing for treatment.

It will take a personal meeting to decide whether a therapist is right for you. Besides checking out a therapist's basic professional qualifications, you will need to know whether you feel comfortable with his or her personality, values and belief system, and psychological orientation. Does the therapist seem like a warm, intelligent person who would be able and interested in helping you? Is the therapist willing to talk about the techniques she or he uses? Does the therapist make sense to you? If the first therapist you see seems all right, there is no need to look further; but if you feel at all uncomfortable, it's worthwhile setting up one-shot consultations with one or two others before you make up your mind. If you're not in need of emergency care, spend as much time shopping for the right therapist as you would for anything else that is important to you. If you can afford only free or low-cost treatment, your options may be limited.

The number and frequency of sessions depends on the type of therapy. Psychological therapies focusing on specific problems may require eight or ten sessions at weekly intervals. Therapies aiming for psychological awareness and personality change can last months or years with one to four sessions per week. Treatment with medication usually starts with weekly sessions; after the best medication and optimal dose is found, the frequency of sessions is reduced. For schizophrenia or bipolar disorder, medication may have to be continued for years.

Whomever you choose to help you, respect your own judgment as to whether you are actually being helped. Although too much "shopping around" may be a way of avoiding the resolution of problems, you certainly have the right to change therapists if therapy is not helpful after a reasonable period of time. First, ask yourself whether you are displeased because your therapy is raising difficult, painful issues you don't want to deal with. Then express your dissatisfaction to your therapist and deal with it in your session. Finally, if you are convinced that your therapy isn't working or is harmful, find another therapist.

Personal Insight If you were feeling depressed or anxious or were having trouble in your relationship, would you be tempted to see a counselor or therapist? Why or why not?

SUMMARY

What Mental Health Is Not

- Mental health encompasses more than normality. Psychological diversity is valuable.

- Getting professional help does not necessarily indicate mental illness. Neither symptoms nor appearances are reliable indicators of mental health.

What Mental Health Is

- Maslow's definition of mental health is centered on self-actualization, the highest level of his hierarchy of needs. Self-actualized people have high self-esteem and are inner-directed, authentic, capable of emotional intimacy, and creative.

Meeting Life's Challenges

- A crucial part of mental wellness is to grow up psychologically. A personal identity—a sense of who you are and what you're capable of—develops as people interact with the world.

- A sense of self-esteem develops during childhood as a result of giving and receiving love and learning to accomplish goals. Self-concept is challenged every day; healthy people adjust their goals to their abilities if they fail.

- Fighting demoralization requires recognizing and testing negative thoughts. It's possible to develop rational responses through practice in logical thinking.

- Using defense mechanisms to cope with problems can make finding solutions much harder. Analyzing thoughts and behavior can help people develop less defensive and more effective ways of coping.

- Honest communication requires recognition of what needs to be said and the ability to say it clearly. Assertiveness allows people to insist on their rights and to participate in the give-and-take of good communication.

Psychological Disorders

- People who suffer from psychological disorders have symptoms severe enough to interfere with daily living.

- Anxiety refers to a fear that is not directed toward any definite threat. Anxiety disorders include simple phobias, social phobias, panic disorder, obsessive-compulsive disorder, and post-traumatic stress disorder.

- Depression is a common mood disorder; loss of interest or pleasure in things seems to be its most universal symptom.

- Severe depression carries a high risk of suicide, and suicidally depressed people must seek professional help.

- Symptoms of mania include exalted moods with unrealistically high self-esteem, little need for sleep, and rapid speech. Elation gives way to depression in bipolar disorders.

- Schizophrenia is characterized by disorganized thoughts, inappropriate emotions, delusions, auditory hallucinations, and deteriorating social and work performance. Schizophrenia may be accompanied by depression, and suicide is a possibility.

Getting Help

- Behavioral and cognitive approaches are useful in self-help. Books are available for guidance; talking to friends or relatives and joining self-help groups are ways to start treatment.

- Professional help is necessary if problems interfere with performance or interpersonal relationships; if suicide is considered or attempted; if hallucinations, delusions, memory loss, or other severe symptoms occur; or if alcohol or drug abuse impairs normal functioning.

- Mental health workers have various forms of training and play different roles in treatment. Several problems can probably be treated best by an interdisciplinary team. It helps to take time choosing a therapist and to continually review the benefits of therapy, changing therapists if necessary.

1. Investigate the mental health services provided on your campus and in your community. What services are available? Think about which ones you would feel comfortable using, for either yourself or someone else, should the need ever arise.

2. Many colleges and communities have peer counseling programs, hot-line services (for both general problems and specific issues such as rape, suicide, drug abuse, parental stress, and so on), and other kinds of emergency counseling services. Some of these programs are staffed by volunteers trained in listening, helping, and providing information. Investigate such programs in your school (through the health clinic or student services) or community (look in the yellow pages), and consider volunteering for one. The training and experience can give you invaluable assistance in understanding both yourself and others.

3. Being assertive rather than passive or aggressive is a valuable skill that everyone can learn. To improve your ability to assert yourself appropriately, sign up for a workshop or class in assertiveness training on your campus or in your community.

JOURNAL ENTRY

1. Do you remember incidents or moments from childhood that stand out as wonderful or horrible? Write a short essay about two such incidents, including what your feelings were and what you think you learned from them. Then include a description of what you would do now in the same situations and why.

2. *Critical Thinking:* In the past, some political candidates have dropped out of a race or been defeated after it was revealed that they had undergone psychiatric treatment or some other form of mental health therapy. Do you think that a person who has been treated for a mental illness should be excluded from holding a public office or from any other profession? Why or why not? Does your position depend on the type of illness or the treatment the individual received? In your health journal, write a brief essay outlining your position.

3. Think about a person you admire. Describe that person in writing, listing the qualities that you admire in him or her. Do you have any of those qualities? What does your list say about the kind of person you want to be?

DEALING WITH SOCIAL ANXIETY

Everyone is lonely at times, but some people have a harder time meeting new people, initiating friendships, and establishing romantic relationships than others do. In some cases, the problem is social anxiety—also known as shyness, social inhibition, or interpersonal anxiety.

To evaluate your own level of social anxiety, examine the following list of statements made by college students identified as lonely in a study conducted at Stanford University. These students said that it was difficult for them to:

• Make friends in a simple, natural way
• Introduce themselves to others at parties
• Make phone calls to others to initiate social activity
• Participate in groups
• Get pleasure out of a party
• Get into the swing of a party
• Relax on a date and enjoy themselves
• Be friendly and sociable with others
• Participate in playing games with others
• Get buddy-buddy with others

These statements suggest a level of social anxiety and inhibition that interferes with dating and making friends. If they describe you, consider looking into a shyness clinic or treatment program on your campus. You have nothing to lose and everything to gain.

Programs usually begin with a self-monitoring phase in which all facets of a person's daily routine are noted in a journal format. The Social Activity Journal shows how a coding scheme (noted in the key) can be used to help keep track of the pattern of social contacts, the amount of time spent in effective studying, and the amount of time wasted each day. These patterns are monitored for at least one week so that general trends can be identified.

Depending on the particular program, the shy person is then told to make better use of "wasted time" and to begin to practice some of the skills he or she has learned in the class or clinic in the least troublesome (anxiety-producing) situations. This tactic might be translated into an assignment to initiate brief, nonthreatening conversations with classmates on an academic topic. Once these conversations are successfully accomplished, then the next phase of the program could encourage practice of discussions that involve more personal subjects. Later assignments might involve social gatherings. The individual steps would form a type of hierarchy, incorporating topics, people, and places, from least to most difficult. The person increases social skills and confidence levels, at the same time decreasing anxiety, until social interactions can be sustained with comfort and enjoyment.

Social Activity Journal
KEY
P = Social phone call
I = Social interaction (at least 5 minutes)
A = Social activity
S = Study time
W = Wasted time

		DATE:	11/16	DATE:		DATE:	
		AM	PM	AM	PM	AM	PM
12			I,I,W				
1			AW				
2			S				
3			S				
4			S				
5			I,I				
6			W				
7			W				
8			S				
9			S,P,P				
10		I,I,S	S				
11		S	W				

SELECTED BIBLIOGRAPHY

American Psychiatric Association. 1987. *Diagnostic and Statistical Manual of Mental Disorders,* 3rd ed., revised (DSM-III-R). Washington, D.C.: American Psychiatric Association Press.

Antidepressants. 1994. *Mayo Clinic Health Letter.* July.

Beck, A. T., A. J. Rush, B. F. Shaw, and G. Emery. 1987. *Cognitive Therapy of Depression: A Treatment Manual.* New York: Guilford Press.

Cowley, G. 1991. The bold and the bashful: Even the terminally shy sometimes triumph on their own terms. *Newsweek Special Issue,* summer.

Duncan, D. D. 1987. Creativity and mental wellness. *Health Values* 2:3–7.

Erikson, E. 1963. *Childhood and Society.* New York: W. W. Norton.

Hatton, C. L., and S. M. Valente, eds. 1984. *Suicide: Assessment and Intervention,* 2nd ed. Norwalk, Conn.: Appleton-Century-Crofts.

Kohut, H. 1971. *The Psychology of the Self.* New York: International Universities Press.

Kramer, P. D. 1993. *Listening to Prozac.* New York: Viking.

Maslow, A. H. 1968. *Toward a Psychology of Being,* 2nd ed. Princeton, N.J.: Van Nostrand Reinhold.

Newman, B. M., and P. R. Newman. 1991. *Development Through Life: A Psychosocial Approach,* 5th ed. Pacific Grove, Calif.: Brooks/Cole.

Nicholi, A. M., Jr. 1988. *The New Harvard Guide to Psychiatry.* Cambridge, Mass.: Harvard University Press.

Turner, S. M., K. S. Calhoun, and H. E. Adams, eds. 1992. *Handbook of Clinical Behavior Therapy,* 2nd ed. New York: John Wiley.

Vaillant, G. E. 1977. *Adaptation to Life.* Boston: Little, Brown.

Winokur, G., and D. W. Black. 1992. Suicide—what can be done? *New England Journal of Medicine* 327:490–92.

RECOMMENDED READINGS

Beck, A. T. 1989. *Love Is Never Enough.* New York: HarperCollins. *Subtitled "How couples can overcome misunderstandings, resolve conflicts, and solve relationship problems," this book was written by a pioneer in the field of cognitive psychotherapy.*

Burns, D. D. 1989. *The Feeling Good Handbook.* New York: Penguin Books. *A self-help book with cognitive techniques for handling depression and anxiety.*

Davison, G. C., and J. M. Neale. 1993. *Abnormal Psychology,* 6th ed. New York: John Wiley. *This classic textbook is a good place to find more detailed descriptions of psychological disorders.*

Jeffers, S. 1987. *Feel the Fear and Do It Anyway.* New York: Fawcett Columbine. *This practical self-help book describes a variety of cognitive strategies and techniques for working through fears, irrational ideas, and self-defeating beliefs.*

Papolos, D. F., and J. Papolos. 1992. *Overcoming Depression,* rev. ed. New York: HarperCollins. *Its subtitle explains its contents: "For the millions who suffer depression and manic depression and for the families affected by these recurring disorders."*

Patterson, C. H. 1990. *Theories of Counseling and Psychotherapy,* 4th ed. New York: Harper and Row. *This book summarizes the basic principles of a variety of psychological treatments.*

Seligman, M. E. P. 1993. *What You Can Change and What You Can't.* New York: Fawcett Columbine. *A well-documented book about what treatments make sense for problems with anxiety, anger, depression, eating, alcohol, and sex.*

Torrey, E. F. 1988. *Surviving Schizophrenia: A Family Manual,* rev. ed. New York: Harper and Row. *This book is a detailed and intelligent account of what schizophrenia is and how to cope with it.*

Zimbardo, P. G. 1977. *Shyness—What It Is, What to Do About It.* Reading, Mass.: Addison-Wesley. *Students and their interpersonal problems are the focus of the research and therapy techniques reported in this book.*

4

Intimate Relationships

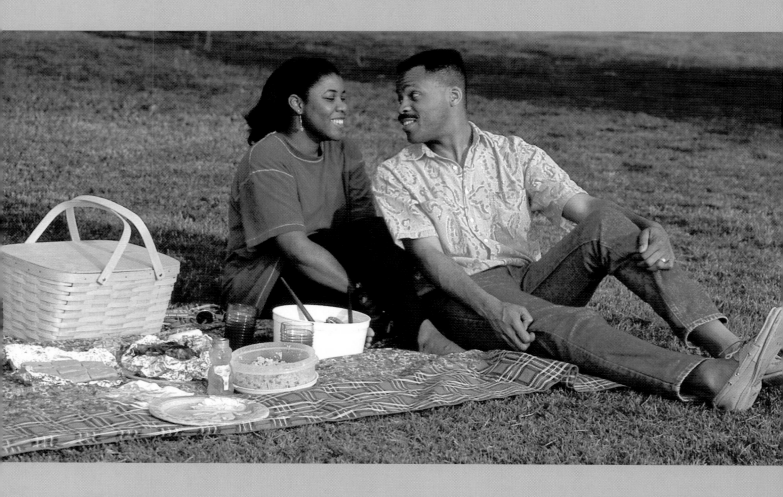

CONTENTS

Human beings need social relationships; people cannot thrive as solitary creatures. Nor could the human species survive if adults didn't cherish and support each other, if they didn't form strong mutual attachments with their infants, and if they didn't create families in which to raise children. Simply put, people need people.

Although people are held together in relationships by a variety of factors, the foundation of many relationships is love. Love in its many forms—romantic, passionate, platonic, parental—is the wellspring from which much of life's meaning and delight flows. In our culture, it binds us together as partners, parents, children, and friends. People devote tremendous energy to seeking mates, nurturing intimate relationships, keeping up friendships, maintaining marriages—all for the pleasure of loving and being loved.

Many human needs are satisfied in intimate relationships—needs for approval and affirmation, for companionship, for meaningful ties and a sense of belonging, for sexual satisfaction. Many of society's needs are fulfilled by relationships too, most notably the need to nurture and socialize children. Overall, intimate relationships are an important contributor to human well-being.

DEVELOPING INTIMATE RELATIONSHIPS

People who develop successful intimate relationships believe in themselves and in the people around them. They are willing to give of themselves—to share their ideas, feelings, time, needs—and to accept what others want to give them.

Self-Image and Self-Esteem

The principal thing that we all bring to our relationships is our *selves*. To have successful relationships, we must first accept and feel good about ourselves. A positive **self-image** and high **self-esteem** help us to love and respect others. How and where do we acquire a positive sense of self?

The roots of our sense of identity and self can be found in childhood, in the relationships we had with our parents and other family members. We're likely, as adults, to have a sense that we're basically lovable, worthwhile people and that others are trustworthy if, as babies and children, we felt loved, valued, and respected; if adults responded to our needs in a reasonably appropriate way; and if they gave us the freedom to explore and develop a sense of being separate individuals.

Our sense of personal identity isn't fixed or frozen. According to psychologist Erik Erikson, it continues to develop as we encounter and resolve various crises at each stage of life. The fundamental tasks of early childhood are the development of trust during infancy and of **autonomy** during toddlerhood. From these experiences and interactions we construct our first ideas about who we are. (For a more detailed discussion of Erikson's theory, see Chapter 3.)

Another thing we learn in early childhood is **gender role**—the activities, abilities, and characteristics our culture deems appropriate for us based on whether we're male or female. In our society, men have traditionally been expected to work and provide for their families; to be aggressive, competitive, and power-oriented; and to use thinking and logic to solve problems. Women have been expected to take care of home and children; to be cooperative, supportive, and nurturing; and to approach the world emotionally and intuitively. Although much more egalitarian gender roles are emerging in our society, the stereotypes we absorb in childhood tend to be deeply ingrained and resistant to change.

Our ways of relating to others may also be rooted in childhood. Some researchers have suggested that our adult styles of loving may be based on the style of **attachment** we established in infancy with our mother, father, or other primary caregiver. According to this view, people who are secure in their intimate relationships may have had a secure, trusting, mutually satisfying attachment to their mother or other parenting figure. As adults they find it relatively easy to get close to others. They don't worry about being abandoned or having someone get too close to them. They feel that others like them and are generally well-intentioned.

Even if people's earliest experiences and relationships were less than ideal, however, they can still establish satisfying relationships in adulthood. Humans are resilient and flexible. They have the capacity to change their ideas, beliefs, and patterns of behavior. They can learn ways to raise their self-esteem; they can become more trusting, accepting, and appreciative of others; and they can acquire the communication and conflict resolution skills needed to maintain successful relationships. It helps to have a good start in life, but it may be more important to start from where you are.

Friendship

The first relationships we form outside the family are friendships. Whether with members of the same or the other sex, friendships give people the opportunity to

---

Self-image   The idea or conception one has of oneself or one's role.

Self-esteem   Feelings about one's own value and worth.

Autonomy   Independence; the sense of being self-directed.

Gender role   A culturally expected pattern of behavior and attitudes determined by whether a person is male or female.

Attachment   The emotional tie between an infant and his or her caregiver, or between two people in an intimate relationship.

TERMS

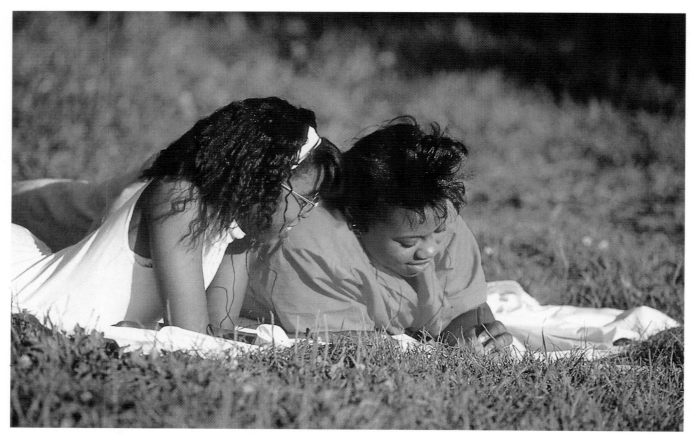

Close relationships without a sexual component are more common than those with
sexual activity. Friendship satisfies the human needs for affection, affirmation, sharing,
and companionship.

share themselves and discover others. Friendships are
reciprocal relationships between equals, held together
with ties of respect, affection, trust, tolerance, and loyalty.
Friends typically have interests and values in common,
enjoy each other's company, and accept each other's indi-
viduality. When they are together, they feel comfortable,
spontaneous, and authentic.

Friendship is like love in many ways, but love has additional characteristics. Love usually includes sexual desire, a greater demand for exclusiveness, and deeper levels of caring. But friendships are often seen as more stable
and longer lasting than love relationships and less capable
of "breaking up." Friends are more accepting and less critical than lovers, probably because their expectations are
different. Like love relationships, friendships bind society
together, providing people with emotional support and
buffering them from stress.

Love, Sex, and Intimacy

Love is one of the most basic and profound human emotions. It is a powerful force in all our intimate relationships. Love encompasses opposites—affection and anger,
excitement and boredom, stability and change, bonds

and freedom. Love does not give us perfect happiness,
but it does give our lives meaning.

For most people, love, sex, and commitment are
closely linked ideals in intimate relationships. Love reflects the positive factors that draw people together and
sustain them in a relationship. It includes trust, caring, respect, loyalty, interest in the other, and concern for the
other's well-being. Sex brings excitement and passion to
the relationship. It tends to intensify the relationship and
add fascination and pleasure. Commitment, the determination to continue, reflects the stable factors that help
maintain the relationship. Responsibility, reliability, and
faithfulness are characteristics of commitment. Although
love, sex, and commitment are related, they are not necessarily connected. One can exist without the others. Despite the various permutations of the three, most of us
long to be part of a special relationship that contains them
all.

Other elements can be identified as features of love,
such as euphoria, preoccupation with the loved one, ide-
alization of the loved one, and so on, but these tend to be
peripheral. As relationships progress, the central aspects
of love and commitment become more characteristic of
the relationship than the peripheral ones.

Even when they begin with the best of intentions, intimate relationships may not last. Sometimes a couple is mismatched to begin with; other times the relationship doesn't thrive and partners turn elsewhere for satisfaction. Ending an intimate relationship is usually difficult and painful. Both partners often feel attacked and abandoned, but feelings of distress are likely to be more acute for the rejected partner. If you are involved in a breakup, following a few simple guidelines can make the ending easier:

- Give the relationship the best chance you can before breaking up. If it still is not working, you'll know you did everything you could.

- Be fair and honest. If you are the one initiating the breakup, don't try to make your partner feel responsible.

- Be tactful and compassionate. You can leave the relationship without deliberately damaging your partner's self-esteem. Emphasize your mutual lack of fit and admit your own contributions to the problem.

- If you are the rejected person, give yourself time to resolve your anger and pain. You may go through a process of mourning the relationship, experiencing disbelief, anger, sadness, and finally acceptance. Despite all the romantic talk about your "one and only," remember that there are actually many potential candidates with whom you can have an intimate relationship.

- Find the value in the experience. Ending a close relationship can teach you valuable lessons about your needs, preferences, strengths, and weaknesses. Use your insights to increase your chances of success in your next relationship.

The Pleasure and Pain of Love   The experience of intense love has confused and tormented lovers throughout history. They live in a tumultuous state of excitement, subject to wildly fluctuating feelings of joy and despair. They lose their appetites, can't sleep, and can think of nothing but the loved one. Is this happiness, misery, or both?

The contradictory nature of passionate love can be understood by realizing that human emotions have two components—physiological arousal and an emotional explanation for the arousal. (For a discussion of the biochemical and hormonal processes involved in arousal, see the description of the stress response in Chapter 2). Love is just one of many emotions accompanied by physiological arousal. Numerous unpleasant emotions can also generate physiological arousal, including fear, rejection, frustration, and challenge. Although experiences like attraction and sexual desire are pleasant, extreme excitement is similar to fear and is unpleasant. For this reason, passionate love may be too intense to enjoy. Over time the physical intensity and excitement of such a relationship tend to diminish. When this happens, pleasure may actually increase.

The Transformation of Love   All human relationships change over time, and love relationships are no exception. At first, love is likely to be characterized by high levels of passion and rapidly increasing intimacy. In time, passion decreases as we become habituated to it and to the person.

The disappearance of romance or passionate love is often experienced as a crisis in a relationship. If a more lasting love fails to emerge, the relationship will likely break up and each person will search for another who will once again ignite his or her passion. But love does not necessarily have to be passionate. When intensity diminishes, partners often discover a more enduring love. They can now move from absorption in each other to a relationship that includes external goals and projects, friends, and family. In this kind of intimate, more secure love, satisfaction comes not just from the relationship but also from achieving other creative goals, such as work or child rearing. The key to successful relationships isn't in love's intensity but in transforming passion into an intimate love, based on closeness, caring, and the promise of a shared future.

Personal Insight   What are your expectations of love? How much are your expectations shaped by movies and magazines, by what your friends expect, by what you've observed of your parents' relationship? Are there any contradictions among these views? If so, can you reconcile them?

PAIRING AND SINGLEHOOD

Although most people eventually marry, all spend some time as singles, and nearly all make some attempt—conscious or unconscious—to find a partner. Relationships are as important for singles as for couples.

Choosing a Partner

Most men and women select partners for stable relationships through a fairly predictable process, although they may not be consciously aware of it. Most people pair with someone who lives in the same geographical area and who is similar in racial, ethnic, and socioeconomic background, educational level, lifestyle, physical attractiveness, and other traits. In simple terms, people select partners like themselves.

First attraction is based on easily observable characteristics—looks, dress, social status, and reciprocated interest. Once the euphoria of romantic love winds down, personality traits and behaviors become more significant factors in how the partners view each other. Through sharing and self-disclosing, they gradually gain a deeper knowledge of each other. The emphasis shifts to basic values, such as religious beliefs, political persuasion, sexual attitudes, and future aspirations regarding career, family, and children. At some point, they decide whether the relationship feels viable and is worthy of their continued commitment. If they are compatible, many people gradually discover deeper, more enduring forms of love.

When people are choosing intimates, perhaps the most important question they can ask is, How much do we have in common? Although differences add interest to a relationship, similarities increase the chances of a relationship's success. If there are major differences, partners should ask, first, How accepting of differences are we? and second, How well do we communicate? Acceptance and communication skills go a long way toward making a relationship work, no matter how different the partners. Areas in which differences can affect the relationship include values, religion, race, attitudes toward sexuality and gender roles, socioeconomic status, familiarity with the other's culture, and interactions with the extended family.

Dating

Every society has some rituals for pairing and finding mates. Parent-arranged marriages are still popular in many cultures. They are often very stable and permanent; divorce is unheard of, except for infertility. Although American culture emphasizes personal choice in courtship, the popularity of dating services suggests that many individuals do want assistance in finding suitable mates.

Most Americans—whether single, divorced, widowed, or gay—find romantic partners through some form of dating. They narrow the field through a process of getting to know each other. Dating often revolves around a mu-

tually enjoyable activity, such as seeing a movie or having dinner. In the traditional male-female dating pattern, the man takes the lead, initiating the date, while the woman waits to be called. In this pattern, casual dating might evolve into steady or exclusive dating, then engagement and finally marriage.

For many young people today, traditional dating has given way to a more casual form of "getting together." Greater equality between the sexes is at the root of this change. People may meet in groups rather than go out as couples, with each person paying his or her way. A man and woman may begin to spend more time together, but often in the group context.

Living Together

According to the U.S. Census Bureau, over 3.5 million heterosexual couples were living together in the United States in 1993. Additionally, an estimated 1.5 million gay and lesbian couples (who cannot legally marry) were living together. Living together, or **cohabitation,** is one of the most rapid and dramatic social changes that has ever occurred in our society. It seems to be gaining acceptance as part of the normal mate selection process. By age 30, about half of all men and women will have cohabited. The only thing separating those who cohabit from those who don't is degree of religiousness.

For those who choose it, living together has certain advantages over marriage. For one thing, it can give the partners a greater sense of autonomy. They don't feel bound by the social rules and expectations that are part of marriage. They may find it easier to keep their identity and more of their independence, and they don't incur the same obligations that marriage brings. If things don't work out, they may find it easier and less complicated to leave a relationship that hasn't been legally sanctioned.

But living together has some liabilities, too. In most cases, the legal protections of marriage are absent; these include health insurance benefits and property and inheritance rights. These considerations can be particularly serious if the couple has children, from either former relationships or the current partnership. Since social acceptance of cohabitation is not universal, couples may feel pressure from family members or others to marry or otherwise change their living arrangements, especially if they have young children. The general trend, however, is toward legitimizing single relationships, whether gay or heterosexual. For example, some employers and communities now extend benefits to domestic partners.

Although many people choose cohabitation as a kind of trial marriage, there is little evidence as yet that people who live together before getting married have happier or longer-lasting marriages. Statistically, people who cohabit before marrying are just as likely to divorce as are those who don't cohabit. One study found slightly less marital satisfaction among married couples who had cohabited.

TERMS

Cohabitation   Living together in a sexual relationship without being married.

Gay and Lesbian Partnerships

Regardless of **sexual orientation,** most people are looking for love in a close, satisfying, committed relationship. Gay and lesbian (or **homosexual**) couples have many similarities with **heterosexual** couples. According to one study, most gay men and lesbians have experienced at least one long-term relationship with a single partner. Like heterosexual relationships, gay and lesbian partnerships provide intimacy, passion, and security.

One difference among gay, lesbian, and heterosexual couples is that gay and lesbian couples tend to adopt "best friend" roles in their relationship rather than traditional gender roles. Domestic tasks are shared or split, and both partners usually support themselves. Another difference is that gay and lesbian couples often have to deal with societal hostility toward their relationships (in contrast to the approval given to heterosexual couples). Consequently, the community may be more important as a source of identity and social support than it is for heterosexuals. Community support has been particularly important since the advent of the HIV/AIDS crisis. Gay men and lesbians have played an important role in the development of education and counseling programs, research foundations, and outreach programs for people infected with HIV.

Singlehood

Despite the prevalence and popularity of marriage, a significant proportion of adults in our society are unmarried. In 1990 nearly 72.6 million Americans were single. They are a diverse group, encompassing young people who have not married yet but plan to in the future, people who are living together, whether gay or heterosexual, and people of all ages who would like to marry but haven't found a suitable mate. In other words, the category includes people of all ages who are single both by choice and by chance.

Several factors contribute to the growing number of single people. One is the changing view of singlehood, which is increasingly being viewed as a legitimate option to marriage. Education and career are delaying the age at which young people are marrying. More young people are living with their parents as they complete their education, seek jobs, or strive for financial independence. High rates of divorce and cohabitation (among both heterosexuals and homosexuals) also contribute to the growing number of single people.

Being single doesn't mean that people don't have close relationships, however. They may date and enjoy active and fulfilling social lives. Other advantages of being single include more opportunities for personal and career development without concern for family obligations and more freedom and control in making life choices. Disadvantages of being single include loneliness and lack of companionship as well as economic hardships (mainly for single women). Single people, both male and female, experience some discrimination and often are pressured to get married.

Nearly everyone has at least one episode of being single in adult life, whether it's prior to marriage, between marriages, following divorce or the death of a spouse, or for the entire adult life span. How enjoyable and valuable this single time is depends on several factors, including how deliberately the person has chosen it; how satisfied the person is with social relationships, standard of living, and job; how comfortable the person feels when alone; and how resourceful and energetic the person is about creating an interesting and fulfilling life.

MARRIAGE

Although half of all marriages in our society now end in divorce, the popularity of marriage itself hasn't diminished. Marriage fulfills a number of basic needs. There are many important social, moral, economic, and political aspects of marriage, all of which have changed over the years. In the past, people married mainly for practical reasons, such as raising children or forming an economic unit. Today, people marry more for personal, emotional reasons. This shift places a greater burden on marriage to fulfill needs and expectations. People may assume that all their emotional needs will be met by their partner, or they may simply expect to "live happily ever after." When people enter marriage with such preconceptions, it may be harder for them to appreciate the benefits that marriage really offers.

Personal Insight   What are your ideas and beliefs about marriage? Do you think it should last forever? What influences your views of marriage?

Benefits of Marriage

The primary functions and benefits of marriage are those of any intimate relationship: affection, personal affirmation, companionship, sexual fulfillment, emotional growth. Marriage also provides a setting in which to raise children, although a growing number of couples choose

Sexual orientation   Sexual attraction to individuals of the opposite sex, same sex, or both.

Homosexual   Sexual orientation toward and preference for the same sex.

Heterosexual   Sexual orientation toward and preference for the opposite sex.

TERMS

Alone on the banks of Walden Pond, Henry David Thoreau enjoyed a life of simplicity and solitude. But is the solitary lifestyle healthy? Recent research indicates that it's not. Studies underscore the importance of strengthening your family and social ties to help maintain your mental and physical health. Living alone, or simply feeling alone, can have a negative effect not only on your state of mind but on your physical health as well.

Two studies published in the January 1992 issue of the *Journal of the American Medical Association* showed that social isolation is a risk factor for people with heart problems. The first study looked at the effects of living alone on people who had had a heart attack. Those living alone had a 15.8 percent chance of having a second serious nonfatal or fatal heart attack, compared to 8.8 percent for those not living alone. The second study looked at people with severe narrowing of at least one major heart vessel. Those who were unmarried and without one close friend or confidant were "over three times more likely to die of a heart problem within five years than married patients or unmarried patients who did report having a confidant."

Similar evidence has been found for people with cancer. A long-term study of over 6,000 adults in California showed that women who had no or few social contacts were twice as likely to die of cancer. These women also were more than five times as likely to die of smoking-related cancers.

Another study at Stanford University Medical Center was conducted to evaluate the psychological effect of emotional support groups on cancer patients. Eighty-six women who were receiving treatment for breast cancer were randomly divided into two groups. One group took part in weekly discussions in which they shared their feelings and learned simple techniques to reduce stress. After a year, the women in the support group were less depressed, felt less pain, and had a more positive outlook than did the women who received only conventional treatment. To the surprise of the researchers, the women in the support group also survived nearly twice as long as the women in the control group. Researcher David Spiegel said, "Believe me, if we'd seen these results with a new drug, it would be in use in every cancer hospital in the country today."

What is it about social relationships that supports people's health? Researchers aren't sure, but they suggest that intimate relationships, and especially living with a loving partner, have both physical and emotional benefits. When you're sick, a partner can cook, bring you food, and make your life easier and more comfortable. Partners encourage and reinforce healthy habits, such as eating well, smoking and drinking less, and taking fewer risks. (Women generally have healthier lifestyles than men, so when people marry, men's health improves more significantly than women's.) Partners also help identify problems and encourage each other to rest, treat illnesses, see a physician, and so on. These are probably some of the reasons that married people live longer, have fewer illnesses, and report a higher sense of well-being than do their unmarried peers.

But it's not just the physical support that helps people get and stay well. Although married people have better emotional health than unmarried people, this is true only if the marriage is happy. Unhappily married people have *more* emotional distress than unmarried people. And when partners are unsupportive or unfair, sick people often feel depressed or demoralized.

Clearly, emotional support is a crucial element in physical health. When someone cares and listens, it helps reduce depression, anxiety, and other psychological problems. Feeling loved, esteemed, and valued brings comfort at a time of vulnerability. Being connected with others helps mitigate the damaging effects of stress. In general, improved emotional well-being improves physical health and survival ability.

Although solitude may have helped Thoreau achieve his purposes (he returned to life in Boston after two years at Walden Pond), prolonged isolation is a strain for most human beings. To protect your health over your whole life span, stay connected with people, maintain your social ties, and take good care of your intimate relationships.

Adapted from "Living Alone," *Mayo Clinic Health Letter,* September 1992; and P. Jaret, "Mind over Malady," *Health,* November/December 1992.

to remain childless and people can also choose to raise children without being married. Marriage is also important for its provision for the future. By committing themselves to the relationship, people provide themselves with lifelong companions as well as some insurance for their later years.

Issues in Marriage

Although we would all like to believe otherwise, love is not enough to make a successful marriage. Couples have to have strengths; they have to be successful in their relationship before marriage. Problems in relationships are magnified rather than solved by marriage. The following relationship characteristics appear to be the best predictors of a happy marriage:

- The partners have realistic expectations about their relationship.
- Each feels good about the personality of the other.
- They communicate well.
- They have effective ways of resolving conflicts.

- When you want to have a serious discussion with your partner, you need to find an appropriate time and place. Choose a block of time when you will not be interrupted or rushed and a place that will afford you privacy.
- Face your partner and maintain eye contact. Use nonverbal feedback to show that you are interested and involved in the communication process.

When you are the speaker . . .

- State your case as clearly as you can.

- Use "I" messages—statements about how *you* feel—rather than statements beginning with "You," which tell another person how *you* think he or she feels. When you use "I" messages, you are taking responsibility for your feelings. "You" statements are often blaming or accusatory and are likely to elicit a defensive or resentful response. The statement "I feel unloved," for example, sends a clearer, less blaming message than the statement "You don't love me."

- Focus on behavior rather than on the person. People are able to change their behavior much more readily than they can change themselves. Be specific about the behavior you like or don't like. Avoid generalizations that begin "You always" or "You never." Such statements make people feel defensive.

- Make constructive requests. Beginning your request with "I would like" keeps the focus on your needs rather than your partner's supposed deficiencies.

- Avoid blaming, accusing, and belittling. Even if you are right, you have little to gain by putting your partner

down. Studies have shown that when people feel criticized or attacked, they are less able to think rationally or solve problems correctly.

- Ask for action ahead of time, not after the fact. Tell your partner what you would like to have happen in the future—don't wait for him or her to blow it and then express anger or disappointment.

When you are the listener . . .

- Provide appropriate nonverbal feedback (nodding, smiling, and so on).

- Don't interrupt.

- Develop the skill of reflective listening. Don't judge, evaluate, analyze, or offer solutions (unless asked to do so). Your partner may just need to have you there in order to sort out feelings. By jumping in right away to "fix" the problem, you may actually be cutting off communication.

- Don't give unsolicited advice. Giving advice implies that you know more about what a person needs to do than he or she does; therefore, it often evokes anger or resentment.

- Clarify your understanding of what your partner is saying by restating it in your own words and asking if your understanding is correct.

- Be sure you are really listening, not off somewhere in your mind rehearsing your reply. Try to tune into your partner's feelings as well as the words.

- Let your partner know that you value what he or she is saying and want to understand. Respect for the other person is the cornerstone of effective communication.

- They agree on religious/ethical values.

- They have an egalitarian role relationship.

- They have a good balance of individual versus joint interests and leisure activities.

Once they're married, couples have a number of adjustments to make. In addition to providing each other with emotional support, they have to negotiate and establish marital roles; establish domestic and career priorities; manage their budget and finances; make sexual adjustments; manage boundaries and relationships with their extended family; and participate in the larger community.

The area of marital roles and responsibilities has probably undergone the most change in recent years. Many couples no longer accept traditional assumptions about roles, such as that the husband is solely responsible for supporting the family and the wife is solely responsible

for domestic work. Today, many husbands share domestic tasks and many wives work outside the home. In fact, over 50 percent of married women are in the labor force, including women with babies under one year of age. Although women still take most of the responsibility for home and children even when they work, and although men still suffer more job-related stress and health problems than women do, the trend is toward an equalization of duties and responsibilities.

Coping with all these challenges requires that couples be committed to remaining married through the inevitable ups and downs of the relationship. They will need to be tolerant of each other's imperfections, keep their sense of perspective and their sense of humor, and put energy into retaining sufficient levels of intimacy, sexual satisfaction, and commitment. The most important skills they bring to these challenges are their communication and conflict resolution skills.

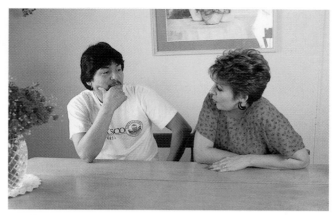

Conflict is an inevitable part of any intimate relationship. Couples need to develop constructive ways of resolving conflicts to maintain a healthy relationship.

Communication Skills

The key to developing and maintaining an intimate relationship is good **communication.** Most of the time, we don't think about communicating—we simply talk and act in natural ways. But when problems arise—when we feel others don't understand us or when someone accuses us of not listening—we become aware of our limitations or, more commonly, what we think are other people's limitations. Miscommunications create frustration and distance us from our friends and partners.

As much as 65 percent of face-to-face communication is nonverbal. Even when we're silent, we're communicating. We send messages when we look at someone or look away, lean forward or sit back, smile or frown. Especially important forms of nonverbal communication are touch, eye contact, and proximity. If someone we're talking to touches our hand or arm, looks into our eyes, and leans toward us when we talk, we get the message that the person is interested in us and cares about what we're saying. If a person keeps looking around the room while we're talking or takes a step backward, we get the impression that the person is uninterested or wants to end the conversation. The ability to interpret nonverbal messages correctly is important to the success of relationships. It's also important, when sending messages, to make sure our body language agrees with our words. When our verbal and nonverbal messages are incongruent with each other, we send a confusing mixed message.

Three keys to good communication in relationships are self-disclosure, listening skills, and feedback. Self-disclosure involves revealing personal information that we ordinarily wouldn't reveal because of the risk involved. It usually increases feelings of closeness and allows the relationship to move to a deeper level of intimacy. Friends often disclose the most to each other, sharing feelings, experiences, hopes, and disappointments; married couples sometimes share less because they think they already know everything there is to know about each other.

Listening is the second component of good communication, and it is a rare skill. Good listening skills require that we spend more time and energy trying to fully understand another person's "story" and less time judging, evaluating, blaming, advising, analyzing, or trying to control. Empathy, warmth, respect, and genuineness are qualities of skillful listeners. Attentive listening encourages friends or partners to share more and, in turn, to be attentive listeners. To connect with other people and develop real emotional intimacy, listening is essential.

Self-disclosing and good listening both build trust in a relationship. The third component of good communication is feedback—a constructive response to another's self-disclosure. Giving positive feedback means acknowledging that the friend's or partner's feelings are valid—no matter how upsetting or troubling—and offering self-disclosures in response. If, for example, your partner discloses unhappiness about your relationship, it is more constructive to say that you're concerned or saddened by that and want to hear more about it than to get angry, to blame, to try to inflict pain, or to withdraw. Self-disclosure and feedback can open the door to change, where other responses block communication and change.

Some of the difficulties people encounter in relationships can be traced to common gender differences in communication. Many authorities believe that, because of the way they've been raised, men as a group and women as a group approach conversation and communication differently. (This doesn't mean that there aren't individual exceptions.) According to this view, men tend to use conversation in a competitive way, perhaps hoping to establish dominance in relationships. When male conversations are over, men often find themselves in a one-up or a one-down position. Women tend to use conversation in a more **affiliative** way, perhaps hoping to establish friendships. They negotiate various degrees of closeness, seeking to give and receive support. Men tend to talk more—though without disclosing more—and listen less. Women tend to use good listening skills like eye contact, frequent nodding, focused attention, and relevant questions.

Although these are generalized patterns, they can translate into problems in specific conversations. Even when a man and a woman are talking about the same subject, their unconscious goals may be very different. The woman may be looking for understanding and closeness while the man may be trying to demonstrate his competence by giving advice and solving problems. Both styles are valid; the problem comes when differences in styles result in poor communication and misunderstanding.

Sometimes communication is not the problem in a relationship—the partners understand each other all too well. The problem is that they're unable or unwilling to change or compromise. Good communication can't salvage a bad relationship, but it does allow people to see their differences and make more informed decisions.

Conflict and Conflict Resolution

Conflict is natural in intimate relationships. No matter how close two people become, they still remain separate individuals with their own wants, needs, past experiences, and ways of seeing the world. In fact, the closer the relationship, the more differences will be discovered and the more opportunities for conflict will arise. Conflict itself isn't dangerous to intimate relationships; it may simply indicate that the relationship is growing. But if it isn't handled in a constructive way, it will damage—or destroy—the relationship.

Conflict is often accompanied by anger, a natural enough emotion but one that can be difficult to handle. If we vent anger, we run the risk of creating distrust, fear, and distance; if we act it out without thinking things through, we can cause the conflict to escalate; if we suppress it, it turns into resentment and low-level hostility. The best way to handle anger in a relationship is to recognize it as a symptom of something that requires attention and needs to be changed. When they are angry, the partners should back off until they calm down, then come back to the issue later and try to resolve it rationally. Negotiation will help to dissipate anger so that the conflict can be resolved.

Sources of conflict for couples change over time but revolve mainly around the basic task of living together— how housework is divided, how much time and attention are given to each other, how money is handled. Sexual interaction is a source of disagreement for many couples.

There are many theories on and approaches to conflict resolution, but there are some basic strategies that are generally useful in successfully negotiating with a partner:

- Clarify the issue. Take responsibility for thinking through your feelings and discovering what is really bothering you. Agree that one partner will speak first and have the chance to speak fully while the other listens. Then reverse the roles. Try to understand the other's position fully by repeating what you've heard and asking questions to clarify or elicit more information. Agree to talk only about the topic at hand and not get distracted by other issues. Sum up what your partner has said.

- Find out what each person wants. Ask your partner to express his or her desires. Don't assume you know what your partner wants and speak for him or her. Clarify and summarize.

- Identify various alternatives for getting each person what he or she wants. Practice brainstorming to generate a variety of options.

- Decide how to negotiate. Work out some agreements or plans for change, such as agreeing that if one partner will do one task, the other will do another task or that a partner will do a task in exchange for being able to do something else he or she wants.

- Solidify the agreements. Go over the plan verbally and write it down if necessary to ensure that you both understand and agree to it.

- Review and renegotiate. Decide on a time frame for trying out the new plan and set a time to discuss how it's working. Make adjustments as needed.

To resolve conflicts, partners have to feel safe in voicing disagreements. They have to trust that the discussion won't get out of control, that they won't be abandoned by the other, and that the partner won't take advantage of their vulnerability. Partners should follow some basic ground rules when they argue, such as avoiding ultimatums, resisting the urge to give the silent treatment, refusing to "hit below the belt," and not using sex to smooth over disagreements.

Marital and Family Violence and Abuse

Conflict resolution skills are just part of what's missing in relationships that become abusive or violent.

Violence against wives, or battering, occurs at every level of society but is more common at lower socioeconomic levels. It also occurs more frequently in marriages with a high degree of conflict—and an apparent inability to resolve arguments through negotiation and compromise. There are no figures on how many battered women there are in the United States, but battering is probably one of the most common and underreported crimes in the country.

Communication The process by which we establish contact and exchange information with others.

Affiliative Relating to connections, associations, or relationships.

TERMS

At the root of abusive behavior is the need to control another person: Abusive partners are controlling partners. They not only want to have power over another person; they believe they are entitled to it, no matter what the cost to the other person. Abuse can be defined as a pattern of coercive control that one person exercises over another, whether or not the relationship includes physical violence. Abuse includes behavior that physically harms, arouses fear, prevents a person from doing what she wants, or compels her to behave in ways she does not freely choose.

Controlling people use a variety of psychological, emotional, and physical tactics to keep their partners bound to them, including the following:

Criticizing

Using moodiness, anger, or threats

Being overprotective and "caring"

Denying the other person's perceptions

Ignoring the other person's needs and opinions

Making all the decisions

Controlling money

Shifting responsibility for everything to the other person

Limiting contact with other people

Using physical intimidation

Using sexual humiliation

Using physical and sexual violence

Early in a relationship, a person's tendency to be controlling may not be obvious. If you are a woman concerned about whether a man you are dating has the potential to be abusive, observe his behavior. There are no sure ways to tell, but there are warning signs that you can look for. Ask yourself these questions:

- What is this person's attitude toward women? How does he treat his mother and his sister? How does he work with female colleagues or a female boss? How does he treat your women friends?
- What is his attitude toward your autonomy? Does he respect the work you do and the way you do it? Or does he put it down, or tell you how to do it better, or encourage you to give it up? Does he tell you he'll take care of you?
- How self-centered is he? Does he want to spend leisure time on your interests or his? Does he listen to you? Does he remember what you say?
- Is he possessive or jealous? Does he want to spend every minute with you? Does he cross-examine you about things you do when you're not with him?
- What happens when things don't go the way he wants them to? Does he blow up? Does he always have to get his way?
- Is he moody, mocking, critical, or bossy? Do you feel as if you're "walking on eggshells" when you're with him?
- Do you feel you have to avoid having an argument with him?
- Does he drink too much or use drugs?

- Does he refuse to use condoms or take other safe-sex precautions?

Experts summarize their advice to women this way: Listen to your own uneasiness and stay away from any man who disrespects women, who wants or needs you intensely and exclusively, and who has a knack for getting his own way almost all the time.

If you are in a serious relationship with a controlling person, you may already have experienced abuse. Consider the questions on the following list.

- Does your partner constantly criticize you, blame you for things that are not your fault, or verbally degrade you?
- Does he humiliate you in front of others?
- Is he suspicious or jealous? Does he accuse you of being unfaithful or monitor your mail or phone calls?
- Does he "track" all your time? Does he discourage you from seeing friends and family?
- Does he prevent you from getting or keeping a job or attending school? Does he control your shared resources or restrict your access to money?
- Has he ever pushed, slapped, hit, kicked, bitten, or restrained you? Thrown an object at you? Used a weapon on you?
- Has he ever destroyed or damaged your personal property or sentimental items?
- Has he ever forced you to have sex or to do something sexually you didn't want to do?
- Does he anger easily when drinking or taking drugs?
- Has he ever threatened to harm you or your children, friends, pets, or property?
- Has he ever threatened to blackmail you if you leave?

If you answered yes to one or more of these questions, you may be experiencing domestic abuse. If you believe you or your children are in imminent danger, look in your local telephone directory for a women's shelter or call 911. If you want information, referrals to a program in your area, or assistance, contact one of these organizations:

National Coalition Against Domestic Violence, P.O. Box 18749, Denver, CO 80218, (303) 839-1852

National Family Violence Helpline, (800) 222-2000

National Clearinghouse for the Defense of Battered Women, 125 S. 9th Street, Suite 302, Philadelphia, PA 19107, (215) 351-0010

If you are a man concerned about abusive or violent relationships, contact

Emerge: A Men's Counseling Service on Domestic Violence, 18 Hurley Street, Suite 100, Cambridge, MA 02141, (617) 422-1550

Adapted from A. Jones and S. Schechter. 1992. *When Love Goes Wrong.* New York: HarperCollins; A. Jones. 1994. *Next Time She'll Be Dead.* Boston: Beacon Press; and "How to Tell If You Are in an Abusive Situation." *San Francisco Chronicle,* June 24, 1994.

Husbands may also rape wives. Strong evidence suggests that one of every seven American women who have ever married has been raped by her husband or ex-husband. One study found that 60 percent of 430 battered women had been raped by their husbands. A charge of mate rape can now be taken to court in over half the states.

In these relationships, the man usually has a history of violent behavior, traditional beliefs about gender roles, and problems with alcohol abuse. He has low self-esteem and seeks to raise it by dominating and imposing his will on another person. Research has revealed a three-phase cycle of battering, consisting of a period of increasing tension, a violent explosion and loss of control, and a period of contriteness, in which the man begs forgiveness and promises it will never happen again.

Battered women often stay in violent relationships for years. They may be economically dependent on their husbands, believe their children need a father, or have low self-esteem themselves. They may love or pity their husbands, or they may believe they'll eventually be able to stop the violence. They usually leave the relationship only when they become determined that the violence must end. Battered women's shelters offer them physical protection, counseling, support, and various types of survival assistance.

Many battering husbands are arrested, prosecuted, and imprisoned. Treatment programs for men focus on stress management, communication and conflict resolution skills, behavior change, and individual and group therapy. A crucial factor in changing men's violent behavior seems to be their partners' adamant insistence that the abuse stop.

Violence is also directed against children. At least 1 million American children are physically abused by their parents every year. Parental violence is one of the five leading causes of death for children aged 1 to 18.

Children are also vulnerable to sexual abuse, which is a sexual act imposed on a minor. Adults and older adolescents are able to coerce a child into sexual activity because of their authority and power over children; threats, force, or the promise of friendship or material rewards may be used to manipulate a child. Sexual abuse is often unreported. Recent surveys suggest that as many as 27 percent of women and 16 percent of men were sexually abused as children. Child sexual abuse can leave lasting scars, and adults who were abused as children are more likely to suffer from low self-esteem, depression, anxiety, eating disorders, self-destructive tendencies, sexual problems, and difficulties in intimate relationships.

Parents who abuse children tend to have low self-esteem, to believe in physical punishment, to have a poor marital relationship, and to have been abused themselves (although many people who were abused as children do not grow up to abuse their own children). Poverty, unemployment, and social isolation are characteristics of families in which children are abused. Single parents, both men and women, are at especially high risk for abusing their children. Very often, one child, whom the parents consider different in some way, is singled out for violent treatment.

When government agencies intervene in child abuse situations, their goals are to protect the victims and to assist and strengthen the families. The most successful programs are those that stress education and early intervention, such as home visits to high-risk first-time mothers. Educational efforts focus on stress management, money management, job-finding skills, and information about child behavior and development. Parents may also receive counseling and be referred to alcohol or drug abuse programs. Support groups like Parents Anonymous are effective for parents committed to changing their behavior.

Separation and Divorce

The high rate of divorce in the United States doesn't indicate that Americans don't believe in marriage any more. Instead, it reflects our extremely high expectations for emotional fulfillment and satisfaction in marriage. It also indicates that we no longer believe in the permanence of marriage.

The process of divorce usually begins with an emotional separation. Often one partner is unhappy and looks beyond the relationship for other forms of validation. Dissatisfaction increases until the unhappy partner decides that he or she can no longer go on. Physical separation follows, although it may take some time for the relationship to be over emotionally.

Except for the death of a spouse, divorce is the greatest stress-producing event in life. Both men and women experience turmoil, depression, and lowered self-esteem during and after divorce. People experience separation distress and loneliness for about a year and then enter on a one- to three-year-long recovery period. During this time they gradually construct a postdivorce identity along with a new pattern of life. Most people are surprised by how long it takes to recover from divorce. Children are especially vulnerable to the trauma of divorce, and sometimes counseling is appropriate to help them adjust to the changes in their lives.

Despite the distress of separation and divorce, the negative effects are usually balanced sooner or later by the possibility of finding a more suitable partner, constructing a new life, and developing new aspects of the self. About three-quarters of all people who divorce remarry, often within five years. One result of the high divorce and remarriage rate is a growing number of stepfamilies (also known as "blended" families), a trend discussed in the next section.

American families are very different today than they were even a few decades ago. Currently, about half of all families are based on a first marriage; nearly 30 percent are headed by a single parent; the remainder are remarriages or involve some other arrangement. Despite the tremendous variation apparent in American families, certain patterns can still be discerned.

For many young adults, the family life cycle begins with marriage. This first stage, when newlyweds are learning how to live together, ends abruptly if and when they have a baby. New parents have a new set of responsibilities, and their roles change profoundly and irreversibly—no more spontaneous outings to see a movie or leisurely Sunday mornings sipping coffee and browsing through the paper. The third member of the family, the new infant, demands round-the-clock attention.

Deciding to Become a Parent

Many factors have to be taken into account when couples consider parenthood. The following are some questions partners should ask themselves and some issues they should consider when making this decision. Some issues are relevant to both men and women; others apply only to women.

- Their physical health and age. Are they in reasonably good health? If not, can they improve their health by changing their lifestyle, perhaps by modifying their diet or giving up cigarettes or drugs? Does the woman have physical conditions, such as being overweight or having diabetes, that will require extra care and medical attention during pregnancy? Does either partner have a family history of genetic problems that a baby might inherit? Does the mother's age place her or her baby at risk? (Teenagers and women over 35 have a higher incidence of some problems.) The birth of a healthy baby depends in part on the mother's general health and well-being *before* conception. The U.S. Public Health Service has recommended that all women receive health care to help them prepare for pregnancy. **Preconception care** should include assessment of health risks, promotion of healthy lifestyle behaviors, and any treatments necessary to reduce risk.

- Their financial circumstances. Can they afford a child? Will their health insurance cover the costs of pregnancy, prenatal tests, delivery, and medical attention for mother and baby before and after the birth, including physicians' fees and hospital costs? Supplies for the baby are expensive too—diapers, bedding, cribs, strollers, car seats, clothing, food and medical supplies, and child care.

- The couple's relationship. Is it stable, and do both of them want a child? Are their views compatible on such issues as child-rearing goals, the distribution of responsibility for the child, and work and housework?

- Their educational, career, and child care plans. Have they completed as much of their education as they want right now? Have they sufficiently established themselves in careers, if that is something they want to do? Have they investigated parental leave and company-sponsored child care? Do both partners agree on child care arrangements, and does such child care exist in their community? Some child development experts advise against full-time child care for babies under 1 year of age because it can disrupt their attachment to their parents. The child care issue, which some people consider the most difficult one in parenting, requires a great deal of thought.

- Their emotional readiness for parenthood. Are they prepared to have a helpless being completely dependent on them 24 hours a day? Do they have the emotional reserves to care for and nurture an infant? Are they willing to change their lifestyle to provide the best conditions for a baby's development, both before and after birth?

- Their social support system. Do they have a network of family and friends who will help them with the baby? Are there community resources that they can call on for additional assistance? A family's social support system is one of the most important factors affecting their ability to adjust to a baby and cope with new responsibilities.

- Their personal qualities, attitudes toward children, and aptitude for parenting. Do they like infants, young children, and adolescents? Do they think time with children is time well spent? Do they feel good enough about themselves to love and respect others? Do they have safe ways of handling anger, frustration, and impatience?

Emotional Responses to Pregnancy

A woman's feelings during pregnancy will vary dramatically depending on her circumstances—her self-image, how she feels about pregnancy and motherhood, whether the pregnancy was planned, what type of relationship she has with her partner, whether she has a secure home situation, and many other factors. A first pregnancy is especially important because it has traditionally symbolized the transition to maturity and is a major developmental milestone in the lives of mothers—and fathers as well.

Pregnancy is likely to change a couple's relationship. Communication is especially important because people may have preconceived ideas about how they and their partners should feel. Both partners may have fears about the approaching birth, their ability to be good parents, and the ways in which the baby will affect their own relationship. These concerns are normal, and sharing them can deepen and strengthen a relationship. For a woman without a partner or whose partner is not supportive, it's important that she find other sources of support, perhaps from friends, family members, or support groups. The relationships that parents-to-be have with their own parents may also change. Impending parenthood may allow them to assert their independence from their parents but may also allow them to identify with their parents' own experience of pregnancy, childbirth, and parenting.

Becoming a Parent

Few new parents have any preparation for the job of parenting, yet they have to assume that role literally overnight. They have to learn quickly how to hold a baby, how to change it, how to feed it, how to interpret its cries. No wonder the birth of the first child is one of the most stressful transitions for any couple.

Marital satisfaction often declines after the birth of the first child but marital dissatisfaction is not inevitable. Couples who successfully weather the stresses of a new baby seem to have three characteristics in common: They had developed a strong relationship before the baby was born; they had planned to have the child and want it very much; and they communicate well about their feelings and expectations.

Parenting and the Life Cycle of the Family

Sometimes being a parent is a source of unparalleled pleasure and pride—the first smile (at you), the first word, the first home run. But at other times, parenting can seem like an overwhelming responsibility. How can you be sure that you're not making some mistake that will stunt your child's physical or emotional growth? Child-rearing experts all seem to agree that (1) it's virtually impossible to stop a child's physical growth and development and (2) children's emotional health and self-esteem depend above all on their feeling that their parents want them, accept them, and love them, although there's no one right way to raise children that will ensure that they will become happy and productive adults.

At each stage of the family life cycle, the relationship between parents and children changes. And with those changes come new challenges. The parents' primary responsibility to a small, helpless baby is to ensure its physical well-being round the clock. As babies grow into toddlers and begin to crawl and walk and talk, they begin to

Preconception care   Health care to prepare for pregnancy.

TERMS

be able to take care of some of their own physical needs. For parents, the challenge at this stage is to strike a balance between giving their children the freedom to explore and setting limits that will keep their children safe and secure. As children grow toward adolescence, parents need to allow them increasing independence and finally be willing to step back and let them risk success or failure on their own.

Marital satisfaction for most couples is low while their children are in school. There are several reasons, including the financial and emotional pressures of a growing family and the increased job and community responsibilities for parents in their thirties, forties, and fifties. Once the last child has left home, marital satisfaction usually increases because the couple have time to enjoy each other once more.

Single Parents

Chances are good that you know a number of families who haven't followed the traditional family life cycle, or perhaps you are a member of such a family. In 1993, according to U.S. Census Bureau statistics, nearly 30 percent of all families with children under 18 were one-parent families. And more than one-third of women who were in their late twenties in 1984 could expect to be single parents at some point in their life.

Economic difficulties are the primary problem for single mothers, especially for unmarried mothers who have not finished high school and have difficulty finding work. Divorced mothers usually experience a sharp drop in income the first few years on their own, but if they have job skills or education, they are usually able eventually to support themselves and their children adequately. Other problems for single mothers are the often-conflicting demands of playing both father and mother and the difficulty of filling their own needs for adult companionship and affection.

Financial pressures are also a complaint of single fathers, but they do not experience them to the extent that single mothers do. Because they are likely to have less practice than mothers in juggling parental and professional roles, they often worry that they do not spend enough time with their children. Because single fatherhood is so rare, however, the men who choose it are likely to be stable, established, and strongly motivated to be with their children.

Research on the effect on children of growing up in a single-parent family is not conclusive; however, evidence seems to indicate that children from single-parent families tend to have less success in school and in their careers than do children from two-parent families. Nevertheless, two-parent families are not necessarily better if one of the parents spends little time relating to the children or is physically or emotionally abusive.

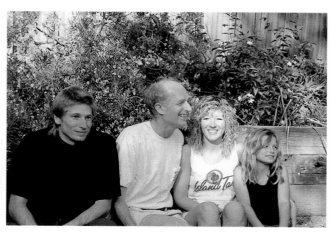

Almost one out of every five American families is a stepfamily, in which parents bring children from a previous marriage into a new family unit.

Stepfamilies

Overall, almost half of the marriages in the United States are remarriages for the husband, the wife, or both. If either brings children from a previous marriage into the new family unit, a stepfamily is formed.

Stepfamilies are significantly different from intact families and should not be expected to duplicate the emotions and relationships of an intact family. Research has shown that healthy stepfamilies are less cohesive and more adaptable than healthy intact families; they have a greater capacity to allow for individual differences and accept that biologically related family members will have emotionally closer relationships. Stepfamilies gradually gain more of a sense of being a family as they build a history of shared everyday experiences and major life events.

Successful Families

Family life can be extremely challenging. A strong family isn't a family without problems; it's a family that copes successfully with stress and crisis. Although there is tremendous variation in American families, researchers have proposed that six major qualities or themes appear in strong families.

- *Commitment.* The family is very important to its members; sexual fidelity between partners is included in commitment.

- *Appreciation.* People care about one another and let one another know it. The home is a positive place.

- *Communication.* People spend time listening to one another and enjoying one another's company. They talk about disagreements and attempt to solve problems.

- *Time together.* People do things together, often simple activities that don't cost money.

- *Spiritual wellness.* The family promotes sharing, love, and compassion for other human beings.
- *Coping with stress and crisis.* When faced with illness, death, marital conflict, or other crisis, family members pull together, seek help, go with the flow, and use other coping strategies to meet the challenge.

It may surprise some people that members of strong families are often seen at counseling centers. They know that the smartest thing to do in some situations is to get help. Many resources are available for individuals and families seeking counseling; people can turn to physicians, clergy, marriage and family counselors, psychologists, or other trained professionals.

Families—and intimate relationships of all kinds—are essential to our health and well-being. A fulfilling life nearly always involves other people; no one can be happy completely isolated. Whether we're single or married, young or old, heterosexual or gay, we continue to need meaningful relationships throughout life.

SUMMARY

- Intimate relationships are important to people's health and well-being. Many intimate relationships are held together by love.

Developing Intimate Relationships

- Successful relationships begin with a positive sense of self and reasonably high self-esteem.
- Friendships are reciprocal relationships between equals, held together by common interests, mutual acceptance, and feelings of respect and affection.
- Love, sex, and commitment are closely linked ideals in intimate relationships. Love includes trust, caring, respect, and loyalty. Sex brings excitement, fascination, and passion to the relationship. Commitment reflects the stable factors that help maintain the relationship.
- Intense love is usually accompanied by physiological arousal, a state that may be too extreme to be enjoyed.
- Love changes over time, with passion decreasing, intimacy increasing and then leveling off, and commitment increasing or decreasing.

Pairing and Singlehood

- People usually choose partners like themselves. If partners are very different, acceptance and good communication skills are necessary to maintain the relationship.
- Most Americans find partners through dating or through "getting together."
- Cohabitation is a growing social pattern that allows partners to get to know each other intimately without being married.
- Gay and lesbian partnerships are similar to heterosexual relationships, with some differences. Partners are technically single, since they're not allowed to marry legally; they don't follow traditional gender roles; and they often experience hostility rather than approval toward their partnerships from society.
- Singlehood is a growing option in our society. Advantages include greater opportunities in personal and career development and more freedom in making life decisions; disadvantages include loneliness and possible economic hardship, especially for single women.

Marriage

- Marriage fulfills many functions for individuals and society. It can provide people with affection, affirmation, and sexual fulfillment; a setting for child rearing; and the promise of lifelong companionship.
- Love isn't enough to ensure a successful marriage. Partners have to be realistic, feel good about each other, have communication and conflict resolution skills, share values, and have a balance of individual and joint interests.
- Marital tasks include providing each other with emotional support, establishing domestic and career priorities, managing finances, making sexual adjustments, managing boundaries with parents and extended family, and participating in the community. The most rapidly changing area is marital roles, which are tending to become more egalitarian.
- Communication skills are essential to successful relationships. The keys to good communication in relationships are self-disclosure, listening skills, and feedback.
- Conflict is inevitable in intimate relationships; partners need to have constructive ways to negotiate their differences.
- Domestic violence is a serious problem in American society. Wife battering and child abuse occur at every socioeconomic level. The core issue is the abuser's need to control other people.
- When problems can't be worked out, people often separate and divorce. Divorce is traumatic for all involved, especially children. The negative effects are usually balanced in time by positive ones. About three-quarters of all people who divorce remarry.

Family Life

- The family life cycle usually begins with marriage; the next stage begins with the arrival of a baby. Becoming a parent profoundly changes the relationship between the partners.
- Factors couples should consider when deciding if and when to have a child include (1) physical health and age, (2) financial circumstances, (3) relationship between partners, (4) educational, career, and childcare plans, (5) emotional readiness for parenthood, (6) social support system, and (7) personal qualities, attitudes toward children, and aptitude for parenting.
- At each stage of the family life cycle, relationships change. Marital satisfaction is often low during the child-rearing years and higher later.
- Many families today are single-parent families. Problems for single parents include economic difficulties, conflicting demands, and time pressures.
- Stepfamilies are formed when single or divorced people remarry and form new family units. Stepfamilies gradually gain more of a sense of being a family as they build a history of shared everyday experiences.
- Important qualities of successful families include commitment to the family, appreciation of family members, communication, time spent together, spiritual wellness, and effective methods of dealing with stress and crisis. Strong families use outside resources when they need help dealing with problems.

TAKE ACTION

1. Take an informal survey among your friends of what they find attractive in a member of the opposite sex and what they look for in a romantic partner. Are there substantial differences among different people? Do men and women look for different things?
2. Ask your parents what their experiences of dating and courtship were like. How are they different from your experiences? What do your parents think of current customs?

JOURNAL ENTRY

1. What are you looking for in an intimate relationship? In your health journal make a list of the needs you would like to have met by a partner. Are they needs that you can realistically expect to have satisfied in a relationship?

2. *Critical Thinking:* What approach do you take when it comes to communicating your feelings and needs to your friends and partners? Think of a particular issue that has been bothering you and write down the statements you would make if you were discussing it. Examine your statements to see if unrelated feelings or issues are coming through in them. Devise a strategy for dealing with the issue, using the guidelines given in this chapter on conflict resolution.

SELECTED BIBLIOGRAPHY

Arond, M., and S. L. Panker. 1987. *The First Year of Marriage.* New York: Warner Books.

Bader, E., R. Riddle, and C. Sinclair. 1981. *Family Therapy News.* Washington, D.C.: American Association for Marital and Family Therapy.

Borcherdt, B. 1989. *Think Straight! Feel Great!* Sarasota, Fla.: Professional Resource Exchange.

Crosby, J. 1991. *Illusion and Disillusion.* Belmont, Calif.: Wadsworth.

DeMaris, A., and G. Leslie. 1984. Cohabitation with the future spouse: Its influence upon marital satisfaction and communication. *Journal of Marriage and the Family* 46(1): 77–84.

DiMona, L., and C. Herndon, eds. 1994. *The 1995 Information Please® Women's Sourcebook.* Boston: Houghton Mifflin.

Fehr, B. 1988. Prototype analysis of the concepts of love and commitment. *Journal of Personality and Social Psychology* 55(4): 557–79.

Gelles, R. J., and J. R. Conte. 1991. Domestic violence and sexual abuse of children: A review of research in the eighties. In *Contemporary Families: Looking Forward, Looking Back,* ed. A. Booth. Minneapolis: National Council on Family Relations.

Gelles, R. J., and C. P. Cornell. 1990. *Intimate Violence in Families,* 2nd ed. Beverly Hills, Calif.: Sage.

Jack, B. W., and L. Culpepper. 1990. Preconception care: Risk reduction and health promotion in preparation for pregnancy. *Journal of the American Medical Association* 264(9): 1147–49.

Jones, A. 1994. *Next Time She'll Be Dead.* Boston: Beacon Press.

Jones, A., and S. Schechter. 1992. *When Love Goes Wrong.* New York: HarperCollins.

Levine, L., and L. Barbach. 1983. *The Intimate Male.* New York: Signet.

Lewis, R. A., E. B. Kozac, R. M. Milardo, and W. A. Grosnick. 1981. Commitment in same-sex love relationships. *Alternative Lifestyles* 4(1): 22–42.

Lips, H. 1992. *Sex and Gender,* 2nd ed. Mountain View, Calif.: Mayfield.

Olson, D., and J. DeFrain. 1994. *Marriage and the Family.* Mountain View, Calif.: Mayfield.

Olson, D., H. McCubbin, H. Barnes, A. Larsen, A. Muxem, and M. Wilson. 1983. *Families: What Makes Them Work?* Beverly Hills, Calif.: Sage.

Peplau, Letitia. 1988. Research on homosexual couples. In *Gay Relationships,* ed. J. DeCecco. New York: Haworth Press.

Raschke, H. 1987. Divorce. In *Handbook of Marriage and the Family,* ed. M. Sussman and S. Steinmetz. New York: Plenum Press.

Rice, F. P. 1993. *Intimate Relationships, Marriages, and Families,* 2nd ed. Mountain View, Calif.: Mayfield.

Shaver, P., and others. 1988. Love as attachment: The integration of three behavioral systems. In *The Psychology of Love,* ed. R. Sternberg and M. Barnes. New Haven: Yale University Press.

Stein, P., and M. Fingrud. 1985. The single life has more potential for happiness than marriage and parenthood for both men and women. In *Current Controversies in Marriage and the Family,* ed. H. Feldman and M. Feldman. Beverly Hills, Calif.: Sage.

Sternberg, R., and M. Barnes, eds. 1988. *The Psychology of Love.* New Haven: Yale University Press.

Stinnett, N., and J. DeFrain. 1986. *Secrets of Strong Families.* Boston: Little, Brown.

Straus, M., R. Gelles, and S. Steinmetz. 1980. *Behind Closed Doors.* Garden City, N.Y.: Anchor Books.

Strong, B., and C. DeVault. 1992. *The Marriage and Family Experience.* St. Paul, Minn.: West.

Strong, B., C. DeVault, and B. Sayad. 1996. *Core Concepts in Human Sexuality.* Mountain View, Calif.: Mayfield.

Stuart, R. B. 1983. *Improving Communication.* Champaign, Ill.: Research Press.

Vaughan, D. 1986. *Uncoupling: Turning Points in Intimate Relationships.* New York: Oxford University Press.

Walker, L. 1979. *The Battered Woman Syndrome.* New York: Harper and Row.

The World Almanac and Book of Facts. 1995. Mahwah, N.J.: Funk & Wagnalls.

Strong, B., C. DeVault, and B. Sayad. 1996. *Core Concepts in Human Sexuality.* Mountain View, Calif.: Mayfield. *A comprehensive, up-to-date textbook covering all aspects of love, intimacy, and sexuality.*

Tannen, D. 1990. *You Just Don't Understand: Women and Men in Conversation.* New York: William Morrow. *This discussion of gender differences in language shows how men and women use language differently; it also provides many helpful ideas about how to improve communication in relationships.*

RECOMMENDED READINGS

Alberti, R. E., and M. L. Emmons. 1983. *Your Perfect Right: A Guide to Assertive Living.* San Luis Obispo, Calif.: Impact. *This effective guide is designed to help individuals develop their assertiveness skills.*

Buscaglia, L. F. 1984. *Loving Each Other: The Challenge of Human Relationships.* Thorofare, N.J.: Charles B. Slack. *A university professor and popular public speaker, Buscaglia is witty and energetic on his favorite topic, the nature of love.*

DeFrain, J., J. Fricke, and J. Elmen. 1987. *On Our Own: A Single Parent's Survival Guide.* Lexington, Mass.: D. C. Heath. *This practical guide is based on interviews with 900 single parents from around the country.*

Hochshild, A. 1989. *The Second Shift.* New York: Viking. *The author, a sociologist, describes the dilemma of women who work outside the home and find themselves still putting in a "second shift" of spousal, parental, and household duties in the evening.*

Jones, A. 1994. *Next Time She'll Be Dead.* Boston: Beacon Press. *An in-depth look at battering by a survivor; includes an important section on what we as individuals and as a society can and must do.*

Lerner, H. G. 1985. *The Dance of Anger.* New York: Harper and Row. *In this best-selling book, the author describes different styles of handling anger and suggests ways that people can balance them in their relationships.*

5

Sexuality, Pregnancy, and Childbirth

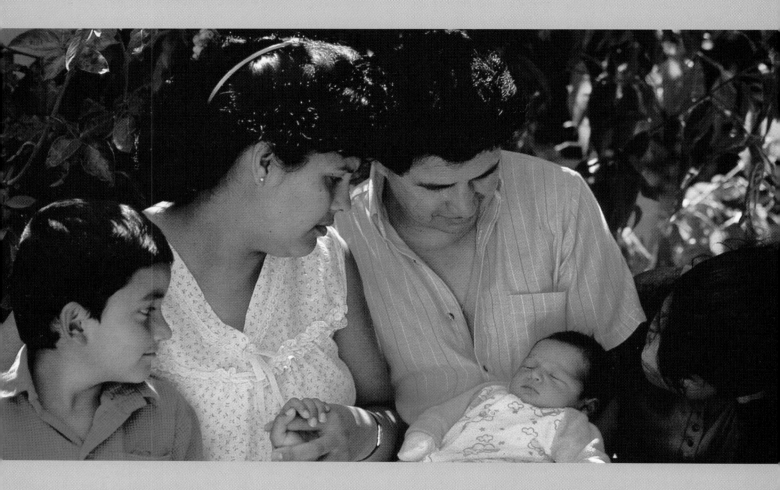

CONTENTS

Sexuality is an important part of being human. Sexual activity is a central ingredient in many of our intimate emotional relationships and, of course, the key to the reproduction of our species. Sexuality is a complex and interacting group of inborn, biological characteristics and acquired behaviors people learn in the course of growing up in a particular family, community, and society.

Because of the important role sexuality plays in human life, communication about sexuality is emotionally charged. Sexual expression is usually regulated with restrictions and taboos—written and unwritten laws specifying which functions and behaviors are acceptable and "normal" and which are unacceptable and "abnormal." Young people growing up in the United States are bombarded with conflicting messages about sexuality from parents, educators, television, movies, magazines, and popular music. Confusion and fear are often the result.

Decisions about sexuality have far-reaching consequences. Understanding the basic facts about sexuality, pregnancy, and childbirth will help you make intelligent, informed decisions that are right for you.

SEXUAL ANATOMY AND HORMONES

In spite of their different appearance, the sexual organs of men and women arise from the same structures and fulfill similar functions. Each person has a pair of **gonads:** ovaries are the female gonads; testes are the male gonads. The gonads produce **germ cells** and **sex hormones.** The female germ cells are ova (eggs); the male germ cells are sperm. Ova and sperm are the basic units of reproduction; their union can lead to the creation of a new life.

Female Sex Organs

The external sex organs, or genitals, of the female are called the vulva ("covering") and are illustrated in Figure 5-1a. The mons pubis, a rounded mass of fatty tissue over the pubic bone, becomes covered with hair during puberty. Below it are two paired folds of skin called the labia majora and the labia minora. Enclosed within are the **clitoris,** the clitoral hood **(prepuce)**, the opening of the urethra, and the opening of the vagina. The clitoris is highly sensitive to touch and plays an important role in female sexual arousal and orgasm in many women.

The female's urethra leads directly from the urinary bladder to its opening between the clitoris and the opening of the vagina; it conducts urine from the bladder to the outside of the body. Unlike the male's urethra, it is independent of the genitals.

The vaginal opening is partially covered by the hymen. This membrane can be stretched or torn during athletic activities or when a woman has sexual intercourse for the first time. The idea that an intact hymen is the sign of a virgin is a myth.

The vagina is the passage that leads to the internal reproductive organs (Figure 5-1b). It is the female organ for sexual intercourse and serves as the birth canal during childbirth. Its soft, flexible walls are normally in contact with each other.

Projecting into the upper part of the vagina is the neck of the uterus, called the cervix. It is inside the pear-shaped uterus, which slants forward above the bladder, that the fertilized egg is implanted and grows into a fetus.

The pair of fallopian tubes (or oviducts) leads out from the top of the uterus. The fringed end of each tube surrounds an ovary and guides the mature ovum down into the uterus after the ovum bursts from its follicle on the surface of the ovary.

Male Sex Organs

A man's external sexual organs, or genitals, are the penis and the **scrotum** (Figure 5-2a and 5-2b). The penis consists of spongy tissue that becomes engorged with blood during sexual excitement, causing the organ to enlarge and become erect. The scrotum is a pouch that contains a pair of testes. The purpose of the scrotum is to maintain the testes at a temperature approximately 5° F below that of the rest of the body—that is, at about 93.6° F. The process of sperm production is extremely heat-sensitive. In hot temperatures the muscles in the scrotum relax, and the testes move away from the heat of the body. Conversely, in cold temperatures the muscles of the scrotum contract, and the testes move upward toward the body, where they can maintain their 5-degree temperature difference.

The smooth, rounded tip of the penis is the **glans** penis. It is a sensitive part of the penis and an important source of sexual arousal. It is partially covered by the foreskin, or prepuce, a retractable fold of skin that is removed by circumcision in about 60 percent of newborn males in the United States. Circumcision is performed for cultural, religious, and hygienic reasons, and rates of circumcision vary widely among different groups.

Through the entire length of the penis runs a passage

TERMS

Sexuality   A dimension of personality shaped by biological, psychosocial, and cultural forces and concerning all aspects of sexual behaviors.

Gonads   Primary reproductive organs that produce germ cells and sex hormones; ovaries and testes.

Germ cells   Sperm and ova.

Sex hormones   Chemical substances that stimulate and promote the development of sexual characteristics.

Clitoris   Highly sensitive female genital structure.

Prepuce   Foreskin of the penis or clitoris.

Scrotum   The loose sac of skin and muscle fibers that contains the testes.

Glans   Rounded head of the penis or of the clitoris.

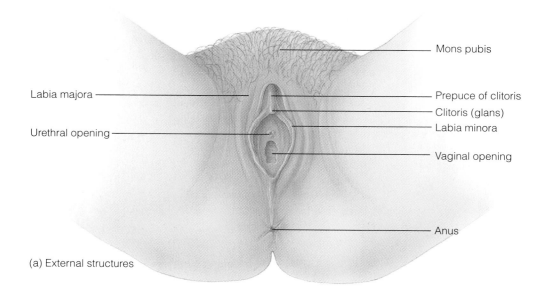

(a) External structures

Mons pubis

Labia majora

Urethral opening

Prepuce of clitoris

Clitoris (glans)

Labia minora

Vaginal opening

Anus

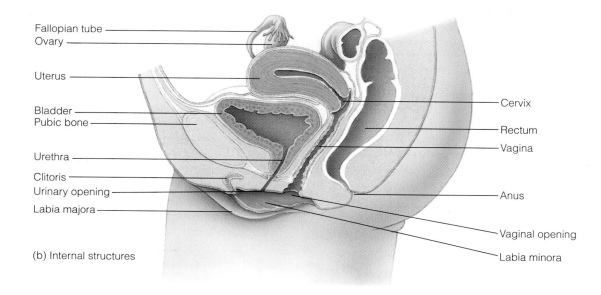

Fallopian tube

Ovary

Uterus

Bladder

Pubic bone

Urethra

Clitoris

Urinary opening

Labia majora

(b) Internal structures

Cervix

Rectum

Vagina

Anus

Vaginal opening

Labia minora

Figure 5-1   *Female sex organs.*

called the urethra, which can carry both urine and semen to the opening at the tip of the glans. Although urine and semen share a common passage, they are prevented from mixing together by muscular sphincters that control their entry into the urethra.

The testes contain tightly packed seminiferous ("sperm-bearing") tubules within which sperm are produced. These tubules end in a maze of ducts that flow into a single storage tube called the epididymis, on the surface of each testis. This tube leads to the vasa deferentia (singular: vas deferens), two tubes that rise into the ab-

dominal cavity and, inside the prostate gland, join the ducts of the two seminal vesicles, whose secretions provide nutrients to semen. The prostate gland produces some of the fluid in semen that nourishes and transports sperm. The tubes of the seminal vesicle and the vas deferens on each side lead to the ejaculatory duct, which joins the urethra. The Cowper's glands are two small structures flanking the urethra. During sexual arousal, these glands secrete a clear, mucuslike fluid that appears at the tip of the penis. The purpose of this preejaculatory fluid is not known, but it may contain a few sperm in some men.

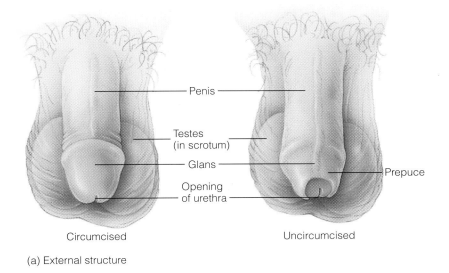

Penis

Testes
(in scrotum)

Glans

Prepuce

Opening
of urethra

Circumcised

Uncircumcised

(a) External structure

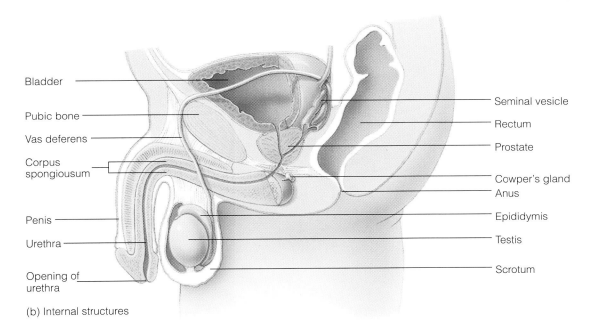

Bladder

Pubic bone

Vas deferens

Corpus
spongiousum

Penis

Urethra

Opening of
urethra

Seminal vesicle

Rectum

Prostate

Cowper's gland

Anus

Epididymis

Testis

Scrotum

(b) Internal structures

Figure 5-2 *Male sex organs.*

Personal Insight Do you ever wonder if you're sexually "normal"? Do you worry about the size, shape, or appearance of any part of your body? Where do you think your ideas of "normal" come from?

Hormones and the Reproductive Life Cycle

There are many powerful cultural and personal factors that shape the expression of your sexuality. But biology also plays a role, particularly through the action of hor-mones, chemical messengers that are secreted directly into the bloodstream by **endocrine glands.** The sex hor-mones produced by the ovaries and testes greatly influ-ence the development and function of the reproductive system throughout life.

Endocrine glands Glands that produce hormones.

TERMS

Many people think of circumcision—the surgical removal of the foreskin of the penis—as a standard medical procedure, but it is equally a cultural practice, varying among different national, ethnic, and religious groups, among people of different educational and income levels, and even from one historical period to another.

Worldwide, groups who circumcise their males have always been in the minority. It is estimated that only about 15 percent of the world's population practices circumcision. Most groups do not, including most Europeans, Asians, South and Central Americans, and Africans. Jews and Muslims are the major groups who circumcise for religious reasons. For both groups, the practice derives from the biblical account of Abraham's "covenant" with God to have all his male descendants circumcised.

In the United States, circumcision was widely accepted from the early 1940s to the mid-1970s as a routine procedure that promoted hygiene and prevented genital disease. Educated middle-class parents almost always had their newborn sons circumcised. In the late 1960s, however, the practice began to be questioned, and in 1971 the American Academy of Pediatrics (AAP) took a stand against it as an unnecessary procedure. A strong anticircumcision movement grew, led by the same kind of affluent, well-educated, suburban parents who had originally supported the practice. Between 1974 and 1984, the rate of circumcision in the United States fell from 85 to 70 percent.

Ironically, as public sentiment against circumcision has grown over the last 20 years, evidence of its medical benefits has mounted. Research indicates that uncircumcised infants have higher rates of urinary tract infections, which can lead to serious kidney damage. In 1988 the AAP reconsidered the issue and took a neutral position on circumcision, stating that it does carry some risks but also has some benefits. The rate of circumcision began climbing again in the late 1980s, and in 1993 it was estimated that 80 percent of all newborns were circumcised.

What are the advantages and disadvantages of this five-minute procedure, and why is it so variable across cultures? Proponents of circumcision advocate it for several reasons, the two most notable being cleanliness and disease prevention. Bacteria and secretions can be trapped under the foreskin, and uncircumcised boys have to be taught good hygiene to prevent infection. Circumcision removes this potential source of trouble. Men who develop infection or inflammation of the penis sometimes have to be circumcised later in life, when the operation is more difficult.

Recently, evidence has indicated that uncircumcised infants have a much higher incidence of urinary tract infections, which can lead to very serious kidney damage. These are the findings that led the AAP to adopt its current neutral position on routine circumcision. There is also some evidence that circumcision may help reduce the spread of sexually transmitted diseases, including HIV infection, among young men. Finally, circumcised men are less likely to develop cancer of the penis, a rare disease that occurs almost exclusively in uncircumcised men. At one time it was thought that the female sexual partners of uncircumcised men had a higher risk of developing cervical cancer, but new findings indicate that the incidence of cervical cancer depends on many factors.

Opponents of routine circumcision assert that it is the "leading unnecessary surgery" performed in the United States. They point to its medical disadvantages, which include pain to the infant, the possibility of irritation of the penis, and the risk of complications and surgical errors. (Recent research that would help to counter the pain argument showed that if the foreskin is wrapped with a bandage soaked in a pain killer prior to circumcision, infants showed fewer signs of discomfort and pain such as crying and wiggling.)

Although discussions of circumcision tend to focus on its medical advantages and disadvantages, most parents make their decision about circumcision mainly for social or cultural reasons. Fathers want their sons to look like them and their peers. Concern about the emotional impact of "being different" apparently outweighs any medical or health concerns. In many parts of the world, parents simply follow their traditional practices. In a country with wide cultural and socioeconomic differences like the United States, there is likely to be variation from one group to another and even from one family to another. Some parents don't hesitate to have their sons circumcised, while others decide against it. Although circumcision is still the majority practice in most parts of the United States, either decision may be the right one for a particular family, depending on a variety of religious, social, personal, and medical factors.

Adapted from E. J. Schoen. 1990. "The Status of Circumcision of Newborns." *The New England Journal of Medicine* 322(18): 1308–11.

The sex hormones made by the testes are called **androgens,** the most important of which is testosterone. The female sex hormones, produced by the ovaries, belong to two groups—**estrogens** and **progestins,** the most important of which is progesterone. The cortex of the **adrenal glands** (located at the top of the kidneys) also produces androgens in both sexes.

The hormones produced by the testes, the ovaries, and the adrenal glands are regulated by the hormones of the **pituitary gland,** located at the base of the brain. This gland in turn is controlled by hormones produced by the **hypothalamus** in the brain. Sex hormones exert their primary developmental influences first in the embryo stage, where they control the development of a male or female reproductive system, and later during the individual's adolescence.

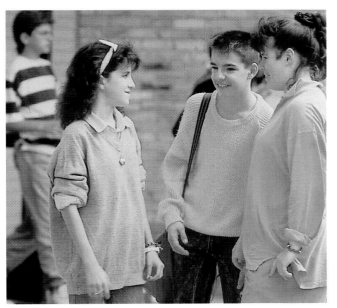

The physical changes of puberty usually begin between the ages of 8 and 13 for girls and 10 and 14 for boys. Once they reach puberty, these adolescents are biologically adults; however, it will take another five to ten years for them to become adults in social and psychological terms.

Reproductive Maturation Although human beings are fully sexually differentiated at birth, the differences between males and females are accentuated at **puberty.** The reproductive system matures, secondary sexual characteristics develop, and the bodies of males and females come to appear more distinctive. Female puberty usually begins at about age 8 to 13; the reproductive maturation of boys lags about two years behind that of girls. The physical changes of female puberty include breast development, rounding of the hips and buttocks, growth of hair in the pubic region and the underarms, and the start of menstruation (discussed in the next section). For boys, physical changes include enlargement of the testes, development of pubic hair, growth of the penis, the onset of ejaculation (usually at about age 11 or 12), deepening of the voice, the appearance of facial hair, and a period of rapid growth. The physical changes of puberty are brought about by estrogens and progestins from the ovaries, testosterone from the testes, and androgens from the adrenal glands.

The Menstrual Cycle A major landmark of puberty among females is the onset of the **menstrual cycle**, the monthly ovarian cycle that leads to menstruation (loss of blood and tissue lining the uterus) in the absence of pregnancy. The first menstrual period, or menarche, occurs at the average age of 12.8 years in the United States, but it may also normally start several years earlier or later.

The menstrual cycle can be divided into four phases: (1) menses, (2) the estrogenic phase, (3) ovulation, and (4) the progestational phase (Figure 5-3). Day 1 of the cycle is considered to be the day of the onset of bleeding. For the purposes of our discussion, a cycle of 28 days will be used; however, normal cycles vary in length.

During the menses, characterized by the menstrual flow, hormones from the ovaries and anterior pituitary gland are found in relatively low amounts. This phase of the cycle usually lasts from day 1 to about day 5.

The estrogenic phase of the cycle begins when the menstrual flow ceases, and the anterior pituitary gland begins to produce increasing amounts of two **gonadotropic hormones—follicle-stimulating hormone (FSH)** and **luteinizing hormone (LH).** Under the influence of FSH, an egg-containing ovarian follicle begins to mature and to produce increasingly higher and higher amounts of estrogens. Stimulated by estrogen, the uterine lining, called the endometrium, thickens with large numbers of blood vessels and uterine glands.

A surge of a potent estrogen called estradiol from the follicle causes the anterior pituitary gland to release a large burst of LH and a smaller amount of FSH. The high concentration of LH stimulates the developing follicle to release its ovum. This event is known as ovulation. After ovulation, the follicle is transformed into the **corpus luteum,** which produces progesterone and estrogen. Ovula-

TERMS

Androgens Male sex hormones produced by the testes in males and by the adrenal glands in both sexes.

Estrogens A class of female sex hormones, produced by the ovaries, that bring about sexual maturation at puberty and maintain reproductive functions.

Progestins A class of female sex hormones, produced by the ovaries, that sustain reproductive functions.

Adrenal glands Endocrine glands, located over the kidneys, that produce androgens (among other hormones).

Pituitary gland An endocrine gland at the base of the brain that produces gonadotropic (FSH and LH) and other hormones.

Hypothalamus A region of the brain above the pituitary gland whose hormones control the secretions of the pituitary and that is also involved in the nervous control of sexual functions.

Puberty The period of biological maturation during adolescence.

Menstrual cycle Monthly ovarian cycle controlled by pituitary and ovarian hormones; in the absence of pregnancy, menstruation occurs.

Gonadotropic hormones Follicle-stimulating hormone (FSH) and luteinizing hormone (LH), produced by the pituitary gland in both sexes.

Follicle-stimulating hormone (FSH) The pituitary hormone that stimulates maturation of the ovum in the female and sperm production in the male.

Luteinizing hormone (LH) The pituitary hormone that causes ovulation and stimulates the production of progestins in the female and androgens in the male.

Corpus luteum The part of the ovarian follicle left after ovulation, which secretes hormones during the second half of the menstrual cycle.

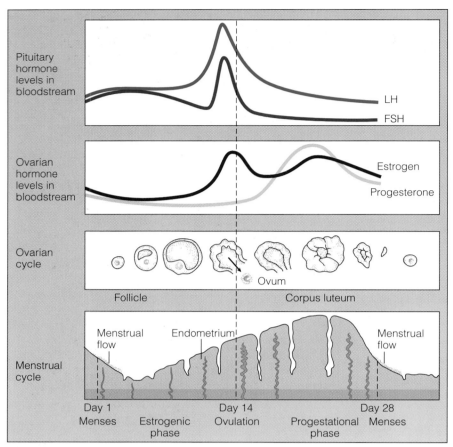

Figure 5-3 *The menstrual cycle.*
The anterior pituitary releases FSH and LH, which stimulate the ovarian follicle to develop and release a mature egg. The ovarian follicle releases estrogen and progesterone, which stimulate the endometrium to continue to develop so that it will be ready to receive and nourish a fertilized egg. Unless pregnancy occurs, ovarian hormone levels fall and the endometrium sloughs off (menses).

tion usually occurs about 14 days prior to the onset of menstrual flow.

During the progestational phase of the cycle, the amount of progesterone secreted from the corpus luteum increases and remains high until the onset of the next menses. Under the influence of estrogen and progesterone, the endometrium continues to develop, readying itself to receive and nourish a fertilized ovum. When pregnancy occurs, the fertilized egg produces a hormone called human chorionic gonadotropin (HCG), which maintains the corpus luteum. Thus, levels of ovarian hormones remain high and the uterine lining is preserved, preventing menses.

If pregnancy does not occur, the corpus luteum degenerates and levels of estrogen and progesterone gradually fall. Below certain hormonal levels, the endometrium can no longer be maintained, and it begins to slough off, initiating menses. As the levels of ovarian hormones fall, a slight rise in LH and FSH occurs, and a new menstrual cycle begins.

Menstruation is a normal biological process, but it may cause distressing physical or psychological symptoms in some women. Two common problems are dysmenorrhea and premenstrual tension. Dysmenorrhea ("painful menstruation") is characterized by cramps in the lower abdomen, backache, a bloated feeling, nausea, vomiting, diarrhea, and loss of appetite. Some of these symptoms can be attributed to uterine muscular contractions (spasms), which are caused by chemicals called prostaglandins that are released from the uterine lining as it is shed during menstruation. Any drug such as aspirin or ibuprofen that blocks the effects of prostaglandins will usually be effective in alleviating some of the symptoms of dysmenorrhea.

Premenstrual tension involves negative mood changes and physical symptoms associated with the time immediately preceding the onset of menses (hence the name "premenstrual"). A more serious condition known as **premenstrual syndrome (PMS)** is experienced by a smaller number of women.

Premenstrual syndrome (PMS) is characterized by a diverse group of physical, emotional, and behavioral symptoms that occur after ovulation but usually cease before menstruation. Many women experience mild physical and emotional changes prior to their menstrual periods, but a few—about 10 percent of menstruating women—experience more severe symptoms. Sufferers have reported a wide variety of symptoms associated with PMS, including tension, fluid retention, breast swelling and tenderness, constipation, craving for sweets or salty foods, dizziness, fainting spells, headache, joint pain, sensitivity to light and noise, increased appetite, anxiety, depression, decreased self-esteem, and sleep disturbances. Some women with PMS become virtually incapacitated for several days or weeks each month. For a woman with severe PMS, the physical and emotional symptoms that precede menstruation may dominate her life, leading her to plan her activities around the time she knows she'll be experiencing them.

Despite decades of study, researchers still don't understand exactly what causes PMS or why some women are more vulnerable to it than others. Research has focused on a variety of substances in the body that may fluctuate with the menstrual cycle, including progesterone, prostaglandins, certain vitamins and minerals, and a naturally occurring opiate known as beta-endorphin. Some clinicians think that PMS is not a single disorder, but a group of entities with different symptoms. The majority opinion is that until PMS is

better defined and its causes more clearly understood, any treatment is experimental.

There are no proven therapies for PMS, but many different treatments are under investigation: oral contraceptives; light therapy (exposing women to fluorescent lights for several hours each day prior to menstruation); antidepressants; antianxiety agents; antiprostaglandins; drugs that elevate levels of beta-endorphin; and other drugs that improve mood and diminish appetite. Over-the-counter medications for PMS commonly contain a diuretic (to compensate for water retention), an analgesic (for pain), and an antihistamine; women with mild PMS may obtain relief from some of their symptoms by using these medications.

Women can take a few behavioral steps to treat the symptoms of PMS: Eat a nutrient-rich diet; get adequate sleep; decrease intake of alcohol, caffeine, nicotine, sugar, and salt to lessen nervousness, depression, and bloating (the number and severity of symptoms have been shown to have a strong relationship to the amount of caffeine consumed); and increase exercise to stimulate relaxation. A regular program of aerobic exercise for a minimum of 30 minutes, three to four times per week, especially during the premenstrual time, is recommended. Finally, relaxation response techniques like those described in Chapter 2, practiced 15 minutes, two times daily, have been shown to reduce PMS symptoms by 58 percent. These approaches are sensible and safe and may help relieve the discomfort of PMS.

Personal Insight   Think back to adolescence and try to recall your feelings about your sexuality as you went through puberty. Did you feel anxious or overwhelmed by the changes in your body or any emotions—worry, guilt, excitement—you felt about your sexuality? Do you still have any of the feelings about your sexuality that you had then? Are you satisfied with the adjustment to sexuality that you've made so far in your life?

Aging and Human Sexuality   Changes in hormone production and sexual functioning occur as we age. As a woman approaches age 50, her ovaries gradually cease to function and she enters the **menopause** (cessation of menstruation). For some women, the associated drop in hormone production causes a set of symptoms that are troublesome.

Among the most common physical symptoms of menopause are hot flashes (or flushes), consisting of a sensation of warmth rising to the face from the upper chest with or without perspiration and chills. Other symptoms include headaches, dizziness, palpitations, and joint pains. Osteoporosis can develop (that is, bones can

become more porous), making older women more liable to suffer fractures. Some menopausal women become moody, even markedly depressed, and they may also complain of tiredness, irritability, and forgetfulness. Estrogen replacement therapy significantly improves most of these symptoms, but it may increase some women's risk of gallbladder disease and certain types of cancer.

Some women have a difficult time making the psychological adjustment to this stage of life, associating it with a loss of youth and sexual attractiveness. Others welcome it as a time of increased personal freedom, an opportunity for inner growth and repose. Menopause is seen as signaling the end of one phase of life and the beginning of another, equally meaningful one.

In men, testosterone production declines gradually with age. As they get older, men depend more on direct

Premenstrual syndrome (PMS)   A disorder characterized by physical discomfort, psychological distress, and behavioral changes that begin after ovulation and cease when menstruation begins.

Menopause   Cessation of menstruation in middle-aged women.

TERMS

physical stimulation for sexual arousal. They take longer to get an erection and find it more difficult to maintain; orgasmic contractions are less intense.

Many men go through a period of reassessment and readjustment in middle age (sometimes popularly referred to as "midlife crisis"), which may have repercussions for their sexuality. As with women, sexual activity can continue to be a source of pleasure and satisfaction for men as they grow older. When problems do arise, they are more often due to psychological reactions to bodily changes than to the physical changes themselves.

SEXUAL FUNCTIONING

In this section, we discuss sexual physiology—how the sex organs function during sexual activity—and problems that can occur with sexual functioning.

Sexual Stimulation

Sexual excitement can come from many sources, both physical and psychological. Although physical stimuli have an obvious and direct effect, some people believe psychological stimuli—thoughts, fantasies, desires, perceptions—are even more powerfully erotic. Regardless of the source of erotic stimuli, all stimulation has a physical basis, which is given meaning by the brain.

Physical Stimulation   Physical stimulation comes through the senses: People are aroused by things they see, hear, taste, smell, and feel. The most obvious and effective physical stimulation involves touching. Even though culturally defined practices vary and individual people have different preferences, most sexual encounters eventually involve some form of touching with hands, lips, and body surfaces. Kissing, caressing, fondling, and hugging are as much a part of sexual encounters as they are of expressing affection.

Sexually sensitive areas, or **erogenous zones,** are especially susceptible to sexual arousal for most people, most of the time. Often, though, it's not *what* is touched but how, for how long, and by whom that determines the response. Under the right circumstances, touching any part of the body can arouse someone sexually.

Psychological Stimulation   Sexual arousal also has an important psychological component, regardless of the nature of the physical stimulation. Fantasies, ideas, memories of past experiences, general "mood"—all can generate excitement. Erotic thoughts may be linked to an imagined person or situation or to a sexual experience from the past.

Arousal is also powerfully influenced by emotions. How you feel about a person and how the person feels about you matters tremendously in how sexually respon-

sive you are likely to be. Even the most direct forms of physical stimulation carry emotional overtones. Kissing, caressing, and fondling express affection and caring. The emotional charge they give to a sexual interaction is at least as significant to sexual arousal as the purely physical stimulation achieved by touching.

Sexual Response

Noted sex researchers William Masters and Virginia Johnson were the first to describe in detail the human sexual response cycle. Men and women respond physiologically with a predictable set of reactions, regardless of the nature of the stimulation.

Two physiological mechanisms explain most genital and bodily reactions of men and women during sexual arousal and orgasm. These mechanisms are **vasocongestion** and **myotonia.** Vasocongestion is the engorgement of tissues that results when more blood flows into an organ than is flowing out. Myotonia is increased muscular tension, which culminates in rhythmical muscular contractions during **orgasm.**

Four stages characterize the sexual response cycle. In the *excitement phase,* the penis becomes erect as its tissues become congested with blood. The testes expand and are pulled upward within the scrotum. In women, the clitoris and the labia are similarly congested with blood, and the vaginal walls become moist with lubricant fluid.

The *plateau phase* is an extension of the excitement stage. Reactions become more marked: In men, the penis becomes harder, and the testes larger. In women the lower part of the vagina swells, while its upper end expands and vaginal lubrication increases.

In the *orgasmic phase,* rhythmical contractions occur along the man's penis, urethra, prostate gland, seminal vesicles, and muscles in the pelvic and anal regions. These involuntary muscular contractions lead to ejaculation of semen, which consists of sperm cells from the testes and secretions from the prostate gland and seminal vesicles. In women, contractions occur in the lower part of the vagina and in the uterus, as well as in the pelvic region and the anus.

In the *resolution phase,* all the changes initiated during the excitement phase are reversed. Excess blood drains from tissues, the muscles in the region relax, and the genital structures return to their unstimulated state. After ejaculation, men enter a *refractory period* during which they cannot be restimulated to orgasm. Women do not have a refractory period; immediate restimulation is possible.

More general bodily reactions accompany the changes in the genital organs in both sexes. Beginning with the excitement phase, the nipples of both sexes become erect, the woman's breasts begin to swell, and in both sexes the skin of the chest becomes flushed; all these changes are more marked among women. The heart rate doubles by the plateau phase, and respiration becomes faster. During orgasm, breathing becomes irregular and the person may moan or cry out. A feeling of warmth leads to increased sweating during the resolution phase. Deep relaxation and a sense of well-being pervade the body and the mind.

Sexual Disorders and Dysfunctions

Both psychological and physical problems can interfere with normal sexual functioning. If you are not in good physical health, for example, or if you are experiencing high levels of stress or anxiety, your sexual functioning might very well be negatively affected. Sexual problems caused mainly by biological or physical conditions are referred to as **sexual disorders**; problems of psychological origin are called **sexual dysfunctions**.

Common Sexual Disorders Sexual disorders may be physiological in origin, but they may also be the result of infections, which can be prevented. Sexual disorders that affect women include the following:

- *Vaginitis* is inflammation of the vagina and can be caused by a variety of organisms, including *Candida* (yeast infection), *Trichomonas* (trichomoniasis), and *Gardnerella* (nonspecific vaginitis).
- *Endometriosis* is the growth of endometrial tissue (tissue normally found lining the uterus) outside of the uterus, which can cause pain and scarring or blockage of the oviducts.
- *Pelvic inflammatory disease* (PID) is an infection of the uterus, oviducts, or ovaries, caused by microorganisms (usually transmitted sexually) that spread to these areas from the vagina; PID can cause illness, pain, and scarring of the oviducts.

Sexual disorders among men include the following:

- *Prostatitis* is inflammation or infection of the prostate gland, a disorder more common in men over 40.
- *Testicular cancer* occurs most commonly in men in their twenties and thirties. (It is a rare cancer and has a very high cure rate if detected early.)

Sexual Dysfunctions The term *sexual dysfunction* encompasses disturbances in sexual desire, performance, or satisfaction. Although a wide variety of physical conditions and drugs may interfere with sexual functions (for instance, diabetes may interfere with the blood and nerve supply to the sex organs), sexual dysfunctions more often result from psychological causes and problems in intimate relationships. The same two mechanisms—vasocongestion and myotonia—that are the basis of the sexual response cycle are also at the root of the main forms of sexual disturbance: inability to become aroused and problems with orgasm.

Common Sexual Dysfunctions Common sexual dysfunctions in men include **erectile dysfunction** (previ-

ously called impotence), which is the inability to have or maintain an erection that is sufficient for sexual intercourse; **premature ejaculation**, which is ejaculation before or just on penetration of the vagina; and **retarded ejaculation**, the inability to ejaculate once an erection is achieved. Many men will experience occasional difficulty in achieving an erection or ejaculating because of excessive alcohol consumption, fatigue, or stress.

Two sexual dysfunctions in women are **vaginismus**, in which the woman experiences painful involuntary muscular spasms when sexual intercourse is attempted, and **orgasmic dysfunction**, which is the inability to experience orgasm. Vaginismus is a conditioned reflex probably related to fear of intercourse. Orgasmic dysfunction has been the subject of a great deal of discussion over the years as people debated the nature of the female orgasm and what constitutes dysfunction in women. Many women experience orgasm but not during intercourse, or they experience orgasm during intercourse only if the clitoris is directly stimulated at the same time. Do these patterns of response reflect normal female sexual functioning, or are they forms of orgasmic dysfunction? In general, the inability to experience orgasm under certain circumstances is a problem only if the woman considers it a problem. If a woman does believe that she has a problem—for example, if she has never experienced orgasm under any circumstances—then she is considered to have orgasmic dysfunction.

Treating Sexual Dysfunction Most forms of sexual dysfunction can be treated. The first step is to treat any underlying medical condition. Diabetes and heart disease, for example, may cause erectile dysfunction. Medications and drugs, especially depressants such as alcohol, may also inhibit sexual responses. Anyone experiencing sexual difficulties should have a thorough physical examination.

If no physical problem is found, the problem may be psychosocial in origin. Psychosocial causes of dysfunction include troubled relationships, lack of sexual skills, irrational attitudes and beliefs, anxiety, and psychosexual trauma, such as sexual abuse or rape. Many of these problems can be addressed by sex therapy methods, which often highlight the fact that sex is not merely a mechanical body response. Sexual problems are closely tied in with emotional and psychological concerns and with a person's thoughts, perceptions, beliefs, values, and relationships with others.

SEXUAL BEHAVIOR

Many behaviors stem from sexual impulses, and sexual expression takes a variety of forms. Sexual behavior is a product of many factors, including genetics, physiology, psychology, and social and cultural forces. Our behavior is shaped by the interplay of our biological predispositions and our learning experiences throughout life.

Adult Sexuality

Early adulthood is a time when people make important life choices, a time of increasing responsibility in terms of interpersonal relations and family life. According to psychologist Erik Erikson, developing the capacity for intimacy is a central task for young adults. In mature love relationships, people ideally are able to integrate all the aspects of intimacy so that sexuality is a deeply meaningful part of how they express love.

Most people express their sexuality in a variety of ways, although health considerations and religious and moral beliefs may lead some people to practice **celibacy.** Human sexual behaviors include the following:

- *Autoeroticism and masturbation.* The most common autoerotic sexual activity is **erotic fantasy,** mental experiences that arise in the imagination. **Masturbation,** self-stimulation to obtain sexual arousal and orgasm, may be used as a substitute for coitus or as part of sexual activity with a partner.

- *Touching.* Tactile stimulation—touching—is integral to sexual experiences, whether in the form of massage, kissing, fondling, or holding. Touching can convey a variety of messages, including affection, comfort, and a desire for further sexual contact.

- *Oral-genital stimulation.* Cunnilingus (the stimulation of the female genitals with the lips and tongue) and fellatio (the stimulation of the penis with the mouth) are common practices, either as part of foreplay or as

a sex act culminating in orgasm. Like all acts of sexual expression between two people, oral sex requires the cooperation and consent of both partners.

- *Anal intercourse.* Anal stimulation and penetration by the penis or a finger is a less common but well known practice. About 10 percent of heterosexuals and 50 percent of homosexual males regularly practice anal intercourse. Anal intercourse carries a greater risk of transmission of certain diseases, including HIV infection, so special care and precaution should be exercised if anal sex is practiced.

- *Sexual intercourse.* For most adults, most of the time, **sexual intercourse** is the ultimate sexual experience. Men and women engage in coitus—make love—to fulfill both sexual and psychological needs. The most common practice involves the man placing his erect penis into the woman's dilated and lubricated vagina after sufficient arousal.

People can continue to enjoy sexual activities throughout their entire lives, varying and expanding the scope of their experiences as they gain more understanding of their own and their partners' needs and desires.

Personal Insight   What sexual practices are acceptable to you and what ones are unacceptable? What influences your feelings about them? Are there sexual practices that you object to but find arousing anyway? Remember, there's a big difference between what you think and what you do.

Problematic and Coercive Sexual Behaviors

In our society, a wide variety of sexual behaviors are accepted. However, some types of sexual expression are considered unacceptable or harmful. The term **sexual variations** refers to less common types of sexual behaviors that are usually considered undesirable by others. These include adult behaviors such as exhibiting one's genitals in public, peeping uninvited into strangers' homes, child sexual abuse, and rape. The effects of these behaviors on others range from minor upset to serious physical and emotional harm. The use of force and coercion in sexual relationships is one of the most serious problems in human interactions. The most extreme manifestation of **sexual coercion**—forcing a person to submit to another's sexual desires—is rape, but coercion occurs in many subtler forms, including sexual harassment.

A person who repeatedly and persistently prefers certain unusual behaviors for sexual gratification is classified as a **sex offender** if his or her sexual activity violates moral and legal codes, offends the public sense of decency, or threatens others. Almost all sex offenders are

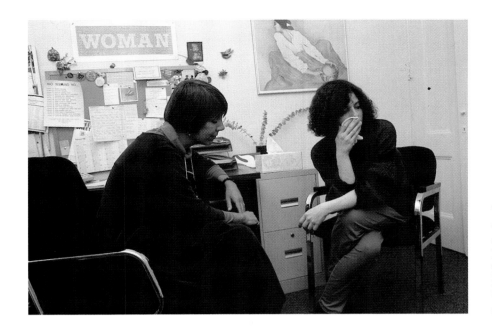

Victims of acquaintance rape usually don't suffer physical injury, but the psychological pain may be severe. Professional counseling may help this young woman overcome the shock, anxiety, depression, and feelings of self-blame typically experienced by victims of rape.

men, though occasionally a woman is cited for sexual harassment or sexual abuse of children.

Sexual Harassment   Sexual pressuring of someone in a vulnerable or dependent position—a youth, employee, or student, for example—is termed **sexual harassment.** Employers, professors, or other people in authority may use their ability to control or influence jobs or grades to coerce people into sexual relations, or to punish them if they refuse. In extreme cases, a person may be threatened with being fired or being given a bad grade if he or she will not submit to the harasser's demands. Men are usually, but not always, the offenders, partly because they are more often in positions of power.

Sexual harassment can take a variety of forms, including verbal abuse, sexual remarks about clothing or appearance, touching or pinching, and demands for sexual favors. It may be accompanied by implied or overt threats concerning the victim's job or grades. Victims often do not report the abuse, in part because they may fear they will be ignored or blamed. In a recent survey of 17,000 federal employees, 42 percent of women and 15 percent of men reported being sexually harassed.

If you have been the victim of sexual harassment, you can take action to stop it. Be assertive with anyone who uses language or actions you find inappropriate. If it's emotionally possible for you, confront your harasser either in writing, over the telephone, or in person, informing him or her that the situation is unacceptable to you and you want the harassment to stop. If that doesn't work, assemble a file or log documenting the harassment, noting the details of each incident along with any witnesses who may be able to support your claims. You may discover others who have been harassed by the same person, which will strengthen your case. Then file a grievance with the harasser's supervisor or employer, such as someone in the dean's office if you are a student or someone in the personnel office if you are an employee.

If your attempts to deal with the harassment internally aren't successful, you can file an official complaint with your city or state Human Rights Commission or Fair Employment Practices Agency or with the federal Equal Employment Opportunity Commission. You may also wish to pursue legal action under the Civil Rights Act or under local laws prohibiting employment discrimination. Very often the threat of a lawsuit is enough to stop the harasser.

Sexual Assault: Rape   Sexual coercion that relies on the threat and use of physical force or takes advantage of circumstances that render a person incapable of giving

---

Celibacy   Continuous abstention from sexual activities.

Erotic fantasy   Sexually arousing thoughts and daydreams.

Masturbation   Self-stimulation to obtain sexual arousal and orgasm.

Sexual intercourse   Sexual relations involving genital union; coitus; also called "making love."

Sexual variations   Atypical sexual behaviors considered undesirable by others.

Sexual coercion   Use of physical or psychological force or intimidation to force a person to submit to sexual demands.

Sex offender   One who engages in sexual behaviors prohibited by law.

Sexual harassment   Sexual pressuring of someone in a vulnerable or dependent position, such as a youth, student, or employee.

TERMS

To reduce the risk of being raped, try not to let yourself get into vulnerable situations; specifically

- Avoid dark, lonely city streets or parks.
- Stay aware of your surroundings and notice if anyone is following you.
- Have your keys out in your hand as you approach your car or house so you can get inside quickly, and lock the door behind you.
- Avoid showing that you are alone in a house or apartment.
- Find out with certainty who is at the door before opening it.
- Try to look confident, strong, and purposeful when you're out by yourself.
- Try to remain as cool as possible in all situations.
- Think out in advance what you would do if you were threatened with rape.

When asked what to tell women who found themselves facing a rapist, an experienced counselor responded:

Please be very careful about giving specific advice on what to do. There is great disagreement on the subject. Some rapists say that if a woman had screamed or resisted loudly, they'd have run; others report they'd have killed her. Self-defense training is valuable in that it helps a woman feel and act more assertively, but it is risky in that none of us really knows how we would use it when scared to death—and badly or ineffectively used active self-defense could get us killed. Some say it is best to seem to give in quietly so as to avoid being injured or killed, and to try to calm the rapist, to win time, so that escape is more likely should the opportunity arise. The trouble with telling a woman she *should* resist and yell is that she adds to her already large burden of guilt if she does not do so, and it plays into the hands of prosecutors and those who insist (against the law) that a woman isn't really raped unless she is beaten up or shows signs of struggle. I think it is best to give various options and then say that each woman and each rapist and each situation are unique, and the woman should respond in whatever way she thinks best.

If you are threatened by a rapist and decide to fight back, here is what Women Organized Against Rape (WOAR) recommends:

- *USE YOUR VOICE!* Yell and keep yelling. (This may sound obvious but you would be surprised how few people have ever really yelled. It takes practice and you should do it today.) Yelling will clear your head and start your adrenalin going. It may scare your attacker and also bring help.
- If you just throw your hands out for striking, they can be grabbed by an attacker and used to get you down.
- If an attacker grabs you from behind, use your *elbows* for striking the neck or his sides, or even his stomach to take him by surprise.
- Don't forget that a rapist also feels pain and is also afraid of pain, plus he is afraid of getting caught. Try to use this weakness to get away.
- Your legs are the strongest part of your body—they have been carrying you around all of your life. Your kick is longer than his reach and a series of hard, fast kicks should keep him away from you. Always kick with your rear foot and with the toe of your shoe. Aim low to avoid losing your balance.
- His most vulnerable spot is his *knee*; it's low, difficult to protect, and easily knocked out of place. The most effective kick is a glancing one across his kneecap.
- Don't try to kick a rapist in the crotch. He has been protecting this area all of his life. In addition, he may grab your foot, knocking you off balance.
- Trust your gut feelings. If you feel you are in danger, don't hesitate to run and scream. It is better to feel foolish than to be raped. In any situation, screaming and a general uproar are strongly recommended.

---

consent (such as when drunk) constitutes **sexual assault** or **rape.** When the victim is younger than the legally defined "age of consent," the act constitutes **statutory rape,** whether or not coercion is involved. Coerced sexual activity in which the victim knows or is dating the rapist is often referred to as **acquaintance** or **date rape.**

Any woman—or man—can be a rape victim. It is conservatively estimated that at least 3.5 million females are raped annually in the United States. Some men are raped by other men, perhaps 10,000 annually. Rape victims suffer both physical and psychological injury. For most, physical wounds are not severe and heal within a few weeks. Psychological pain may endure and be substantial.

Men who commit forcible rape may come from any social class and be any age. Some rapists are exploiters in the sense that they rape on the spur of the moment and want immediate gratification. Some attempt to compensate for feelings of sexual inadequacy and inability to obtain satisfaction otherwise. Others are more hostile and sadistic and are interested not in sex but in hurting and humiliating a particular woman or women in general.

Most women are in much less danger of being raped by

- Remember that ordinary rules of behavior don't apply. It's OK to vomit, act "crazy," or claim to have a sexually transmissible disease.

- When you do decide to fight, always accompany it with a strong bellowing war cry.

- Don't ever expect a single blow to end the fight. Don't give up, keep fighting. Your objective is to get away, and to get away as soon as you can.

- If a rapist is carrying a weapon, you shouldn't fight unless absolutely necessary.

If you are raped, WOAR gives the following advice:

- Tell what happened to the first friendly person you meet.

- Call the police. Use the emergency number. Give your location and tell them you were raped.

- Try to remember as many facts as you can about your attacker: clothes, height, weight, age, skin color, etc. Try to remember his car, license number, the direction in which he went, etc. Write all this down right away.

- *Don't* wash or douche before the medical exam, or you destroy important evidence. *Don't* change your clothes, but bring a new set with you if you can.

- At the hospital you will have a complete exam, including a pelvic exam. Show the doctor any bruises, scratches, etc.

- Tell the police simply but exactly what happened. Try not to get flustered. Have a friend or relative accompany you if possible. Be honest and stick to your story.

- If you do not want to report the rape to the police, see a doctor as soon as possible. Make sure you are checked for pregnancy and venereal disease.

- Contact an organization with skilled counselors so you can talk about the experience. Look in the telephone directory under "Rape" or "Rape Crisis Center" for a hotline number to call or a local chapter of WOAR.

To avoid date rape:

- Believe in your right to control what you do. Set limits and communicate these limits clearly, firmly, and early. Say "no" when you mean "no."

- Be assertive with someone who is sexually pressuring you. Often men interpret passivity as permission.

- If you are unsure of a new acquaintance, go on a group or double date. If possible, have your own transportation.

- Remember that some men assume sexy dress and a flirtatious manner mean a desire for sex.

- Remember that alcohol and drugs interfere with clear communication about sex.

- Use the statement that has proven most effective in stopping date rape: "This is rape and I'm calling the cops."

Guidelines for men:

- Be aware of social pressure. It's OK not to "score."

- Understand that "no" means "no." Don't continue making advances when your date resists or tells you she wants to stop. Remember that she has the right to refuse sex.

- Don't assume sexy dress and a flirtatious manner are invitations to sex, that previous permission for sex applies to the current situation, or that your date's relationships with other men constitute sexual permission for you.

- Remember that alcohol and drugs interfere with clear communication about sex.

Adapted from L. Dimona and C. Herndon, eds. 1994. *The 1995 Information Please® Women's Sourcebook.* (New York: Houghton Mifflin), p. 454; D. Goleman. 1989. "When the Rapist Is Not a Stranger." *New York Times,* 29 August, B1, B11; and M. S. Calderone and E. W. Johnson. 1989. *The Family Book About Sexuality.* (New York: Harper and Row), pp. 176–77.

a stranger than of being sexually assaulted by a man they know or date. Surveys suggest that as many as one woman in four has had experiences in which the man she was dating persisted in trying to force sex on her despite her pleading, crying, screaming, or resisting. One of every 6 to 15 women has been raped by a man she knew or was dating. Most cases of date rape are never reported to the police, partly because of the subtlety of the crime. Usually no weapons are involved and direct verbal threats may not have been made. Rather than being terrorized, the victim usually is attracted to the man at first. Victims of

date rape tend to shoulder much of the responsibility for the incident, questioning their own judgment and behavior rather than blaming the aggressor.

Sexual assault   Use of force to gain sexual access to someone.

Rape   Coercing a person into sexual relations by threats or use of force.

Statutory rape   Sexual interaction with someone below the legal age of consent.

Acquaintance or date rape   Sexual assault by someone the victim knows or is dating.

TERMS

Sexual Behavior in the 1990s

The sexual behaviors and attitudes of Americans were recently explored in two of the largest sex surveys since Alfred Kinsey's work in the late 1940s and early 1950s. More than 6,000 men and women aged 18 years and older volunteered information about their sexual activities and their attitudes toward important social issues such as marriage, divorce, and parenthood. Along with other recent research findings, these surveys provide a snapshot of sexual behavior in America in the 1990s. Some of the more interesting, and in some cases surprising, findings are presented below.

- *Sexual peak among males.* The popular myth that males reach their sexual peak in their teens was found to be false. The frequency of sexual activity (with a partner or through self-stimulation) was higher among men between the ages of 27 and 64 than it was for men between the ages of 18 and 26.

- *Sexual experience before marriage.* For men, sexual experience before marriage was rated as important or very important by 56 percent of men and 52 percent of women. Forty-six percent of both men and women felt it was important or very important for a woman to be sexually experienced before marriage.

- *Gender roles.* Traditional gender roles were supported by people of all age groups and marital status categories. However, divorced people were the least supportive of traditional gender roles. This may be due to their experiences with the breakup of the family unit and the necessity of performing both male and female roles.

- *Masturbation.* In a change from the past, about two-thirds of all men and women surveyed viewed masturbation as a natural part of their sexual lives. As in the past, men masturbate more than women.

- *Coercive sex.* Almost 23 percent of all women surveyed stated that they had been forced to have some type of sex, usually by someone they knew well, were in love with, or were married to. In contrast, only 3 percent of all men stated that they had ever forced a woman to have any type of sex. This great discrepancy may be explained by under-reporting by the men and by the fact that men may not know how coercive their behaviors are to women.

- *Motivations for sex.* Motivations for sex among college-aged males involve physical reasons such as pleasure and physical gratification, whereas women in this same age group engage in sex for emotional reasons. As men and women enter their 30s and beyond, however, many women are motivated to engage in sex for physical reasons and many men engage in sex for emotional reasons. Perhaps with age, men and women feel more secure with their sexuality and go against the typical gender stereotypes regarding reasons for engaging in sex.

- *Preferred sexual practices.* College-aged men were found to prefer intercourse, while college-aged women preferred foreplay. This pattern is reversed for people in their 30s. As men and women age, men may need more physical stimulation and women may feel more free to express their sexuality and their sexual needs.

In terms of preferences for specific sexual activities, respondents to a recent sex survey were asked to rate different activities. The table below summarizes some of the responses for people aged 18 to 44.

Activity	Percentage of people aged 18–44 who rated the activity as "very appealing"	
	Women	Men
Vaginal intercourse	78	83
Watching partner undress	30	50
Receiving oral sex	33	50
Giving oral sex	19	37
Group sex	1	14
Sex with a stranger	1	5

Adapted from E. Laumann and others. 1994. *The Social Organization of Sexuality: Sexual Practices in the United States.* (Chicago: University of Chicago Press); S. Janus and C. Janus. 1993. *The Janus Report on Sexual Behavior.* (New York: John Wiley and Sons); and J. Sprague and D. Quadagno. 1989. "Gender and Sexual Motivation." *Journal of Psychology and Human Sexuality.* Vol. 2: 57–76.

Responsible Sexual Behavior

Healthy sexuality is an important part of adult life. It can be a source of pleasurable experiences and emotions and an important part of intimate partnerships. But sexual behavior also carries many responsibilities, and you need to make choices about your sexuality that contribute to your well-being and your partner's well-being. Sexual responsibility includes the following:

- Open, honest communication about intentions. Each partner needs to clearly indicate what sexual involvement means to him or her. Does it mean love, fun, a permanent commitment, or something else?

- Sexual activities that both partners agree upon and are comfortable with. No one should pressure or coerce a partner. Sexual behaviors should be consistent with the sexual values and preferences of

both partners. Everyone has the right to refuse sexual activity at any time.

- The use of contraception during sexual intercourse (if partners wish to avoid pregnancy). Both partners need to take responsibility for protecting against unwanted pregnancy. Partners should discuss contraception before sexual involvement begins.

- The use of safer sex practices to guard against HIV infection and other sexually transmissible diseases (STDs). Many sexual behaviors carry the risk of STDs, including HIV infection. Partners should be honest about their medical condition and work out a plan for protecting themselves from STDs.

- Taking responsibility for the consequences of sexual behavior. Everyone should be aware of the physical and emotional consequences of their sexual behavior and accept responsibility for them. These consequences include pregnancy, STDs, and emotional changes in the relationship between partners.

UNDERSTANDING FERTILITY

Conceiving is a highly complex process. Although many couples conceive readily, others can testify to the difficulties that can be encountered.

Conception

The process of **conception** involves the fusion of an egg (ovum) from a woman's ovary with a sperm from a man. Every month during a woman's fertile years, her body prepares itself for conception and pregnancy. In one of her ovaries an egg ripens and is released from its **follicle.** The egg—about the size of a pinpoint, 1/250 inch in diameter—is then drawn into an oviduct (or fallopian tube) through which it travels to the uterus. The journey takes three to four days. The lining of the uterus has already thickened to assist the implantation of a **fertilized egg,** or zygote. If the egg is not fertilized, it lasts about 24 hours and then disintegrates. It is expelled along with the uterine lining during menstruation.

Sperm cells are produced in the man's testes and ejaculated from his penis into the woman's vagina during sexual intercourse. Sperm cells are much smaller than eggs (1/8000 inch in diameter). The typical ejaculate contains millions of sperm, but only a few complete the long journey through the uterus and up the fallopian tube to the egg. Of those that reach the egg, only one will be allowed to penetrate the hard outer layer of the egg. As sperm approach the egg, they release enzymes that soften the outer layer of the egg. The first sperm cell that bumps into a spot that is soft enough can swim into the cell. It then merges with the nucleus of the egg and **fertilization** occurs.

The ovum carries the hereditary characteristics of the mother and her ancestors; sperm cells carry the hereditary characteristics of the father and his ancestors. Together they contain the **genetic code,** a set of instructions for development. Each parent cell—egg or sperm—contains 23 chromosomes, and each of these chromosomes contains many genes, so small that they cannot be seen through a microscope. These genes are packages of chemical instructions for designing every part of a new baby. They specify that the infant will be human; what its sex will be; whether it will tend to be (depending also on its environment) short, tall, thin, fat, healthy, or sickly; and hundreds of other characteristics. Together, they provide the blueprint for a new and unique person.

The usual course of events at conception is that one egg and one sperm unite to produce one fertilized egg and one baby. But if the ovaries release two (or more) eggs during ovulation, and if both eggs are fertilized, two babies will develop. These twins will be no more alike than will be siblings born from different pregnancies, because each came from a different fertilized egg. Twins who develop this way are referred to as **fraternal twins;** they may be the same sex or different sexes. Twins can also develop from the division of a single fertilized egg into two cells that develop separately. Because these babies share all genetic material, they will be **identical twins.**

Infertility

Although the main concern for many women and men, especially if they are young and single, is how *not* to get pregnant, the reverse is true for millions of couples who have difficulty conceiving. **Infertility** is usually defined as the inability to conceive after trying for a year or more. About 1 out of 13 American couples are unable to have the children they want. Over a million couples seek treat-

TERMS

Conception   The formation of a zygote (fertilized egg), the cell resulting from the fusion of ovum and sperm, and in normal conditions capable of survival and maturation in the uterus.

Follicles   The thousands of protecting, enclosing spherical bubbles in the ovaries in which ova mature. Each follicle contains a liquid supplied with estrogen.

Fertilized egg   The egg after it has been penetrated by a sperm; a zygote.

Fertilization   The initiation of biological reproduction, as, for example, when the sperm and ovum unite to form a zygote (fertilized egg).

Genetic code   Master blueprint message directing the body's growth and cell differentiation, contained in genetic material.

Fraternal twins   Twins who develop from separate fertilized eggs; not genetically identical.

Identical twins   Twins who develop from the division of a single zygote; genetically identical.

Infertility   The inability to conceive after trying for a year or more.

The genetic inheritance that each of us receives from our parents—and that our children receive from us—contains more than just physical characteristics such as eye and hair color. Heredity also contributes directly to our risk of developing certain diseases and disorders.

For certain uncommon diseases such as hemophilia and sickle cell anemia, heredity is the primary cause; if your parents give you the necessary genes, you'll almost always get the disease. But heredity plays a subtler role in many other diseases, which are caused at least in part by "environmental" influences such as infection, cancer-causing chemicals, or an artery-clogging diet. While your genes alone will not produce those diseases, they can determine how susceptible you are. Researchers have found a genetic influence in many common disorders, including coronary heart disease, diabetes, certain forms of cancer, depression, and alcoholism.

Knowing that a specific disease runs in your family can save your life. It allows you to watch for early warning signs and get screening tests more often than you otherwise would. Changing health habits, too, can be valuable for people with a family history of certain diseases. A smoker with a close relative who had lung cancer, for example, is 14 times more likely to get the disease than other smokers.

In general, the more relatives that had a genetically transmitted disease and the closer they are to you, the greater your risk. However, nongenetic facts such as health habits can also play a role. Signs of strong hereditary influence include early onset of the disease, appearance of the disease largely or exclusively on one side of the family, onset of the same disease at the same age in more than one relative, and disease despite good health habits.

You can put together a simple family tree by compiling a few key facts on your primary relatives: siblings, parents, aunts and uncles, and grandparents. Those facts include the date of birth, major diseases, health-related conditions and habits, and, for deceased relatives, the date and cause of death. (For a free family-medical-history form and guide-

lines on what to ask, write The March of Dimes Birth Defects Foundation, 1275 Mamaroneck Avenue, White Plains, NY 10605.) Once you've collected the information you want, create a tree using the example here as a guide. Then show your tree to your physician to get a full picture of what the information means for your or your children's health.

A Sample Family Health Tree and What It Means

In this sample family tree, the prostate cancer that killed the man's father means that he should be tested for a prostate tumor at a younger age and more frequently than is generally recommended.

His sisters may need to have earlier, more frequent mammograms because of their mother's breast cancer. If they're overweight, they can reduce their risk by losing weight.

One grandmother and one uncle each died of a heart attack. There are several reasons not to worry too much about that: The two relatives were from different sides of the family; both had the attack at a relatively old age; both had two other major risk factors for coronary heart disease—smoking and either diabetes or obesity; and neither of the man's parents had any apparent heart trouble. He should check to see whether either relative had highly elevated cholesterol levels, a possible sign of familial hypercholesterolemia.

The colon cancer that struck another grandmother and uncle is a different story. Two factors suggest a possible hereditary link: They were mother and son, and they both developed the disease at nearly the same comparatively young age. So the man should be screened early and often.

Finally, alcoholism seems to run in the family. The man should be aware that such a history could indicate a hereditary susceptibility to the problem, though the habit might simply have been passed down by example.

Source: "What's Lurking in Your Family Tree?" *Consumer Reports on Health,* September 1992.

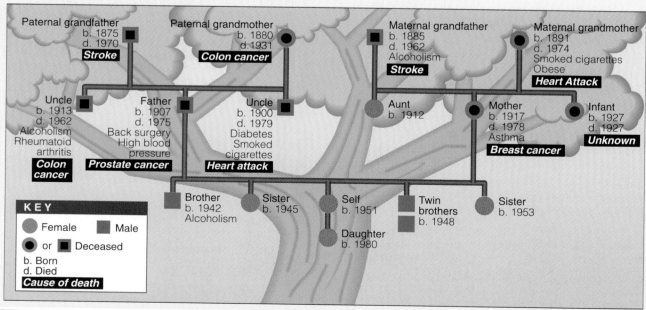

ment for infertility each year. Although the focus is often on women, about 40 to 50 percent of the factors contributing to infertility are male and in about 15 percent of infertile couples both partners have problems.

Female Infertility   The leading cause of infertility among women is blocked fallopian tubes, usually the result of pelvic inflammatory disease (PID). Most occurrences of PID are due to untreated cases of chlamydia or gonorrhea; unsterile abortions, abdominal surgery, and certain types of older IUDs are other possible causes of PID. The second leading cause of infertility in women is endometriosis, in which uterine tissue grows outside the uterus and may block the oviducts. Other causes include benign growths in the uterus, hormonal imbalances that prevent ovulation, and exposure to toxic substances. Evidence also indicates that the daughters of mothers who were prescribed **diethylstilbestrol (DES)** have a significantly higher infertility rate. (DES was prescribed regularly from 1945 until 1960 to prevent miscarriage, but later research linked the drug to problems such as increased rates of infertility and certain cancers in the children of women who took it.) Age is another factor—beginning around age 30, women's fertility naturally begins to decline.

Male Infertility   The leading causes of infertility among men are low sperm count, lack of sperm motility (the ability to move spontaneously), or blocked passageways between the testes and the urethra. Some studies indicate that men's sperm counts have dropped by as much as 50 percent over the last 30 years. Evidence suggests that toxic substances, such as lead, chemical pollutants, and radiation, are responsible for this decrease in sperm counts. Smoking, prenatal exposure to DES, and certain prescription and illegal drugs also affect the number and quality of sperm. Other causes of sperm problems include injury of the testicles, infection (especially from mumps during adulthood), birth defects, or subjecting the testicles to high temperatures, such as those produced by hot baths or tight-fitting underwear. In many cases, affected men's fertility can be increased by removing the causative factor.

Treating Infertility   Some kinds of infertility can be treated; others cannot. About 90 percent of infertile couples receive a physical diagnosis for their condition; for the remaining 10 percent, the cause of the infertility remains unexplained. Surgery can sometimes repair oviducts, clear up endometriosis, and correct anatomical problems in both men and women. Fertility drugs can help a woman ovulate, although they carry the risk of causing multiple births.

If these procedures don't work, more advanced techniques may help. Male infertility can sometimes be overcome by collecting and concentrating the man's sperm

and introducing it mechanically into the woman's vagina or uterus, a procedure known as **artificial or intrauterine insemination.** The sperm can be provided by the woman's partner or, if there are severe problems with his sperm, by a donor. Intrauterine insemination has a success rate of about 60 percent for infertile couples.

Some kinds of female infertility can be bypassed with **in vitro fertilization.** In this procedure, eggs are removed from the woman's ovary and fertilized in a laboratory dish by her partner's sperm. One or more of the resulting embryos is implanted in the woman's uterus. If one partner is infertile, a donor can supply the sperm or egg. In vitro fertilization is a costly procedure and usually has to be repeated a number of times before a viable pregnancy results; success rates are usually between 12 and 20 percent.

The most controversial of all approaches to infertility is surrogate motherhood. This practice involves a contract between a fertile woman who agrees to carry a fetus and a couple who wishes to have a child but cannot because the woman is infertile. The surrogate mother agrees to be artificially inseminated by the father's sperm, carry the baby to term, and give it to the couple at birth. In return, the couple pays her for her services. Some people question the morality of paying a woman to carry a baby. Experience has shown, too, that some surrogate mothers have a very difficult time giving up the baby and are unwilling to fulfill the contract after the birth, causing emotional trauma for themselves and the couple.

All these treatments for infertility are expensive and emotionally draining, and their success is uncertain. Some infertile couples choose not to try to have children, while others turn to adoption, which can also be difficult and expensive. One measure that you can take now to avoid infertility is to protect yourself against STDs and to treat promptly any diseases you do contract.

Personal Insight   How do you think you would feel if you discovered that you were infertile? Would you consider extraordinary measures—artificial insemination or in vitro fertilization, for example—in order to become a parent? Would you consider adoption?

Diethylstilbestrol (DES)   A synthetic hormone that produces the effects of natural estrogen. In the past, it was given to women to prevent miscarriage, but its use was discontinued when it was linked to health problems.

Artificial (intrauterine) insemination   The introduction of semen into the vagina by artificial means, usually a syringe.

In vitro fertilization   Combining ovum and sperm outside the body, usually in a laboratory dish, for the purpose of fertilization.

TERMS

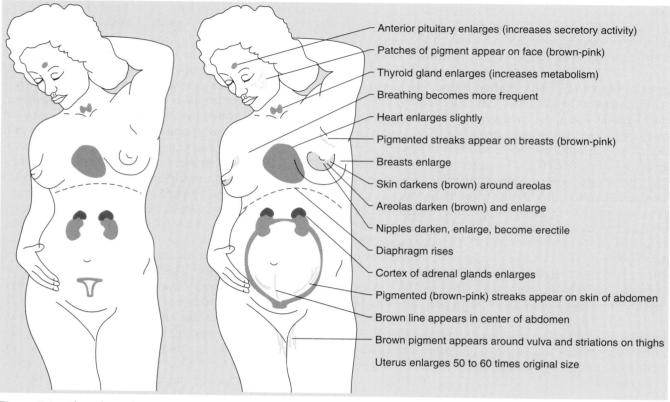

Figure 5-4 *Physiological changes during pregnancy.*
(Left) the female body at the time of conception; (right) development after 30 weeks of pregnancy.

The following labels appear in the figure:

- Anterior pituitary enlarges (increases secretory activity)
- Patches of pigment appear on face (brown-pink)
- Thyroid gland enlarges (increases metabolism)
- Breathing becomes more frequent
- Heart enlarges slightly
- Pigmented streaks appear on breasts (brown-pink)
- Breasts enlarge
- Skin darkens (brown) around areolas
- Areolas darken (brown) and enlarge
- Nipples darken, enlarge, become erectile
- Diaphragm rises
- Cortex of adrenal glands enlarges
- Pigmented (brown-pink) streaks appear on skin of abdomen
- Brown line appears in center of abdomen
- Brown pigment appears around vulva and striations on thighs
- Uterus enlarges 50 to 60 times original size

PREGNANCY

Pregnancy is usually discussed in terms of **trimesters**—three periods of about three months (or 13 weeks) each. During the first trimester, the mother experiences a few bodily changes and some fairly common symptoms. During the second trimester, often the most peaceful time of pregnancy, the mother gains weight, looks noticeably pregnant, and may experience a general sense of well-being if she is happy about having a child. The third trimester is the hardest for the mother because she must breathe, digest, excrete, and circulate blood for herself and the growing fetus. The weight of the **fetus,** the pressure of its body on her organs, and its increased demands on her system cause discomfort and fatigue and may make the mother increasingly impatient to give birth.

Pregnancy Tests

The earliest tests for pregnancy are chemical tests designed to detect the presence of **human chorionic gonadotropin (HCG),** a hormone produced by the implanted fertilized egg. Home pregnancy test kits are sold over the counter in drugstores; if the directions are followed carefully, these tests are 85–95 percent reliable.

Changes in the Woman's Body

Hormonal changes begin as soon as the egg is fertilized, and for the next nine months the woman's body nourishes the fetus and adjusts to its growth. Let's take a closer look at the changes of early, middle, and late pregnancy (Figure 5-4).

Early Signs and Symptoms   Early recognition of pregnancy is important, especially for women with physical problems and nutritional deficiencies. The following symptoms of pregnancy are not absolute indications of pregnancy, but they are reasons to visit a gynecologist for an examination.

- Missed menstrual period. If an egg has been fertilized and implanted in the uterine wall, the uterine lining is retained to nourish the embryo. A woman who misses a period after having unprotected intercourse may be pregnant.

- Slight bleeding. Slight bleeding may follow the implanting of the fertilized egg in the uterine wall, about 11 or 12 days after fertilization. Because this happens about the time a period is expected, the bleeding is sometimes mistaken for menstrual flow. It usually lasts only a few days.

- Nausea. About two-thirds of pregnant women feel nauseated, probably as a reaction to increased levels of progesterone and other hormones. The nausea is often called morning sickness, but some women have it all day long. It frequently disappears by the twelfth week but can last thoughout pregnancy.
- Breast tenderness. Some women experience breast tenderness, swelling, and tingling, usually described as different from the tenderness experienced before menstruation.
- Sleepiness, fatigue, and emotional upset. These symptoms result from hormonal changes.

Chemical tests for pregnancy can be done within weeks of fertilization. The first reliable physical signs of pregnancy can be distinguished about four weeks after a woman misses her menstrual period. (At this point the woman would be considered to be eight weeks pregnant because physicians calculate pregnancy from the time of the woman's last menstrual period rather than from the time of actual fertilization, since the latter date is often difficult to determine.) A softening of the uterus just above the cervix, called **Hegar's sign,** and other changes in the cervix and pelvis are apparent during a pelvic examination. The labia minora and the cervix may take on a purple color rather than their usual pink hue.

Continuing Changes in the Woman's Body The most obvious changes during pregnancy occur in the reproductive organs. The uterus enlarges to many times its nonpregnant size, placing pressure on other organs and causing the woman's abdomen to protrude. The breasts enlarge, become more sensitive, and may tingle or throb. After the tenth week, **colostrum,** a thin milky fluid, may be squeezed from the mother's nipples, but actual secretion of milk is prevented by high levels of estrogen and progesterone.

Early in pregnancy, the muscles and ligaments attached to bones begin to soften and stretch. The joints between the pelvic bones loosen and spread, making it easier to have a baby but harder to walk. The circulatory system and lungs become more efficient, the rib cage widens, and the heart pumps more rapidly. Blood volume increases by 50 percent, and the mother inhales up to 40 percent more air.

Women of normal weight gain an average of 18 to 25 percent of their initial weight during pregnancy: 23 to 32 pounds for a woman weighing 128 pounds. About 60 percent of weight gained relates directly to the baby—the weight of the fetus, placenta, amniotic fluid, and heavier breasts and uterus. The remainder accumulates over the mother's entire body as fluid (blood) and fat. As the mother's skin stretches to accommodate her changing shape, small breaks may occur in the elastic fibers of the lower layer of skin, producing "stretch marks" on her abdomen, hips, breasts, or thighs.

Changes of the Later Stages of Pregnancy By the end of the sixth month, the increased needs of the fetus place a burden on the mother's lungs, heart, and kidneys. Her back may ache from the pressure of the baby's weight and from having to throw her shoulders back to keep her balance while standing. Her body retains up to three extra quarts of fluid. Her legs, hands, ankles, or feet may swell, and she may be bothered by leg cramps, heartburn, or constipation. Despite discomfort, both her digestion and her metabolism are working at top efficiency.

The uterus prepares for childbirth throughout pregnancy with preliminary contractions, called **Braxton Hicks contractions.** Unlike true labor contractions, these are usually short, irregular, and painless. The mother may only be aware that at times her abdomen is hard to the touch. These contractions become more frequent and intense as the delivery date approaches.

In the ninth month, the baby settles into the pelvic bones, usually head down, fitting snugly. This process, called **lightening,** allows the uterus to sink down about two inches, producing a visible change in the mother's profile. Pelvic pressure increases and pressure on the diaphragm lightens. Breathing becomes easier; urination becomes more frequent. Sometimes, after a first pregnancy, the baby doesn't settle down into the pelvis until **labor** begins.

Fetal Development

Now that we've seen what happens to the mother's body during pregnancy, let's consider the development of the fetus. By the end of the first trimester, the anatomy of the fetus is almost completely formed; further refinements are made during the second trimester; and needed fat and pounds are added during the third trimester (Figure 5-5).

TERMS

Trimester One of the three 13-week periods of pregnancy.

Fetus Developmental stage of a human from the ninth week after conception to the moment of birth.

Human chorionic gonadotropin (HCG) A hormone produced by the fertilized egg that can be detected in the urine or blood of the mother within a few weeks of conception.

Hegar's sign A softening of the uterus just above the cervix that may be an early indication of pregnancy.

Colostrum The thin, milky fluid secreted by the mammary glands around the time of childbirth until milk comes in, about the third day.

Braxton Hicks contractions Uterine contractions that occur periodically throughout pregnancy.

Lightening A labor process in which the uterus sinks downward about 2 inches because the baby's head, or other body part, settles far down into the pelvic area.

Labor The act or process of giving birth to a child, expelling it with the placenta from the mother's body by means of uterine contractions.

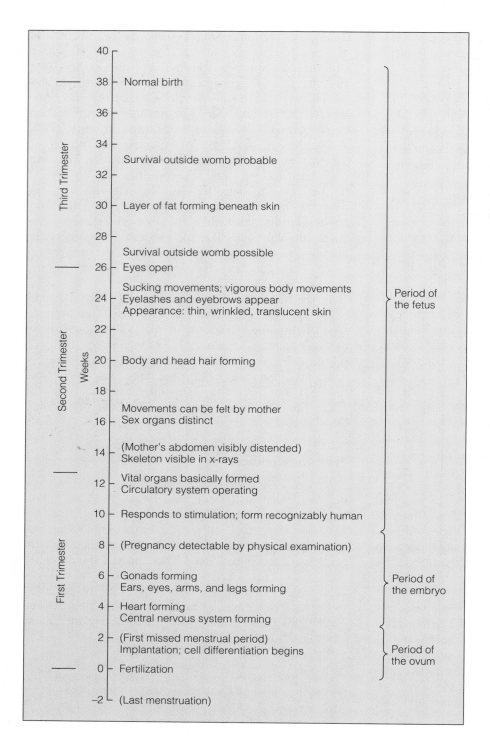

Figure 5-5 *Chronology of milestones in prenatal development.*
Source: Judith Schickedanz, David Schickedanz, Karen Hansen, and Peggy Forsyth. 1993. *Understanding Children.* 2nd ed. (Mountain View, Calif.: Mayfield), p. 86.

First Trimester About 30 hours after the egg is fertilized the cell reproduces itself by dividing in half. The process of cell division repeats many times. On about the fourth day after fertilization, the cluster, now about 64 to 128 cells and hollow, arrives in the uterus. In this form it is known as a **blastocyst.** On the sixth or seventh day, the blastocyst burrows into the uterine lining, usually along the upper curve. One week after conception the cells number over 100, and the cluster is now considered an

embryo. It begins to draw nourishment from the **endometrium,** the uterine lining.

The outermost shell of blastocyst cells becomes the **placenta,** umbilical cord, and **amniotic sac.** A network of roots called **chorionic villi** sprouts from the blastocyst and eventually forms the placenta. The human placenta is a two-way street, allowing the transfer of some materials between the mother and the fetus. The placenta brings oxygen and nutrients to the fetus and transports waste

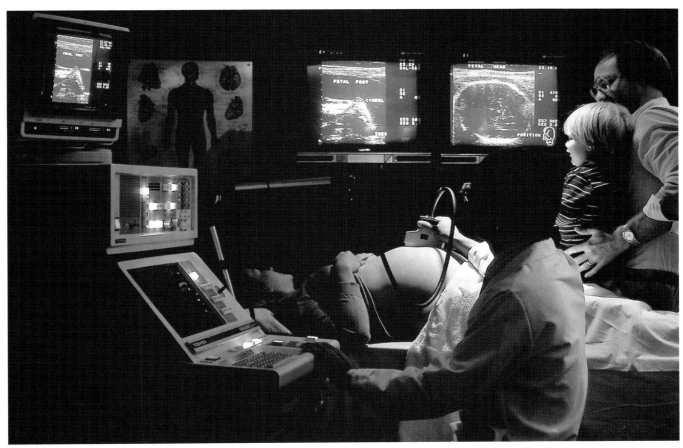

Ultrasound provides information about the position, size, and physical condition of a fetus in the uterus. This couple can see the baby move and perhaps tell its sex by watching it on the screen.

products out. The placenta does not provide a perfect barrier between the fetal circulation and the maternal circulation, however. Some blood cells are exchanged and some substances, such as alcohol, pass freely from the maternal circulation through the placenta to the fetus.

The period between the second and ninth weeks of development is a time of rapid differentiation and change. All the major body structures are formed during this time, including the heart, brain, liver, lungs, and sex organs; the eyes, nose, ears, arms, and legs also appear. Some organs begin to function—the heart begins to beat, the liver starts producing blood cells, and the testes produce sex hormones. Because body structures are forming during this period, the developing organism is vulnerable to damage from environmental influences such as drugs and infections (discussed in greater detail below).

By the end of the second month, the brain sends out impulses that coordinate the functioning of other organs. The embryo is now considered a fetus, and most further bodily changes will be in the size and refinement of working parts. In the third month the fetus begins to be quite active. By the end of the first trimester, the fetus is about 4 inches long and weighs 1 ounce.

Second Trimester To achieve its growth during the second trimester—to about 14 inches and 2 pounds—the fetus must have large amounts of food, oxygen, and water, which come from the mother through the placenta. All body systems are operating, and the fetal heartbeat can be heard with a stethoscope. Fetal movements can be

Blastocyst A stage of human development, lasting only from about the sixth to the fourteenth day, during which the cell cluster divides into the embryo and the placenta.

Embryo The developing cluster of cells from the end of the first week to the end of the eighth week following conception.

Endometrium The mucous membrane that forms the inner lining of the cavity of the uterus.

Placenta The organ through which the fetus receives nourishment and empties waste via the mother's circulatory system; after birth, the placenta is expelled from the uterus.

Amniotic sac Fluid-filled membrane pouch enclosing and protecting the fetus.

Chorionic villi Threadlike blood vessels that sprout from the blastocyst into the mother's vessels to draw out blood and nourishment.

TERMS

felt by the mother beginning in the fourth or fifth month. Against great odds, a fetus born prematurely at the end of the second trimester might survive.

Third Trimester The fetus gains most of its birth weight during the last three months. Some of the weight is fatty tissue under the skin that insulates the fetus and supplies food. The fetus must obtain large amounts of calcium, iron, and nitrogen from the food the mother eats. Some 85 percent of the calcium and iron she consumes goes into the fetal bloodstream.

Although the fetus may live if it is born during the seventh month, it needs the fat layer acquired in the eighth month and time for the organs, especially the respiratory and digestive organs, to develop. It also needs the immunities that the mother's blood supplies in the last three months. Her blood protects the fetus against many of the diseases to which she has acquired immunity. These immunities wear off within six months after birth, but they can be replenished by the mother's milk if the baby is breastfed.

Diagnosing Abnormalities of the Fetus Information about the health and sex of a fetus can be obtained before it's born through prenatal testing. **Ultrasound** examinations use high-frequency sound waves to create a visual image (**sonogram**) of the fetus in the uterus. Sonograms show the position of the fetus; its size, its gestational age, and sometimes its sex; and the presence of certain anatomical problems, such as cleft palate.

Alpha-fetoprotein (AFP) is a protein produced by the fetus and present in the amniotic fluid and in the mother's blood. **Alpha-fetoprotein (AFP) screening,** usually done between 15 and 20 weeks into the pregnancy, involves analysis of AFP levels in a sample of the mother's blood. Although not foolproof, high levels of AFP may indicate the presence of neural tube defects such as anencephaly (absence of part or all of the brain) and spina bifida. A low level of AFP sometimes indicates a chromosomal defect, such as Down's syndrome.

Amniocentesis involves the removal of fluid from the uterus with a long, thin needle inserted through the abdominal wall. It is usually performed at about 16 weeks of gestation. A genetic analysis of the fetal cells contained in the fluid can reveal the presence of possible birth defects and the sex of the fetus. Amniocentesis carries a slight risk (a 0.5 to 2 percent chance of fetal death) and is usually performed only in cases where the fetus is at increased risk for a particular defect.

A newer alternative to amniocentesis is **chorionic villus sampling (CVS),** which can be performed between the ninth and eleventh weeks of gestation. This procedure involves removal through the cervix (by catheter) or abdomen (by needle) of a tiny piece of the chorionic villi, which contains fetal cells that can be analyzed. CVS also carries a slight risk of fetal death.

Genetic counselors explain the results of the different tests so that parents can understand their implications.

The Importance of Prenatal Care

Adequate prenatal care—appropriate diet, exercise, and rest, avoidance of drugs, and regular medical evaluation—is essential to the health of both mother and baby. The pregnant woman cannot help but be responsible for the condition of the baby she carries. Everything she eats, drinks, and does affects the fetus to one degree or another. The fetus gets its nutrients and oxygen from the mother's bloodstream and has its wastes removed the same way. Many harmful substances can also be passed on to the fetus via the placenta and umbilical cord. For these reasons, taking care of her health during pregnancy is a lifelong investment in her child's health.

Regular Checkups In the woman's first visit to her obstetrician, she will be asked for a detailed medical history of herself and her family. The physician or midwife will note especially any hereditary conditions that may assume increased significance during pregnancy. The tendency to develop gestational diabetes (diabetes during pregnancy only), for example, can be inherited. Appropriate treatment during pregnancy reduces the risk of serious harm from the condition, if it does develop.

The woman is given a complete physical exam and is informed about appropriate diet. She returns for regular checkups throughout the pregnancy, during which her blood pressure and weight gain are measured and tracked and the size and position of the fetus are monitored. Regular prenatal visits also give the mother a chance to discuss her concerns and to assure herself that everything is proceeding normally. Early advice from physicians, midwives, health educators, and teachers of childbirth classes provides the mother with invaluable information.

Blood Tests A blood sample is taken during the initial prenatal visit to reveal blood type, anemia, and Rh incompatibilities. The Rh factor is a protein found in the blood. If an Rh-positive father and an Rh-negative mother conceive an Rh-positive baby, the baby's blood will be incompatible with the mother's. If some of the baby's blood enters the mother's bloodstream during delivery, she will develop antibodies to it just as she would toward a virus. If she has subsequent Rh-positive babies, the antibodies in the mother's blood, passing through the placenta, will destroy the fetus's red blood cells, possibly leading to jaundice, anemia, mental retardation, or death. This condition is completely treatable with a serum called Rh-immune globulin, which destroys Rh-positive cells as they enter the mother's body and prevents her from forming antibodies to them. (Blood tests can also reveal the presence of some sexually transmissible diseases, discussed later in the chapter.)

Prenatal Nutrition An appropriate diet throughout pregnancy is essential for both the fetus and the mother. Not only does the baby get all its nutrients from the mother, but it also competes with her for nutrients not sufficiently available to meet both their needs. When a woman's diet is low in iron or calcium, the fetus receives most of it and the mother may become deficient in it. To meet the increased nutritional demands of her body, a pregnant woman shouldn't just eat more; she should make sure that her diet is adequate in all the basic nutritional categories. In the early weeks of pregnancy, high intake of the B vitamin folic acid has been shown to decrease the risk of neural tube defects, including spina bifida. In the second and third trimesters, requirements increase for calories and most nutrients, including protein, calcium, the B vitamins, vitamins A, C, D, and E, iodine, iron, magnesium, and zinc. With the possible exception of iron, for which some authorities recommend a supplement, all these nutrients can be obtained from a sensible, varied diet designed for a healthy pregnancy.

Avoiding Drugs and Other Environmental Hazards

In addition to the food the mother eats, the drugs she takes and the chemicals she is exposed to affect the fetus. Everything the mother ingests may eventually reach the fetus in some proportion. Some drugs harm the fetus but not the mother because the fetus is in the process of developing and because the proper dose for the mother represents a massive dose for the fetus.

During the first trimester, when basic body structures are rapidly forming, the fetus is extremely vulnerable to environmental factors such as viral infections, radiation, drugs, and other **teratogens,** any of which can cause **congenital malformations** (birth defects). The most susceptible body parts are those growing most rapidly at the time of exposure. The rubella (German measles) virus, for example, can cause malformation of a delicate system such as the eyes or ears, leading to blindness or deafness, if exposure occurs during the first trimester, but it does no damage later in the pregnancy. Other agents can cause damage throughout prenatal development.

Prenatal exposure to psychoactive drugs, including tobacco, alcohol, and cocaine, are serious and growing problems. Cigarette smoking is associated with severe adverse conditions in newborns, including low birth weight. Infants whose parents smoke are unusually susceptible to pneumonia and bronchitis during their first year. A high level of alcohol consumption during pregnancy is associated with miscarriages, stillbirths, and, in live babies, **fetal alcohol syndrome (FAS).** A baby born with FAS is likely to suffer from mental retardation, low birth weight, abnormal smallness of the head, unusual facial characteristics, congenital heart defects, defective joints, and abnormal behavior patterns. Babies exposed to cocaine are likely to be born prematurely, to have small heads, and to have problems in early physical and emotional development. During pregnancy, total abstinence from tobacco, alcohol, and other psychoactive drugs is recommended to help ensure the health of the fetus.

Prescription and over-the-counter drugs can also harm the fetus and should be used only under medical supervision. Infections, including those that are sexually transmitted, are another serious problem for the fetus if contracted either before or during birth. Syphilis, gonorrhea, hepatitis B, herpes simplex, and HIV are among the most dangerous infections for the fetus. (Women at risk for HIV infection should be tested before or during pregnancy because the AIDS drug AZT has been shown to dramatically reduce the rate of transmission of the virus to the fetus during pregnancy.)

Prenatal Activity and Exercise

Prenatal Activity and Exercise Physical activity during pregnancy contributes to mental and physical well-being. Women can continue working at their jobs until late in their pregnancies provided the work isn't so physically demanding that it jeopardizes their health. At the same time, pregnant women need more rest and sleep to maintain their own and the fetus's well-being. They become fatigued more easily because the energy demands on their bodies are so great.

The prospective mother can and should continue all reasonable exercising that she is accustomed to, such as tennis, swimming, low-impact aerobics, or dancing, unless or until her pregnancy inhibits movement. The amniotic sac protects the fetus so that normal activities will not harm it. More strenuous activities that could result in a fall, such as skiing, skating, or horseback riding, are best delayed until after the birth. A pregnant woman who hasn't been exercising and wants to start should first consult with her physician. Additional recommendations for

Ultrasound A method of viewing the fetus in the uterus by reflecting high-frequency sound waves off it; also called ultrasonography.

Sonogram The visual image of the fetus produced through the use of ultrasound.

Alpha-fetoprotein (AFP) screening Tests of the level of alpha-fetoprotein in a pregnant woman's blood that can reveal the possible presence of fetal abnormalities.

Amniocentesis A process in which amniotic fluid is removed to detect possible birth defects.

Chorionic villus sampling Surgical removal of a tiny piece of chorionic villi to be analyzed for genetic defects.

Teratogen An agent or influence that causes physical defects in a developing embryo.

Congenital malformation A physical defect existing at the time of birth, either inherited or caused during gestation.

Fetal alcohol syndrome A combination of birth defects caused by excessive alcohol consumption by the mother during pregnancy.

TERMS

exercise during pregnancy from the American College of Obstetricians and Gynecologists (ACOG) include the following: Don't exercise strenuously for more than 15 minutes; keep heart rate below 140 beats per minute and body temperature below 100.4° F (38° C); avoid exercising in hot, humid weather or while you have a fever; don't hold your breath; avoid jarring movements or exercises that require deep flexion or extension of joints; and drink plenty of fluids before, during, and after exercise.

Prenatal exercise classes are valuable because they teach exercises that tone the body muscles involved in birth, especially those of the abdomen, back, and legs. Toned-up muscles aid delivery and help the body regain its nonpregnant shape afterward.

Preparing for Birth   As hospital childbirth practices have been increasingly challenged over the last 20 years, many women have chosen to learn techniques in childbirth preparation classes that help them deal with the discomfort of labor and delivery without pain-relieving drugs. Childbirth classes are almost a routine part of the prenatal experience for both mothers and fathers these days. The mother learns and practices a variety of techniques so she can choose what works best for her during labor. The father typically acts as a coach, supporting the mother emotionally and helping her with her breathing and relaxing. He remains with the mother throughout labor and delivery, even when a cesarean section is performed. It can be an important and fulfilling time for the parents to be together.

Complications of Pregnancy and Pregnancy Loss

Pregnancy usually proceeds without major complications. Sometimes, however, complications may prevent full-term development of the fetus or affect the health of the infant at birth. As discussed earlier in the chapter, exposure to harmful substances, such as alcohol and cocaine, can harm the fetus. Other complications in the development of the fetus are caused by physiological problems or genetic abnormalities.

Ectopic Pregnancy   In **ectopic pregnancy,** the fertilized egg implants itself and begins to develop outside the uterus, usually in an oviduct. Ectopic pregnancies usually occur because the tube is blocked, most often as a result of pelvic inflammatory disease. The embryo may spontaneously abort or the embryo and placenta may continue to expand until they rupture the oviduct.

Spontaneous Abortion   A **spontaneous abortion** or **miscarriage** is a pregnancy that ends before the twentieth week of gestation. Although the exact frequency of spontaneous abortion is unknown, it is estimated that 10–40 percent of pregnancies end this way, some without the woman's awareness that she was pregnant. Most miscar-

riages occur between the sixth and eighth weeks of pregnancy, and most—about 60 percent—are due to chromosomal abnormalities in the fetus. Certain occupations that involve exposure to chemicals may increase the likelihood of spontaneous abortions.

Toxemia   A potentially serious condition that occasionally develops in the later months of pregnancy (usually not before the twentieth week) is **toxemia,** characterized by high blood pressure and fluid retention. The early stages of toxemia, known as **preeclampsia,** can usually be treated through nutritional means. However, if left untreated, blood pressure continues to rise, the face and legs swell, and excess protein appears in the urine. In the later stages, known as **eclampsia,** vision blurs and the head aches continuously, leading eventually to convulsions, coma, and even death. Toxemia is not common and it can be prevented or controlled through diet, rest, and sometimes medication.

Low Birth Weight   A **low birth weight (LBW)** baby usually weighs less than 5.5 pounds at birth. LBW babies may be premature (born before the thirty-seventh week of pregnancy) or full-term. Babies who are born small even though they're full-term are referred to as small-for-date babies. Most LBW babies will grow normally, but some will experience disabilities. Although they are at greater risk than bigger babies for complications during infancy, small-for-date babies tend to have fewer problems than premature infants.

The most fundamental problem of prematurity is that many of the infant's organs are not sufficiently developed. Premature infants are subject to respiratory problems and infections. They may have difficulty eating because they may be too small to suck a breast or bottle and their swallowing mechanism may be underdeveloped. As they get older, premature infants may have problems such as low intelligence, learning difficulties, poor hearing and vision, and physical awkwardness.

Low birth weight affects about 7 percent of infants born each year in the United States. About half of all cases of LBW are related to teenage pregnancy, cigarette smoking, poor nutrition, and poor health of the mother. One study found a sixfold increase in the risk of LBW if the mother had financial problems during the pregnancy. Adequate prenatal care is the best means of preventing LBW.

Infant Mortality   The rate of **infant mortality** (the death of a child of less than one year of age) in the United States is at its lowest point ever; however, it remains far higher than that of most of the developed world. Many of these deaths are due to poverty and lack of adequate health care. Poverty-related infant mortality could be reduced by making sure that all pregnant women receive prenatal care and that all infants and young children receive adequate health care and immunizations.

Although many infants die of poverty-related conditions, others die from congenital problems, infectious diseases, injuries, and other causes. About 1 out of every 375 infant deaths is due to **sudden infant death syndrome (SIDS),** in which an apparently healthy infant dies suddenly while sleeping.

Coping with Loss   Parents form a deep attachment to their children even before birth, and parents who lose an infant before or during birth usually experience a deep grief reaction. Initial feelings of shocked disbelief and numbness may give way to sadness, anger, crying spells, and preoccupation with the loss. Experiencing the pain of loss is part of the healing process, which can take up to a year or more. Keeping active with work or travel can help renew interest in life. Support groups or professional counseling is also often helpful. Planning the next pregnancy, with a physician's input, can be an important step toward recovery, as long as the mind and body are given time to heal. If future pregnancies are ruled out, couples can consider other options, including adoption.

CHILDBIRTH

By the end of the ninth month of pregnancy, most women are tired of being pregnant; both mother and father are impatient to start a new phase of their lives. Most couples find the actual process of birth to be an exciting and positive experience.

Choices in Childbirth

Many couples today can choose the type of practitioner and the environment they want for the birth of their child. A high-risk pregnancy is probably best handled by a specialist physician in a hospital with a nursery, but for low-risk births, a wide variety of options is available.

Parents can choose to have their baby delivered by a physician (an obstetrician or family practitioner) or by a certified nurse-midwife. Most babies in the United States are delivered in hospitals or in freestanding alternative birth centers. Many hospitals have introduced alternative birth centers in response to criticisms of traditional hospital routines. Alternative birth centers provide a comfortable, emotionally supportive environment in close proximity to up-to-date medical equipment.

Couples preparing for childbirth may have other options to choose from, including type of room and bed or chair for labor and delivery, drugs and equipment used, and under what circumstances some medical procedures will be carried out. It's important for parents-to-be to discuss all aspects of labor and delivery with their physician or midwife beforehand, so they can learn what to expect and, where appropriate, can state their preferences.

Labor and Delivery

The birth process occurs in three stages (Figure 5-6). Labor starts when hormonal changes in both the mother and the baby cause strong, rhythmic uterine **contractions** to begin. These contractions exert pressure on the cervix and cause the lengthwise muscles of the uterus to pull on the circular muscles around the cervix, causing effacement (thinning) and dilation (opening) of the cervix. The contractions also pressure the baby to descend into the mother's pelvis, if it hasn't already. The entire process of labor and delivery usually takes from 2 to 36 hours, depending on the size of the baby, the baby's position in the uterus, the size of the mother's pelvis, and other factors. The length of labor is generally shorter for second and subsequent births.

The first stage of labor averages about 13 hours for a first birth, although there is a wide variation among women. Contractions usually last about 30 seconds and come every 15 to 20 minutes at first, more often later. The prepared mother relaxes as much as possible during these contractions to allow labor to proceed without being blocked by tension. Early in the first stage, a small amount of bleeding may occur as a plug of slightly bloody mucus that blocked the opening of the cervix during pregnancy is expelled. In some women, the amniotic sac ruptures and the fluid rushes out—sometimes referred to as "breaking of the waters."

The end of the first stage of labor, called **transition,** is characterized by strong and frequent contractions, much

TERMS

Ectopic pregnancy   A pregnancy in which the embryo develops outside the uterus, most typically in the fallopian tube.

Spontaneous abortion (miscarriage)   Termination of pregnancy when the uterine contents are expelled; causes vary, but can include an abnormal uterus, insufficient hormones, and genetic or physical fetal defects.

Toxemia   A condition of pregnancy characterized by high blood pressure and edema; preeclampsia and eclampsia.

Preeclampsia   Early stage of toxemia characterized by increasingly high blood pressure, edema, and protein in the urine.

Eclampsia   Severe form of toxemia characterized by convulsions, coma, and possibly death (in addition to the symptoms of preeclampsia).

Low birth weight (LBW)   Weighing less than 5 pounds at birth, often the result of prematurity.

Infant mortality   Death of a child of less than 1 year of age.

Sudden infant death syndrome (SIDS)   Sudden death of an apparently healthy infant during sleep.

Contraction   (uterine) Shortening of the muscles in the uterine wall, which causes effacement and dilation of the cervix and assists in expelling the fetus.

Transition   The final phase of the first stage of labor during which the cervix becomes fully dilated, characterized by intense and frequent contractions.

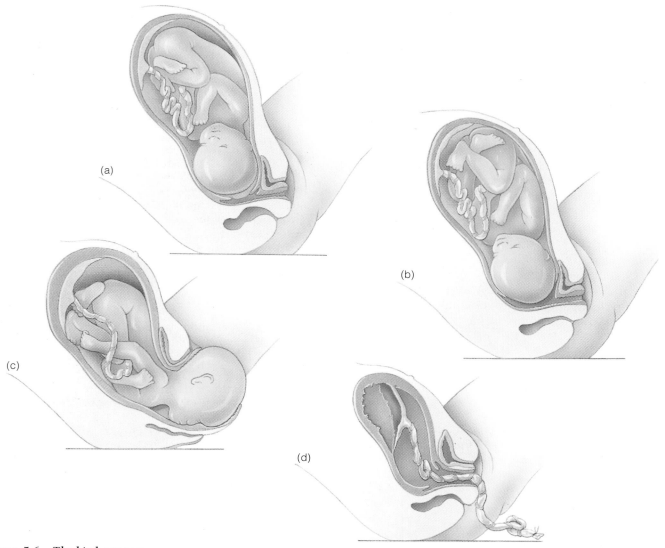

Figure 5-6 *The birth process.*
(a) early stages of labor; cervix begins to dilate; (b) second stage of labor; cervix completely dilated;
(c) late stage of labor; baby's head is completely turned; head begins to emerge; (d) final stage of
labor; delivery of the placenta.

more intense than in the early stages of labor. Contractions may last 60 to 90 seconds and occur every 1 to 3 minutes. It is during transition that the cervix opens completely, to a diameter of about 10 centimeters. Since the head of the fetus usually measures between 9 and 10 centimeters, once the cervix has dilated completely, the head can pass through. Many women report that transition, which normally lasts about 30 minutes to an hour, is the most difficult part of labor. The mother may become angry or fearful and will need the support of her helpers.

The second stage of labor begins when the baby's head moves into the birth canal and ends when the baby is born. The baby is slowly pushed down, through the bones of the pelvic ring, past the cervix, and into the vagina, which it stretches open. The mother bears down with the contractions to help push the baby down and out. Some women find this the most difficult part of labor, while others find that the contractions and bearing down bring a sense of euphoria. The baby's back bends, the head turns to fit through the narrowest parts of the passageway, and the soft bones of the baby's skull move together and overlap as it is squeezed through the pelvis. When the top of the head appears at the vaginal opening, the baby is said to be crowning.

As the head of the baby emerges, the physician or midwife will remove any mucus from the mouth and nose, wipe the baby's face, and check to ensure that the umbilical cord is not around the neck. With a few more contractions, the baby's shoulders and body emerge. As the baby is squeezed through the pelvis, cervix, and vagina,

The number of **cesarean sections** performed in the United States has risen dramatically in the past 30 years, causing concern among both parents and medical personnel. In 1970, 5.5 percent of American babies were delivered by cesarean section; today, nearly one out of every four babies—close to 25 percent—is delivered by cesarean. Yet according to national health statistics, there is no clear evidence that maternal and child health has improved as a result of this increase. Why are babies delivered by cesarean section, and why is the number of such operations increasing? What can be done to lower the rate of cesarean deliveries in the United States?

Cesarean sections are necessary when a baby can't be delivered vaginally. If the baby's head is bigger than the pelvic girdle of the mother, the baby may need to be delivered by cesarean. If the baby is in an unusual position—feet down, buttocks down, or lying sideways across the uterus—instead of in the usual head-down position, vaginal birth is more difficult. If the mother has a serious health condition such as kidney or heart disease, diabetes, high blood pressure, or toxemia, she may need to have a cesarean to avoid the stress of a long labor and a vaginal delivery. Sometimes a woman is unable to sustain labor, and a physician may perform a cesarean to reduce the risk of infection to the newborn. If a woman has an active vaginal herpes infection, a cesarean is performed to protect the baby from becoming infected. Other reasons for cesarean delivery include abnormal or difficult labor and fetal distress.

A substantial part of the increase in cesarean births is due to repeat cesarean deliveries. In the United States, fewer than about 10 percent of women who have had a cesarean in the past deliver subsequent babies vaginally; in other countries, the rate of vaginal birth after cesarean section is closer to 50 percent. The American College of Obstetricians and Gynecologists now recommends that low-risk women who have had one previous cesarean birth be encouraged to attempt labor and vaginal delivery in their current pregnancy.

Cesarean sections are major surgery and carry some risk themselves, although much less than in the past. Improved medical care—including better antibiotics and better use of anesthesia—make the procedure relatively safe. A local anesthetic may be used so the woman remains conscious during the operation. The father may be present in the delivery room during a cesarean. Advocates of increased reliance on cesareans claim that the procedure makes birth safer for mothers and babies in some situations. They point to reduced rates of maternal and neonatal mortality and the better health of newborns.

Critics of increased reliance on cesarean deliveries, including many physicians, believe that cesareans are often performed unnecessarily. They claim that American medical personnel don't manage labor very well and cannot always interpret signs of fetal distress or abnormal labor accurately. They suggest that cesareans are often performed more for the convenience of the physician than out of consideration for the mother's or baby's health. They point to studies that indicate that cesareans carry a risk of maternal death 2 to 26 times higher than that of vaginal delivery. And they note that other countries with rates of maternal and infant death as low as those in the United States have much lower rates of cesarean section.

The U.S. Department of Health and Human Services has set a goal for reducing the rate of cesarean delivery to no more than 15 percent by the year 2000. Several strategies have been suggested to help lower this rate.

- *Addressing malpractice concerns.* Physicians may perform cesareans because they are afraid of being sued if something goes wrong.

- *Eliminating financial incentives for physicians and hospitals.* Cesareans are more lucrative than vaginal deliveries. Statistics indicate that for-profit hospitals have higher rates of cesarean section than nonprofit hospitals. In addition, a woman with private insurance is more likely to have a cesarean than is a woman who is without insurance or covered by Medicaid. Reimbursing vaginal and cesarean deliveries equally would eliminate any financial incentive.

- *Publishing cesarean delivery rates of individual physicians and hospitals.* Increasing public awareness would alert people to differences in practice and allow them to make informed choices about practitioners.

- *Increasing training in normal labor and vaginal deliveries.* Current training tends to emphasize high-risk care and the reliance on advanced technological devices to assess and manage labor. Older, more experienced physicians perform significantly fewer cesarean sections for difficult labor and unusual fetal position. The use of secondary tests to confirm a diagnosis of fetal distress based on electronic fetal monitoring has also been shown to lower rates of cesarean delivery.

the fluid in the lungs is forced out by the pressure on the baby's chest. Once this pressure is released as the baby emerges from the vagina, the chest expands and the lungs fill with air for the first time. The baby will still be connected to the mother via the umbilical cord, which is not cut until it stops pulsating. The baby will appear wet and often is covered with a milky substance. The baby's head may be oddly shaped at first, due to the molding of the soft plates of bone during birth, but it usually takes on a normal appearance within 24 hours.

In the third stage of labor, the uterus continues to contract until the placenta is delivered. This stage usually takes 5 to 20 minutes. If the placenta does not come out on its own, the physician or midwife may exert gentle pressure on the abdomen to help with its delivery. It is important that the entire placenta be expelled; if part remains in the uterus, it may cause infection or bleeding. Breastfeeding soon after delivery helps control uterine bleeding because it stimulates the secretion of a hormone that makes the uterus contract; massaging the abdomen may also help. (It usually takes 6 or 8 weeks for a woman's reproductive organs to return to their prebirth condition.)

In the meantime, the physical condition of the baby will be assessed: Heart rate, respiration, color, reflexes, and muscle tone are individually rated with a score of 0 to 2. The total, called an **Apgar score,** will be at least 7 if the child is healthy. The baby is then usually wrapped tightly in a blanket and returned to the mother, who may begin to nurse the baby right away.

> *Personal Insight*   If you are a woman and want to have a child, what kind of birth experience do you want to have? If you are a man, do you want to participate and have a role in your partner's birth experience, or would you rather just leave it to her? Where do you think your ideas come from?

The Postpartum Period

The three or so months following childbirth are considered the **postpartum period,** a time of critical family adjustments. Parenthood—a job that goes on around the clock—occurs literally overnight, and the transition can cause considerable physical and emotional stress.

Lactation—the production of milk—begins about three days after childbirth. Prior to that time (sometimes as early as the second trimester), a yellowish liquid called colostrum is secreted by the nipples. Colostrum contains antibodies that help protect the newborn from infectious diseases and is also high in protein. The American Academy of Pediatricians recommends breastfeeding for a baby's first six months. In general, breastfeeding is pre-

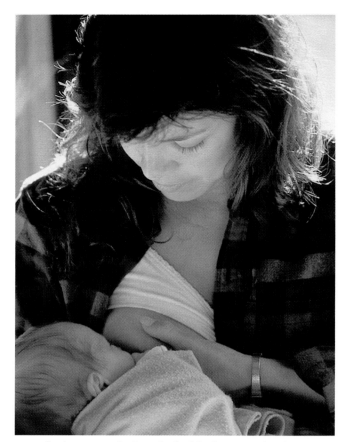

Breastfeeding is an ideal method of feeding an infant because the mother's milk contains antibodies against disease and is perfectly suited to the baby's nutritional needs. But women who choose bottlefeeding can still experience the physical contact and emotional closeness that are such an important part of the parent-child relationship.

ferred to bottlefeeding because human milk is perfectly suited to the baby's nutritional needs and digestive capabilities and because it supplies the baby with antibodies. Breastfeeding is also beneficial to the mother, because it stimulates contractions that help the uterus return to normal more rapidly. It may also contribute to weight loss after pregnancy. Nursing also provides a sense of closeness and emotional well-being for mother and child. For women who want to breastfeed but who have problems, help is available from support groups, books, or a lactation consultant.

For some women, physical problems such as tenderness or infection of the nipples can make breastfeeding difficult. If a woman has an illness or requires drug treatment, she may have to bottlefeed her baby because drugs and infectious agents may show up in breast milk. Some parents choose bottlefeeding because breastfeeding can be restrictive—mothers may not be able to leave the baby for more than a few hours at a time. Companies rarely provide part-time employment or nursing breaks for their female employees, so bottlefeeding or the use of a breast pump (to express milk for use while the mother is away from her infant) may be the only practical alternatives. Bottlefeeding makes it easier to tell how much milk an infant is taking in and bottlefed infants tend to sleep longer. Bottlefeeding also allows the father or other caregiver to share in the nurturing process. Both breastfeeding and bottlefeeding can be part of loving, secure parent-child relationships.

Many women experience fluctuating emotions during the postpartum period as hormone levels change. The physical stress of labor, as well as dehydration, blood loss, and other physical factors, contribute to lowering the woman's stamina. About 50–80 percent of new mothers experience "baby blues," characterized by episodes of sadness, weeping, anxiety, headache, sleep disorders, or irritability. She may feel lonely and anxious about caring for her infant. About 10 percent of new mothers experience **postpartum depression,** a more disabling syndrome characterized by despondency, mood swings, guilt, and occasional hostility. Rest, sharing feelings and concerns with others, and relying on supportive relatives and friends for assistance are usually helpful in dealing with mild cases of the baby blues or postpartum depression, which generally lasts only a few weeks. If the depression is serious, professional treatment may be needed. Some men also seem to get a form of postpartum depression, characterized by anxiety about their changing roles and feelings of inadequacy. Both mothers and fathers need time to adjust to their new roles as parents.

SUMMARY

Sexual Anatomy and Hormones

- Female external sex organs are called the vulva; the clitoris plays an important role in sexual arousal and orgasm. The vagina leads to the internal sex organs, including the uterus, oviducts, and ovaries.

- Male external sex organs are the penis and the scrotum; the glans penis is an important source of sexual arousal. Internal sexual structures include the testes, vasa deferentia, seminal vesicles, and prostate gland.

- The testes and adrenal glands produce androgens; the ovaries produce estrogens and progestins.

- Hormones initiate the changes that occur during puberty: The reproductive system matures, secondary sexual characteristics develop, and the bodies of males and females become more distinctive.

- The menstrual cycle is divided into four phases: menstruation, the estrogenic phase, ovulation, and the progestational phase.

- Ovaries cease to function as women approach 50, and they enter menopause. The pattern of male sexual responses changes with age, and testosterone production gradually decreases.

Sexual Functioning

- Sexual activity consists of a stimulus and a response. Stimulation may be physical or psychological.

- Vasocongestion and myotonia are the primary physiological mechanisms of sexual response.

- The sexual response cycle has four stages: excitement, plateau, orgasm, and resolution. Specific genital changes accompany each stage, as do more general body reactions.

- Sexual disorders include vaginitis, endometriosis, and pelvic inflammatory disease in women and prostatitis and testicular cancer in men.

- In men, dysfunctions include erectile dysfunction, premature ejaculation, and retarded ejaculation. Dysfunction in women includes vaginismus and orgasmic dysfunction.

- Treatment for sexual dysfunction first addresses any underlying medical conditions and then looks at psychosocial problems.

Sexual Behavior

- Developing the capacity for intimacy is an important task of young adults.

- Human sexual behaviors include celibacy, erotic fantasy, masturbation, touching, cunnilingus, fellatio, anal intercourse, and coitus.

- Sexual harassment is sexual pressuring of someone in a vulnerable position.

- Rape victims suffer both physical and psychological pain. Most rape victims are women and most know their attackers.

- Responsible sexuality includes open, honest communication about intentions; sexual activities both partners agree upon; the use of contraception; safe sex practices; and taking responsibility for the consequences of sexual behavior.

Understanding Fertility

- Fertilization is a complex process culminating when a sperm penetrates the membrane of the egg released from the woman's ovary.

- Infertility affects about 1 out of every 13 American couples. Surgery and drugs can cure some problems; more advanced techniques include in vitro fertilization and artificial insemination.

- One way to avoid some forms of infertility is to protect oneself against STDs and to get treatment for any disease contracted.

Pregnancy

- Pregnancy is usually divided into trimesters based on fetal development.

- Early signs and symptoms include a missed menstrual period; slight bleeding; nausea; breast tenderness; sleepiness, fatigue, and emotional upset; and a softening of the uterus just above the cervix.

- During pregnancy, the uterus enlarges until it pushes up into the rib cage; the breasts enlarge and may secrete colostrum; the muscles and ligaments soften and stretch; and the circulatory system, lungs, and kidneys become more efficient.

- The fetal anatomy is almost completely formed in the first trimester and is refined in the second; needed fats and pounds are added during the third trimester.

- Information about the health and sex of a fetus can be obtained through prenatal tests such as ultrasound, alpha-fetoprotein screening, amniocentesis, and chorionic villus sampling.

- Important elements of prenatal care include regular checkups; good nutrition; avoiding drugs, alcohol, tobacco, infections, and other harmful conditions; regular physical activity; and childbirth classes.

- Pregnancy usually proceeds without major complications. Problems that can occur include ectopic pregnancy, spontaneous abortion, toxemia, and low birth weight.

Childbirth

- The first stage of labor begins with contractions that exert pressure on the cervix, causing effacement and dilation. The period of transition is characterized by frequent and intense contractions.

- The second stage of labor begins when the cervix is dilated to about 10 centimeters. The baby is pushed down into the vagina, and the mother bears down until the baby emerges.

- The third stage of labor is delivery of the placenta. The umbilical cord is cut and the baby takes its first breath.

- During the postpartum period, the mother's body begins to return to its prepregnancy state, and she may begin to breastfeed.

TAKE ACTION

1. There are many reputable self-help books about sexual functioning available in libraries and bookstores. If you're not satisfied with your level of knowledge and understanding, do some reading.

2. Investigate the resources on campus and in your community that deal with acquaintance rape. Are any education programs offered to help prevent acquaintance rape? What types of services are available for victims of acquaintance rape?

3. Interview your parents to find out what your birth was like. What were the cultural conditions like at the time, and what were their personal preferences? Find out as much as you can about hospital procedure, use of anesthesia, length of hospital stay, and so on. Did your father have a role in your birth? If possible, interview your grandparents or someone of their generation. How was their experience different from your parents'?

4. Investigate the childbirth facilities in your community. If possible, visit the maternity wing of a hospital and an alternative birth center. What do you like about them, and what do you not like? What types of childbirth preparation classes do they offer? Which of these do you feel most comfortable with and why?

JOURNAL ENTRY

1. Sexual myths and misconceptions are common in our culture. In your health journal, make a list of statements about sexuality that you've heard but are not sure are accurate. Find out the facts by consulting resources mentioned here or available through your school health center or library.

2. *Critical Thinking:* Many states have laws prohibiting certain sexual behaviors. How much control do you think society should have over an individual's sexual practices? What types of behaviors do you think should be regulated and why? What behaviors should be left up to the discretion of the individual? Write an essay outlining your position.

3. *Critical Thinking:* There have been many legal cases involving the status of sperm or embryos frozen as part of an infertility treatment such as artificial insemination or in vitro fertilization. Research one or more of these cases and write an essay outlining some of the moral and legal implications of this technology. What guidelines would you suggest for regulating the use and status of frozen sperm and embryos? What evidence can you give to support your position?

SELECTED BIBLIOGRAPHY

American Academy of Pediatrics. 1989. Report of the task force on circumcision. *Pediatrics* 84:388–91.

American College of Obstetricians and Gynecologists. 1985. *Exercise During Pregnancy and the Postnatal Period (ACOG Home Exercise Programs)*. Washington, D.C.: ACOG.

AZT Limits Spread of HIV to Fetuses. 1994. *San Francisco Chronicle*, 21 February.

Carroll, J. 1990. Tracing the causes of infertility. *San Francisco Chronicle*, 5 March.

Chuong, C., and W. Gibbons. 1990. Premenstrual syndrome: Update on therapy. *Medical Aspects of Human Sexuality* 24:58–66.

Gray, M. J., and others. 1991. *The Woman's Guide to Good Health*. Yonkers, N.Y.: Consumers Union.

Hatcher, R. A., and others. 1994. *Contraceptive Technology*. New York: Irvington.

Hilts, P. 1990. Growing concern over pelvic infection in women. *New York Times*, 11 October.

Laumann, E., J. Gagnon, R. Michael, and S. Michaels. 1994. *The Social Organization of Sexuality: Sexual Practices in the United States*. Chicago: University of Chicago Press.

Laurent, S. L., and others. 1992. An epidemiologic study of smoking and primary infertility in women. *Fertility and Sterility* 57(3): 565–72.

Lizza, E., and R. Cricco-Lizza. 1990. Impotence—Finding the cause. *Medical Aspects of Human Sexuality* 24:30–40.

Masters, W. H., and V. E. Johnson. 1986. *Human Sexual Response*. Boston: Little, Brown.

Morales, K., and C. B. Inlander. 1991. *Take This Book to the Obstetrician with You: A Consumer's Guide to Pregnancy and Childbirth*. Reading, Mass.: Addison-Wesley.

Mueller, B. A., and others. 1992. Risk factors for tubal infertility: Influence of history of prior pelvic inflammatory disease. *Sexually Transmitted Diseases* 19(1): 28–34.

Myers, S. A., and N. Gleicher. 1988. A successful program to lower cesarean-section rates. *New England Journal of Medicine* 319(23): 1511–16.

Notzon, F. C. 1990. International differences in the use of obstetric interventions. *Journal of the American Medical Association* 263(24): 3286–91.

Olshansky, E. F. 1992. Redefining the concepts of success and failure in infertility treatment. *Naacogs Clinical Issues in Perinatal and Women's Health Nursing* 3(2): 343–46.

Our Vitamin Prescription: The Big Four. 1994. *University of California at Berkeley Wellness Letter*, January.

Pear, R. 1992. The U.S. reports rise in low-weight births. *New York Times*, 22 April.

Schickedanz, J., and others. 1993. *Understanding Children*. 2nd ed. Mountain View, Calif.: Mayfield.

Stafford, R. S. 1991. The impact of nonclinical factors on repeat cesarean section. *Journal of the American Medical Association* 265(1): 59–63.

Weiss, P. 1992. The bond of mother's milk. *San Jose Mercury News*, 18 August, 1–2E.

Wilson, C., and W. Kaye. 1992. Premenstrual syndrome. In *Pediatric and Adolescent Gynecology*, ed. S. Carpenter and A. Rock. New York: Raven Press.

Ziporyn, T. 1992. Postpartum depression: True blue? *Harvard Health Letter*, February.

RECOMMENDED READINGS

Boston Women's Health Book Collective. 1992. *The New Our Bodies, Ourselves*. New York: Simon and Schuster. *A very readable book concerned with all aspects of female sexuality.*

Denney, N., and D. Quadagno. 1992. *Human Sexuality*. 2nd ed. St. Louis: Times-Mirror Mosby. *A human sexuality textbook with a complete discussion of all of the biological aspects of human sexuality that are presented in this chapter.*

Dunham, C. (The Body Shop Staff). 1992. *Mamototo: A Celebration of Birth*. New York: Viking Penguin. *An exploration of childbirth in many cultures using text and photos.*

Eisenberg, A., and others. 1991. *What to Expect While You're Expecting*. Rev. 2nd ed. New York: Workman. *A highly readable guide to pregnancy, childbirth, and the postpartum period.*

Janus, S., and C. Janus. 1993. *The Janus Report on Sexual Behavior*. New York: John Wiley and Sons. *An excellent sexual survey that is easy to read and full of fascinating insights on sexual behaviors and attitudes in the 1990s.*

Michael, R., J. Gagnon, E. Laumann, and G. Kolata. 1994. *Sex in America: A Definitive Survey*. Boston: Little, Brown. *Based on recent research and written for the general public, this book contains a wealth of information about the sex lives of Americans.*

Nilsson, L., and L. Hamberger. 1990. *A Child Is Born*. New York: Delacorte/Seymour Lawrence. *The story of birth, beginning with fertilization, told in stunning photographs with additional text.*

Rosenberg, H. S., and Y. M. Epstein. 1993. *Getting Pregnant When You Thought You Couldn't*. New York: Warner Books. *A useful, sensitive resource for infertile couples.*

Sears, W., and M. Sears. 1994. *The Birth Book: Everything You Need to Know to Have a Safe and Satisfying Birth*. Boston: Little, Brown. *A practical guide to many aspects of childbirth, including preparation for labor and the use of technology.*

Sherokee, I. 1990. *Empty Arms: Coping After Miscarriage, Stillbirth, and Infant Death*. Maple Plain, Miss.: Wintergreen. *A sensitive guide to dealing with the grief involved in miscarriages, stillbirths, and infant deaths.*

Strong, B., C. DeVault, and B. Sayad. 1996. *Core Concepts in Human Sexuality*. Mountain View, Calif.: Mayfield. *A comprehensive introduction to human sexuality with special emphasis on sexual wellness.*

6

Contraception and Abortion: Current Issues

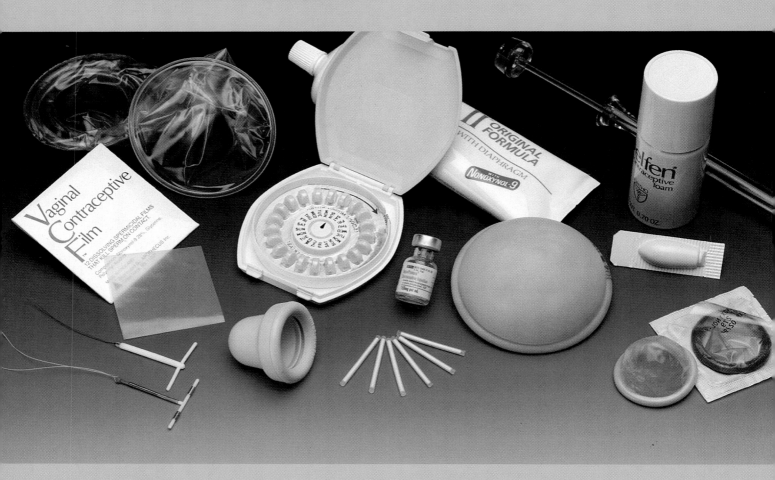

CONTENTS

In her lifetime, the ovaries of an average woman release over 400 eggs, one a month for about three and a half decades. Each is capable of developing into a human being if fertilized by one of the millions of sperm a man produces in every ejaculate. Furthermore, unlike most other mammals, human beings are capable of sexual activity at any time of the month or year. These facts help explain why people have always had a compelling interest in controlling fertility and in preventing unwanted pregnancies.

Today, people have many choices when they're making decisions about sexual and contraceptive behavior. And because the prevention of unintended pregnancies and **sexually transmissible diseases (STDs)** is such a crucial element in lifelong health and well-being, these decisions are among the most significant people can make.

PRINCIPLES OF CONTRACEPTION

The underlying principle of **contraceptives** used today is to block the female's ovum (egg) from uniting with the male's sperm (**conception**), thereby preventing pregnancy. A variety of approaches has proven effective in preventing conception; these approaches are based on different principles of birth control. Barrier methods work by physically blocking the sperm from reaching the egg. Diaphragms, condoms, and several other methods are based on this principle. Hormonal methods alter the biochemistry of the woman's body, preventing ovulation and producing changes that make it more difficult for the sperm to reach the egg if ovulation does occur. Birth control pills operate on this principle. A variety of so-called natural methods of contraception are based on the fact that egg and sperm have to be present at the same time if fertilization is to occur. Finally, surgical methods—female and male sterilization—more or less permanently prevent transport of the sperm or eggs to the site of potential conception.

All the contraceptive methods have advantages and disadvantages that make them appropriate for some people but not for others or at one period of life but not at another. Factors that affect the choice of method include effectiveness, convenience, cost, reversibility, side effects and risk factors, and protection against STDs.

Effectiveness, one of the factors listed above, requires further explanation. Contraceptive effectiveness is partly determined by the reliability of the method itself—the failure rate if it were always used exactly as directed. This rate cannot be accurately measured, but it can be inferred from studying the most successful users. Effectiveness is also determined by characteristics of the user, including fertility of the individual, frequency of intercourse, and, more importantly, how consistently and correctly the method is used. Because the "method" and "user" variables are difficult to separate out, one overall failure rate reflecting all variables is generally used. This **contracep-**

tive failure rate is based on studies that directly measure the percentage of women experiencing an accidental pregnancy in the first year of contraceptive use. Another measure of effectiveness is provided by the **continuation rate**—the percentage of people who continue to use the method after a specified period of time. This measure is important because many unintended pregnancies occur when a method is stopped and not immediately replaced with another. Thus, a contraceptive with a high continuation rate would be more effective at preventing pregnancy than one with a low continuation rate.

We turn now to a description of the various contraceptive methods, discussing first those that are reversible and then those that are permanent.

REVERSIBLE CONTRACEPTIVES

Reversibility is an extremely important consideration for young adults when they choose a contraceptive method, since most people either plan to have children or at least want to keep their options open until they're older. In this section we discuss the reversible contraceptives, beginning with the hormonal methods, then moving to the barrier methods, and finally covering the natural methods.

Oral Contraceptives—The Pill

During pregnancy, the **corpus luteum** secretes **progesterone** and **estrogen** in amounts high enough to suppress **ovulation**. **Oral contraceptives** (OCs), or birth control pills, prevent ovulation by mimicking the hormonal ac-

---

Sexually transmissible diseases (STD) Any of several contagious diseases such as chlamydia and gonorrhea contracted through intimate sexual contact.

Contraceptive Any agent that can prevent conception. Condoms, diaphragms, intrauterine devices, and oral contraceptives are examples.

Conception The fusion of ovum and sperm, resulting in a zygote (fertilized egg).

Contraceptive failure rate The percentage of women using a particular contraceptive method who experience an accidental pregnancy in the first year of use.

Continuation rate The percentage of women who continue to use a particular contraceptive after a specified period of time.

Corpus luteum A gland in the ovary that forms after ovulation; secretes progesterone. If the ovum is not fertilized, the corpus luteum degenerates each month, which causes the shedding of the uterine lining (menstruation).

Progesterone A hormone produced by the corpus luteum and, during pregnancy, by the placenta. Used in oral contraceptives to prevent ovulation.

Estrogen A hormone produced by the ovaries. An active ingredient in birth control pills.

Ovulation The release of the egg (ovum) from the ovaries.

TERMS

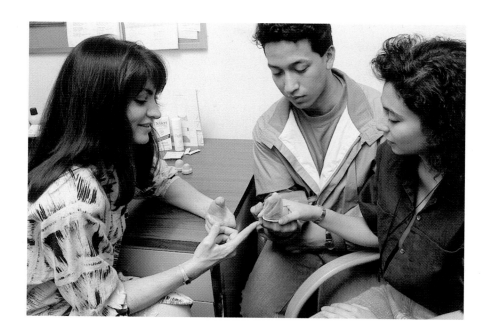

To be effective, contraceptives should be used in exactly the right way. A careful explanation by a health care professional will help this couple use the method they've chosen more effectively.

tivity of the corpus luteum. The active ingredients in OCs are estrogen and progestins, laboratory-made compounds that are closely related to progesterone.

In addition to preventing ovulation, the birth control pill has other backup contraceptive effects. It hampers the movement of sperm by thickening the cervical mucus, alters the rate of ovum transport by means of its hormonal effects on the oviducts, and may inhibit implantation by changing the lining of the uterus, in the unlikely event that a fertilized ovum reaches that area.

Today, the birth control pill is the most widely used form of contraception among unmarried women and is second only to sterilization among married women. The most common type of pill is the combination pill. Each one-month packet contains three weeks of pills that combine varying types and amounts of estrogen and progesterone. Most packets also include one week of inactive pills; others instruct the woman to simply take no pills at all for one week before starting the next cycle. During the week in which no hormones are taken, a light menstrual period occurs. The overall trend has been toward lower-dose pills, which offer the same high effectiveness rate with fewer unwanted side effects.

Advantages   The main advantage of the oral contraceptive is its high degree of effectiveness in preventing pregnancy. Nearly all unplanned pregnancies result because the user did not take the pill as directed. The pill is rela-

tively simple to use and does not require any interruptions that could hinder sexual spontaneity. Most women also enjoy the predictable regularity of periods, as well as the decrease in cramps and blood loss. For young women, its reversibility is especially important; fertility (ability to reproduce) returns after the pill is discontinued, although not always immediately. The medical advantages include a decreased incidence of benign breast disease, iron-deficiency anemia, pelvic inflammatory disease (PID), ectopic pregnancy, endometrial cancer (of the lining of the uterus), and ovarian cancer.

Disadvantages   Although oral contraceptives do lower the risk of pelvic inflammatory disease, they do not protect against HIV infection or other STDs in the lower reproductive tract. OCs have been associated with increased cervical chlamydia. Regular condom use is recommended for an OC user unless she is in a long-term, mutually monogamous relationship with an uninfected partner.

Oral contraceptives can cause a variety of minor side effects, including nausea, weight gain, and swollen breasts during the first few months of use. Serious side effects of pill use have been reported in a small number of women. These include blood clots, stroke, and heart attack, concentrated mostly in older women who smoke or have a history of circulatory disease. Pill users also show a slight increase in the incidence of high blood pressure, which is usually quickly reversed on discontinuation of the pill, and of benign liver tumors.

Some studies have shown an increased risk of cervical cancer for oral contraceptive users, a risk that may rise with increased duration of OC use. Other behaviors linked to cervical cancer include sexual relationships at an early age, sexual relationships with many partners, and

TERMS   **Oral contraceptive (OC)**   Any of various hormone compounds in pill form taken by mouth. Oral contraceptives prevent conception by preventing ovulation.

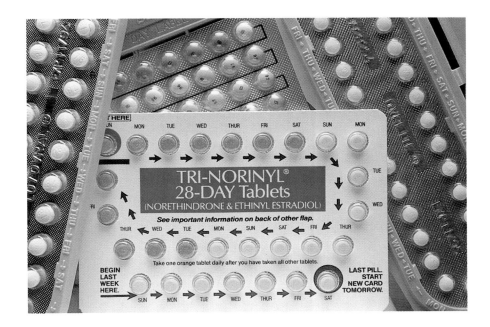

Oral contraceptives are the most popular reversible method of birth control among American women. When used correctly, oral contraceptives are highly effective.

smoking. Regular Pap smears for the detection of early cervical changes are especially important in pill users. Also, because other temporary cervical changes found in some women on OCs may contribute to an increased susceptibility to the STDs chlamydia and gonorrhea, regular screening for those diseases is also recommended, especially when condoms aren't being used.

In trying to decide whether to use oral contraceptives, each woman needs to weigh the benefits against the risks. To make an informed decision, she should seek the help of a health care professional in evaluating the risk variables that are known and that apply to her. A woman can take a number of steps to lower her risk from OC use:

- Request a low-dosage pill.
- Stop smoking.
- Follow the pill-taking instructions carefully and consistently.
- Be alert to preliminary danger signals (severe headaches, problems with vision, severe pain in the abdomen, chest, or legs).
- Have regular checkups of her blood pressure, weight, and urine and have an annual examination of the thyroid, breasts, abdomen, and pelvis.

For most women, the known, directly associated risk of death from use of the pill is much lower than the risk of death from pregnancy.

Effectiveness As explained earlier, the effectiveness of a contraceptive is determined by user failures as well as true method failures. Therefore, the commonly used figures represent the failure rate experienced by average people under average circumstances; they include pregnancies that result from erratic pill taking, as well as those that occur when a woman stops taking pills and she and her partner fail to use another method of contraception. A typical first-year failure rate is 3 percent. The continuation rate for OCs averages 72 percent after one year.

Norplant Implants

A contraceptive implant, another method of hormonal birth control for women, was approved by the FDA and is becoming widely available in the United States. Norplant and other similar implants have been used for more than a decade in various countries, including several in South America, Asia, and Scandinavia.

Norplant consists of six flexible, matchstick-sized capsules, each containing progestin, a synthetic progesterone, released in steady doses for up to five years. The capsules are placed under the skin, usually on the inside of a woman's upper arm in a fan-shaped configuration. The procedure can be done in less than 15 minutes, with a local anesthetic and only one very small incision. No stitches are required.

The progestin in Norplant has several contraceptive effects: Hormonal shifts may inhibit ovulation and affect development of the uterine lining; thickening of cervical mucus hampers the movement of sperm; and transport of the egg through the tubes may be slowed down. This method seems especially suited for women who wish to have continuous and long-term protection against pregnancy.

Advantages Norplant is the most effective reversible method of contraception now available. After insertion of the implants, no further action is required for up to five years of protection; at the same time, contraceptive effects are quickly reversed upon removal. Because Norplant,

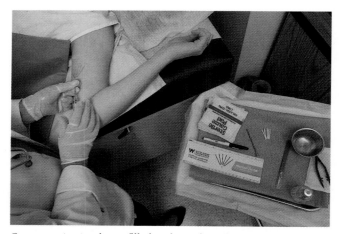

Contraceptive implants, filled with synthetic hormones and inserted under the skin on the arm or leg, can provide five years of protection against pregnancy.

unlike the combination pill, contains no estrogen, it carries a lower risk of certain side effects, such as blood clots and other cardiovascular complications, and has fewer contraindications. The thickened cervical mucus resulting from Norplant use has a protective effect against PID.

Disadvantages   Although the implants are barely visible, their appearance may be bothersome to some women. The initial cost of Norplant can be high. Removal is sometimes difficult, especially if insertion of the implants is deep. Both insertion and removal of implants are procedures that can be done only by specially trained practitioners.

The most common side effects of Norplant use are menstrual irregularities, including longer menstrual periods, spotting between periods, or having no bleeding at all. The menstrual cycle usually becomes more regular after one year of use. The more serious health concerns are similar to those associated with the oral contraceptive, but they are less common with Norplant. As with the pill, Norplant gives no protection against HIV infection and other STDs of the lower reproductive tract.

Effectiveness   Typical failure rates are very low (0.09 percent) in the first year of use, increasing slowly with each additional year of use. The cumulative failure rate at the end of five years of use is about 3.7 percent. Some studies have shown slightly higher failure rates for women who weigh more than 154 pounds. A key factor contributing to Norplant's high effectiveness is its steady release of progestin, allowing for a fairly constant hormone level. The continuation rate after one year of use is about 85 percent.

Depo-Provera Injections

A contraceptive injection utilizing a long-acting progestin is available in the United States under the name Depo-

Provera. Injected in the arm or buttocks, Depo-Provera is usually given every 12 weeks. As another progestin-only contraceptive, it prevents pregnancy in the same ways as Norplant.

Advantages   The advantages of Depo-Provera are similar to those of Norplant: It is highly effective, requires little action on the part of the user, and has no estrogen-related side effects. In addition, Depo-Provera requires only periodic injections, rather than the minor surgical procedures of implant insertion and removal. Because the injections leave no trace and involve no ongoing supplies, they allow women almost total privacy in their decision to use contraception.

Disadvantages   Users of Depo-Provera must visit a health care facility every three months to receive the injections. Its side effects and contraindications are similar to those associated with Norplant use. After discontinuing use of Depo-Provera, women often experience temporary infertility for up to 12 months. Depo-Provera gives no protection against HIV infection and other STDs.

Effectiveness   Typical failure rates reported with Depo-Provera have been 0.3 percent.

The Postcoital Pill for Emergency Contraception

A much less commonly used hormonal method of contraception is the "morning after" or postcoital pill. Postcoital contraceptives work primarily by preventing uterine implantation of a fertilized egg, should one be present.

The postcoital pill most often used today is a combination of estrogen and progesterone. It has been approved in western Europe for emergency situations such as rape. This same pill, although approved by the FDA as a prescription drug for other uses, has not been approved specifically for postcoital purposes in the United States. Studies regarding effectiveness have reported a wide range of results. One overall analysis of the data concludes that the expected risk of pregnancy is reduced by more than 75 percent.

The Intrauterine Device (IUD)

The **intrauterine device (IUD)** is a plastic device that is placed in the uterus as a contraceptive. IUD use has declined since the 1970s, mostly due to the publicity about the increased risk of serious infections associated with the popular Dalkon Shield and its withdrawal from the market. Today, only two IUDs are available in the United States: the hormone-releasing Progestasert, which requires replacement every year, and the newer Copper T-380A (also known as the ParaGard), which gives protection for up to eight years. A third, the Levonorgestral IUD, may be approved for use in the near future.

No one knows exactly how IUDs work. They may cause biochemical changes in the uterus, such as the production of specific cells that destroy the egg and/or sperm; they may immobilize sperm in the uterus or shorten the normal travel time of the egg in the fallopian tube; or they may interfere with the implantation of eggs in the uterus.

Advantages   Intrauterine devices are highly reliable and are simple and convenient to use, requiring no attention except for a periodic check of the threads that are attached to the device and normally extend 1 to 1½ inches into the upper vagina. In the absence of complications, their effects are considered fully reversible. In most cases fertility resumes as soon as the IUD is removed.

Disadvantages   By far the most common complaint is abnormal menstrual bleeding. The menstrual flow tends to appear sooner, last longer, and become heavier after insertion of an IUD. Bleeding and spotting between periods may also occur. Another common complaint is pain, particularly uterine cramps and backache, side effects that seem to occur most often in women who have never been pregnant.

Spontaneous expulsion of the IUD happens in 5 to 10 percent of all users within the first year after insertion, most commonly during the first months after insertion. For this reason, it is important to check occasionally that the device is in place by locating the threads.

A serious complication sometimes associated with IUD use is **pelvic inflammatory disease (PID)**. Most pelvic infections among IUD users are relatively mild and can be treated successfully with antibiotics. However, early and adequate treatment is critical, for a smoldering infection can lead to tubal scarring and subsequent infertility.

IUDs should be removed only by a trained professional. Most physicians advise against the use of IUDs by young women who have never been pregnant. Early IUD danger signals that the user should be alert to are abdominal pain, fever, chills, foul vaginal discharge, irregular menstrual periods, and other unusual vaginal bleeding. An annual checkup is important.

Effectiveness   The typical failure rate of IUDs during the first year of use is 1 to 2 percent. Many of these pregnancies are due to undetected partial or complete expulsion of the device. The continuation rate of IUDs is about 80 percent after one year of use.

Male Condoms

The **male condom** is a thin sheath, usually made of latex, designed to cover the penis during sexual intercourse. It prevents sperm from entering the vagina and provides protection against disease. Condoms are the most widely used **barrier method** and the third most popular of all birth control methods used in the United States, exceeded only by the pill and sterilization.

Sales of condoms have increased dramatically in recent years, primarily because condom use provides some protection against all STDs and is the only method that gives substantial protection against HIV infection. At least one-third of all male condoms are bought by women. This figure will probably increase as more women become aware of the serious risks associated with STDs and assume the right to insist on condom use. Women are more likely to contract an STD from an infected partner than vice versa. Women also face additional health risks from STDs, including cervical cancer, pelvic inflammatory disease, ectopic pregnancy (which is potentially life-threatening), and tubal infertility.

The user or his partner must put the condom on the penis before it is inserted into the vagina, because the small amounts of fluid that may be secreted unnoticed prior to **ejaculation** often contain sperm capable of causing pregnancy. The rolled-up condom is placed over the head of the erect penis and unrolled down to the base of the penis, leaving a half-inch space (without air) at the tip to collect semen. Some brands of condoms have a reservoir tip designed for this purpose. If the user has not been circumcised, he must first pull back the foreskin of the penis. He and his partner must be careful not to damage the condom with fingernails, rings, or other rough objects. When the man loses his erection after ejaculating, the condom loses its tight fit. To avoid spilling semen, the condom must be held around the base of the penis as the penis is withdrawn.

Some condoms are sold already lubricated. If the users wish, they can lubricate their own condoms with contraceptive foam, creams, or jelly or water-based preparations. All products that contain mineral oil—including baby oil and Vaseline petroleum jelly—should never be used; studies have shown that they cause latex condoms to begin to disintegrate within 60 seconds, thereby markedly increasing their chances of breaking.

Prelubricated condoms are now available containing nonoxynol-9, the same spermicidal agent found in many of the contraceptive foams and creams that women use.

Worldwide, more than 40 million couples use male condoms for contraception. Two-thirds of them live in developed countries, with Japan accounting for about 25 percent of all condom sales. In the United States, women now purchase about 40 percent of all condoms sold. Condoms are recommended for a number of reasons:

- They are readily accessible and can be purchased without a prescription in drugstores, convenience stores, supermarkets, campus dormitories, student unions, hotels, and so on.

- They are relatively inexpensive compared with the pill, the IUD, and the diaphragm.

- They are moderately effective when used correctly as a contraceptive, especially in conjunction with spermicide. Effectiveness can be increased if condoms are combined with another method, such as the diaphragm.

- They help prevent the transmission of HIV infection and other STDs (latex condoms only). They are not 100 percent effective (only abstinence is), but careful and consistent use can improve your chances of avoiding disease.

- They may slow or reduce the development of cervical abnormalities that could lead to cancer.

Despite their growing popularity, many people, especially teenagers, continue to view the use of condoms as an intrusion into their sexual activity, interfering with spontaneity. This attitude—that intercourse must be spontaneous to be an expression of love—needs to be replaced with more practical and realistic ideas. Condoms don't have to interfere with sexual arousal or pleasure. They come in an array of styles, shapes, colors, thicknesses, and textures, and their use can be integrated into sexual activities before intercourse. Use them properly by following these guidelines:

- Buy latex. If you're allergic to rubber, try wearing a lambskin condom under a latex one.

- Buy fresh. Don't use it if it's more than a year old (most have a date stamped near the rim). Don't remove the condom from its individual sealed wrapper until you're ready to use it. Don't use it if it's gummy, dried out, or discolored.

- Store it right. Too much heat or cold can damage a condom. Don't leave it in your wallet longer than overnight.

- Practice. Condoms aren't hard to use, but practice helps. Take one out of its wrapper—examine it and stretch it to see how strong it is. Practice by yourself and with your partner.

- If you use a lubricant, choose one that is water-based, preferably one that also contains a spermicide.

- Use it right. Air bubbles and insufficient lubrication are the biggest reasons why condoms break. Use a new condom every time you have intercourse.

Adapted from San Francisco AIDS Foundation. 1994. *Just for Men.* San Francisco: Impact AIDS, Inc.; and Bernard Goldstein. 1989. "Condoms—On a Roll!" *Healthline,* August.

Since the **spermicide** kills many of the sperm soon after ejaculation, its addition may significantly decrease contraceptive failure associated with breakage and the spilling of semen. The use of spermicide can greatly increase the use effectiveness of a condom.

Advantages   Condoms are easy to purchase and are available without prescription or medical supervision. They are simple to use and allow increased male participation in contraception. Condoms are immediately and completely reversible and are free from most medical side effects. Rubber condoms (not the lambskin type) help to protect against STDs and related consequences. Except for abstinence, condoms offer the most reliable protection available against transmission of HIV infection.

Disadvantages   The two most nearly universal complaints about condoms are that they diminish sensation and interfere with spontaneity. Although some people find these drawbacks serious, others consider them only minor disadvantages.

Effectiveness   In actual use, the failure rate of condoms varies considerably. First-year rates among typical users average about 12 percent. At least some of these pregnancies happen because the condom is used carelessly. Some may also happen because of a break or a tear, which is estimated to occur one to two times in every 100 instances. Because heat destroys rubber, condoms should not be stored for long periods in a wallet or in the glove compartment of a car.

Personal Insight   How do you feel about buying contraceptives at the drugstore? About asking for a prescription contraceptive at your health clinic or from your physician? Why do you feel the way you do? Have your feelings changed as you've grown older?

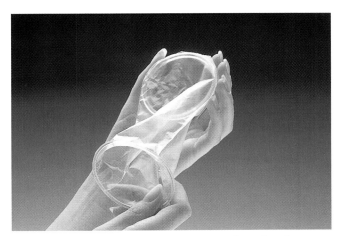

The Reality female condom is held in position by a closed ring placed at the cervix and an open ring that hangs outside the body.

Female Condoms

A female condom is a latex or polyurethane pouch that a woman or her partner inserts into her vagina. One brand, Reality, was approved in May 1993 for use in the United States. Reality consists of a soft, loose-fitting polyurethane sheath with two flexible rings. The directions that accompany it should be followed closely. The condom can be inserted up to 8 hours before intercourse and should be used with the supplied lubricant or a spermicide. Following intercourse, the user should remove the condom immediately, before standing up. By twisting and squeezing the outer ring, she can prevent spillage of semen.

Advantages   For many women, the greatest advantage of the female condom is the control it allows them to have over contraception and STD prevention. Female condoms can be inserted before intercourse and are thus less disruptive than male condoms. Because the outer part of the condom covers the area around the vaginal opening, it offers potentially better protection against some STDs. However, conclusive research is not yet available. Male condoms are still recommended as the safest protection against STDs.

Disadvantages   As with the traditional condom, interference with spontaneity is likely to be a common complaint. For many couples, initial awkwardness and difficulty is largely eliminated after a few weeks' use. Female condoms, like male condoms, are made for one-time use and cost about three times as much.

Effectiveness   The typical first year failure rate is 21 percent.

The Diaphragm with Spermicide

The **diaphragm** is a dome-shaped cup of thin rubber stretched over a collapsible metal ring. When correctly used with spermicidal cream or jelly, the diaphragm covers the cervix, blocking sperm from entering the uterus (Figure 6-1). A diaphragm must be carefully fitted to ensure that it will be both effective and comfortable, and only a trained person can make these adjustments. The fitting should be checked with each routine annual medical examination and after any change in health status.

The diaphragm must not be inserted more than six hours before intercourse. Additional cream or jelly should be inserted into the vagina before any additional act of coitus. The diaphragm must be left in place for at least six hours after the last act of coitus to give the spermicide enough time to kill all the sperm. The diaphragm should be washed and examined for holes or cracks after each use.

Advantages   Diaphragm use is less intrusive than condom use because a diaphragm can be inserted up to six hours before intercourse. Its use can be limited to times of sexual activity only, and it allows for immediate and total reversibility. The diaphragm is free of medical side effects (other than rare allergic reactions). When used along with spermicidal jelly or cream, it offers significant protection against gonorrhea and perhaps chlamydia. Diaphragm use can also protect the cervix from semen infected with the human papillomavirus, which has been implicated as an important factor in cellular changes in the cervix that can lead to cancer. However, the diaphragm is unlikely to protect against HIV infection, genital herpes, and syphilis.

Disadvantages   Diaphragms must always be used with a spermicide, and therefore a user must keep both of these somewhat bulky supplies with her whenever she anticipates sexual activity. Diaphragms require extra attention, since they must be cleaned and stored with care to preserve their effectiveness. Diaphragm use has also been associated with a slightly increased risk of **toxic shock syndrome (TSS)**, an occasionally fatal bacterial infection. To diminish the risk of TSS, women should wash their hands carefully with soap and water before inserting or removing the diaphragm, should not use the diaphragm during menstruation or whenever there is an

Spermicide   An agent that kills sperm.

Diaphragm   A contraceptive device consisting of a flexible, dome-shaped cup that covers the cervix. The diaphragm prevents sperm from entering the uterus.

Toxic shock syndrome (TSS)   A disease whose major symptoms include high fever, vomiting, diarrhea, headache, sore throat, and rash. Although primarily associated with menstruating women who use tampons, the disease has also been reported in men. It is usually caused by the bacterium *Staphylococcus aureus*. Mortality rate has decreased from 10–15 percent to 3 percent or less due to earlier recognition and treatment.

TERMS

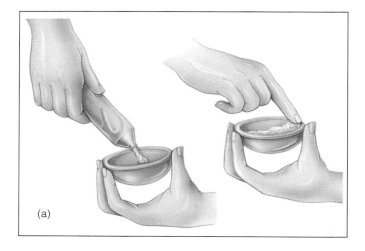

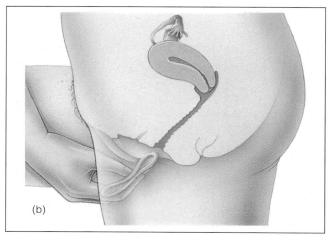

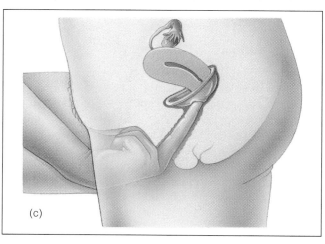

Figure 6-1 *Use of the diaphragm.*
(a) Place about one tablespoon of spermicidal jelly in the concave side of the diaphragm and spread it around the inside of the diaphragm and around the rim. (b) Press the diaphragm firmly between the thumb and forefinger and insert it in the vagina; push it along the back wall of the vagina as far as it will go. (c) Check the position of the diaphragm to make sure that the cervix is completely covered and that the front rim of the diaphragm is tucked behind the pubic bone.

abnormal discharge, and should never leave the device in place for more than 24 hours.

Effectiveness The effectiveness of the diaphragm is highly dependent on user factors, including proper insertion, consistent use, and accurate fitting. Typical failure rates for the diaphragm are 18 percent during the first year of use.

The Cervical Cap

The **cervical cap** is another barrier device. It consists of a thimble-shaped rubber or plastic cup that fits snugly over the cervix and is held in place by suction. The cap comes in various sizes and must be fitted by a trained clinician. It is used in a manner similar to the diaphragm, a small amount of spermicide being placed in the cup before each insertion.

Advantages Advantages of the cervical cap are similar to those associated with diaphragm use and include partial STD protection. In addition, it may be left in place for up to 48 hours, and it does not require reintroduction of spermicide with repeated intercourse.

Disadvantages Along with most of the disadvantages associated with the diaphragm, difficulty with insertion and removal is more common for cervical cap users. In addition, studies indicate that women who use the cap rather than the diaphragm initially have a higher rate of abnormal Pap smears. Because there may be a slightly increased risk of TSS with prolonged use, the cap should not be left in place more than 48 hours.

Effectiveness Cervical cap effectiveness is about 18 percent for women who have never had children and 36 percent for women who have given birth.

The Sponge

The contraceptive sponge, an over-the-counter alternative to the diaphragm and cervical cap, is no longer available. An FDA inspection found unacceptably high levels of bacteria in the water and air of the New Jersey plant where the sponges were made. Citing the time and cost involved in upgrading the plant, the manufacturer announced in January of 1995 that it was discontinuing the product. At that time, about 1.1 percent of women using contraception were using the sponge.

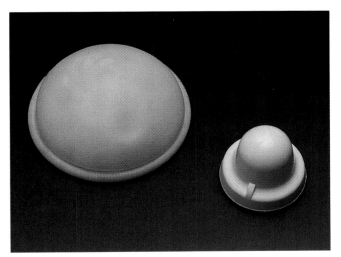

The diaphragm and cervical cap work by covering the mouth of the cervix, blocking sperm from entering the cervix. Both require professional fitting.

Vaginal Spermicides

In recent years spermicidal compounds developed for use with a diaphragm have been adapted for use without a diaphragm by combining them with a bulky base. Foams, creams, jellies, and vaginal suppositories are all available. Foams, creams, and jellies must be placed deep in the vagina near the cervical entrance and must not be inserted more than one-half hour before intercourse. Because body heat is needed to dissolve and activate suppositories, they should be inserted at least 10 minutes before intercourse. After an hour, their effectiveness is drastically reduced, and a new applicatorful must be inserted. Another application is also required before each repeated act of coitus. If the woman wants to **douche**, she should wait for at least eight hours after the last coitus to make sure that there has been time for the spermicide to kill all the sperm.

Advantages The use of vaginal spermicides is relatively simple and can be limited to times of sexual activity. They are readily available in most drugstores and do not require a prescription or a pelvic examination. Spermicides allow for complete and immediate reversibility. Vaginal spermicides may offer limited protection against some STDs, but should never be used instead of condoms for reliable protection, especially when there is a risk of HIV infection.

Disadvantages When used alone, vaginal spermicides must be inserted shortly before intercourse, so their use may be seen as an annoying disruption. Some women find the slight increase in vaginal fluids after spermicide use unpleasant. Spermicides can alter the balance of bacteria in the vagina and may increase the risk of urinary tract infections.

Effectiveness The reported effectiveness rates of vaginal spermicides cover a wide range, again depending partly on how consistently and carefully instructions are followed. The typical failure rate is about 21 percent during the first year of use.

Abstinence, Fertility Awareness, and Withdrawal

Millions of people throughout the world do not use any of the methods we have described. Either they will not because of religious conviction or cultural prohibitions or they cannot because of poverty or lack of information and supplies. If they use any method at all, they are likely to use one of the following relatively "natural" methods of attempting to prevent conception.

Abstinence The decision not to engage in sexual intercourse for a chosen period of time, or **abstinence**, has been followed by human beings throughout history for a variety of reasons. Until relatively recently, many people abstained because they had no other birth control measures. Today, with other methods available, about 5 percent of all American women who use birth control rely on periodic abstinence as a birth control method. Concern regarding possible side effects, STDs, and unwanted pregnancy may be factors. Intercourse may also be temporarily avoided because of medical reasons such as recent illness or surgery. In other cases, abstinence may be seen as the wisest choice in terms of personal emotional needs.

Fertility Awareness Method (FAM) The basis for **FAM** is abstinence from coitus during the fertile phase of a woman's menstrual cycle. Ordinarily only one egg is released by the ovaries per month, and it lives about 24

Cervical cap A thimble-shaped cup that fits over the cervix, to be used with spermicide.

Douche To apply a stream of water or other solutions to a body part or cavity such as the vagina; not a contraceptive technique.

Abstinence Avoidance of sexual intercourse. This is one method of birth control.

Fertility Awareness Method (FAM) A method of preventing conception based on avoiding coitus during the fertile phase of a woman's cycle.

TERMS

hours unless it is fertilized. Sperm deposited in the vagina are apparently on the average capable of fertilizing an egg for about six to seven days; so conception theoretically can only occur during eight days of any cycle. Predicting *which* eight days these are is difficult. It is done either by the calendar method or by the temperature method. Information on cyclical changes of the cervical mucus has also been helpful in determining the time of ovulation.

The *calendar method* is based on the knowledge that the average woman releases an egg 14 to 16 days before her next period begins. Few women menstruate with complete regularity, so a record of the menstrual cycle must be kept for 12 months, during which time some other method of birth control must be used. The first day of each period is counted as Day 1. To determine the first fertile, or "unsafe" day of the cycle, subtract 18 from the number of days in the shortest cycle (Figure 6-2). To determine the last unsafe day of the cycle, subtract 11 from the number of days in the longest cycle.

The *temperature method* is based on the knowledge that a woman's body temperature drops slightly just before ovulation and rises slightly after ovulation. A woman using the temperature method records her basal, or resting, body temperature (BBT) every morning before getting out of bed and before eating or drinking anything, since the activities may alter the results. Once the temperature pattern can be seen (usually after about three months), the period unsafe for coitus can be calculated as the interval from Day 5 (Day 1 is the first day of the period) until three days after the rise in BBT. To arrive at a shorter unsafe period, some women combine the calendar and the temperature methods, calculating the first unsafe day from the shortest cycle of the calendar chart and the last unsafe day as the third day after a rise in the BBT.

The *mucus method* (or Billings method) is based on changes in the cervical secretions throughout the menstrual cycle. During the estrogenic phase, cervical mucus increases and is clear and slippery. At the time of ovulation some women can detect a slight change in the texture of the mucus and find that it is more likely to form an elastic thread when stretched between thumb and finger. After ovulation these secretions become cloudy and sticky and decrease in quantity. Infertile, safe days are likely to occur during the relatively dry days just before and after menstruation. These additional clues have been found helpful by some couples who rely on the Fertility Awareness Method. One possible problem that may interfere with this method is that vaginal infections or vaginal products or medication can also change cervical mucus.

FAM is not recommended for women who have very irregular cycles. The failure rate is high—approximately 20 percent among typical users during the first year of use.

Withdrawal Probably the oldest known method of contraception is **withdrawal.** In this method, the male removes his penis from the vagina just before he ejaculates. Withdrawal has three advantages: It is free, it requires no preparation, and it is always available. For many people, these advantages are far outweighed by the disadvantages: The male has to overcome a powerful biological urge. A man may also have difficulty judging when to withdraw. The fear that withdrawal may be too late can detract from sexual pleasure for both partners. Also, since many women take longer than men do to reach orgasm, withdrawal before the woman's orgasm is likely and can leave the couple frustrated if she relies on coitus for satisfaction. The typical failure rate for withdrawal is 18 percent. One key factor in the high failure rate is the degree of self-control necessary. In addition, preejaculatory fluid, which may contain viable sperm, is commonly secreted unnoticed before actual ejaculation occurs.

Figure 6-3 summarizes the use effectiveness of eleven reversible contraceptive methods.

Combining Methods

Couples can choose to combine the preceding methods in a variety of ways, both to add STD protection and/or to increase contraceptive effectiveness. For example, condoms are strongly recommended along with pill use whenever there is a risk of STDs. Foam may be added to condom use to increase protection against both STDs and pregnancy. For many couples, and especially for many women, the added benefits will far outweigh the extra effort and expense.

PERMANENT CONTRACEPTION— STERILIZATION

Sterilization is permanent, and it provides complete protection. For these reasons, it is becoming an increasingly popular method of birth control. At present it is the most commonly used method in the United States and in the world. It is especially popular among couples who have been married 10 or more years, as well as among couples who have had all the children they intend. Sterilization provides no protection against STDs.

An important consideration in choosing sterilization is that, in most cases, it cannot be reversed. Although the chances of restoring fertility are being increased by mod-

TERMS

Withdrawal   Purposely interrupting sexual intercourse by withdrawing the penis before ejaculation (to avoid conception)

Sterilization   Surgically altering the reproductive system to prevent pregnancy. Vasectomy is the procedure in males, tubal sterilization or hysterectomy in females.

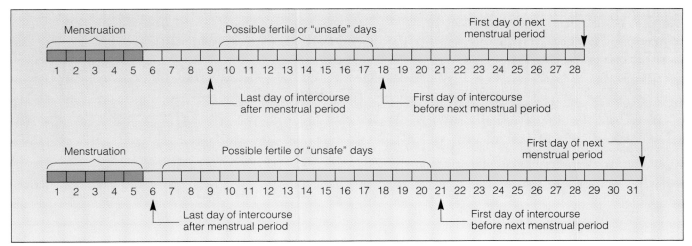

Figure 6-2 The Fertility Awareness Method of contraception, showing the safe and unsafe days for a woman with a regular 28-day cycle (top), and a woman with an irregular cycle, ranging from 25 to 31 days (bottom).

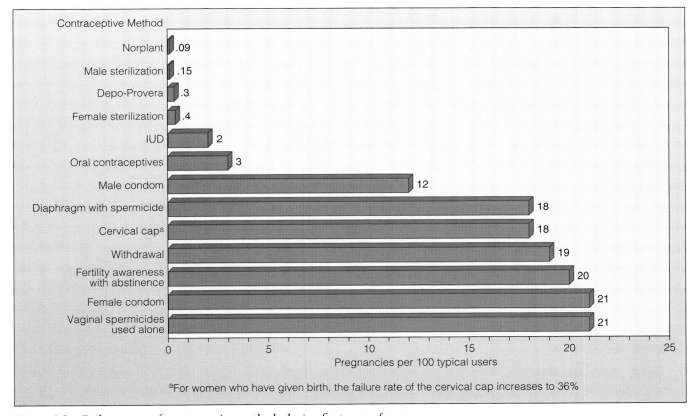

Figure 6-3 *Failure rates of contraceptive methods during first year of use.*

ern surgical techniques, such operations are costly and pregnancy can never be guaranteed. Some couples choosing male sterilization are using sperm banks as a way of extending the option of childbearing.

Some recent studies have indicated that male sterilization is preferable to female sterilization in a variety of ways. The overall cost of a female procedure is about four times that of a male procedure, and women are much more likely than men to experience both minor and major complications following the operation. Furthermore, regret seems to be somewhat higher in women than in men after sterilization.

Many potential solutions have been proposed to deal with the problems of unintended pregnancy and the spread of sexually transmissible diseases. Abstinence, the avoidance of sexual intercourse, is a solution that is appropriate for some people. Anyone can practice abstinence at any time, including people who are not yet sexually active, those who are beginning a relationship with a new partner, and those who are not currently in a relationship. Consider the following reasons for choosing abstinence and the guidelines for making sexual decisions to determine whether abstinence is an appropriate choice for you.

Reasons for Choosing Abstinence

People may choose abstinence for a variety of reasons. The most obvious is that avoiding sexual intercourse is the only sure way to prevent pregnancy and exposure to STDs. Even consistent condom use may fail because condoms can break and they may not always cover all infected surfaces.

For some people, the most important reason for choosing abstinence is a moral one, based on cultural or religious beliefs or strongly held personal values. Individuals may feel that sexual intercourse is appropriate only for married couples or for people in serious, committed relationships. Abstinence may also be seen as the wisest choice in terms of an individual's emotional needs. A period of abstinence may be chosen as a time to focus energies on other aspects of interpersonal or personal growth.

Abstinence is chosen by some couples to allow their relationships to grow before they face the emotions and stresses that go along with sexual intimacy. This gives them time to get to know and trust each other; to share experiences, thoughts, and feelings; and to become good friends. Couples who choose not to have intercourse are still free to express affection in a variety of ways.

Whatever the reason for choosing abstinence, a person's decision should be respected. What may seem "right" and highly desirable for one person may be unacceptable for another. External pressure alone, either from individuals or from society at large, is not a satisfactory reason for engaging in intercourse. Assertiveness and communication skills are keys to making appropriate choices and sticking to them.

Making Decisions About Sex

Choosing to have sex can change a relationship and an individual's life. It makes sense to think about it and to talk about it. Ask yourself the following questions:

- What are my moral and religious views about sex before marriage? How will I feel if I go against my beliefs?

- Who am I doing this for? Am I doing this to make my partner happy? Am I trying to prove something?

- Do I feel pressured to have sex? Where are those pressures coming from?

- How do I feel about my partner? Do I respect and trust my partner? Does my partner respect and trust me?

- Have we talked about this decision? Does each of us know what the other is thinking?

- If we decide to have sexual intercourse, what method of contraception will we use? How will we protect ourselves from STDs?

- Am I being honest with myself about my feelings and about my relationship with my partner?

Sticking to Your Decision

If you decide that abstinence is the right choice for you at this time, you may be faced with situations that make it difficult to stick with your decision. First, it is important you talk with your partner. Plan what you will say ahead of time and choose a good time to talk. Explain your feelings and then listen to what he or she has to say.

Think about the situations in which you are likely to be tempted to go further sexually than you really want to—for example, getting drunk together or spending private time together in your partner's bedroom. If you are serious about abstinence, you should consider avoiding situations in which the temptation to have intercourse may be greater than you can handle. Find other ways to be with your partner. Spend time with friends and in public activities getting to know one another.

Using alcohol or other drugs can also make it difficult to stick to your decision. Being drunk or high greatly affects judgment and may lead to actions that you'll regret later, such as having sex or engaging in unsafe sex. Don't mix alcohol and drugs with sexual situations.

Remember, your sexuality is yours—to be enjoyed when you decide the time is right. If you choose not to have sex right now, it doesn't mean you will not have a close sexual relationship with your partner. It does mean that you will move at your own pace and find your own "right time." When you make choices about sex based on self-respect and physical, emotional, and spiritual considerations, you will be more likely to feel good about your decisions—now and in the future.

Adapted from B. Strong, C. DeVault, and B. Sayad. 1996. *Core Concepts in Human Sexuality* (Mountain View, Calif.: Mayfield); Boston Women's Health Book Collective. 1992. *The New Our Bodies, Ourselves* (New York: Simon and Schuster); and J. Hiatt. 1986. *The Choice to Abstain* (Network Publications, P.O. Box 1830, Santa Cruz, CA 95061).

Although some physicians will perform surgery for sterilization on request, most require a thorough discussion with both partners before the operation. Most physicians also recommend that people who have religious conflicts, psychiatric problems related to sex, or unstable marriages not be sterilized. Young couples with one or two children, who might later change their minds and want more, are also frequently advised not to undergo sterilization.

Male Sterilization—Vasectomy

The procedure for male sterilization, **vasectomy,** involves severing the vasa deferentia, two tiny ducts that transport sperm from the testicles to the seminal vesicles. The testicles continue to produce sperm, but the sperm are absorbed into the body. Since the testicles contribute only about one-tenth of the total seminal fluid, the actual quantity of ejaculate is only slightly reduced. Hormone output from the testicles continues with very little change, and secondary sex characteristics are not altered.

Vasectomy is ordinarily done in the physician's office and takes about 30 minutes. A local anesthetic is injected into the skin of the scrotum and near the vasa. Small incisions are made at the upper end of the scrotum where it joins the body, and the vas deferens on each side is exposed, severed, and tied off or coagulated with electrocautery. The incisions are then closed with sutures, and a small dressing is applied.

Vasectomy is highly effective. In a small number of vasectomies, a severed vas rejoins itself, and sperm can again travel up through the duct and be ejaculated in the semen. The overall failure rate for vasectomy is 0.15 percent. Although some surgeons report pregnancy rates of about 80 percent for partners of men who have their vasectomies reversed within 10 years of the original procedure, most studies report figures in the 50 percent range.

Female Sterilization

The most common method of female sterilization involves severing or in some manner blocking the oviducts, thereby preventing the egg from reaching the uterus and the sperm from entering the tubes. Ovulation and menstruation continue, but the unfertilized eggs are released into the abdominal cavity and absorbed. Although progesterone levels in the blood may decline slightly, in general hormone production by the ovaries and secondary characteristics are not affected.

One method of **tubal sterilization** is accomplished by making a small incision in the abdominal wall, locating each oviduct, bringing it into view, severing it, removing a small section, and tying or stapling shut the two ends. Tubal sterilization can also be done by a method called **laparoscopy,** in which a tube containing a tiny light is inserted through a small abdominal incision. The surgeon looks through the laparoscope to locate the oviducts, which are cauterized (sealed off) by electrocautery. Either a regional or general anesthetic can be used, and the operation usually takes about 15 to 30 minutes. The patient can often go home the same day.

About 7 percent of the patients experience problems after the operation, arising mainly from wound infection or bleeding. Serious complications are rare, and the death rate is low, particularly when regional rather than general anesthesia is used. (Because of the higher risks involved, **hysterectomy,** removal of the uterus, is the preferred method of sterilization for only a small number of women, usually women with preexisting gynecologic problems.)

The failure rate for tubal ligations and laparoscopy is about 4 out of every 1,000 cases. Reversibility rates are 50–70 percent.

NEW METHODS OF CONTRACEPTION

Even with all the improvements of recent years, the best of the present methods of contraception have drawbacks. The search still continues for the ideal method, the one that will be more effective, safer, cheaper, easier to use, more readily available, easily reversible, and acceptable to more people.

Many people place a high priority specifically on an increase in contraceptive alternatives for males. Throughout history, the responsibility for birth control has been assumed predominantly by women, partly because women have greater personal investment in preventing pregnancy, with its many risks, and childbearing, with the many demands that fall mostly on women. Some women in some settings see complete control as crucial. More birth control options have been available for female use, because there are more ways to intervene in the female reproductive system. Another factor may be the continuing underrepresentation of women in medicine, scientific research, pharmaceutical management, the FDA, and other political forces. Participation by women and an emphasis on their needs regarding birth control has been limited in these areas.

After years of diminishing contraceptive choice in the United States, several new methods have been approved and are now being marketed. Many new birth control

---

Vasectomy   Surgical severing of the ducts that carry sperm to the ejaculatory duct.

Tubal sterilization   Severing or in some manner blocking the oviducts. This prevents ova (eggs) from reaching the uterus.

Laparoscopy   Examining the internal organs by inserting a tube containing a small light through an abdominal incision.

Hysterectomy   Total or partial surgical removal of the uterus.

TERMS

About half of all the world's couples of reproductive age currently use some form of contraception. Worldwide, sterilization is the most commonly used method followed by IUDs, oral contraceptives, condoms, and natural family planning methods. But striking differences exist from one country to another in both the rates of contraceptive use and method chosen. These differences reflect a variety of factors, including the following:

- *Access to services.* How far people have to travel for contraceptive services and how long they have to wait once they get there are important factors in contraceptive use. Geographical barriers can be significant, particularly in developing countries or isolated rural areas. For example, a study of contraceptive use in rural Bangladesh revealed that the presence of paved roads was as much a factor as the location of facilities.

- *Availability.* Not all methods are available in every country. In the United States, for example, access to IUDs is limited, and Norplant and Depo-Provera have only recently become available. IUDs and injectables are more available—and more widely used—in Mexico than in the United States. In Japan, oral contraceptives are available only in high dosages and only for a few women; this may be one reason why condom use is high there.

- *Cost.* Studies have shown that people are willing to pay moderate amounts for contraceptive supplies; but for many people, the price threshold is fairly low. Furthermore, many methods have hidden costs, such as the purchase of spermicide for use with a diaphragm.

Methods that require the replenishing of supplies are less likely to be used in developing nations.

- *Political, cultural, and religious factors.* Government policies can have a strong impact on contraceptive use. The Chinese government limits family size to one child and penalizes families who have additional children. China has one of the highest rates of contraceptive use in the world. Cultural influences are important too. A woman seeking contraceptives may encounter opposition from her peer group, husband, or extended family. A large family may be valued as a source of labor, a symbol of virility or fertility, or a form of "social security" in old age. In some countries, religious traditions and doctrines prohibit contraceptive use. Roman Catholics have opposed national family planning efforts in Mexico, Kenya, and the Philippines. Muslim fundamentalists have done the same in Iran, Egypt, and Pakistan.

Although Americans tend to think of contraceptive use as a matter of personal choice, it is clearly bounded by numerous physical and cultural constraints, even in the United States. In many societies, most individuals may have very little choice in which, if any, contraceptive they use. On a worldwide scale, lack of contraceptive use is associated with rapid population growth, poverty, and high mortality rates from unsafe conditions of childbirth, risky illegal abortions, and sexually transmissible diseases. This is why family planning is sure to be one of the most pressing—and complex—issues that nations will face in the twenty-first century.

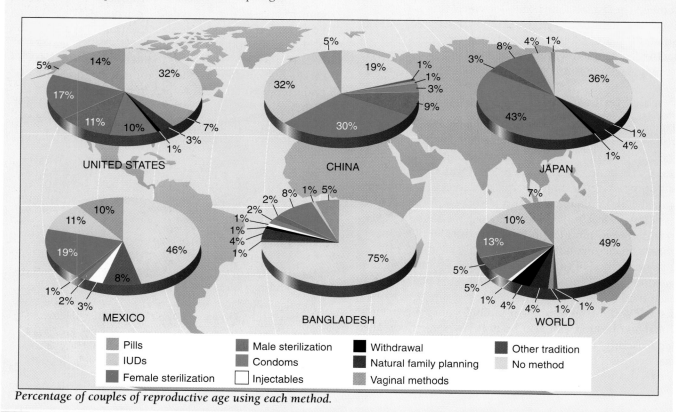

Percentage of couples of reproductive age using each method.

methods are used widely in other countries long before they become available in the United States. This delay is due in part to higher costs of preclinical safety testing, greater liability risk for manufacturers, and lower levels of government funding for contraceptive research.

WHICH CONTRACEPTIVE METHOD IS RIGHT FOR YOU?

If you are sexually active, you need to use the contraceptive method that will work best for you. The process of choosing and using a contraceptive method can be complex and varies greatly from one couple to another. Each individual must consider many variables in deciding which method is most acceptable and appropriate for her or him. Important considerations include:

1. *Individual health risks of each method in terms of personal and family medical history.* IUDs are not recommended for any young woman without children, because of an increased risk of pelvic infection and subsequent infertility. Hormonal methods should be used only after a clinical evaluation of one's medical history. Other methods have only minor and local side effects.

2. *Implications of unwanted pregnancy and therefore the importance of effectiveness.* Hormonal methods, when used correctly, offer by far the best protection against pregnancy. Condoms, diaphragms, and cervical caps should be combined with a spermicide and used with every intercourse. Neither FAM nor withdrawal is very effective and should never be relied upon when pregnancy prevention is important.

3. *Possible risks of sexually transmissible diseases.* Condom use, preferably with foam, is of critical importance whenever any risk of STD is present. This is especially true when you are not in an exclusive, long-term relationship or when you are taking the pill, because cervical changes occurring during hormone use may lead to increased vulnerability to certain diseases. Abstinence or activities that don't involve intercourse or any other exchange of body fluids can be a satisfactory alternative for some people.

4. *Convenience and comfort of the method as viewed by each partner.* The hormonal methods are generally ranked high in this category unless there are negative side effects and health risks or if forgetting to take pills is a problem with OC use. Some users think condom use disrupts spontaneity and lowers penile sensitivity. (Creative approaches to condom use and improved quality can decrease these complaints.) The diaphragm, cap, and spermicides can be inserted before intercourse begins, but are still considered a significant bother by some.

5. *Type of relationship.* The barrier methods require more motivation and a sense of responsibility from *each* partner than hormonal methods do. When the method depends on the cooperation of one's partner, assertiveness is necessary, no matter how difficult. This is especially true in new relationships, when condom use is most important. When sexual activity is infrequent, a barrier method may make more sense than an IUD or one of the hormonal methods.

6. *Ease and cost of obtaining and maintaining each method.* With OC use, an annual pelvic exam and periodic clinic checks are required and important. In addition, the cost of the pills themselves tends to be higher than barrier supplies for most couples, although insurance plans will sometimes cover pill expense. The initial cost of Norplant may be high, and use of Depo-Provera involves an injection every 12 weeks. Diaphragms and cervical caps also require an initial exam and fitting.

7. *The method's acceptability in terms of religious or other philosophical beliefs.* According to the religious beliefs of some individuals, abstinence is the only acceptable form of sexual behavior in all premarital relationships.

THE ABORTION ISSUE

In the United States today, few issues are as complex and emotion-filled as abortion. While most public attention has focused on legal definitions and restrictions, the most difficult aspects of abortion actually take place at a much more personal level. On campuses today, as in our society at large, many powerful forces (including the great emphasis on sexuality and on the "good times" that follow alcohol consumption) contribute to the high rate of unintended pregnancy and abortion. At all school levels and in the general public, there is simultaneously great resistance to confronting these related issues openly and honestly—resulting in a lack of programs to deal with the problem at a preventive level.

With their inside vantage point, college students are in a key position to understand and to address the contributing factors as well as the broad effects of unintended pregnancies and abortion. Instead of simply attempting to legislate certain behaviors, they can choose to grapple with the complex human factors that go into the prevention as well as the "treatment" of unintended pregnancy.

The word **abortion,** by official or strict definition,

Abortion The premature expulsion or removal of an embryo or fetus from the uterus.

TERMS

means the expulsion of a fetus from the uterus before it is sufficiently developed to survive. As commonly used, however, *abortion* refers only to those expulsions that are artificially induced by mechanical means or drugs, and *miscarriage* is the word generally used for a spontaneous abortion, one that occurs naturally with no causal intervention. In this chapter, the word *abortion* is used to mean a deliberately induced abortion.

History of Abortion in the United States

For more than two centuries, abortion policy in the United States followed English common law, which made the practice a crime only when performed after "quickening" (fetal movement that begins at about 20 weeks). There was little public objection to this policy until the early 1800s when an anti-abortion movement began, led primarily by physicians who questioned the doctrine of quickening and who objected to the growing practice of abortion by untrained persons (in part because it weakened their control of medical services).

This anti-abortion drive gained minimal attention until the mid-1800s, when newspaper advertisements for abortion preparations became common and concern grew that women were using abortion as a means of birth control (and perhaps to cover up extramarital activity). There was much discussion about the corruption of morality among women in the United States, and by the 1900s, virtually all states had anti-abortion laws. These laws stayed in effect until the 1960s, when courts began to invalidate them on the grounds of constitutional vagueness and violation of right to privacy.

Current Legal Status

In 1973, the abortion issue was thrust to the center of legal debate when the U.S. Supreme Court made abortion legal in the landmark case of *Roe vs. Wade*. To replace the restrictions most states still imposed at that time, the justices devised new standards to govern abortion decisions. They divided pregnancy into three parts, or trimesters, giving a pregnant woman less choice about abortion as she advances toward full term. In the first trimester, the abortion decision must be left to the judgment of the pregnant woman and her physician. During the second trimester, similar rights remain but a state may regulate factors that protect the health of the woman, such as type of facility where an abortion may be performed. In the third trimester, when the fetus is viable (capable of survival outside of the uterus), a state may regulate and even bar all abortions except those considered necessary to preserve the mother's life or health.

In July 1989, another legal milestone was reached, when the Supreme Court handed down its decision in *Webster vs. Reproductive Health Services*. The Court did not overturn *Roe*, but did let stand several key restrictions on abortions enacted by the Missouri legislature in 1986. The two most severe restrictions forbid the use of all public facilities, resources, and employees for abortion services and require costly and time-consuming tests to determine fetal viability whenever the doctor estimates the fetus to be 20 weeks or older. In June 1992, another major Court decision was handed down in *Planned Parenthood of Southeastern Pennsylvania vs. Casey*. Although this ruling continues to uphold a woman's basic right to abortion, it gives the state further powers to regulate abortion throughout pregnancy, as long as it does not impose an "undue burden" on women seeking the procedure. The Court decided that the following provisions of the Pennsylvania law do not constitute "undue burden" and therefore let these restrictions stand: Women seeking abortion must be told about fetal development and alternatives to ending their pregnancies; they must wait at least 24 hours after receiving that information; minors must get permission from a parent or judge; and physicians are required to keep detailed records, subject to public disclosure. The Court turned down a requirement that married women must notify their husbands of their intention to have an abortion.

While not banning abortion outright, the addition of these various regulations will seriously restrict accessibility to abortion for many women, especially those with limited resources. For example, the indigent and the young will be most affected by any prohibitions placed on public facilities and funding. These are the same women who will be most affected by legal changes necessitating travel for a legal abortion and laws requiring additional tests in the case of late abortion (since they make up the bulk of those having late abortion). Concerns have been expressed that the new regulations may result in a two-tiered health care system, one for women with means and another for those without. In addition, since the *Webster* and *Casey* decisions gave few guidelines (other than that further state restrictions will probably be upheld), great disparities in the availability of legal abortion are likely to exist from one area of the country to another.

The complete overturning of *Roe vs. Wade* by the Supreme Court may occur as numerous new test cases are brought for its consideration. Such a reversal would permit, but not require, states to prohibit all abortion. In the absence of federal legislation, differences in availability, cost, and timing of abortion would continue to exist from one state to another, depending on each one's laws and court interpretations. Both pro-choice and pro-life groups will most likely move to the national level, seeking federal legislation, the former to ensure abortion rights (as found in the Freedom of Choice Act) and the latter to make abortion a federal crime (laws pertaining to the health care provider and/or the woman having the abortion).

Attention is also being focused on political campaigns and the backing of candidates with well-defined views on abortion. In the foreseeable future, heated debate is likely to continue.

> ***Personal Insight*** Some people believe that teenagers should have their parents' permission before they can have an abortion and married women should have their husband's permission before they can have an abortion. How do you feel about these restrictions?

Moral Considerations

Along with the legal debates have come ongoing arguments between "pro-life" and "pro-choice" groups regarding the ethics of abortion, what is right and what is wrong in a moral sense. Central to the pro-life position is the belief that the fertilized egg must be valued as a human being from the moment of conception and that abortion at any time is equivalent to murder. This group holds that any woman who has sexual intercourse knows that pregnancy is a possibility, and should she willingly have intercourse and get pregnant she is morally obligated to carry the pregnancy through. Pro-life followers encourage adoption for women who feel they are unable to raise the child and point out how many couples are seeking babies for adoption. Pro-lifers do not see the availability of legal abortion as essential to women's well-being, but view it instead as having an overall destructive effect on our traditional morals and values.

By contrast, the pro-choice viewpoint holds that distinctions must be made between the stages of fetal development and that preserving the fetus of early gestation is not always the ultimate moral concern. Members of this group maintain that women must have the freedom to decide whether and when to have children; they argue that pregnancy can result from contraceptive failure or other factors out of a woman's control. When pregnancy does occur, pro-choice individuals believe that the most moral decision possible must be determined according to each individual situation and that in some cases greater injustice would result if abortion were not an option. If legal abortions were not available, some pro-choice supporters say, "back-alley shops" and do-it-yourself techniques, with their many health risks, as well as the births of unplanned children, would again grow in number. Others argue that discrimination in health care would result, since wealthy women could more easily make the travel arrangements necessary for a legal abortion elsewhere. Still others emphasize that some physicians, because of their strong personal convictions regarding abortion rights, would feel forced into becoming lawbreakers.

Some individuals strongly identify exclusively with either the pro-life or the pro-choice stance, but many people have moral beliefs that are blurred, less defined, and in some cases a mixture of the two. A common assumption is that all religious organizations and individuals adhere to the pro-life position. This notion can be misleading. Although some generalizations can be made, moral positions regarding abortion can vary widely among religious believers just as they can differ markedly among individuals who consider themselves nonreligious.

> ***Personal Insight*** How do you define life? When do you think it begins? How does your answer affect your position on abortion?

Public Opinion

In general, U.S. public opinion on abortion is somewhat flexible and seems to change depending on the specific situation. Many individuals approve of legal abortion as an option when destructive health or welfare consequences could result from continuing pregnancy, but they do not advocate abortion as a simple way out of an inconvenient situation. Overall, most adults in the United States continue to approve of legal abortion and are opposed to overturning the basic right to abortion established in *Roe vs. Wade*. But the amount of public support will vary considerably, depending on the circumstances surrounding the abortion request. Most people see many areas of ambiguity in the abortion issue.

For example, people who feel that abortion should be available in early pregnancy often question at which stage in later pregnancy the fetus's rights should take precedence over the woman's rights. The 1973 U.S. Supreme Court decision considered viability the key criterion in establishing the point beyond which a woman's right to choose abortion becomes markedly restricted. In 1973, viability was generally considered to be about 26 to 28 weeks. Today it is about 24 weeks, with isolated cases of survival at 23 weeks. Although neonatal intensive care units continue to advance technologically, most experts feel that viability cannot ever be expected beyond this limit.

Other individuals associate fetal rights not with viability but with earlier developmental characteristics such as onset of heartbeat, brain size, and nervous system maturity. Still other individuals argue that the embryo becomes a human being at the point of individuation or twinning, which occurs about two weeks after conception. (Before that time, the embryo has not yet differentiated into either a single or an identical twin pregnancy.) Others believe that the moment of conception is the only critical point to consider. For them, all other developmental stages are irrelevant to the abortion debate. As can be seen from such wide variation of opinion, objective measures of humanness and clear-cut guidelines regarding fetal rights are elusive, and decisions ambiguous.

Although opinions vary as to whether, or when, in

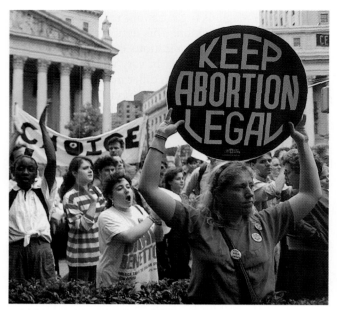

Pro-choice groups believe that the decision to end or continue a pregnancy is a personal matter that should be left up to the individual.

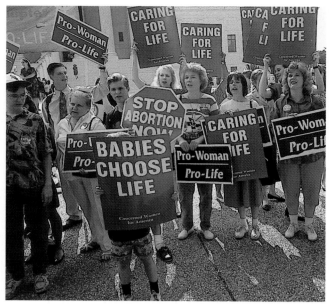

Pro-life groups oppose abortion on the basis of their belief that life begins at the moment of conception.

pregnancy, abortion rights should be tightly regulated by law, most people agree that abortions done later in pregnancy present more difficulties in personal, medical, philosophical, and social terms. Who are the women who have late abortions? Of all abortions done after the twelfth week of gestation, more than 35 percent are performed on teenagers. Possible explanations include teenagers' ignorance, denial, fear, and lack of supportive family or friends. Other typical recipients of late abortions include low-income women who may have more difficulty finding suitable facilities as well as necessary funds, and premenopausal women who fail to recognize a delayed period as pregnancy. Another small group of women who may seek late abortion are those who have learned through amniocentesis (the withdrawal and analysis of amniotic fluid) that the fetus is suffering from a specific abnormality, such as Down's syndrome. Because the results of this test are usually not available until the sixteenth week of pregnancy, abortion, if chosen, is necessarily delayed. Chorionic villus sampling can be

performed in the first trimester, but this technique does not diagnose neural tube defects and also carries slightly more risk of miscarriage. (See Figures 6-4 and 6-5 for information about women who choose abortion.)

Current Trends

Clearly, all responses to unintended pregnancy can be difficult, including abortion and especially late abortion. Fortunately, with the increased accessibility to legalized abortion following the mid-1970s, the rate of late abortions dropped steadily, until fewer than 1 percent of all abortions were performed at more than 20 weeks and fewer than 10 percent at more than 12 weeks by the early 1990s. Also, the overall abortion *rate*, which rose during most of the 1970s and leveled off around 1980, fell gradually between 1982 and 1992 (Figure 6-6).

The effects of legal restrictions are hard to predict. Women seeking abortions usually do so with very strong motivation and determination and are not likely to be deterred easily. However, studies have shown that the mandatory delay law passed in August 1992 in Mississippi did have an effect: Some women had abortions later in pregnancy and others never completed their stated desire for pregnancy termination. The effect of the mandatory delay may have been compounded by increased travel demands. Research into possible effects of legal barriers in other states is underway, and new findings may help to establish which restrictions do, indeed, constitute an "undue burden" for women seeking abortions. Adding to the legal restrictions is the growing scarcity of physicians willing to provide abortion services. This diminish-

> *Personal Insight* Women choose abortion for a wide variety of reasons: The pregnancy threatens their health; having a child would interfere with their educational or career plans; the pregnancy resulted from rape or incest; they can't afford to have a child; they don't want to be single parents; prenatal tests reveal fetal abnormalities; and so on. Under what circumstances (if any) do you think abortion is justified?

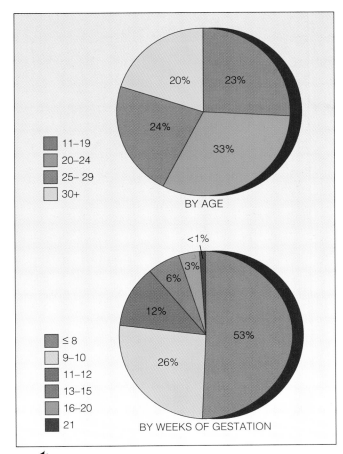

BY AGE

11–19
20–24
25–29
30+

<1%
3%
6%
12%
53%
26%

≤ 8
9–10
11–12
13–15
16–20
21

BY WEEKS OF GESTATION

VITAL STATISTICS
Figure 6-4   *Percentage distribution of all women who had abortions in 1992.*

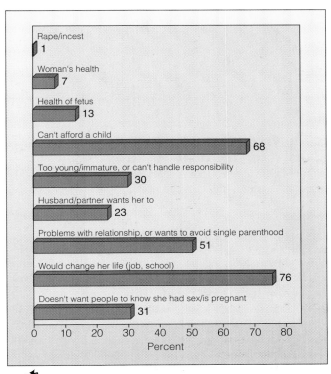

Rape/incest 1
Woman's health 7
Health of fetus 13
Can't afford a child 68
Too young/immature, or can't handle responsibility 30
Husband/partner wants her to 23
Problems with relationship, or wants to avoid single parenthood 51
Would change her life (job, school) 76
Doesn't want people to know she had sex/is pregnant 31

Percent

VITAL STATISTICS
Figure 6-5   *The reasons women choose abortions (respondents could give more than one answer).*

ing number is due in part to increased anti-abortion protests and violence, including the murders of several physicians and clinic workers. If the constitutional right to abortion is maintained, these obstacles need to be considered carefully and dealt with effectively.

There is also growing speculation regarding the possible impact of the new "abortion pill," RU-486, now approved for use in several countries. U.S. drug trials of RU-486 are scheduled to be completed by the spring of 1995, and the drug may become available to U.S. physicians beginning in 1996. In addition, university researchers have been studying two other inexpensive, generic drugs that may prove to be equally effective at ending very early pregnancies. Federal officials and university researchers are urging physicians to wait for the final results from these studies before using any drugs for abortion. Many worry about the dangers of women obtaining these drugs outside responsible medical channels. Taken incorrectly, these agents could damage the fetus instead of causing an abortion or, in some cases, be life-threatening for the woman taking them.

Unless coupled with attention to the prevention of unwanted pregnancy, especially among the young and single women who make up the majority of those seeking abortions, legal changes alone will probably not reduce the number of abortions dramatically.

Abortion Complications

In recent years, several studies have focused on both physical and psychological concerns; slowly, more information is being gathered on this important subject.

Possible Physical Effects   The incidence of immediate problems following abortion (infection, bleeding, trauma to the cervix or uterus, and incomplete abortion requiring repeat curettage) varies widely. The overall incidence is significantly reduced with good patient health, early timing of abortion, use of the suction method and local anesthesia, performance by a well-trained clinician, and availability and use of prompt follow-up care. All patients should thoroughly understand the postabortion danger signs and should not hesitate to report any concerns.

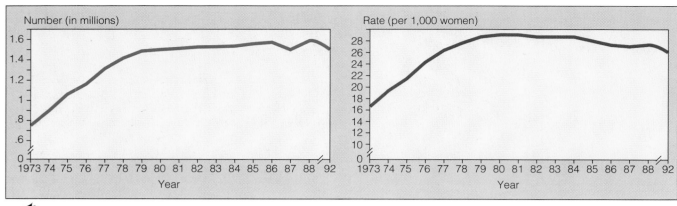

VITAL STATISTICS

Figure 6-6 *Abortion in the United States.*
(a) Number of legal abortions. (b) Rate of abortions per 1,000 women aged 15–44

Studies on long-term complications (subsequent infertility, spontaneous second abortions, premature delivery, and babies of low birth weight) have not revealed any major risks with the most common abortion methods. The risk of mortality associated with childbirth is about 11 times as high as that associated with abortion. The risk of death associated with abortion increases with the length of pregnancy, from 1 death for every 500,000 abortions at 8 weeks or less to 1 per 30,000 at 16 to 20 weeks and 1 per 8,000 at 21 or more weeks.

Possible Psychological Effects After an exhaustive review completed in 1988, then–Surgeon General C. Everett Koop concluded that the available evidence failed to demonstrate either a negative or positive long-term impact of abortion on mental health. The psychological side effects of abortion are less clearly defined than the physical ones. Responses vary and depend on the individual woman's psychological makeup, family background, current personal and social relationships, surrounding cultural attitudes, and many other factors. A woman who has specific goals with a somewhat structured life pattern may incorporate her decision to abort as the unequivocally "best" and acceptable decision more easily than may a woman who feels uncertain about her future.

Although many women experience great relief after abortion and virtually no negative feelings, some go through a period of ambivalence. Along with relief, they often feel a mixture of other responses, such as guilt, regret, loss, sadness, and/or anger. When a woman feels she was pressured into sexual intercourse or into the abortion, she may feel bitter. If she has strongly believed abortion to be immoral, she may wonder if she is still a good person. Many of these feelings are strongest immediately after abortion, when hormonal shifts are occurring; such feelings often pass quite rapidly. Others take time and

fade only slowly. It is important for a woman to realize that such a mixture of feelings is natural, enabling her to accept all her reactions and to share them with others.

For a woman who does experience painful feelings, talking freely with a close friend or family member who is understanding and trustworthy can be very helpful. Supportive people can help her feel positive about herself and her decision. Although a legal and common procedure in the United States, abortion is still treated very secretively in most of our society, so it is easy for a woman to feel unique, isolated, and alone. Some women may specifically seek out other women who have had an abortion. Many clinical centers that offer abortions make such peer counseling available. Other women find they can identify with case histories in books written on abortion, which can help them deal with their own reactions. In a few cases, unresolved emotions may persist, and a woman should seek more professional counseling.

SUMMARY

Principles of Contraception

- Barrier methods of contraception physically prevent the sperm from reaching the egg; hormonal methods are designed to prevent ovulation, fertilization, and/or implantation; and surgical methods permanently block the movement of sperm or eggs to the site of potential conception. The concept of effectiveness includes failure rate and continuation rate.

Reversible Contraceptives

- In oral contraceptives (OCs), a combination of estrogen and progestins, laboratory-made compounds that prevent ovulation, hinders the movement of

Adoption: How Viable an Alternative?

Many people encourage women to deal with unwanted pregnancies through adoption rather than through abortion. But adoption is much less commonly chosen than the other alternatives—abortion or keeping the baby—and adoption rates are falling. The proportion of married or once-married women who adopted a child in 1987 was 1.7 percent, down from 2.2 percent in 1982. And according to figures from the National Center for Health Statistics, only 200,000 women sought to adopt a child in 1988, about one-tenth the number expected. Why is adoption not a more attractive alternative to marriage, single parenthood, or abortion, and why are adoption rates falling?

One reason for this change is that many more women are keeping their babies than in the past. Thirty years ago, about 50 percent of single white women under 25 who became pregnant routinely gave up their babies for adoption. Today, partly because of the diminished social stigma attached to unmarried pregnancy, many young women are choosing to be single mothers rather than relinquish their babies.

Another reason is the current prevailing assumption that children are better off with their biological parents under almost any circumstances. Government policies and laws provide financial incentives—in the form of food stamps, food supplements, Aid to Families with Dependent Children, and other assistance—for biological families to stay together. The effect of such policies is to discourage adoption.

These and other factors have worked together to produce a smaller pool of babies placed for adoption each year—at least the babies most in demand, who are healthy, white newborns. Many more babies and children are in need of homes but are less likely to be adopted, including older children, siblings who must be adopted together, children with disabilities, babies born to drug-addicted mothers, babies with HIV infection, and children with physical, mental, emotional, or behavioral problems.

Additionally, cross-racial adoptions are often discouraged, reducing the chances that minority children will be adopted, since many more potential adoptive parents are white than black. Finally, financial factors can be barriers to adoption. In 1990 the average fee for receiving a child, not including some legal costs, was $8,500.

A factor that may change this pattern of falling adoption rates is the trend toward "open" adoptions. In the past, adoptions were usually conducted in secrecy. Mothers unable to care for their children handed them over to adoption agencies and stepped out of the picture, supposedly forever. Records were sealed, preventing any future contact between biological parents and children. But in the 1970s many adults who had been adopted began searching for their biological mothers, and many mothers acknowledged that they were unable to forget the child they had given up. Awareness of these difficulties has contributed to the movement toward open adoptions, in which names, addresses, health records, family histories, and other information are available to all parties involved.

Today, between 60 and 90 percent of all adoptions are open. Couples seeking a baby may put personal ads in newspapers and send letters to lawyers, obstetricians, and clergy across the nation in the hope of finding a pregnant woman willing to relinquish her baby. They usually pay the mother's medical expenses and sometimes her living expenses before and after the baby is born. The biological mother has the opportunity to choose the adoptive family and in many cases to keep in touch with them and her child.

Although open adoption can ease the difficult transition during which the baby passes from biological mother to adoptive parents, adoption is never carefree. Even for women who choose their child's adoptive parents, the transition can be accompanied by intense feelings of loss, grief, and regret. For other women, however, adoption may be the best of all possible solutions.

Adapted from "Abortion and the Adoption Option," *Washington Post Health*, 15 August 1989, p. 607; "Where Have All the Babies Gone?" *Money*, December 1988, pp. 164–76; "The Adoption Option," *American Demographics*, October 1989, p. 11; "Project Provides Help, Hope," *San Francisco Chronicle*, 7 July 1987; "Joys and Fears of Adopting a Child," *San Francisco Chronicle*, 6 March 1990, pp. B3–B5; "Quiet Revolution in U.S. Adoption," *San Francisco Chronicle*, 24 September 1992.

---

sperm, and affects the uterine lining so that implantation of the egg is inhibited.

- Norplant consists of six hormone-filled capsules that are inserted under the skin. They release steady doses of synthetic progesterone that provide contraceptive protection for up to five years.

- Depo-Provera injections contain a long-acting progestin that protects against pregnancy for a period of three months.

- The postcoital pill prevents implantation of the fertilized embryo. No postcoital contraceptives currently have FDA approval.

- How intrauterine devices work is not clear; they may cause biochemical changes in the uterus, immobilize sperm in the uterus, shorten the travel time of the egg in the oviduct, or interfere with the implantation of the egg in the uterus.

- Male condoms are the most popular barrier method,

and their use has increased dramatically, partly because of their effectiveness against STDs.

- Female condoms consist of a polyurethane or latex sheath that can be inserted well before intercourse.

- When used correctly, with spermicidal cream or jelly, the diaphragm covers the cervix and blocks sperm from entering. Diaphragms require a prescription, and a careful fitting is necessary.

- The cervical cap is a rubber or plastic cup that adheres to the cervix through suction.

- Vaginal spermicides come in the form of foams, creams, jellies, and suppositories. They must be inserted less than one-half hour before intercourse.

- The Fertility Awareness Method (FAM) is based on avoiding coitus during the fertile phase of a woman's menstrual cycle. A calendar method, a basal body temperature method, and a mucus method may be used to determine the fertile period.

- When withdrawal is used, the male must remove his penis from the vagina just before he ejaculates.

- Combining methods can increase contraceptive effectiveness and help protect against STDs.

Permanent Contraception—Sterilization

- Sterilization is permanent, and no further contraceptive action is needed. Reversibility can never be guaranteed. Male sterilization may be preferable to female sterilization because it's associated with fewer costs and complications.

- Vasectomy—male sterilization—involves severing the vasa deferentia. Female sterilization involves severing or blocking the oviducts so that the egg cannot reach the uterus.

New Methods of Contraception

- New contraceptive techniques are under investigation, but the high cost of research, greater liability risk, and lack of government funding may delay progress.

Which Contraceptive Method Is Right for You?

- Issues to be considered in choosing a contraceptive include (1) individual health risks of each method, (2) importance of effectiveness in terms of implications of unwanted pregnancy, (3) possible risk of sexually transmissible diseases, (4) convenience and comfort of the method as viewed by each partner, (5) type of relationship, (6) cost and ease of maintaining each method, (7) acceptability in terms of religious or philosophical beliefs.

The Abortion Issue

- The common use of the word *abortion* refers only to artificially induced expulsion of the fetus (using drugs or mechanical means).

- Until the mid-1800s abortion in the United States was legal if it took place before the twentieth week; more restrictive laws passed by the various states remained in effect until they began to be invalidated by courts in the 1960s.

- The 1973 *Roe vs. Wade* Supreme Court case devised new standards to govern abortion decisions; it was based on the trimesters of pregnancy and limited a woman's choices as she advanced through pregnancy. Recent decisions by the Court have given the states some power to regulate abortion.

- The controversy between pro-life and pro-choice movements centers on the issue of when life begins. Pro-life groups believe that a fertilized egg is a human life from the moment of conception and that any abortion is a murder. Pro-choice groups distinguish between stages of fetal development and argue that the woman and not government regulations should determine the final decision regarding her pregnancy.

- Overall public opinion in the United States supports legal abortion and opposes overturning *Roe vs. Wade*. Opinion changes according to individual situations.

- Physical complications following abortion can be reduced with good patient health, early timing, use of the suction method and local anesthesia, a well-trained physician, and follow-up care. The risk of postabortion complications is very low.

- Psychological side effects of abortion vary with the individual. Many women go through a period of ambivalence; the strongest feelings usually occur immediately after the abortion. Having a supportive partner, friend, and family can be helpful.

TAKE ACTION

1. Make an appointment with a physician or other health care provider to review the health risks of different contraceptive methods as they apply to you. For each contraceptive method, determine if any risk factors associated with its use apply to you or your partner.

2. Visit a local drugstore and make a list of the contraceptives they sell and their prices. Next, investigate the costs of prescription contraceptive methods by contacting your physician, medical clinic,

and/or pharmacy. Estimate the yearly cost of regular use of each method and rank the methods from most to least expensive.

3. Devise a public service campaign that will encourage men to become more involved in contraception. Your campaign might use techniques such as TV and print advertisements, radio announcements, and posters. Look at other public service campaigns and advertisements for ideas. What sorts of images do you think would be motivational? What sort of tone and message do you think would be most effective?

4. Survey your classmates about their position on the abortion issue. How many people consider themselves pro-choice and how many pro-life? How strong are their opinions? What, if anything, might cause them to change their minds? Do opinions seem to depend on age, gender, or any other factor?

JOURNAL ENTRY

1. Consider the different methods of contraception described in this chapter. In your health journal, rank the methods according to how they suit your particular lifestyle. Take into account such considerations as how often you have sexual intercourse, convenience, and cost.

2. In your health journal, list the positive behaviors and attitudes that help you adhere to your beliefs about contraception (for example, not drinking alcohol or drinking only in moderation makes it unlikely that you would make an unwise choice because you had had too much to drink). Are there ways you can strengthen these behaviors? Then list behaviors and attitudes that might interfere with your effective use of contraception. Can you do anything to change or improve any of these?

3. *Critical Thinking:* Write a one-page essay presenting your personal opinion on the abortion issue. Include arguments to refute the points typically made by the opposing side. Then write an essay presenting a convincing case for the opposite position. Make sure your arguments are clearly stated and that you can defend them, where appropriate, with facts.

SELECTED BIBLIOGRAPHY

Abortion: Where are the doctors? (editorial). 1994. *New York Times,* 13 October, A16.

Althaus, F. A., and S. K. Henshaw. 1994. The effects of mandatory delay laws on abortion patients and providers. *Family Planning Perspectives* 26(5): 228–231.

Baulieu, E. E. 1994. RU 486: A compound that gets itself talked about. *Human Reproduction* 9 (supplement 1): 1–6.

Chi, I.C. 1994. A bill of health for the IUD: Where do we go from here? *Advances in Contraception* 10(2): 121–31.

Congleton, G. K., and L. G. Calhoun. 1993. Post-abortion perceptions: A comparison of self-identified distressed and nondistressed populations. *International Journal of Social Psychiatry* 39(4): 255–65.

Darney, P. D. 1994. Hormonal implants: Contraception for a new century. *American Journal of Obstetrics and Gynecology* 170(5): 1536–43.

DiPierri, D. 1994. RU 486, mifepristone: A review of a controversial drug. *Nurse Practitioner* 19(6): 59–61.

Earl, D. T., and D. J. David. 1994. Depo-Provera: An injectable contraceptive. *American Family Physician* 49(4): 891–4, 897–8.

Eilers, G. M., and T. K. Swanson. 1994. Women's satisfaction with Norplant as compared with oral contraceptives. *Journal of Family Practice* 38(6): 596–600.

Frank, P., and others. 1993. The effect of induced abortion on subsequent fertility. *British Journal of Obstetrics and Gynaecology* 100(6): 575–80.

Goldzieher, J. W. 1994. Are low-dose oral contraceptives safer and better? *American Journal of Obstetrics and Gynecology* 171(3): 587–90.

Grimes, D. A. 1994. The morbidity and mortality of pregnancy: Still risky business. *American Journal of Obstetrics and Gynecology* 170(5, pt. 2): 1489–94.

Haspels, A. A. 1994. Emergency contraception: A review. *Contraception* 50(2): 101–8.

Heath, C. B. 1993. Helping patients choose appropriate contraception. *American Family Physician* 48(6): 1115–24.

Henshaw, S. K. 1994. Recent trends in the legal status of induced abortion. *Journal of Public Health Policy* 15(2): 165–72.

International Medical Advisory Panel (IMAP). 1994. IMAP statement on barrier methods of contraception. *International Planned Parenthood Federation Medical Bulletin* 28(2): 1–2.

Kaunitz, A. M. 1994. Long-acting injectable contraception with depot medroxyprogesterone acetate. *American Journal of Obstetrics and Gynecology* 170(5): 1543–9.

Ketting, E., and A. P. Visser. 1994. Contraception in the Netherlands: The low abortion rate explained. *Patient Education and Counseling* 23(3): 161–71.

Meier, K. J., and D. R. McFarlane. 1994. State family planning and abortion expenditures: Their effect on public health. *American Journal of Public Health* 84(9): 1468–72.

Only Manufacturer Discontinues Sponge for Contraception. 1995. *New York Times,* 11 Jan.

Roberts, S. V. 1994. Unveiling the face of abortion politics. *U.S. News & World Report,* 19 Sept., p. 10.

Rookus, M. A., and F. E. Leeuwen. 1994. Oral contraceptives and risk of breast cancer in women aged 20–54 years. *Lancet* 344(8926): 844–51.

Rosenberg, L., and others. 1994. The relation of vasectomy to the risk of cancer. *American Journal of Epidemiology* 140(5): 431–8.

Sparrow, M. J., and K. Lavill. 1994. Breakage and slippage of condoms in family planning clients. *Contraception* 50(2): 117–29.

Tornbom, M., and others. 1994. Evaluation of stated motives for legal abortion. *Journal of Psychosomatic Obstetrics and Gynaecology* 15(1): 27–33.

Trussell, J., and others. 1994. Comparative contraceptive efficacy of the female condom and other barrier methods. *Family Planning Perspectives* 26(2): 66–72.

Westrom, L. V. 1994. Sexually transmitted diseases and infertility. *Sexually Transmitted Diseases* 21(2, supplement): S32–7.

RECOMMENDED READINGS

Hatcher, R. A., and others. 1992. *Safely Sexual.* New York: Irvington. *Detailed coverage of how to plan for a safer sexual lifestyle. Realistic recommendations regarding the prevention of unplanned pregnancy, as well as HIV infection and other sexually transmissible infections.*

Hatcher, R. A., F. J. Guest, F. H. Stewart, G. K. Stewart, J. Trussell, S. Cerel, and W. Cates. 1994. *Contraceptive Technology.* 16th ed. New York: Irvington. *A compact, reliable source of up-to-date information on contraception, with a focus on the technological aspects, rather than the psychological. The information is geared toward health care providers, but suitable for all readers. Many references and sources of information are included. Updated every two to three years.*

Henshaw, S. K., and J. Van Vort, eds. 1992. *Abortion Factbook— 1992 Edition: Readings, Trends, and State and Local Data to 1988.* New York: Alan Guttmacher Institute. *A collection of articles and tables that depict abortion in the United States today, including medical services, political phenomena, and related issues.*

Mohr, J. C. 1978. *Abortion in America: The Origins and Evolution of National Policy, 1800–1900.* New York: Oxford University Press. *A historical perspective of views on abortion within American society. Includes a discussion of the powerful role that physicians played in the formation of public opinion and related legal decisions.*

Rosenblatt, R. 1992. *Life Itself: Abortion in the American Mind.* New York: Random House. *The author, who is pro-choice, describes the schism in American society over the abortion issue. He argues that Americans can repair the rift by learning to live with conflicting feelings on the issue, as we have done on other issues.*

Stewart, F. H., and others. 1987. *Understanding Your Body.* New York: Bantam Books. *A broad and inclusive guide to women's gynecological health. Discusses common problems and everyday health care, as well as methods of contraception.*

Zilbergeld, B. 1993. *The New Male Sexuality.* New York: Bantam Books. *An update of the popular* Male Sexuality *(1978). A practical discussion of common issues in male sexuality; includes a chapter on sexual behavior and the single man.*

Tobacco and Alcohol

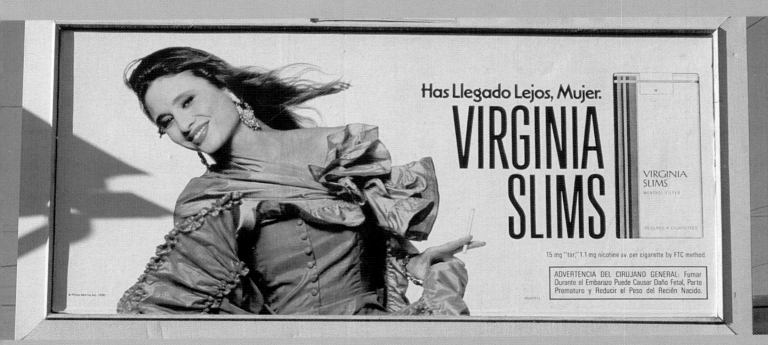

CONTENTS

When we hear about the dangers of drugs and drug abuse, most of us think of illicit drugs like marijuana, cocaine, heroin, and methamphetamine. Stories of violence and deaths related to the sale and use of illegal drugs often appear on the evening news. Far less attention is given to the drugs that are actually responsible for the most injuries and deaths in the United States—**tobacco** and **alcohol.** Indeed, tobacco and alcohol are seldom even thought of as drugs. The truth is that both **nicotine** (the **psychoactive drug** in tobacco products) and alcohol are powerful drugs that can have a devastating impact on health.

Although the proportion of cigarette smokers among American adults has dropped over the last four decades, tobacco use remains widespread and is the leading preventable cause of death in this country. About one in four American adults smokes. Every day about 1,100 people die from tobacco-related heart and lung diseases. Nonsmokers subjected to the smoke of others also suffer: Exposure to **environmental tobacco smoke (ETS)** causes more than 35,000 deaths each year, and smoking by pregnant women is responsible for up to 10 percent of all infant deaths in this country.

Two-thirds of Americans over the age of 15 drink alcohol in some form. Many people think of alcohol the way it's portrayed in advertisements, on television, and in movies—as part of a good time, an integral ingredient of celebrations and special events. However, like other drugs, alcohol can impair functioning in the short term and cause devastating damage in the long term. Through automobile crashes and other injuries, alcohol is the leading cause of death among people between the ages of 15 and 24.

Avoiding tobacco and using alcohol wisely, if at all, are important parts of a healthy lifestyle. This chapter explores the reasons people use tobacco and alcohol, how these drugs affect health, and how people can make healthy and responsible choices about the role of tobacco and alcohol in their lives.

WHY PEOPLE USE TOBACCO

If the United States is to become a tobacco-free society, the problem of tobacco use needs to be addressed not just in terms of cure but also in terms of prevention.

Nicotine Addiction

The primary reason people continue to use tobacco despite the health risks is that they have become addicted to a powerful psychoactive drug—nicotine. Nicotine reaches the brain via the bloodstream seconds after it is inhaled or, in the case of smokeless tobacco, absorbed through membranes of the mouth or nose. Like other psychoactive drugs such as cocaine and heroin, nicotine acts by triggering the release of powerful chemical messengers in the brain, including epinephrine, norepinephrine, and dopamine. But unlike street drugs, most of which are used to achieve a "high," nicotine's primary attraction seems to lie in its ability to modulate everyday emotions.

At low doses, nicotine appears to act as a stimulant: It increases heart rate and blood pressure and can enhance alertness, concentration, rapid information processing, memory, and learning. People type faster on nicotine, for instance. At high doses, on the other hand, nicotine appears to act as a sedative—it can reduce aggression and alleviate the stress response. Tobacco users may be able to fine-tune nicotine's effects and regulate their moods by increasing or decreasing their intake of the drug. Studies have shown that smokers experience milder mood variation than nonsmokers while performing long, boring tasks or while watching emotional movies, for example.

All tobacco products contain nicotine, and use of any of them can lead to addiction. Physicians define an addictive drug as one that produces loss of control; pharmacological tolerance, in which progressively higher doses of a drug are needed in order to produce the same effect; and, when its use is abruptly stopped, a withdrawal syndrome.

Loss of Control   Three out of four smokers want to quit but find they cannot. Of the 60 to 80 percent of people who kick cigarettes at stop-smoking clinics, 75 percent start smoking again within a year—a relapse rate similar to rates for alcoholics and heroin addicts. Some evidence suggests quitting is even harder for smokeless users: In one study, only 1 of 14 smokeless tobacco users who participated in a tobacco-cessation clinic was able to stop for more than four hours.

Regular tobacco users live according to a rigid cycle of

TERMS

Tobacco   The leaves of cultivated tobacco plants (genus *Nicotiana*) prepared for smoking, chewing, or use as snuff.

Alcohol   The intoxicating ingredient in fermented liquors. A colorless, pungent liquid.

Nicotine   A poisonous, addictive substance found in tobacco and responsible for many of the effects of tobacco.

Psychoactive drug   A drug that affects the brain or nervous system.

Environmental tobacco smoke   Smoke that enters the atmosphere from the burning end of a cigarette, cigar, or pipe, as well as smoke that is exhaled by smokers.

Tolerance   A phenomenon in which increased doses of a drug or medication are required to achieve the same effect.

Withdrawal syndrome   A set of physical and psychological symptoms that occur when a person suddenly stops taking a drug to which he or she has been addicted.

Secondary reinforcers   Stimuli that are not necessarily pleasurable in themselves, but have been associated with other stimuli that are pleasurable.

- In 1915, most tobacco was used for pipes, cigars, and chewing tobacco, and cigarette smoking was uncommon. Lung cancer was virtually unknown.

- In 1964 — the year of the first Surgeon General's Report linking smoking with heart disease — 42 percent of adult Americans smoked.

- Today, about 26 percent of the adult population smoke cigarettes. A major goal in the *Healthy People 2000* report is to reduce the proportion of Americans who smoke to 15 percent by decade's end.

- Nearly 20 percent of high school boys use smokeless tobacco. The average age for starting is 10.

- Nearly 70 percent of smokers under age 50 say they would like to quit.

- Half of all smokers began to smoke regularly before the age of 18; every day, 3,000 American teenagers take up cigarettes.

- 1,200 people quit smoking every day — by dying. That is equivalent to two fully loaded jumbo jets crashing every day, with no survivors.

- Smoking by pregnant women accounts for up to 14 percent of preterm deliveries, 20 to 30 percent of low birth weight babies, and 10 percent of all infant deaths each year. Twenty to 25 percent of pregnant American women continue to smoke throughout pregnancy.

- Environmental tobacco smoke causes 3,000 lung cancer deaths and an estimated 35,000 deaths from heart disease in this country each year.

- Tobacco smoke contains over 4,000 chemical compounds, including at least 43 that are carcinogenic (cancer-causing).

- High prices, health concerns, and declining social acceptance of smoking have led to decreased per capita consumption of cigarettes in the United States. However, cigarette exports have jumped by 275 percent since 1985.

- It costs the American economy approximately $68 billion a year to cover cigarette-related health care costs and loss of worker productivity.

- Polls suggest that 30 percent of the American public are unaware that smoking causes heart disease. Nearly 50 percent of women polled did not know that smoking during pregnancy increases the risk of stillbirth and miscarriage.

Sources: American Cancer Society, *Cancer Facts and Figures 1994;* Centers for Disease Control; Coalition on Smoking and Health; Environmental Protection Agency; U.S. Surgeon General.

---

need and gratification. On average, they can go no more than 40 minutes between doses of nicotine; otherwise, they begin feeling edgy and irritable and have trouble concentrating. If ignored, nicotine cravings build until getting a cigarette or some smokeless tobacco becomes a paramount concern, crowding out other thoughts. Tobacco users become adept, therefore, at keeping a steady amount of nicotine circulating in the blood and going to the brain. Smokeless tobacco users maintain bloodstream nicotine levels as high as those of cigarette smokers.

Tolerance and Withdrawal Syndrome   Tobacco use also produces **tolerance.** Where one cigarette may make a beginning smoker nauseated and dizzy, a long-term smoker may have to chain-smoke a pack or more to experience the same effects. For most regular tobacco users, sudden abstinence from nicotine produces a predictable **withdrawal syndrome** as well. Symptoms, which come on several hours after the last dose of nicotine, include severe cravings, insomnia, confusion, tremors, difficulty concentrating, fatigue, muscle pains, headache, nausea, irritability, anger, and depression. Sufferers undergo measurable changes in brain waves, heart rate, and blood pressure, and they perform poorly on tasks requiring sus-

tained attention. While most of these symptoms pass in two to three days, many ex-smokers report intermittent, intense urges to smoke for years after quitting.

Social and Psychological Factors

Why do tobacco users have such a hard time quitting even when they want to? Social and psychological forces combine with physiological addiction to maintain the tobacco habit. Many people, for example, have established habits of smoking while doing something else—while talking, working, drinking, and so on. The smokeless tobacco habit is also associated with certain situations— studying, drinking coffee, or playing sports. It's difficult for these people to break their habits because the activities they associate with tobacco use continue to trigger their urge. Psychologists call such activities **secondary reinforcers;** they act together with the physiological addiction to keep the user dependent on tobacco.

Why Start in the First Place?

Although smoking rates among American youth have declined by about one-third since the late 1970s, children and teenagers still constitute 90 percent of all new smok-

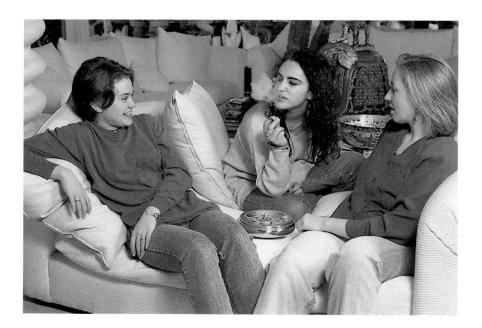

Cigarette smoke contains many toxic and carcinogenic chemicals that affect both the person smoking and the people breathing the environmental tobacco smoke. A growing body of evidence links ETS with lung cancer and respiratory and cardiovascular diseases.

ers in this country: Every day, an estimated 3,000 adolescents become regular cigarette smokers, while hundreds of others take up snuff or chewing tobacco. The average age for starting smokers? Thirteen. For smokeless tobacco users? Ten. Meanwhile, children—especially girls—are beginning to experiment with tobacco at ever-younger ages. The trends are particularly worrisome because the earlier people begin smoking, the more likely they are to become heavy smokers—and to die of tobacco-related disease.

Swayed by seductive advertising or older role models like siblings or sports stars, these young people have decided that the touted benefits of tobacco—sexual attractiveness, slenderness, confidence, and popularity, to name a few—outweigh the risks. Making such a decision requires minimizing or denying both the health risks of tobacco use and the tremendous pain, disability, emotional trauma, family stress, and financial expense involved in tobacco-related diseases such as cancer and emphysema. A sense of invincibility, characteristic of many adolescents and young adults, also contributes to the decision to use tobacco. These young people may persuade themselves they are too intelligent, too lucky, or too robustly healthy to be vulnerable to tobacco's dangers. "I'm not dumb enough to get hooked," they may argue. "I'll be able to quit before I do myself any real harm." Other typ-

ical rationalizations: "My grandmother smoked and she lived to be 80" and "You can get killed just by crossing the street."

Who Uses Tobacco?

In 1991, about 28 percent of men and 24 percent of women smoked cigarettes. Rates of smoking varied, based on gender, age, racial or ethnic group, and education level. Adults with less than a twelfth-grade education were more than twice as likely to smoke as were those with college degrees.

An estimated 20 percent of male high school seniors used smokeless tobacco in 1993. Studies of college students indicate one-fourth to one-half of male varsity and intramural athletes use smokeless tobacco; among major league baseball players, about 34 percent report regular use of smokeless tobacco.

HEALTH HAZARDS

Tobacco adversely affects nearly every part of the body—including brain, stomach, mouth, and reproductive organs.

Tobacco Smoke: A Poisonous Mix

Tobacco smoke contains hundreds of damaging chemical substances. Smoke from a typical unfiltered cigarette contains about 5 billion particles per cubic millimeter—50,000 times as many as are found in an equal volume of smoggy urban air. These particles, when condensed, form the brown, sticky mass called **cigarette tar.**

Some chemicals in tobacco tar are linked to the devel-

Personal Insight Did people in your family smoke when you were growing up? Do you think it has affected your feelings and attitudes about smoking today? If so, how?

opment of cancer. Some, such as benzopyrene and vinyl chloride, are **carcinogens;** that is, they directly cause cancer. Other chemicals, such as formaldehyde and phenol, are **cocarcinogens;** they do not themselves cause cancer but combine with other chemicals to stimulate the growth of certain cancers, at least in laboratory animals. Other substances in tobacco cause health problems because they damage the lining of the respiratory tract or decrease the lungs' ability to fight off infection.

Tobacco also contains poisonous substances, including arsenic. In addition to being an addictive psychoactive drug, nicotine is also a poison and can be fatal in high doses. Many cases of nicotine poisoning occur each year in toddlers and infants who eat tobacco.

Cigarette smoke contains carbon monoxide, the deadly gas in automobile exhaust, in concentrations 400 times greater than is considered safe in industrial workplaces. Not surprisingly, smokers often complain of breathlessness when they require a burst of energy to run across campus for their next class. Carbon monoxide displaces oxygen in red blood cells, depleting the body's supply of life-giving oxygen for extra work. Carbon monoxide also impairs visual acuity, especially at night.

In a cigarette, the unburned tobacco itself acts as a filter. As a cigarette burns down, there is less and less filter. Thus, more chemicals are absorbed into the body during the last third of a cigarette than during the first. A smoker can cut down on absorption of harmful chemicals by not smoking cigarettes down to short butts. Any gains, of course, will be offset by smoking more cigarettes, inhaling deeper, or puffing more frequently.

Some smokers switch to low-tar, low-nicotine, or filtered cigarettes because they believe them to be healthier alternatives that expose the smoker to fewer harmful chemicals. But researchers warn that there is no such thing as a "safe" cigarette. Low-tar or low-nicotine cigarettes may reduce some health risks. However, some smokers who switch to low-tar or low-nicotine cigarettes change their smoking habits to compensate for their change in brands. They smoke more cigarettes and inhale more deeply to meet their craving for nicotine.

Immediate Effects of Smoking

The beginning smoker often has symptoms of mild *nicotine poisoning:* dizziness; faintness; rapid pulse; cold, clammy skin; and sometimes nausea, vomiting, and diarrhea. The seasoned smoker occasionally suffers these effects of nicotine poisoning, particularly after quitting and returning to a previous level of consumption. The effects of nicotine on smokers vary, depending greatly on the size of the nicotine dose and how much tolerance previous smoking has built up. Nicotine can either excite or tranquilize the nervous system, depending on dosage.

Nicotine has many other immediate effects. It stimulates the part of the brain called the **cerebral cortex.** It also stimulates the adrenal glands to discharge adrenalin. And it inhibits the formation of urine, constricts the blood vessels, especially in the skin, increases the heart rate, and elevates blood pressure. Higher blood pressure, faster heart rate, and constricted blood vessels require the heart to pump more blood. In healthy people, the heart can usually meet this demand, but in people whose coronary arteries are damaged enough to interfere with the flow of blood, the heart muscle may be strained.

People who smoke often do not feel as hungry as people who do not. Smoking depresses hunger contractions and causes the liver to release glycogen, which slightly raises the level of sugar in the blood. Smoking also dulls taste buds so that food does not taste as good. People who quit smoking usually notice how much better food tastes. Figure 7-1 summarizes these immediate effects.

Long-Term Effects of Smoking

Smoking is a dangerous habit linked to many deadly and disabling diseases. Research indicates that the total amount of tobacco smoke inhaled is a key factor contributing to disease. People who smoke more cigarettes per day, inhale deeply, puff frequently, smoke cigarettes down to the butts, or begin smoking at an early age run a greater risk of disease than do those who behave more moderately or who do not smoke at all. Although cancer tends to receive the most publicity, one form of cardiovascular disease, **coronary heart disease (CHD),** is actually the most widespread single cause of death for cigarette smokers.

Cardiovascular Disease Cigarette smoking is strongly related to various cardiovascular disorders that involve the heart and blood vessels. CHD is one type and often results from a disease called **atherosclerosis,** in which fatty deposits called **plaques** form on the inner walls of heart arteries, causing them to narrow and stiffen. If a plaque completely blocks the flow of blood to a portion of the heart, it can cause a heart attack. CHD can also interfere with the normal electrical activity of the heart, resulting in

TERMS

Cigarette tar Brown sticky mass created when the chemical particles in tobacco smoke condense.

Carcinogen A substance that causes cancer.

Cocarcinogen A substance that works with a carcinogen to produce cancer.

Cerebral cortex The outer layer of the brain, which controls the complex behavior and mental activity of human beings.

Coronary heart disease (CHD) Heart disease caused by hardening of the arteries that supply oxygen to the heart muscle.

Atherosclerosis Cardiovascular disease caused by the deposit of fatty substances in the walls of the arteries.

Plaque A deposit on the inner wall of blood vessels. Blood can coagulate around plaque and form a clot.

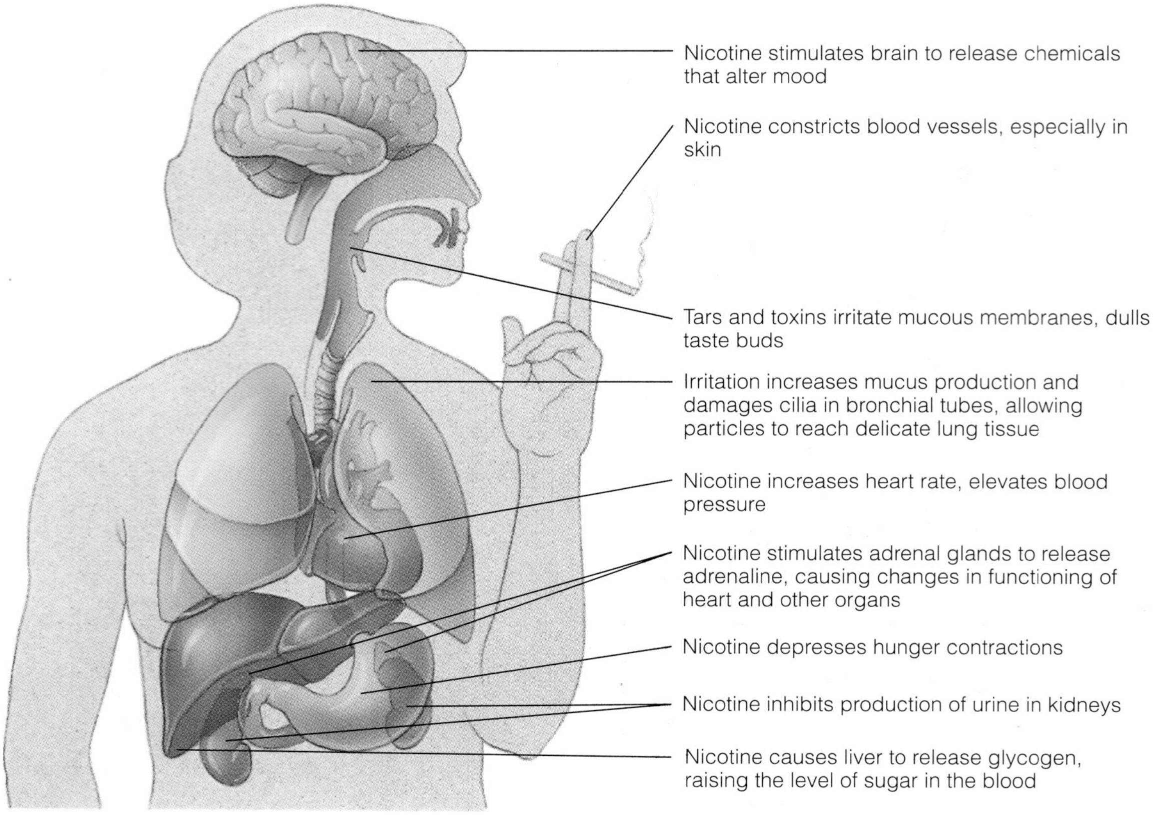
Nicotine stimulates brain to release chemicals that alter mood
Nicotine constricts blood vessels, especially in skin
Tars and toxins irritate mucous membranes, dulls taste buds
Irritation increases mucus production and damages cilia in bronchial tubes, allowing particles to reach delicate lung tissue
Nicotine increases heart rate, elevates blood pressure
Nicotine stimulates adrenal glands to release adrenaline, causing changes in functioning of heart and other organs
Nicotine depresses hunger contractions
Nicotine inhibits production of urine in kidneys
Nicotine causes liver to release glycogen, raising the level of sugar in the blood

Figure 7-1 *How does smoking a cigarette affect your body?*

disturbances of the normal heartbeat rhythm. Sudden and unexpected death is a common result of CHD, particularly among smokers. Smokers have a 70 percent higher death rate from CHD than nonsmokers.

We do not completely understand how cigarette smoking increases the risk of CHD. Researchers, however, are beginning to shed light on the process. Smoking reduces the amount of **HDL** cholesterol (**high-density lipoprotein,** the "good" cholesterol) and thus promotes plaque formation and speeds blood clotting. Smoking may also increase tension in the heart muscle walls, speed up the rate of muscular contraction, and increase the heart rate. The workload of the heart thus increases, as does its need for oxygen and other nutrients. Carbon monoxide produced by cigarette smoking combines with hemoglobin in the red blood cells, displacing oxygen and thus providing less oxygen to the heart.

As suggested earlier, the risks of CHD decrease rapidly when the person stops smoking, particularly for younger smokers whose coronary arteries haven't yet been extensively damaged. Cigarette smoking has also been linked to other cardiovascular diseases, including:

- Stroke, a sudden interference with blood circulation in the brain that destroys brain cells
- Aortic aneurysm, a bulge in the aorta caused by weakening in its walls
- Pulmonary heart disease, a disorder of the right side of the heart, caused by changes in the blood vessels of the lungs

Lung and Other Cancers Cigarette smoking is the primary cause of lung cancer. Those who smoke two or more packs of cigarettes a day have lung cancer death rates 12 to 25 times greater than nonsmokers. The dramatic rise in lung cancer among women clearly parallels the increase of smoking in this group; lung cancer now exceeds breast cancer as the leading cause of cancer deaths among women. The risk of developing lung cancer increases with the number of cigarettes smoked each day, the number of years smoking, and the age at which the person started smoking. The evidence suggests that after a year without smoking the risk of lung cancer decreases substantially. If smoking is stopped before cancer has started, lung tissue tends to repair itself, even if cellular changes that can lead to cancer are already present.

Research has also linked smoking to cancers of the trachea, mouth, pharynx, esophagus, larynx, pancreas, bladder, kidney, cervix, stomach, liver, and colon.

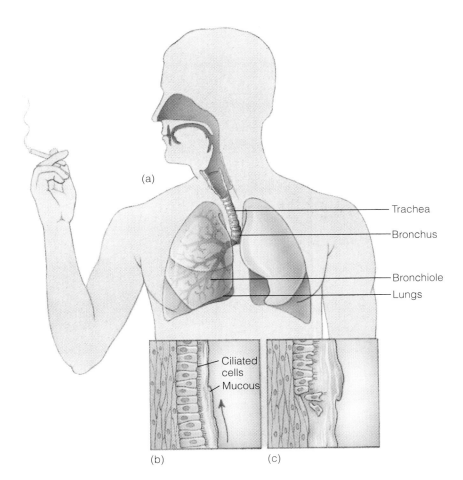

(a)

Trachea

Bronchus

Bronchiole

Lungs

Ciliated cells

Mucous

(b)   (c)

Figure 7-2 *Damage to the lungs caused by smoking.*
(a) The respiratory system.
(b) View of the inside of a bronchiole of a nonsmoker. Foreign particles are collected by a thin layer of sticky mucus and transported out of the lungs, up toward the mouth, by the action of cilia.
(c) View of the inside of a bronchiole of a smoker. Smoking irritates the lung tissue and causes increased mucus production, which can overwhelm the action of the cilia. A smoker develops a chronic cough as the lungs try to rid themselves of foreign particles and excess mucus. Eventually the cilia are destroyed, leaving the delicate lung tissue exposed to injury from foreign substances.

Chronic Obstructive Lung Disease The lungs of a smoker are constantly exposed to dangerous chemicals and irritants, and they must work harder to function adequately. The stresses placed on the lungs by smoking can permanently damage lung function and lead to chronic obstructive lung disease (COLD), also known as chronic obstructive pulmonary disease (COPD). This progressive and disabling disorder consists of several different but related diseases; emphysema and chronic bronchitis are two of the most common.

Emphysema Smoking is the primary cause of **emphysema,** a particularly disabling condition in which the walls of the air sacs in the lungs lose their elasticity and are gradually destroyed. The lungs' ability to obtain oxygen and remove carbon dioxide is impaired. A person with emphysema is breathless, is constantly gasping for air, and has the feeling of drowning. The heart must pump harder and may become enlarged. People with emphysema often die from a damaged heart. There is no known way to reverse this disease. In its advanced stage, the victim is bedridden and severely disabled.

Chronic Bronchitis Chronic bronchitis is persistent, recurrent inflammation of the bronchial tubes. When the

cell lining of the bronchial tubes is irritated, it secretes excess mucus. Bronchial congestion is followed by a chronic cough, which makes breathing more and more difficult. If smokers have chronic bronchitis, they face a greater risk of lung cancer, no matter how old they are or how many (or few) cigarettes they smoke. Chronic bronchitis seems to be a shortcut to lung cancer.

Other Respiratory Damage Even when the smoker shows no signs of lung impairment or disease, cigarette smoking damages the respiratory system. Normally the cells lining the bronchial tubes secrete mucus, a sticky fluid that collects particles of soot, dust, and other substances in inhaled air. Mucus is carried up to the mouth by the continuous motion of the cilia, hairlike structures

High-density lipoprotein (HDL) Blood fats that help keep cholesterol in a watery state and thus protect against cardiovascular diseases.

Emphysema Loss of lung tissue elasticity and breakup of the many small air sacs in the lungs so that fewer, larger, and less elastic air sacs are formed. The progressive accumulation of air causes difficulty in breathing.

TERMS

that protrude from the inner surface of the bronchial tubes (Figure 7-2). If the cilia are destroyed or don't work or if the pollution of inhaled air is more than the system can remove, the protection provided by cilia is lost.

Cigarette smoke first slows, then stops the action of the cilia. Eventually it destroys them, leaving delicate membranes exposed to injury from substances inhaled in cigarette smoke or from the polluted air in which the person lives or works. Special cells of the body, the **macrophages** (literally "big eaters"), also work to remove foreign particles from the respiratory tract by engulfing them. Smoking appears to make macrophages work less efficiently. This interference with the functioning of the respiratory system often leads rapidly to the conditions called smoker's throat and smoker's cough, as well as to shortness of breath. Even smokers of high school age show impaired respiratory function, compared with nonsmokers of the same age.

Although cigarette smoking can cause many respiratory disorders and diseases, the damage is not always permanent. Once a person stops smoking, steady improvement in overall lung function usually takes place. Chronic coughing subsides, phlegm (mucus) production returns to normal, and breathing becomes easier. The likelihood of lung disease drops sharply. People of all ages, even those who have been smoking for decades, improve after they stop smoking. If given a chance, the human body has remarkable powers to restore itself.

Additional Health Hazards
Besides respiratory problems, common physical complaints of smoking include loss of appetite, diarrhea, fatigue, hoarseness, weight loss, stomach pains, and insomnia. These conditions usually disappear in people who stop smoking. People who smoke cigarettes are more likely to develop peptic ulcers than nonsmokers and are more likely to die from them, especially from ulcers of the stomach. Premature skin wrinkling, premature baldness, gum disorders, tooth decay, impotence, and allergies have all been associated with cigarette smoking. Recent research also suggests that smoking may harm the immune system. Further research may link tobacco use to still other disorders.

Cumulative Effects
The cumulative effects of tobacco use fall into two general categories. The first category is reduced life expectancy. A male who takes up smoking before age 15 and continues to smoke is only half as likely to live to age 75 as is a male who never smokes. If he inhales deeply, he risks losing one minute of life for every minute of smoking. Females who have similar smoking habits also have a reduced life expectancy.

The second category involves quality of life. A national health survey begun in 1964 shows that smokers spend one-third more time away from their jobs because of illness than do nonsmokers. Female smokers spend 17 percent more days sick in bed than do female nonsmokers. Lost work days associated with cigarette smoking number in the millions.

> *Personal Insight*   How do you think you would feel if you found your 12-year-old child smoking? Would your feelings depend on whether you yourself were a smoker or a nonsmoker?

Other Forms of Tobacco Use

Many smokers have switched from cigarettes to other forms of tobacco, such as cigars, pipes, clove cigarettes, and smokeless tobacco. However, each of these alternatives is far from safe.

Smokeless Tobacco
In the United States in recent years there has been a disturbing resurgence in the use of all forms of smokeless tobacco, especially among teenage boys and young adult males. The U.S. Centers for Disease Control and Prevention reported in 1994 that 20 percent of male high school seniors used smokeless tobacco.

The nicotine in smokeless tobacco—along with a number of flavorings, additives, and carcinogenic chemicals—is absorbed through the gums and lining of the mouth. The dose of nicotine is comparable to that provided by cigarettes. Because of its nicotine content, smokeless tobacco is highly addictive. Some users keep it in their mouth even while sleeping.

Although not as dangerous as cigarettes, the use of smokeless tobacco carries many health risks. Changes can occur in the mouth after only a few weeks of use: Gums and lips become dried and irritated and may bleed, and precancerous white or red patches may appear inside the mouth. Oral cancers occur several times more frequently among snuff users than among those who don't use tobacco at all. Long-term snuff use may increase the risk of cancer of the cheek and gum by as much as 50 times. Smokeless tobacco may also cause cardiovascular problems and pose risks to developing fetuses in female users who are pregnant.

Cigars and Pipes
Cigar and pipe smoking has declined in recent years, but many people, mostly men, still use

TERMS

Macrophages   Large cells in the body that absorb dead tissue and dead cells.

Mainstream smoke   Smoke that is inhaled by a smoker and then exhaled into the atmosphere.

Sidestream smoke   "Secondhand smoke" that comes from the burning end of a cigarette, cigar, or pipe.

Carboxyhemoglobin   A compound formed when carbon monoxide displaces oxygen from red blood cells; it seriously limits the body's ability to use oxygen.

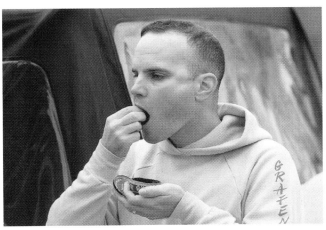

Nearly one out of every five male high school seniors uses smokeless tobacco, a habit linked to oral cancer, dental problems, and possibly cardiovascular problems.

one of these dangerous forms of tobacco. Users of cigars and pipes absorb nicotine through the gums and lining of the mouth. Some cigar and pipe users don't inhale; others do. Those who don't inhale have lower risks for cardiovascular and respiratory diseases than do cigarette smokers; however, their risks are higher than those of nonsmokers. Cigar and pipe smoke is more irritating to the lungs than cigarette smoke, so people who do inhale have even higher rates of respiratory and cardiovascular disease than cigarette smokers. All cigar and pipe smokers face an increased risk for cancers of the lip, mouth, throat, and esophagus.

Clove Cigarettes   Called "kreteks" or "chicartas" and imported primarily from Indonesia, clove cigarettes are made of tobacco mixed with chopped cloves. Despite the addition of cloves, tests show that clove cigarettes deliver more tar, nicotine, and carbon monoxide than ordinary tobacco cigarettes. Clove cigarettes thus offer all the known hazards of tobacco cigarettes plus the unknown hazards of the chemical constituents of cloves. One of the most suspicious of these compounds is eugenol, an anesthetic that may damage the respiratory system's ability to detect and defend against foreign particles. Some individuals may also have severe allergic reactions to eugenol.

THE EFFECTS OF SMOKING ON THE NONSMOKER

In a watershed decision in 1993, the U.S. Environmental Protection Agency (EPA) designated environmental tobacco smoke (ETS) as a Class A carcinogen—an agent known to cause cancer in humans. This designation put ETS in the same category as notorious cancer-causing agents like asbestos. Each year ETS causes thousands of deaths from lung cancer and heart disease and is respon-

sible for hundreds of thousands of respiratory infections in young children.

For the U.S. tobacco industry, the EPA's report was the worst blow since 1964, when the Surgeon General first declared that smoking causes cancer. Tobacco interests went to court to challenge the EPA's designation. Cigarette makers launched a media campaign in an effort to cast doubt on the EPA's science. Despite such efforts, the EPA report gave new momentum to efforts to limit or ban smoking in public and in the workplace.

Environmental Tobacco Smoke

Environmental tobacco smoke consists of mainstream smoke and sidestream smoke. Smoke exhaled by smokers is referred to as **mainstream smoke. Sidestream smoke,** also called secondhand smoke, enters the atmosphere from the burning end of the cigarette, cigar, or pipe. Undiluted sidestream smoke, because it isn't filtered through either a cigarette filter or a smoker's lungs, has significantly higher concentrations of the toxic and carcinogenic compounds found in mainstream smoke. For example, compared to mainstream smoke, sidestream smoke has (1) twice as much tar and nicotine, (2) three times as much benzopyrene, a cancer-causing agent, (3) almost three times as much carbon monoxide, which displaces oxygen from red blood cells and forms **carboxyhemoglobin,** a dangerous compound that seriously limits the body's ability to use oxygen, and (4) three times as much ammonia. Nearly 85 percent of the smoke in a room where someone is smoking comes from sidestream smoke. Sidestream smoke is diffused through the air, so nonsmokers don't inhale the same concentrations of toxic chemicals that the smoker does. Still, the concentrations can be considerable. In rooms where people are smoking, levels of carbon monoxide can exceed those permitted by Federal Air Quality Standards for outside air.

Effects of ETS

Studies show that up to 25 percent of nonsmokers subjected to ETS develop coughs, 30 percent develop headaches and nasal discomfort, and 70 percent suffer eye irritation. Other symptoms range from breathlessness to sinus problems. People with allergies tend to suffer the worst symptoms. Tobacco odor—which clings to skin and clothes—is another unpleasant effect of ETS.

But ETS causes more than just annoyance and discomfort. The EPA estimates that ETS causes 3,000 lung cancer deaths each year. People who live or work among smokers face a 20 to 30 percent increase in lung-cancer risk. ETS also appears to contribute to heart disease. According to the American Heart Association, about 35,000 deaths from heart disease can be attributed to ETS each year. ETS also aggravates asthma, itself an increasing cause of sudden death in otherwise healthy adults.

Everyone knows that smoking is dangerous to your health. It shortens life expectancy and increases the risk of cancer, lung disease, and heart disease. But did you know that smoking carries special risks for women? Many of these risks are associated with reproduction and the reproductive organs. The risk of cervical cancer, for example, is higher in women who smoke than in women who don't. For women trying to become pregnant, smoking may impair fertility. For pregnant women, smoking increases the risk of ectopic (tubal) pregnancy, miscarriage, and stillbirth.

Babies born to women who smoke during pregnancy may suffer from growth retardation in the womb and are typically lower in birth weight than are babies born to nonsmoking women. As a group, they also perform worse on tests in both infancy and childhood. Babies whose mothers smoked during pregnancy are at higher risk for sudden infant death syndrome (SIDS) than are babies of nonsmokers.

Smoking interacts with oral contraceptives in dangerous ways; women who smoke and take birth control pills have a higher risk of developing potentially fatal blood clots than do other women. They are also at greater risk for fatal heart attacks and hemorrhagic strokes.

Smoking increases women's chances of developing osteoporosis, a disease in which bones become thinner and more brittle. Estrogen is often prescribed to prevent this bone loss after menopause, but estrogen works less well in preventing osteoporosis when a woman smokes. Older women who smoke are thus more likely to suffer hip fractures from falls.

Right now, for the first time in U.S. history, teenage girls are taking up smoking in greater numbers than teenage boys. If the trend continues, female smokers will outnumber male smokers in the adult population by the year 2000. We can expect to see a corresponding increase in tobacco-related diseases among women. Already, lung cancer has surpassed breast cancer as the most common cause of cancer death in American women. Unfortunately, we can also expect to see more of these debilitating and life-threatening tobacco-related diseases that are unique to women.

Children and ETS

The EPA estimates that environmental tobacco smoke triggers 150,000 to 300,000 cases of bronchitis, pneumonia, and other respiratory infections in infants and toddlers up to 18 months of age each year, resulting in 7,500 to 15,000 hospitalizations. Older children suffer, too. The EPA has labeled ETS a risk factor for asthma in children who have not previously displayed symptoms of the disease and has blamed ETS for aggravating the symptoms of the 200,000 to 1 million children who already have asthma. ETS is also linked to reduced lung function and to fluid build-up in the middle ear, a contributing factor in middle-ear infections, a leading reason for childhood surgery.

Why are infants and children so vulnerable? Because they breathe faster than adults, they inhale more air—and more of the pollutants in the air. Because they also weigh less, they inhale three times more pollutants per unit of body weight than do adults. And because their young lungs are still growing, this intake can impair optimal development. The problem is widespread. The American Academy of Pediatrics estimates some 9 million American children are exposed to ETS, usually in the home. A mother's smoking has the most impact on a child's health, no doubt because mothers continue to provide more child care than fathers, even when both parents work.

Smoking and Pregnancy

Smoking almost doubles a pregnant woman's chance of suffering a miscarriage, and women who smoke also face an increased risk of ectopic pregnancy. Maternal smoking causes an estimated 4,600 infant deaths in the United States each year, primarily due to premature delivery and smoking-related problems with the placenta, the organ that delivers blood, oxygen, and nutrients to the fetus. Infants whose mothers smoked during pregnancy are also more likely to die from sudden infant death syndrome (SIDS). Maternal smoking causes fetal growth retardation, too. It is a major factor in low birth weight, which puts newborns at high risk for infections and other potentially fatal problems. Babies born to mothers who smoke more than two packs per day perform poorly on developmental tests in the first hours after birth when compared with babies of nonsmoking mothers. Later in life, hyperactivity, short attention span, and lower scores on spelling and reading tests all occur more frequently in children whose mothers smoked throughout pregnancy than in those born to nonsmoking mothers. In addition, animal research suggests certain cancers are more common in animals that were exposed to cigarette smoke as fetuses. Nevertheless, 20 to 25 percent of pregnant Americans continue to smoke throughout pregnancy.

WHAT CAN BE DONE?

Early in 1967, John F. Banzhaf III, outraged by a television commercial that equated smoking with masculinity, fired off a petition to the Federal Communications Commission. In it, Banzhaf, then 26 and fresh out of law school, demanded that foes of cigarettes be given a chance to air their side. On June 2, 1967, the FCC issued a landmark decision agreeing with him. The agency ordered broadcasters to provide "significant" free air time for anti-cigarette announcements. Four years later, Congress banned all cigarette advertising from TV and radio.

In 1993, shortly after he heard that the EPA had declared ETS to be a carcinogen, W. D. "Bill" Landis vowed to stop smoking around his newborn grandson. But he didn't stop there. Landis, a deputy sheriff and city councilman in Pleasanton, California, launched a drive to force others in his town to do the same. He proposed a citywide ban on smoking in all public and private workplaces, including restaurants, and a ban on cigarette vending machines. The ordinance passed unanimously.

In both cases, individuals acted on their own to combat tobacco use, arguably the deadliest plague of our time. Every hour, 50 Americans die from preventable smoking-related diseases. Today there are more avenues than ever before for individual and group action against this major public health threat.

Action at the Local Level

Before the EPA issued its report, most efforts to limit smoking focused on enacting local laws and ordinances. Tobacco interests have been able to block actions at the national and state levels through lobbying and political contributions. However, during the 1980s and early 1990s, tobacco restrictions were passed by local school boards, town councils, and county boards of supervisors, over which the tobacco industry has little or no influence. Local governments also enacted laws that raised cigarette taxes, blocked youth access to cigarette vending machines, tightened enforcement of laws prohibiting cigarette sales to minors, and limiting tobacco advertising. As local no-smoking rules proliferated, evidence also mounted that smoking restrictions encourage smokers to quit. The smoking rate dropped from one in three adults in 1980 to one in four by 1995.

Action at the State and Federal Levels

The EPA report fundamentally changed the politics of tobacco by declaring that smokers not only shorten their own lives, they kill bystanders. It became harder for politicians who are sympathetic to the tobacco industry —and who often accept sizable political contributions from tobacco interests—to argue that anti-tobacco laws constitute unwarranted intrusions into voters' private lives. Smoking also became a clear-cut occupational health issue, subject to the regulatory power of state and federal occupational health agencies. Such agencies can be more independent of the pressure of special interests than are elected lawmakers.

Following the EPA report, a number of state legislatures passed tough new anti-tobacco laws, many of which had met repeated defeat in the same states in the past. For example, Michigan voters approved a 50 percent tax increase on cigarettes in 1994, bringing that state's tax to a national high of 75 cents per pack.

U.S. Food and Drug Administration Commissioner David Kessler raised the prospect of regulating tobacco as an addictive drug, while the House Subcommittee on Health and Environment held hearings on tobacco regulation. Summoned to testify at these hearings, heads of major tobacco companies made national news when they swore they didn't think cigarettes were addictive.

Action in the Private Sector

The EPA report also shook up the private sector, giving employers reason to fear workers' compensation claims based on exposure to workplace smoke. The year after the report was issued, businesses including McDonald's and Taco Bell banned smoking in thousands of their restaurants across the country. By 1995, 70 percent of the nation's shopping malls were smoke free.

Such local, state, and national efforts represent progress, but tobacco industry influence remains strong. As of 1994, smoking laws in 19 states were relatively weak, tobacco-industry backed versions with clauses that prevented stricter local ordinances. Action is especially needed in tobacco-producing states.

Individual Action

When a smoker violates a nonsmoking designation, complain. If your favorite restaurant or shop doesn't have a nonsmoking policy, ask the manager to adopt one. If you see children using cigarette vending machines or buying tobacco in stores, report this illegal activity to the facility manager or the police. Learn more about addiction and tobacco cessation so you can better support the tobacco users you know. Follow local, state, and national politics. Vote for politicians who support anti-tobacco measures. Write to elected officials to let them know your views. Cancel your subscriptions to magazines that carry tobacco advertising; include a note to the publisher or editor explaining your decision. Volunteer with the American Lung Association, the American Cancer Society, or the American Heart Association. These are just some of the many ways individuals can help support tobacco prevention and cessation efforts. Nonsmokers not only have the right to breathe clean air, but they also have the right to take action to help solve this serious public health threat (Figure 7-3 is a Nonsmoker's Bill of Rights).

Checking Tobacco Interests

With their immensely profitable industry shrinking, tobacco companies are concentrating on appealing to narrower and narrower market segments with an ever-increasing array of brands and styles—over 350 in all. As tobacco use has declined among better-educated, wealthier segments of the American population, tobacco compa-

How You Can Help a Tobacco User Quit

The National Cancer Institute recommends a "Four A's" approach for physicians who want to help patients quit tobacco. The approach can be adapted for anyone who wants to help a tobacco user quit.

1. *Ask* about tobacco use. Has your younger brother ever dipped snuff? How long has your roommate smoked? How many cigarettes a day is your friend up to?

2. *Advise* tobacco users to stop. "As your friend, I hate to see you jeopardize your health. I've noticed you cough a lot already and your voice is raspy. You should stop." Studies show the cumulative messages tobacco users get about quitting do help motivate them to stop.

3. *Assist* the tobacco user who is willing to stop. To coincide with your friend's quit date, invite him or her on a camping trip, hike, or other outing far from any stores selling tobacco. Be tolerant if the quitter is

irritable and unpleasant. Introduce the quitter to restaurants that don't allow smoking. Offer to be an exercise partner; exercise can increase a quitter's chance of success. Call the quitter once a day to offer encouragement and help. Bring gifts of low-calorie snacks or crafts that occupy the hands. Offer to take a relaxation course with him or her. If the quitter lapses, be encouraging. A lapse doesn't have to become a relapse.

4. *Arrange* follow-up. Maintaining abstinence is an ongoing process. Every month or so, congratulate quitters again on their success. Note how much better their cars and rooms smell, how they get winded less easily and cough less often, and how much you appreciate not having to breathe their smoke. Continue to engage quitters in exercise and to help them find new ways to enjoy life that don't revolve around tobacco.

---

nies have redirected their marketing efforts toward minorities, the poor, and young women, populations among whom smoking rates are still high. This practice of targeting specific segments of the tobacco market has become extremely controversial. The rise in popularity of smokeless tobacco is one example of targeted marketing. Advertisements for smokeless tobacco associate chewing and dipping with a "macho" image and athletic prowess.

Pressure placed on tobacco companies in response to such targeted marketing campaigns has had an effect, however. The R. J. Reynolds Tobacco Company recently canceled its plans to market Uptown, a brand of cigarettes designed to appeal to African Americans, after the U.S. Secretary of Health and Human Services accused the company of "promoting a culture of cancer." Cigarette companies continue their efforts to appeal specifically to women, however, usually by connecting smoking with thinness (the dominant women's brand is Virginia Slims). In addition, tobacco companies have begun focusing on increasing the export of cigarettes, particularly to developing nations. As companies compete for customers in the years ahead, the need to exercise public pressure to keep the powerful tobacco interests in check will persist.

HOW CAN A TOBACCO USER QUIT?

Giving up tobacco is a long-term, intricate process. Heavy smokers who say they've just stopped "cold turkey" aren't revealing the thinking and struggling and other mental processes that contributed to their final conquest over this powerful addiction. Research shows tobacco users move through predictable stages from being uninterested in stopping, to thinking about change, to making a concerted effort to stop, to finally maintaining abstinence. But most attempt to quit several times before they finally succeed. Relapse is a normal part of the process.

Quitting on Your Own

Some 85 to 95 percent of smokers who quit do so on their own. The National Cancer Institute, the American Cancer Society, and the American Lung Association publish information for would-be quitters on going it alone. But one recent study of solo quitters found that those who used such materials were no more successful than those who didn't. Some factors did seem to increase the chances of success, however. Smokers who quit cold turkey stood a slightly better chance of remaining tobacco-free for seven months than did those who tapered off gradually or switched brands before quitting. Successful quitters were also more likely to have support from others and to exercise. On the other hand, focusing on the negative effects of tobacco use has not proved to be a strategy associated with success. And another study showed that the more alcohol an individual drank, the less likely he or she was to succeed in quitting. The Behavior Change Strategy at the end of the chapter outlines a plan for quitting.

Group Programs

Formal programs are particularly recommended for people who have tried repeatedly to quit on their own without success. The American Cancer Society, the American Lung Association, and the Seventh-day Adventist Church

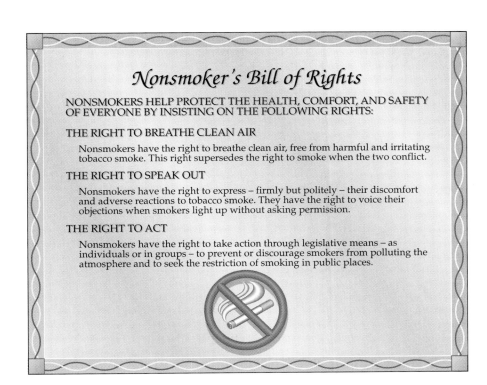

Figure 7-3   *Nonsmoker's Bill of Rights.*

Nonsmoker's Bill of Rights

NONSMOKERS HELP PROTECT THE HEALTH, COMFORT, AND SAFETY OF EVERYONE BY INSISTING ON THE FOLLOWING RIGHTS:

THE RIGHT TO BREATHE CLEAN AIR

Nonsmokers have the right to breathe clean air, free from harmful and irritating tobacco smoke. This right supersedes the right to smoke when the two conflict.

THE RIGHT TO SPEAK OUT

Nonsmokers have the right to express – firmly but politely – their discomfort and adverse reactions to tobacco smoke. They have the right to voice their objections when smokers light up without asking permission.

THE RIGHT TO ACT

Nonsmokers have the right to take action through legislative means – as individuals or in groups – to prevent or discourage smokers from polluting the atmosphere and to seek the restriction of smoking in public places.

all offer well-respected smoking cessation programs. Your college health center or community hospital may also do so. Some programs now are geared specifically to smokeless tobacco users. Some studies have found that as many as 30 percent of the people who enroll in outpatient quit-smoking programs remain tobacco-free a year later. When quitters also use nicotine gum, the success rate can climb as high as 47 percent.

Prescription Help

Physicians can now prescribe nicotine in gum or skin-patch form to help ease quitters' withdrawal symptoms. Clonidine, a drug used to help heroin addicts during withdrawal, is also prescribed to help some smokers quit. Meanwhile, researchers are investigating the usefulness of antidepressants and antianxiety drugs in smoking cessation and are experimenting with nicotine nose drops and sprays.

Benefits of Quitting

Giving up tobacco provides immediate health benefits to men and women of all ages. People who quit smoking find food tastes better. Their sense of smell increases. Circulation improves, heart rate and blood pressure drop, and lung function and heart efficiency increase. People have more "wind," and their capacity for exercise improves. Many ex-smokers report feeling more energetic and alert. They experience fewer headaches. Even their complexions may improve. Quitting also has a positive effect on long-term disease risk.

The younger people are when they stop smoking, the more pronounced the health improvements. And these improvements gradually but invariably increase as the period of nonsmoking increases (Table 7-1). It's never too late to quit, though. According to a 1990 U.S. Surgeon General's report, people who quit smoking, regardless of age, live longer than people who continue to smoke.

THE NATURE OF ALCOHOL

People long ago recognized the power of alcoholic beverages: The "spirit" changed feelings and behavior. Ever since, alcohol has had a somewhat contradictory role in human life. It is associated with good times, cheerfulness, and conviviality, but it is also associated with escape, slow suicide, and self-destructiveness. Many of our slang expressions for **intoxication** reflect its less positive aspects; we say we're "smashed," "bombed," "wasted."

Alcohol is probably the oldest drug in the world. There is evidence that beer and berry wine were used by 6400 B.C., and probably even earlier. Once the **distillation** process was developed (about A.D. 800), the spirit could

Intoxication   The state of being mentally affected by a chemical (literally, a state of being poisoned).

Distillation   The process of heating a mixture and recondensing the vapor. This process intensifies the mixture's properties and eliminates impurities. Distillation is used in manufacturing whiskey and brandy.

TERMS

TABLE 7-1 Benefits of Quitting Smoking

Within 20 minutes of your last cigarette:
- You stop polluting the air
- Blood pressure drops to normal
- Pulse rate drops to normal rate
- Temperature of hands and feet increases to normal

8 hours:
- Carbon monoxide level in blood drops to normal
- Oxygen level in blood increases to normal

24 hours:
- Chance of heart attack decreases

48 hours:
- Nerve endings adjust to the absence of nicotine
- Ability to smell and taste things is enhanced

72 hours:
- Bronchial tubes relax, making breathing easier
- Lung capacity increases

2 to 3 months:
- Circulation improves
- Walking becomes easier
- Lung function increases up to 30 percent

1 to 9 months:
- Coughing, sinus congestion, fatigue, and shortness of breath all decrease
- Cilia regrow in lungs, reduce infection
- Body's overall energy level increases

1 year:
- Heart disease death rate is halfway back to that of a nonsmoker

5 years:
- Heart disease rate drops to the rate for nonsmokers
- Lung cancer death rate decreases halfway back to that of nonsmokers

10 years:
- Lung cancer death rate drops almost to the rate for nonsmokers
- Precancerous cells are replaced
- The incidence of other cancers (mouth, larynx, esophagus, bladder, kidney, and pancreas) decreases

Source: California Medical Association, 1995.

---

be concentrated in a purer and more potent form. It was called *al-kuhl,* an Arabic word meaning "finely divided spirit." Alcohol has been used in religious ceremonies, in feasts and celebrations, and as a medicine for thousands of years. Throughout history, alcohol has been more popular than any other drug in the Western world, despite numerous prohibitions against it. In fact, forbidding the use of alcohol seems only to make it more popular. Even the newer psychoactive drugs have not diminished its popularity.

How does alcohol affect people? Does it affect some people differently than others? Can some people "handle" alcohol? Is it possible to drink a safe amount of alcohol? Many of the misconceptions about the effects of alcohol can be cleared up by examining the chemistry of alcohol and how it is absorbed and metabolized by the body.

The Chemistry of Alcohol

Ethyl alcohol is the common psychoactive ingredient in all alcoholic beverages. Beer, a mild intoxicant brewed from a mixture of grains, usually contains between 3 and 6 percent alcohol by volume. Wines are made by **fermenting** the juices of grapes or other fruits. The concentration of alcohol in table wines is about 9 to 14 percent. *Fortified wines*—so named because distilled alcohol has been added to them—contain about 20 percent alcohol; these include sherry, port, and Madeira. Stronger alco-

holic beverages, called *hard liquors,* are made by distilling brewed or fermented grains or other products. These beverages, including gin, whiskey, brandy, rum, and liqueurs, usually contain from 35 to 50 percent alcohol.

The concentration of alcohol in a beverage is indicated by the **proof value,** which is two times the percentage concentration. For example, if a beverage is 100 proof, it contains 50 percent alcohol. Two ounces of 100-proof whiskey contain one ounce of pure alcohol. When alcohol consumption is discussed, "one drink" refers to the typical 12-ounce bottle of beer, or to a 5-ounce glass of table wine, or to a cocktail with 1½ ounces of liquor. Each of these drinks contains approximately the same amount of alcohol—about 0.6 ounces.

Absorption

When a person ingests alcohol, about 20 percent is rapidly absorbed from the stomach into the bloodstream. About 75 percent is absorbed through the upper part of the small intestine. Any remaining alcohol enters the bloodstream further down the gastrointestinal tract. The rate of absorption is affected by a variety of factors. For example, the carbonation in a beverage like champagne increases the rate of alcohol absorption. Food in the stomach slows absorption, as does drinking concentrated alcoholic beverages such as hard liquor. Remember, though, *all* alcohol consumed is eventually absorbed.

Metabolizing Alcohol: Our Bodies Work Differently

Do you notice that you react differently to alcohol than some of your friends do? If so, you may be noticing genetic differences in alcohol metabolism that are associated with gender or ethnicity. Alcohol is metabolized mainly in the liver, but some alcohol is broken down in the stomach before it can be sent into the bloodstream and on to the liver. Once it's circulating in the bloodstream, alcohol produces the well-known feelings of intoxication. Studies have shown that women metabolize less alcohol in the stomach than men do, so they release more unmetabolized alcohol into the bloodstream. Although the biochemical explanation for this phenomenon is still unknown, the practical implication is that women feel the effect of alcohol sooner and to a greater degree than men do. The same amount of alcohol will have more effect on a woman than on a man.

Other differences in alcohol metabolism are associated with ethnicity. Alcohol is broken down in the liver by an enzyme called alcohol dehydrogenase, producing a by-product called acetaldehyde (see figure). Acetaldehyde is responsible for many of the unpleasant effects of alcohol abuse. Another enzyme, acetaldehyde dehydrogenase, breaks this product down further. Some people, including many of Asian descent, have genetic information that causes them to produce somewhat different forms of the two enzymes that metabolize alcohol. The result is high concentrations of acetaldehyde in the brain and other tissues, producing a host of unpleasant symptoms. When people with these enzymes drink alcohol, they experience a physiological reaction referred to as "flushing syndrome." Their skin feels hot, their heart and respiration rates increase, and they may get a headache, vomit, or break out in hives. Drinking makes them so uncomfortable that it's unlikely they could ever become addicted to alcohol. The body's response to acetaldehyde is the basis for treating alcohol abuse with the drug disulfiram (Antabuse), which inhibits the action of acetaldehyde dehydrogenase. When a person taking disulfiram ingests alcohol, acetaldehyde levels increase rapidly, and he or she develops an intense flushing reaction along with weakness, nausea, vomiting, and other disagreeable symptoms.

How people behave in relation to alcohol is influenced in complex ways by many factors, including social and cultural ones. But in these two cases at least, individual choices and behavior are strongly influenced by a specific genetic/biological characteristic.

Alcohol dehydrogenase

Alcohol (ethanol)

↓

Acetaldehyde

Acetaldehyde dehydrogenase

↓

Smaller molecules and energy

Metabolism and Excretion

Alcohol is quickly transported throughout the body by the blood. Because alcohol easily moves through most biological membranes, it is rapidly distributed throughout most body tissues. The main site of alcohol **metabolism** is the liver, though a small amount of alcohol is metabolized in the stomach.

About 2 to 10 percent of ingested alcohol is not metabolized in the liver or other tissues, but is excreted unchanged by the lungs, kidneys, and sweat glands. Excreted alcohol causes the telltale smell on a drinker's breath and is the basis of breath and urine analyses for alcohol levels. Such analyses do not give precise measurements of alcohol concentrations in the blood (the measure of intoxication), but they do provide a reasonable approximation if done correctly.

Alcohol Intake and Blood Alcohol Concentration

Blood alcohol concentration (BAC) is determined by the amount of alcohol consumed and by individual factors such as body weight and amount of body fat. In most

Fermented   Describes a substance in which complex molecules have been broken down by the action of yeast or bacteria. Fermentation of certain substances produces alcohol.

Proof value   Two times the percentage of alcohol by volume. A beverage that is 50 percent alcohol by volume is 100 proof.

Metabolism   The chemical transformation of food and other substances in the body into energy and wastes.

Blood alcohol concentration (BAC)   The amount of alcohol in the blood in terms of weight per unit volume.

TERMS

TABLE 7-2 Effects of Alcohol

Blood Alcohol Concentrations (Percent)	Common Behavioral Effects	Hours Required for Alcohol to Be Metabolized
0.00–0.05	Slight change in feelings—usually relaxation and euphoria. Decreased alertness.	2–3
0.05–0.10	Emotional lability with exaggerated feelings and behavior. Reduced social inhibitions. Impairment of reaction time and fine motor coordination. Increasingly impaired during driving. Legally drunk at 0.08 in many states and 0.10 in others.	4–6
0.10–0.15	Unsteadiness in standing and walking. Loss of peripheral vision. Driving is extremely dangerous. Legally drunk at 0.15 in all states.	6–10
0.15–0.30	Staggering gait. Slurred speech. Pain and other sensory perceptions greatly impaired.	10–24
More than 0.30	Stupor or unconsciousness. Anesthesia. Death possible at 0.35 and above. Can result from rapid or binge drinking with few earlier effects.	More than 24

cases, a smaller person develops a higher BAC than a larger person after drinking the same amount of alcohol. This is because a smaller person has less overall body tissue into which alcohol can be distributed. A person with a higher percentage of body fat will usually develop a higher BAC than a more muscular person who weighs the same because alcohol does not concentrate as much in fatty tissue as in muscle and most other tissues.

BAC also depends on the balance between the rate of alcohol absorption and the rate of alcohol metabolism. A man who weighs 154 pounds and has normal liver function metabolizes about 0.3 to 0.5 ounces of alcohol per hour—the equivalent of slightly less than a 12-ounce bottle of beer or a 5-ounce glass of wine. The rate of alcohol metabolism varies among individuals and is largely determined by genetics. Contrary to popular myths, this metabolic rate cannot be influenced by exercise, breathing deeply, eating, drinking coffee, or taking other drugs. The rate of alcohol metabolism is the same whether a person is asleep or awake.

ALCOHOL AND HEALTH

The effects of alcohol consumption on health depend on the individual, the circumstances, and the amount of alcohol consumed.

Immediate Effects of Alcohol

At low concentrations, alcohol tends to make people feel relaxed and jovial, but at higher concentrations people are more likely to feel angry, **sedated,** or sleepy. Alcohol is a **central nervous system (CNS) depressant,** and its ef-

fects vary because body systems are affected to different degrees at different BACs (Table 7-2).

The effects of alcohol can first be felt at a BAC of about 0.03 to 0.05 percent. These effects may include lightheadedness, relaxation, and release of inhibitions. Most drinkers experience mild euphoria and become more sociable. When people drink in social settings, alcohol often seems to act as a **stimulant,** enhancing conviviality or assertiveness. This apparent stimulation occurs because alcohol depresses inhibitory centers in the brain.

At higher concentrations, these pleasant effects tend to be replaced by more negative ones—interference with motor coordination, verbal performance, and intellectual functions. The drinker often becomes irritable and may be easily angered or given to crying. When the BAC reaches 0.1 percent, most sensory and motor functioning is reduced, and many people become sedated, or sleepy. Vision, smell, taste, and hearing become less acute. At 0.2 percent, most drinkers are completely unable to function, either physically or psychologically, because of the pronounced depression of the central nervous system, muscles, and many other body systems. Coma usually occurs at a BAC of 0.35 percent, and any higher level can be fatal.

Statistics show that being drunk is hazardous to your health. The combination of impaired judgment, weakened sensory perception, reduced inhibitions, impaired motor coordination, and, often, increased aggressiveness and hostility that characterizes alcohol intoxication can be dangerous or even deadly.

Alcohol causes blood vessels near the skin to dilate, so drinkers often feel warm; their skin flushes, and they may sweat more. Flushing and sweating contribute to loss of

- Drunk drivers as a group are eight times more likely to be involved in a fatal crash than are sober drivers.
- Alcohol use more than triples the chances of fatal accidents during leisure activities such as swimming or boating.
- 69 percent of drowning deaths are alcohol-related.
- Alcohol is involved in up to 50 percent of all fatal falls.
- 35 percent of suicide victims between the ages of 15 and 34 have been drinking.

- Alcohol is related to increased risk of death in a fire.
- Over 50 percent of the perpetrators of murder, assault, and rape were drinking before the crime.
- Alcohol is especially common in "victim-precipitated homicides," in which the eventual victim strikes the first blow.
- Through homicide, automobile crashes, and other incidents, alcohol is the fourth leading killer in the United States.

heat, and so the internal body temperature falls. High doses of alcohol may impair the body's ability to regulate temperature, causing it to drop sharply, especially if the surrounding temperature is low. Drinking alcoholic beverages to keep warm in cold weather does not work, and it can even be dangerous.

Alcohol, particularly in large amounts, definitely changes sleep patterns. Alcohol may facilitate falling asleep more quickly, but the sleep is often light, punctuated with awakenings, and unrefreshing. Even after the habitual drinker stops drinking, his or her sleep may be altered for weeks or months. Users of alcohol frequently awaken with a "hangover"—headache, nausea, stomach distress, and generalized discomfort.

Drinking and Driving

Drunk driving continues to be one of the most serious public health and safety problems in the United States. Every year, about 500,000 people are injured in alcohol-related automobile crashes—an average of one person injured every minute. Over half of the more than 40,000 traffic crash fatalities each year are alcohol-related.

In addition to increased risk of injury and death, driving while intoxicated can have serious legal consequences. Drunk driving is against the law. The legal limit for BAC is 0.10 percent or lower in nearly all states. There are stiff penalties for driving while drunk, and many cities have set up checkpoints where drivers are stopped and checked for intoxication.

Even low doses of alcohol increase the risk of an automobile crash somewhat, especially in crowded conditions; but as the dose increases, the risk increases at a spectacular rate (Figure 7-4). The number of drinks it takes the average person to reach the legal BAC limit is shown in Figure 7-5. Remember that these amounts are approximate, since BACs vary depending on many factors, including gender.

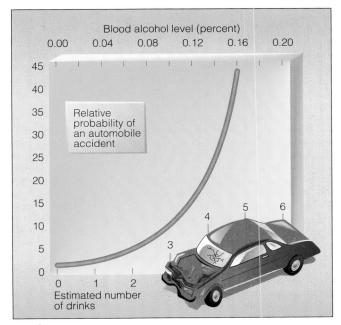

VITAL STATISTICS

Figure 7-4 *The dose-response relationship of alcohol levels and automobile crashes.*

Sedate   To calm by the use of a drug that quiets the activity of the nerves.

Central nervous system depressant   Any chemical that affects the brain or spinal cord and decreases nervous or muscular activity.

Stimulant   Something that increases nervous or muscular activity.

Dose-response relationship   The relationship between the amount of a drug taken and the intensity or type of drug effect.

TERMS

Social drinkers and alcoholics alike are a menace behind the wheel. One-half of all traffic fatalities are associated with alcohol use, and one-third of all alcohol-related traffic accidents involve drivers between the ages of 16 and 24. People who drink and drive are unable to drive responsibly because their judgment is impaired, their reaction time is slower, and their coordination is reduced. No one can drive skillfully and safely when under the influence of alcohol.

What can you do to protect yourself from alcohol-related accidents on the road? If you are out of your home and drinking, follow the practice of having a "designated driver," an individual who refrains from drinking in order to provide safe transportation home for others in the group. The responsibility is rotated, so different people take the role of designated drivers on different occasions. In Sweden and the United Kingdom, where the practice originated, designated drivers place their car keys in their empty beverage glasses so they are not served. In the United States, designated drivers sometimes wear a special button to indicate their role for that evening.

Of course, even if you follow safe practices, you may encounter a drunk driver on the road. To reduce your chances of being involved in a crash caused by someone else, learn to be alert to the erratic driving that signals an impaired driver. Warning signs include the following:

- Unusually wide turns
- Straddling the center line or lane marker
- Driving with one's head out of the window or with the window down in cold weather
- Nearly striking an object or another vehicle
- Weaving or swerving
- Driving on other than the designated roadway

- Stopping with no apparent cause
- Following too closely
- Responding slowly to traffic signals
- Abrupt or illegal turns
- Rapid acceleration or deceleration
- Driving with headlights off at night

If you see any of these warning signs, what should you do?

- If the driver is ahead of you, maintain a safe following distance. Do not try to pass, because the driver may swerve into your car.
- If the driver is behind you, turn right at the nearest intersection. Let the driver pass and then return to your route.
- If the driver is approaching your car, move to the shoulder and stop. Avoid a head-on collision by sounding your horn or flashing your lights.
- When approaching an intersection, slow down and expect the unexpected.
- Make sure your seat belt is fastened, children are in approved safety seats, and keep your doors locked.
- Report suspected impaired drivers to the nearest law enforcement agency by phone. Give a description of the vehicle, license number, location, and direction the vehicle is headed.

Don't become a statistic. Be alert, don't drink and drive, and use a designated driver to make sure you come home alive and safe.

Adapted from "The Designated Driver: Being a Friend." *Healthline*, December 1986.

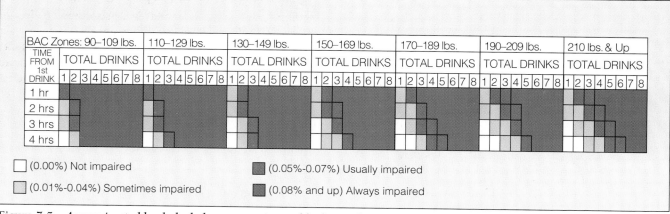

Figure 7-5 *Approximate blood alcohol concentration and body weight.*
A BAC of 0.08 is considered legally drunk in some states and a BAC of 0.10 is considered legally drunk in most others. However, alcohol impairs the user at much lower BACs. This chart illustrates the BAC an average person of a given weight would reach after drinking the specified number of drinks in the time given.
Adapted from California Department of Motor Vehicles.

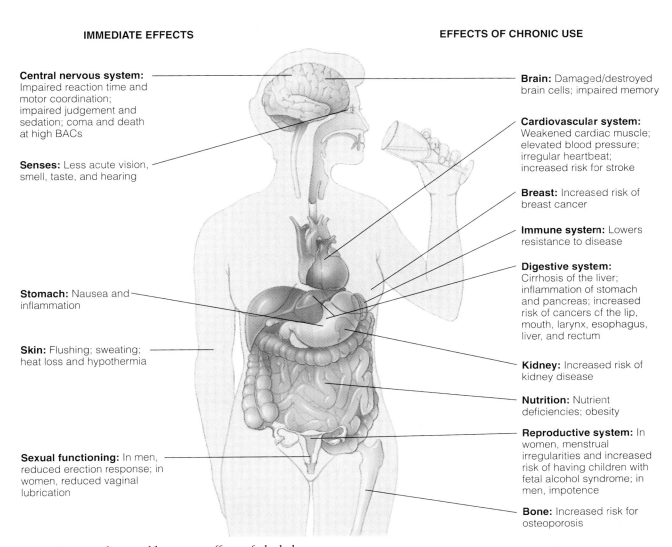

IMMEDIATE EFFECTS

Central nervous system: Impaired reaction time and motor coordination; impaired judgement and sedation; coma and death at high BACs

Senses: Less acute vision, smell, taste, and hearing

Stomach: Nausea and inflammation

Skin: Flushing; sweating; heat loss and hypothermia

Sexual functioning: In men, reduced erection response; in women, reduced vaginal lubrication

EFFECTS OF CHRONIC USE

Brain: Damaged/destroyed brain cells; impaired memory

Cardiovascular system: Weakened cardiac muscle; elevated blood pressure; irregular heartbeat; increased risk for stroke

Breast: Increased risk of breast cancer

Immune system: Lowers resistance to disease

Digestive system: Cirrhosis of the liver; inflammation of stomach and pancreas; increased risk of cancers of the lip, mouth, larynx, esophagus, liver, and rectum

Kidney: Increased risk of kidney disease

Nutrition: Nutrient deficiencies; obesity

Reproductive system: In women, menstrual irregularities and increased risk of having children with fetal alcohol syndrome; in men, impotence

Bone: Increased risk for osteoporosis

Figure 7-6 *Immediate and long-term effects of alcohol use.*

Because alcohol is distributed throughout most of the body, it can affect many different organs and tissues (Figure 7-6). Problems associated with chronic use of alcohol include diseases of the digestive and cardiovascular systems and some cancers. Drinking during pregnancy risks the health of both the woman and the developing fetus.

Digestive System   Even in relatively small amounts, alcohol can alter liver function. With continued use of alcohol, liver cells are damaged and then progressively destroyed. The destroyed cells are often replaced by fibrous scar tissue, a condition known as **cirrhosis of the liver.** As cirrhosis develops, a drinker may gradually lose his or her capacity to tolerate alcohol, because there are fewer and fewer healthy cells remaining in the liver to metabolize it. Alcohol-precipitated cirrhosis is a major cause of death in the United States.

Alcohol can also inflame the pancreas, causing nausea, vomiting, abnormal digestion, and severe abdominal pain. Irritation of the stomach lining by alcohol can cause bleeding and contribute to the formation of ulcers.

Cardiovascular System   The effects of alcohol on the cardiovascular system depend on the amount of alcohol consumed. Moderate doses of alcohol—one or two drinks a day—may reduce slightly the chances of heart attack in some people. The reasons for this finding are poorly understood, but it may be that moderate amounts of alcohol increase blood levels of high-density lipoproteins (HDLs). Red wines may also include a chemical that inhibits blood clotting.

Cirrhosis of the liver   A disease caused by excessive and chronic drinking.

TERMS

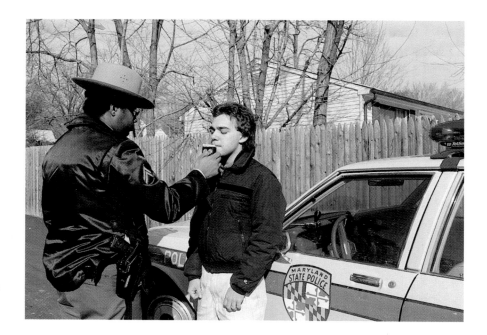

Alcohol interferes with judgment, perception, coordination, and other areas of mental and physical functioning and is a factor in a majority of all fatal automobile crashes. This driver is lucky that he was stopped by a suspicious police officer before a crash occurred. He is being given a breathalyzer test to determine his blood alcohol concentration.

Higher doses of alcohol have harmful effects. In some people, more than two drinks a day will elevate blood pressure, making strokes and heart attacks more likely. Some alcoholics show weakening of the heart muscle, a condition known as **cardiac myopathy.** Cardiac myopathy can be caused by the direct toxic effects of alcohol, or indirectly by the malnutrition and vitamin deficiencies that many alcoholics experience from their poor diets and gastrointestinal disturbances. Although the relationships between alcohol and cardiovascular disease are multiple and complex, it is clear that excessive drinking increases the risk of disease. These health risks progressively increase as the amount of excessive drinking increases.

Mortality An ancient proverb states "Those who worship Bacchus [the god of wine] die young." Modern research supports that statement. In addition to increasing the risk of injury and death, alcohol is associated with early death from cancer. Alcoholics have a cancer rate that is about 10 times higher than would be expected in the general population. They are particularly vulnerable to cancers of the throat, larynx, esophagus, upper stomach, liver, and pancreas. Women who abuse alcohol are at increased risk for breast cancer. Altogether, alcoholics have life spans that are 10 to 12 years shorter than those of nonalcoholics.

Fetal Alcohol Syndrome Alcohol and its metabolic product acetaldehyde quickly cross the placenta. Below-normal birth weights occur when pregnant mothers consume as few as two alcoholic drinks a day. With heavier drinking, a collection of birth defects known as the **fetal alcohol syndrome** becomes increasingly likely. These children have a characteristic mixture of deformities that

include small teeth with faulty enamel; irregular ear lobes; small, wide-set eyes and other facial deformities. They are usually small and may have heart defects. Even with the best of care, their physical and mental growth rate is slower than normal during childhood. In adolescence they sometimes catch up with their age mates in terms of physical size, but not usually in mental abilities. Most remain mentally retarded with IQs in the 40 to 80 range (normal is 90–110). Fetal alcohol effects also include more subtle changes in fine motor coordination and learning problems. There is no precise blood alcohol threshold level above which damage occurs and below which there is no danger. Instead, the frequency and severity of defects progressively increase as the amount of drinking increases.

Any alcohol consumed by a nursing mother quickly enters the breast milk. What impact this has on the child or the mother's milk production is a matter of controversy. Dosage may again be the key issue.

Personal Insight How was alcohol used in your family when you were growing up, and what are your associations with it? Was it used for family celebrations? Was there alcohol abuse in your family? If so, how did you react at the time? How do you feel about it now?

MISUSE OF ALCOHOL

Addiction to alcohol—like addiction to tobacco and other psychoactive drugs—affects more than just the user. Alcoholics can wreak havoc within a family, and children

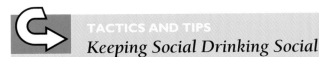
When You're the Guest

- Drink slowly. Learn to sip your drinks rather than gulp them. Avoid drinks made with carbonated mixers, especially if you're thirsty—you'll gulp them down.

- Space your drinks. Learn to drink nonalcoholic drinks at parties or intersperse these with alcoholic drinks.

- Eat before and while drinking to avoid drinking on an empty stomach.

- At a restaurant, order the food first, not a drink. Then if you want a drink you'll probably have time for only one before the meal is served.

- Let your waistline be your incentive. For the same 215 calories in two 7-ounce gin and tonics, you can have a nutritious snack.

- Remember that the pressure to have a drink may often be in your imagination. It is becoming more and more acceptable to say "no thanks" to alcohol.

When You're the Host

- Have plenty of nonalcoholic beverages on hand and make sure they are as accessible and as attractive as the alcoholic drinks.

- Experiment with various juices and beverages until you come up with an alcohol-free concoction all your own. Or stick to traditional punches and blends, but leave out the alcohol.

- If it's a dinner party, try to serve dinner on schedule, before there's time for a second drink.

- Always serve food along with alcohol, and stop serving alcohol an hour or more before people will leave.

- Insist that a guest who had too much to drink take a taxi, ride with someone else, or stay at your house rather than drive.

Adapted from *University of California at Berkeley Wellness Letter*, April 1987.

---

are often those most severely affected. But alcohol can be abused even when there's no true addiction; even though the rate is falling, too many victims of car crashes are actually victims of weekend drinkers.

Alcohol Abuse

According to the fourth edition of the *Diagnostic and Statistical Manual of Mental Disorders* (1994) of the American Psychiatric Association, **alcohol abuse** involves one or more of the following occurring within a 12-month period: (1) recurrent alcohol use resulting in a failure to fulfill major role obligations at work, school, or home; (2) recurrent alcohol use in situations in which it is physically hazardous; (3) recurrent alcohol-related legal problems; and (4) continued alcohol use despite having persistent or recurrent social or interpersonal problems caused by or exacerbated by the effects of alcohol. The term **alcohol dependence,** or **alcoholism,** refers to more extensive problems with alcohol use, usually involving tolerance or withdrawal.

Other authorities use different definitions to describe problems associated with drinking. The important point is that one does not have to be an alcoholic to have problems with alcohol. The person who drinks only once a month, perhaps after an exam, but then drives while intoxicated is an alcohol abuser.

How can you tell if you are beginning to abuse alcohol or if someone you know is doing so? Look for the following warning signs:

1. Drinking alone or secretively.

2. Using alcohol deliberately and repeatedly to perform or get through difficult situations.

3. Feeling uncomfortable on certain occasions when alcohol is not available.

4. Escalating alcohol consumption beyond an already established drinking pattern.

5. Consuming alcohol heavily in risky situations; for example, before driving.

6. Getting drunk regularly or more frequently than in the past.

7. Drinking in the morning or at other unusual times.

TERMS

Cardiac myopathy   Weakening of the heart muscle through disease.

Fetal alcohol syndrome   A characteristic group of birth defects caused by excessive alcohol consumption by the mother, including facial deformities, heart defects, and physical and mental impairments.

Alcohol abuse   The use of alcohol to a degree that causes physical damage, impairs functioning, or results in behavior harmful to others.

Alcohol dependence   Either pathological use of alcohol or impairment in functioning due to alcohol and tolerance or withdrawal; alcoholism.

Alcoholism   Chronic psychological and nutritional disorder from excessive and compulsive drinking; alcohol dependence.

Binge Drinking

Binge drinking is a common form of alcohol abuse on college campuses. In a survey of over 17,000 students on 140 college campuses, 44 percent reported binge drinking, defined as having five drinks in a row for men or four in a row for women on at least one occasion in the two weeks prior to the survey. Binge drinking has a profound effect on students' lives. Frequent binge drinkers were found to be 7 to 10 times more likely than nonbinge drinkers to engage in unplanned sex, to have unprotected sex, to drive after drinking, to get into trouble with campus police, to damage property, and to get injured. Binge drinkers were also more likely to miss classes, get behind in school work, and argue with their friends.

Binge drinking also affects nonbinging students. At schools with high rates of binge drinking, the nonbinging students were up to three times as likely to report being bothered by the drinking-related behaviors of others than students at schools with lower rates of binge drinking. These problems included being pushed, hit, or assaulted; having property damaged; having sleep or studying disrupted; and experiencing unwanted sexual advances. The *Healthy People 2000* report set the goal of reducing binge drinking to 32 percent of college students.

Alcoholism

Alcoholism, or alcohol dependency, is similar to nicotine dependency in its being usually characterized by tolerance to alcohol and withdrawal. Everyone who drinks—even nonalcoholics—develops tolerance to alcohol after repeated use. Tolerance means that a drinker needs more alcohol to achieve intoxication or the desired effect, that the effects of continued use of the same amount of alcohol are diminished, or that the drinker can function adequately at doses or blood levels of alcohol that would produce significant impairment in a casual user. Heavy users of alcohol may need to consume about 50 percent more than they originally needed to experience the same degree of intoxication.

Withdrawal from alcohol occurs when someone who has been using alcohol heavily for several days or more suddenly stops drinking or markedly reduces intake of alcohol. Symptoms of withdrawal can include trembling hands, sweating, and weakness.

Patterns and Prevalence   Alcoholism is found among people of all races, ethnic groups, and socioeconomic classes. The stereotype of the alcoholic skid row bum actually accounts for less than 5 percent of all alcohol-dependent people—and usually represents the final stage of a drinking career that began years earlier. There are different patterns of alcohol dependence, including these four common ones: (1) regular daily intake in large amounts, (2) regular heavy drinking limited to weekends, (3) long periods of sobriety interspersed with binges of daily heavy drinking lasting for weeks or months, and (4) heavy drinking limited to periods of stress.

Among white American men, excessive drinking often begins in the teens or twenties and progresses gradually through the thirties until the individual is clearly identifiable as an alcoholic by the time he is in his late thirties or early forties. Other men remain controlled drinkers until later in life, sometimes becoming alcoholic in association with retirement, the inevitable losses of aging, boredom, illness, or psychiatric disturbances.

The progression of alcoholism in women is usually different. Women tend to become alcoholic at a later age and with fewer years of heavy drinking. It is not unusual for women in their forties or fifties to become alcoholic after years of controlled drinking. Women alcoholics develop cirrhosis and other medical complications somewhat more often than men.

Once established, alcoholism often exhibits a pattern of exacerbations and remissions. The alcoholic may stop drinking and abstain from alcohol for days or months after a frightening problem develops. After a period of abstinence, an alcoholic often attempts controlled drinking, which almost inevitably leads to an escalation in drinking and more problems. Alcoholism is not hopeless, however; many alcoholics do achieve permanent abstinence.

In 1992 the National Council on Alcoholism reported that 13 million Americans were alcoholics. The lifetime risk for alcoholism in the United States is about 10 percent for men and about 3 percent for women.

Causes of Alcoholism   The precise causes of alcoholism are unknown, but a variety of factors is probably involved. Recent studies of twins and adopted children have clearly demonstrated the importance of genetics. However, not all children of alcoholics become alcoholic, so it is clear that other factors are involved. A person's risk of developing alcoholism may be increased by certain personality disorders, having been subjected as a child to destructive child-rearing practices, and imitating the alcohol abuse of peers and other role models. Certain social factors have also been linked with alcoholism, including

TERMS

DTs (delirium tremens)   A state of confusion brought on by reduction of alcohol intake in a person addicted to alcohol. Other symptoms are sweating, trembling, anxiety, and hallucinations.

Hallucinations   False perceptions that do not correspond to external reality. A person who hears voices that are not there or who sees visions is having hallucinations.

Paranoia   A mental disorder characterized by persistent delusions—fixed, false beliefs that would not be accepted by the individual's culture. Hallucinations, if any, are not prominent and intelligence is not impaired.

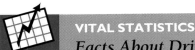
The Scope of College Drinking

- About 9 out of 10 college students drink alcohol. About three-quarters of all college students consume alcohol every month; 4 percent drink every day.

- College students drink less on a daily basis than their noncollege peers, but they are more likely to binge drink. About 44 percent of American college students engage in a bout of binge drinking at least once every two weeks. This pattern indicates that students are more likely to confine their drinking to weekends, but then to drink heavily.

- More than twice as many male students as female students drink daily. On average, fraternity members drink greater quantities than do other college students, drink more frequently, and drink more heavily.

- The average yearly consumption of alcoholic beverages per student is over 34 gallons. Beer is the most commonly consumed beverage; as a group, American college students consume almost 4 billion cans of beer each year.

- Different studies indicate that between 53 and 84 percent of students get drunk at least once a year; between 26 and 48 percent get drunk each month.

The Consequences of College Drinking

- A 1991 survey indicated that approximately 40 percent of students' academic problems and 28 percent of

dropouts were related to alcohol use. Over 7 percent of first-year students drop out of college for alcohol-related reasons.

- Students with high academic standing drink less in almost all contexts than do their peers with low academic standing. There is a negative relationship between college grades and the amount of alcohol consumed.

- Alcohol is involved in two-thirds of college student suicides, in 90 percent of campus rapes, and in 95 percent of violent crime on campus.

- Drinking alcohol increases the risk that a college student will commit a crime and also makes it more likely that he or she will be a crime victim.

- Surveys indicate that one-half to two-thirds of undergraduates have driven while intoxicated or have been a passenger in a car when the driver was intoxicated.

- Of the college students currently enrolled in the United States, approximately the same number will eventually die from alcohol-related causes as will get master's degrees and doctorates combined.

Adapted from L. D. Eigen. 1991. *Alcohol Practices, Policies, and Potentials of American Colleges and Universities: An Office for Substance Abuse Prevention White Paper.* Washington, D.C.: U.S. Department of Health and Human Services, September; H. Wechsler, and others. 1994. Health and behavioral consequences of binge drinking in college. *Journal of the American Medical Association* 272(21): 1672–7.

---

urbanization, disappearance of the extended family, general loosening of kinship ties, increased mobility, and changing religious and philosophical values.

Health Effects of Alcoholism   The main characteristics of alcoholism—tolerance and withdrawal—can have a severe impact on health. When alcoholics stop drinking or sharply decrease their intake, they have withdrawal symptoms. The jitters, or "shakes," are the most common withdrawal symptoms and may continue for as long as two weeks. Seizures, or "rum fits," are less common, but are more serious. Still less common is the severe withdrawal reaction known as the **DTs (delirium tremens)**, a medical emergency characterized by disorientation, confusion, and vivid **hallucinations**, often of vermin and small animals.

Because alcohol is distributed throughout the body's organs and tissues, alcoholism takes a heavy physical and psychological toll. Alcoholics face all the physical health risks associated with intoxication and chronic drinking that were described earlier in the chapter. Some of the damage is worsened by nutritional deficiencies that often

accompany alcoholism. Some people develop alcoholic **paranoia,** characterized by delusions, jealousy, suspicion, and mistrust. Other psychiatric problems associated with alcoholism include profound memory gaps (amnesia), which are sometimes filled by conscious or unconscious lying (confabulation).

Social and Psychological Effects   Alcohol use causes more serious social and psychological problems than all other forms of drug abuse combined. For every person who is an alcoholic, another three or four people are directly affected. In a 1989 Gallup poll, 20 percent of Americans said that drinking had been a cause of trouble in their family.

Excessive drinking interferes with learning the interpersonal and work skills that are required for adult life. Excessive drinkers sometimes narrow their circle of friends to other heavy drinkers and thus limit the range of people they can learn from. Perhaps most important is that people who were excessive drinkers in college are more likely to have social, occupational, and health problems 20 years later.

Treatment Some alcoholics recover without professional help. Most alcoholics, however, require a treatment program of some kind in order to stop drinking. No one treatment works for everyone, so a person may have to try different programs before finding the right one.

One of the oldest and best-known recovery programs is Alcoholics Anonymous. AA consists of self-help groups that meet weekly in most communities and follow a "twelve step" program. Important steps for people in these programs include recognizing that they are "powerless over alcohol" and must seek help from a "higher power" in order to regain control of their lives. By verbalizing these steps, the alcoholic directly addresses the denial that is often prominent in alcoholism and other addictions. Many AA members have a "sponsor" of their choosing who is available by phone 24 hours a day for individual support and crisis intervention.

A companion program to AA is Al-Anon, which consists of groups for families and friends of alcoholics. In Al-Anon spouses and others explore how they "enabled" the alcoholic to drink by denying, rationalizing, or covering up his or her drinking and how they can change this "codependent" behavior. Other self-help programs exist as well. Some of them, like Rational Recovery, Secular Organizations for Sobriety, and Women for Sobriety, deliberately avoid any emphasis on higher spiritual powers.

Other types of programs include inpatient hospital rehabilitation, employee assistance programs, and school-based programs. Chemical treatments for alcoholism include the use of disulfiram, which makes a person violently ill if he or she drinks; naltrexone, which reduces the pleasant effects of alcohol; or some type of chemical substitute for alcohol.

Personal Insight How do you perceive a nondrinker in a social situation where others are drinking? Does it seem like an acceptable choice to you? What is the basis for your attitude?

Helping Someone with an Alcohol Problem

Helping a friend or relative with an alcohol problem requires skill and tact. One of the first steps is making sure you are not an "enabler" or "codependent"—someone who, perhaps unknowingly, allows another to continue excessive use of alcohol. Enabling takes many forms. One of the most common is making excuses or covering up for the alcohol abuser—saying "he has the flu" when it is really a hangover. Whenever you find yourself minimizing or lying about someone's drinking behavior, a warning bell should sound. Often another important step is open, honest labeling—"I think you have a problem with alco-

hol." Such explicit statements usually elicit emotional rebuttals and may endanger a relationship. In the long run, however, you are seldom most helpful to your friends when you allow them to deny their problems with alcohol or other drugs. Even when problems are acknowledged, there is commonly reluctance to obtain help. Your best role might be to obtain information about the available resources and persistently encourage their use.

SUMMARY

- Tobacco and alcohol cause more injuries and deaths than do illicit psychoactive drugs.

Why People Use Tobacco

- Regular tobacco use causes physical dependence on nicotine, characterized by loss of control, tolerance, and the appearance of a withdrawal syndrome when tobacco use ceases. Habits can become associated with tobacco use and trigger the urge for a cigarette or other tobacco product.

- People who begin smoking are usually imitating others or responding to seductive advertising. They often deny or minimize the risks of smoking.

Health Hazards

- Tobacco smoke is made up of particles of several hundred different chemicals, including some that are carcinogenic or poisonous or that damage or irritate the respiratory system.

- Depending on dosage, nicotine acts on the nervous system as a stimulant or a tranquilizer.

- Cardiovascular disease is the most widespread cause of death for cigarette smokers. Cigarette smoking is the primary cause of lung cancer and is linked to many other cancers as well.

- Also associated with smoking are chronic obstructive lung disease, respiratory damage, peptic ulcers, gum disorders, premature skin wrinkling and baldness, impotence, and allergies. Tobacco use leads to lower life expectancy and to a diminished quality of life.

- The use of chewing tobacco or snuff leads to nicotine addiction and is linked to oral cancers. Cigars, pipes, and clove cigarettes are not safe alternatives to cigarettes.

The Effects of Smoking on the Nonsmoker

- Environmental tobacco smoke (ETS) contains high concentrations of toxic chemicals and can cause headaches, eye and nasal irritation, and sinus problems. Long-term exposure to ETS can cause lung cancer and heart disease.

- Babies and young children inhale more air than adults do and so take in more pollutants; children whose parents smoke are especially susceptible to respiratory diseases.
- Smoking during pregnancy increases the risk of spontaneous abortion, stillbirth, congenital abnormalities, premature birth, and low birth weight. Crib death and long-term impairments in physical and intellectual development are also risks.

What Can Be Done?

- Nonsmokers can use social pressure and legislative channels to discourage smokers from polluting the air and assert their rights to breathe clean air.
- The EPA's report on environmental tobacco smoke increased calls for bans on smoking in public and in the workplace.
- Recently tobacco companies have aimed marketing programs at narrower segments of the population in which smoking is still popular.

How Can a Tobacco User Quit?

- Giving up smoking is a difficult and long-term process. Although most ex-smokers quit on their own, some smokers benefit from stop-smoking programs. Prescription medications can ease withdrawal symptoms, and support groups or counseling can help deal with psychological factors.

The Nature of Alcohol

- Ethyl alcohol is the psychoactive ingredient in alcoholic beverages. The proof value of an alcoholic beverage is two times the percentage concentration.
- How long it takes for alcohol to be absorbed into the bloodstream depends on the amount, type, and proof of the beverage, the time taken to drink it, and whether there is food in the stomach.
- After alcohol is absorbed, it is distributed throughout the body via the bloodstream.

Alcohol and Health

- Alcohol helps people relax; in social settings it often acts as a stimulant, probably because it helps people lose their inhibitions. At higher doses, alcohol interferes with motor coordination, intellectual functions, and verbal performance. At very high doses, coma and even death are possible.
- Alcohol affects internal body temperature and changes sleep patterns. Driving under the influence of alcohol, even with BAC below the limit, increases the chances of being involved in an automobile crash.
- Continued alcohol use causes cirrhosis of the liver and other digestive problems.

- Although moderate doses of alcohol may reduce the chances of heart attack, higher doses are associated with cardiovascular problems.
- Alcohol has also been related to certain cancers and abusers have shorter life spans than the average.
- Women who drink while pregnant risk giving birth to children with fetal alcohol syndrome.

Misuse of Alcohol

- Alcohol abuse involves the use of alcohol to a degree that causes social, interpersonal, legal, educational, or professional problems or results in danger to oneself or others.
- Binge drinking is a serious and widespread problem on college campuses that causes problems for both drinkers and nondrinkers.
- Alcohol dependence, or alcoholism, involves more extensive problems with alcohol abuse, usually involving tolerance or withdrawal. Alcoholism affects people from all social and economic classes.
- Some alcoholics recover without professional help; most require some treatment. A variety of approaches to treatment exists.
- Helping someone who abuses alcohol means avoiding being an enabler. The best way to help might be to obtain information about available resources and persistently encourage their use.

TAKE ACTION

1. Make a tour of the public facilities in your community and on your campus, such as movie theaters, auditoriums, business and school offices, and classrooms. What kinds of restrictions on smoking do these places have? In your opinion, are they appropriate? If you feel more or different restrictions are in order, write a letter to the editor of your school or local newspaper making your case. Support it with convincing arguments and appropriate facts.

2. Plan what you will say or do the next time you want to ask a smoker to stop smoking around you. Draw up a list of statements you might make to a smoker in various situations. You'll increase the effectiveness of your statements if they are courteous and don't threaten the person's dignity. Practice saying these statements in a way that is assertive rather than aggressive or passive. The next time you're in an appropriate situation, use one of your statements. If it doesn't have the desired effect, think about why and modify it for the next time.

3. Interview some of your fellow students about their drinking habits. How much do they drink and how often? Are they more likely to drink on certain days

or in certain circumstances? Are there any habits that seem to be common to most students? How do your own drinking habits compare to those of people you interviewed?

4. Plan an alcohol-free party. What would you serve to eat and drink? What would you tell people about the party when you invite them?

JOURNAL ENTRY

1. *Critical Thinking:* Restrictions on smoking are growing in our society. Do you think they're fair? Do they infringe on people's rights? Do they go too far or not far enough? Write a brief essay stating your position on smoking restrictions. Be sure to explain your reasoning. What are the most important factors in your decision? Why do you hold the opinion you do?

2. *Critical Thinking:* Look at advertisements for alcoholic beverages in magazines and on billboards. Analyze several of these ads. What psychological techniques are used to sell the products? What are the hidden messages? Write an essay outlining your opinion of alcohol advertising and marketing. Do you think it's ethical to sell a potentially dangerous substance by appealing to people's desires and vulnerabilities? Do you think liquor manufacturers ought to be held responsible for the damage alcohol inflicts on some people? Explain your reasoning.

3. Make a list of statements you might make to a person you care about whom you think is developing a drinking problem; statements you might make to a person planning to drive under the influence of alcohol, both with and without you in the car; and questions you might ask a friend about your own behavior when you drink. Consider using some of these statements when an appropriate situation arises.

BEHAVIOR CHANGE STRATEGY

KICKING THE TOBACCO HABIT

You can look forward to a longer and healthier life if you join the 39 million Americans who have quit using tobacco. The steps for quitting described below are discussed in terms of the most popular tobacco product in the United States—cigarettes—but they can be adapted for all forms of tobacco use.

Gather Information

Collect personal smoking information in a detailed journal about your smoking behavior. Use your journal to collect two major types of information—cigarettes smoked and smoking urges. Part of the job is to identify patterns of smoking that are connected with routine situations. Use this information to discover the behavior chains involved in your smoking habit.

Set a Target Quitting Date

Choose a date in the near future when you expect to be relatively stress-free and can give quitting the energy and attention it will require. Don't choose a date right before or during finals week, for instance.

Prepare to Quit

One of the most important things you can do to prepare to quit is to develop and practice nonsmoking relaxation methods. It takes time to become proficient at relaxation techniques, so begin practicing before your quit date. Refer to the detailed discussion of relaxation techniques found in Chapter 2.

Other things you can do to help prepare for quitting include the following:

- Make an appointment to see your physician. Ask about some of the new prescription aids for tobacco cessation and whether one might be appropriate for you.

- Make a dentist's appointment to have your teeth cleaned the day after your target quit date.

- Start an easy exercise program if you're not exercising regularly already. Get in the habit of going to bed and getting up at the same time. Don't let yourself become overworked or fall behind at school or on the job.

- Buy some sugarless gum. Stock your kitchen with low-calorie snacks.

- Throw away all your cigarette-related paraphernalia (ashtrays, lighters, and so on).

Quitting

Complete a personal contract for quitting that specifies the day and time when you will stop smoking as well as possible rewards for quitting. Your first few days without cigarettes will probably be the most difficult. It's hard to give up such a strongly ingrained habit, but remember that 39 million Americans have done it—and you can too. Plan and rehearse the steps you will take when you experience a powerful craving. For example, try drinking a glass of water, chewing gum, taking a walk or a shower, going swimming, or practicing a relaxation technique. Avoid or control situations that you know from your journal are powerfully associated with your smoking (see table below). Tell people you've just quit. You may discover many inspiring former smokers who can encourage you and reassure you that it's possible to quit and lead a happier, healthier life.

Maintaining Nonsmoking

The lingering smoking urges that remain once you've quit should be carefully tracked in your smoking journal and controlled to avoid relapses. Watch out for situations and patterns of thinking that can make nonsmoking more difficult. Continue to practice time management and relaxation techniques. Exercise regularly, eat sensibly, and get enough sleep. Focus on the positive aspects of not smoking and give yourself lots of praise—you deserve it.

SELECTED BIBLIOGRAPHY

American Cancer Society. 1994. *Cancer Facts and Figures.* Atlanta, Ga.: American Cancer Society.

———. 1995. *California Cancer Facts and Figures.* Oakland, Calif.: American Cancer Society, California Division.

American Psychiatric Association. 1994. *Diagnostic and Statistical Manual of Mental Disorders* (DSM-IV). 4th ed. Washington, D.C.: American Psychiatric Association.

Blot, W. J. 1992. Alcohol and cancer. *Cancer Research* 52(7 suppl): 2119s–23s.

Centers for Disease Control and Prevention. 1992. Cigarette smoking among adults—United States, 1990. *Morbidity and Mortality Weekly Report* 41(20).

———. 1994. Reasons for tobacco use and symptoms of nicotine withdrawal among adolescent and young adult tobacco users—United States, 1993. *Morbidity and Mortality Weekly Report* 43(41).

Centers for Disease Control and Prevention, Office on Smoking and Health. 1994. *Facts About Second-Hand Smoke.*

Committee on Substance Abuse. 1991. Hazards of clove cigarettes. *Pediatrics* 88(2): 395–96.

Environmental Protection Agency. 1993. *Respiratory Health Effects of Passive Smoking: Fact Sheet.* EPA-43-F-93-003.

Gerace, T. A., and others. 1991. Smoking cessation and change in diastolic blood pressure, body weight, and plasma lipids. *Preventive Medicine* 20:602–620.

Gingiss, P. L., and N. H. Gottlieb. 1991. A comparison of smokeless tobacco and smoking practices of university varsity and intramural baseball players. *Addictive Behaviors* 16:335–40.

Gostin, L. O., and others. 1991. Tobacco liability and public health policy. *Journal of the American Medical Association* 266(22): 3178–82.

Hansen, W. B., A. E. Raynor, and B. H. Wolkenstein. 1991. Perceived personal immunity to the consequences of drinking

Cues and High-Risk Situations	Suggested Strategies
Awakening in morning	Brush your teeth as soon as you wake up. Stay busy and try not to think about smoking.
Drinking coffee	Do something else with your hands. Drink tea or another beverage instead.
Eating meals	Eat in a different location. Sit in nonsmoking sections at restaurants. Get up from the table right away after eating and start another activity. Brush your teeth right after eating.
Driving a car	Have the car cleaned when you quit smoking. Chew sugarless gum or eat a low-calorie snack. Take public transportation or ride your bike.
Socializing with friends who smoke	Suggest nonsmoking events (movies, theater, shopping). Tell them you've quit and ask them not to smoke around you, offer you cigarettes, or give you cigarettes if you ask for them.
Drinking at a bar, restaurant, or party	Try to take a nonsmoker with you or associate with nonsmokers. Let friends know you've just quit. Moderate your intake of alcohol (it can weaken your resolve).
Encountering stressful situations	Practice relaxation techniques. Get out of your room or house. Go somewhere that doesn't allow smoking. Take a shower, chew gum, call a friend, or exercise.

Adapted from *Postgraduate Medicine,* vol. 90, no. 1, July 1991.

alcohol: The relationship between behavior and perception. *Journal of Studies on Alcohol* 14(3): 205–24.

Hymowitz, N., and others. 1991. Baseline factors associated with smoking cessation and relapse. *Preventive Medicine* 20:590–601.

Johnston, L. D., and others. 1994. National survey results on drug use. *The Monitoring the Future Study, 1975–1993.* National Institute on Drug Abuse. NIH Volume 1(61).

Kendler, K. S., A. C. Heath, M. C. Neale, R. C. Kessler, and L. J. Eaves. 1992. A population-based twin study of alcoholism in women. *Journal of the American Medical Association* 268(14): 1877–82.

Lando, H. A., and others. 1991. A comparison of self-help approaches to smoking cessation. *Addictive Behaviors* 16:183–93.

Manley, M., and others. 1991. Clinical interventions in tobacco control. *Journal of the American Medical Association* 266(22): 3172–73.

McGovern, P. G., and H. A. Lando. 1992. An assessment of nicotine gum as an adjunct to freedom from smoking cessation clinics. *Addictive Behaviors* 17:137–47.

McMaster, C., and C. Lee. 1991. Cognitive dissonance in tobacco smokers. *Addictive Behaviors* 16:349–53.

National Center for Health Statistics. 1994. *Healthy People 2000 Review, 1993.* Hyattsville, Md.: Public Health Service.

Pierce, J. P., and others. 1991. Does tobacco advertising target young people to start smoking? Evidence from California. *Journal of the American Medical Association* 266(22): 3154–58.

Roeleveld, N., and others. 1992. Mental retardation associated with parental smoking and alcohol consumption before, during, and after pregnancy. *Preventive Medicine* 21(1): 110–19.

Schatzkin, A., and M. P. Longnecker. 1994. Alcohol and breast cancer. *Cancer Supplement* 74(3): 1101–10.

Transdermal Nicotine Study Group. 1991. Transdermal nicotine for smoking cessation. *Journal of the American Medical Association* 266(22): 3133–38.

The Truth About Secondhand Smoke. 1995. *Consumer Reports,* January, pp. 27–33.

U.S. Public Health Service. 1990. *Seventh Special Report to the U.S. Congress on Alcohol and Health.* Rockville, Md.: National Institute of Alcohol Abuse and Alcoholism.

Volpicelli, J. R., and others. 1992. Naltrexone in the treatment of alcohol dependence. *Archives of General Psychiatry* 49:876–80.

Wechsler, H., and others. 1994. Health and behavioral consequences of binge drinking in college. *Journal of the American Medical Association* 272(21): 1672–77.

RECOMMENDED READINGS

Alcoholics Anonymous, 3rd ed. 1976. New York: Alcoholics Anonymous World Services. *This is the "Big Book," the basic text for AA. It includes the founding tenets of AA and vivid histories of recovering alcoholics.*

Booth, W. 1994. North Carolina watches the gradual fall of King Tobacco. *Washington Post,* 6 June. *A reporter travels into the heart of tobacco country and comes back with a story tracing the changing role of tobacco in America.*

Cahalan, D. 1991. *An Ounce of Prevention: Strategies for Solving Tobacco, Alcohol, and Drug Problems.* San Francisco: Jossey-Bass. *A cogent analysis of proposed solutions to the problem of tobacco and other drug addictions.*

Dorris, M. 1992. *The Broken Cord.* New York: HarperCollins. *A personal story and a current source of information on fetal alcohol syndrome.*

Hilts, P. J. 1994. Embattled Tobacco: Cigarette Makers Debated the Risks They Denied. *New York Times,* 15 June. *A fascinating look behind the congressional hearings on tobacco regulation.*

Krogh, D. 1992. *Smoking: The Artificial Passion.* New York: W. H. Freeman. *Probes the roots of smoking.*

A Lifetime of Freedom from Smoking. 1989. New York: American Lung Association. *Useful for anyone who wants to quit, or wants anyone else to quit.*

Schelling, T. C. 1992. Addictive drugs: The cigarette experience. *Science* 255:430–33. *A fascinating look at addiction and tobacco.*

Vaillant, G. E. 1983. *The Natural History of Alcoholism.* Cambridge: Harvard University Press. *A well-written description of an important longitudinal study of alcoholism.*

Vogel-Sprott, M. 1992. *Alcohol Tolerance and Social Drinking: Learning the Consequences.* New York: Guilford Press. *An interesting book on recent research into behavioral aspects of alcohol use.*

8

The Use and Abuse of Psychoactive Drugs

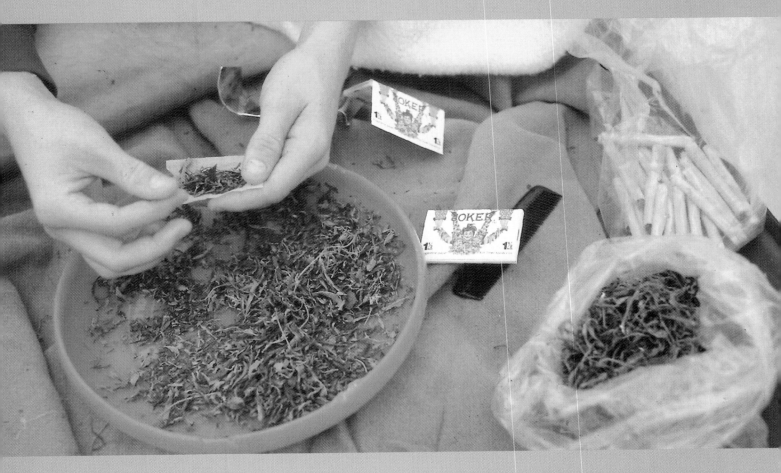

CONTENTS

We live in a drug society. The use of drugs for both medical and social purposes is common and widespread. Too many Americans believe that all problems, large and small, have chemical solutions. They turn to caffeine when they're tired, sedatives when they can't sleep, and alcohol or other recreational drugs when they're anxious, tense, or bored. Advertisements, social pressures, medical research, and our own desires for quick fixes to life's difficult problems all contribute to the prevailing attitude that drugs can ease all physical and emotional complaints.

Drugs are defined as chemicals other than food intended to affect the structure or function of the body. They include prescription medicines, such as antibiotics or tranquilizers; over-the-counter remedies, such as alcohol, tobacco, and caffeine products; and illegal substances, such as cocaine, marijuana, and heroin. This chapter focuses primarily on **psychoactive drugs**, chemicals that can alter a person's experiences or consciousness. Two of the most widely used psychoactive drugs—nicotine and alcohol—were discussed in the last chapter.

THE DRUG TRADITION

Using drugs to alter consciousness is an ancient and universal pursuit. As described in Chapter 7, people have used alcohol to celebrate and intoxicate for thousands of years. Native populations in all parts of the world discovered the psychoactive properties of various local plants, such as the coca plant in South America and the opium poppy in the Middle East and Far East.

In the nineteenth century, chemists were successful in extracting the active elements from medicinal plants, such as morphine from the opium poppy and atropine, a muscle spasm reliever, from belladonna. This was the beginning of *pharmacy,* the art of compounding drugs, and of *pharmacology,* the science and study of drugs. From this point on, a variety of drugs began to be produced, including morphine, cocaine, and heroin (Figure 8-1).

Before their potential for abuse became apparent, these drugs weren't regulated. Many could be purchased without a prescription; even Coca-Cola originally contained a small amount of cocaine, which accounted for the "lift" it provided. Thanks to easy availability, by 1900, many people in Europe and the United States were addicted to drugs. This situation prompted enactment of drug legislation to protect consumers. Over the course of the next 50 years, drug use and addiction dropped sharply.

Recreational drug use expanded in the 1960s and 1970s; it stabilized in the late 1970s and then began to decline slightly. This downward trend lasted through 1991, when researchers noted a resurgence in the use of some illegal drugs, particularly marijuana. This resurgence has been especially marked among younger adolescents. Today, involvement with illicit drugs among high school students and young adults in the United States is

greater than has been documented in any other industrialized nation. The drug scene in the United States remains dominated by a multibillion-dollar criminal drug industry that thrives on the dependencies and recreational habits of large segments of the population.

Personal Insight   What was your family's attitude about drugs when you were growing up? Did your parents discuss drugs with you? Did they set rules or offer advice about how to deal with situations involving drugs? How did their attitudes affect your current values? Do you share your parents' attitudes about drugs or have you adopted a different position?

USE, ABUSE, AND DEPENDENCE

People use drugs for a variety of reasons and in a variety of ways. For some, drug use can lead to the serious problems of abuse and physical and psychological dependence.

Who Uses Drugs?

Use and abuse of drugs occurs at all income and education levels, among all races and ethnic groups, and at all ages. Unborn babies can become involuntary drug users if their mothers use drugs during pregnancy; great-grandmothers can become unintentional abusers of prescription drugs.

But some people are at higher-than-average risk for trying illicit drugs. Risk factors include being male, being an adolescent or young adult, and having frequent exposure to drugs through family members or peers. Risk is also higher for people who come from a single-parent family, for those whose mothers failed to complete high school, for those who are uninterested in school and earn poor grades, and for those who feel lonely or isolated. A risk-taking personality is another factor. People who drive too fast or who don't wear seat belts may have this personality type, which is characterized by a sense of invincibility. Believing themselves invulnerable, such people find it easy to dismiss warnings of danger, whether about drugs or seat belts—"That only happens to other people; it could never happen to me."

What about people who *don't* use drugs? As a group, non-users also share some characteristics. Drug use is less common among young people who attend school regularly, get good grades, have strong personal identities, are religious, have a good relationship with their parents, and are independent thinkers whose actions aren't controlled by peer pressure. Coming from a strong family, one that has a clear policy on drug use and where crises and conflicts are dealt with constructively, is another factor asso-

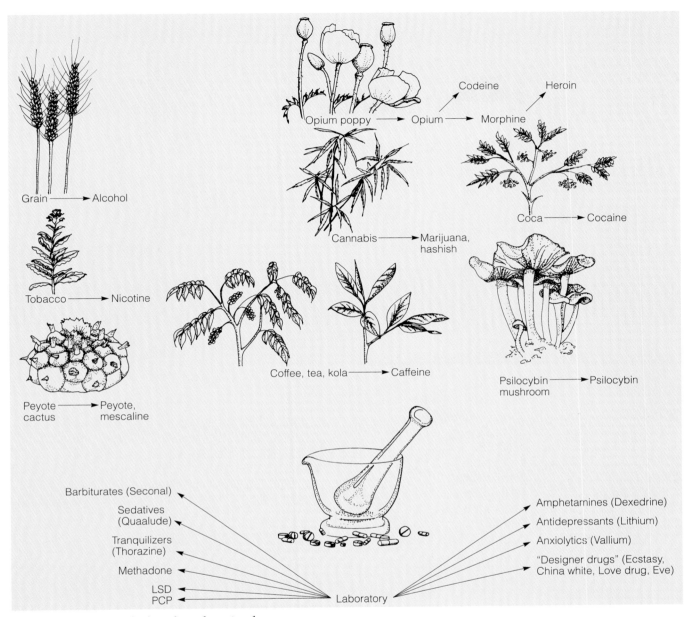

Figure 8-1 *Sources of selected psychoactive drugs.*

ciated with people who don't use drugs. Identifying the personality characteristics and skills that help people resist pressure to use drugs is an important focus of research today.

Why Do People Use Drugs?

The answer to this question depends on both the user and the drug. Young people, especially those from middle-class backgrounds, are frequently drawn to drugs by the allure of the exciting and illicit. They may be curious, rebellious, or vulnerable to peer pressure. They may want to appear to be daring and to be part of the group. They may want to imitate adult models in their lives or in the movies. Most people who have taken illicit drugs have done so on an experimental basis, typically trying the drug one or more times but not continuing beyond that. The main factors in the initial choice of a drug are whether it is available and whether other people around are already using it.

Drugs Chemicals other than food intended to affect the structure or function of the body.

Psychoactive drug Any chemical other than food that, when taken into the body, can alter the user's consciousness.

Although some people use drugs because they have a desire to alter their mood or are seeking a spiritual experience, others are motivated primarily by a desire to escape boredom, anxiety, depression, feelings of worthlessness, or other distressing symptoms of psychological problems. They use drugs as a way to cope with the difficulties they are experiencing in life. The common practice in our society of seeking a drug solution to every problem is a factor in the widespread reliance on both illicit drugs and prescription drugs like Valium.

For people living in poverty in the inner cities, many of these reasons for using drugs are magnified. The problems are more devastating, the need for escape more compelling. The buying and selling of drugs reflect issues of discrimination, prejudice, class, and economics.

> ***Personal Insight*** Have you ever misused or abused a drug, even coffee or an over-the-counter remedy? If so, what were your reasons and motivations? Was it hard to stop? How did the experience affect your current attitudes and behavior?

Drug Abuse

What exactly is **drug abuse?** Many addiction experts describe drug abuse as a maladaptive pattern of use of any substance that persists despite adverse social, psychological, or medical consequences. For example, a person who drinks excessively once a month and then drives is abusing alcohol, even if he or she is not physically dependent. People who continue to smoke marijuana on the weekends even though it makes them feel sluggish and forgetful (and consumes money they should be saving) are abusing the drug.

Drug Dependence

The American Psychiatric Association (APA) defines addiction or **substance dependence** as a cluster of cognitive, behavioral, and physiological symptoms that occur in an individual who continues to use a substance despite suffering significant substance-related problems, leading to significant impairment or distress. Dependence generally follows a pattern of repeated self-administration that results in tolerance, withdrawal, and compulsive drug-taking behavior. The specific criteria the APA uses to diagnose substance dependence are listed below. The first two criteria are associated with **physical dependence**; the final five are associated with compulsive use. To be considered dependent, an individual must experience a cluster of three or more of these seven symptoms during a 12-month period.

1. *Developing tolerance to the substance.* When an individual requires greatly increased amounts of a substance to achieve intoxication or notices a markedly diminished effect with continued use of the same amount, then he or she has developed **tolerance.** For example, heavy heroin users may need to take ten times the amount they took as novices—a dose that would be lethal to a nonuser—in order to achieve the desired effect.

2. *Experiencing withdrawal.* In an individual who has maintained prolonged, heavy use of a substance, a drop in its concentration within the body can result in an unpleasant physical and cognitive **withdrawal syndrome.** For example, nausea, vomiting, and tremors are common withdrawal symptoms for alcohol, opioids, and sedatives.

3. *Taking the substance in larger amounts or over a longer period than was originally intended.* For example, an individual may continue to drink until severely intoxicated despite having set a limit of one drink.

4. *Expressing a persistent desire to cut down or regulate substance use.* This desire is often accompanied by many unsuccessful efforts to cut down on or discontinue use of the substance.

5. *Spending a great deal of time obtaining the substance, using the substance, or recovering from its effects.*

6. *Giving up or reducing important social, school, work, or recreational activities because of substance use.* A dependent person may withdraw from family activities and hobbies in order to use the substance in private or to spend more time with substance-using friends. In some cases, virtually all of a person's daily activities revolve around the substance.

7. *Continuing to use the substance in spite of recognizing that substance use is contributing to a psychological or physical problem.* For example, a person might continue to use cocaine despite recognizing that she is suffering from cocaine-induced depression.

If a drug-dependent person experiences either tolerance or withdrawal, he or she is considered physically dependent. However, dependence can occur without a physical component, based solely on compulsive use. Although drugs are what most people associate with dependency, the loss of control that accompanies drug dependency can also occur with behaviors such as gambling, overeating, and sexual activity (Figure 8-2).

Some people are able to use psychoactive drugs without falling into a pattern of abuse or becoming dependent. Others aren't as lucky. Why do some people become dependent? The answer seems to be in a combination of physical, psychological, and social factors. Some research indicates that some people may be born with certain characteristics of brain chemistry or metabolism that make them more vulnerable to drug dependence. Other research suggests that people who were exposed to drugs

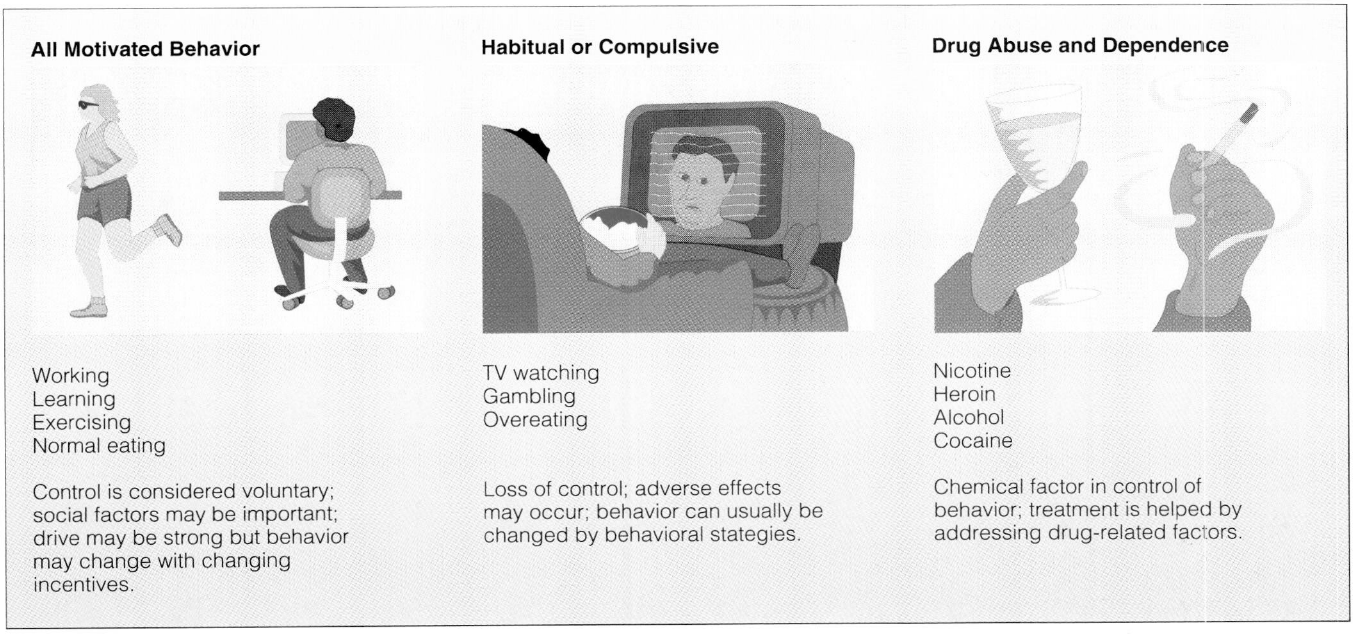

All Motivated Behavior	Habitual or Compulsive	Drug Abuse and Dependence
Working Learning Exercising Normal eating	TV watching Gambling Overeating	Nicotine Heroin Alcohol Cocaine
Control is considered voluntary; social factors may be important; drive may be strong but behavior may change with changing incentives.	Loss of control; adverse effects may occur; behavior can usually be changed by behavioral stategies.	Chemical factor in control of behavior; treatment is helped by addressing drug-related factors.

Figure 8-2 *Behavior control.*
A progression from normal to dependent behavior occurs in some areas of life for some people. The key feature of this progression is loss of control.

while still in the womb may have an increased risk of abusing drugs themselves later in life.

Psychological risk factors for drug dependence include difficulty in controlling impulses and having a strong need for excitement, stimulation, and immediate gratification. Feelings of rejection, hostility, aggression, anxiety, or depression are also associated with drug dependence. Social factors that involve risk for drug dependence include growing up in a family in which a parent or sibling abused drugs, belonging to a peer group that emphasizes and encourages drug abuse, and poverty. Because they have easy access to drugs, health professionals also face an increased risk for drug dependence.

HOW DRUGS AFFECT THE BODY

Like alcohol and tobacco, the psychoactive drugs discussed in this chapter have complex and variable effects. The same drug may affect different users differently or the same user in different ways under different circumstances. The effects of a drug depend on three general categories of factors: (1) drug factors—the properties of the drug itself and differences in how it's used, (2) user factors—the physical and psychological characteristics of the user, and (3) social factors.

Drug Factors

When different drugs or dosages produce different effects, the differences are usually caused by one or more of five different drug factors:

• The **pharmacological properties** of the drug are its overall effects on a person's body chemistry, behavior, and psychology. Of all the millions of chemicals known, only a few have pharmacological properties that lead humans to use and abuse them. These self-administered chemicals are alcohol, nicotine, and the drug groups discussed in this chapter.

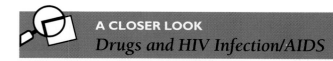
The first wave of HIV infection in the United States primarily struck gay and bisexual men. The second wave, spread by the sharing of contaminated hypodermic needles, affected intravenous (IV) drug users. The third wave of infection is affecting women and children—the sexual partners and children of IV drug users.

The use of contaminated hypodermic needles by intravenous drug users is linked to a third of all cases of AIDS in the United States, including nearly half of the AIDS cases among African Americans and Latinos. Nearly three-quarters of the more than 50,000 AIDS cases among American women that had been diagnosed by early 1995 could be traced to IV drug use or sexual contact with IV drug users. More than 6,000 children with AIDS have been reported to the Centers for Disease Control and Prevention; 90 percent of them acquired the infection from their mothers, either in the womb, at birth, or from breast milk.

No easy solutions are in sight. Education and prevention campaigns, which have succeeded in slowing the spread of HIV through the gay community, are far less effective at changing behavior among IV drug users. Most IV drug users are removed from the social and medical mainstream and lack access to the standard sources of education about health issues. For those dependent on drugs, the physical and psychological cravings for drugs are powerful motivators of behavior; thoughts of safety alone aren't strong enough to change behavior.

Heroin and other injectable opiates are responsible for much of the spread of HIV infection among IV drug users. Crack cocaine, even though it is smoked rather than injected, has also played a major role in the spread of HIV among young heterosexuals. Crack fosters transmission of HIV in two ways. First, many crack users also engage in IV drug use; "speedballs," injected cocaine-heroin mixes, enjoyed an alarming increase in popularity in the late 1980s and early 1990s. Second, crack use frequently leads to increased sexual activity. Many users trade sex for drugs or sex for money to buy drugs. Rates of syphilis and other sexually transmissible diseases have skyrocketed among crack users, also contributing to the spread of HIV. (The presence of genital sores related to STDs greatly increases the likelihood that a person will contract HIV from an infected sexual partner.)

Some public health experts believe free public needle-exchange programs—in which IV drug users turn in a used syringe and get a new, clean one back—could help stem the spread of HIV. By early 1995, there were about 80 needle exchange programs operating in the United States, many in states where they are barred by law. Opponents of exchange programs argue that supplying addicts with syringes gives them the message that illegal drug use is acceptable and could exacerbate the nation's drug program. Some federal health officials have urged linking needle exchange programs to programs that offer AIDS counseling and drug treatment.

People on both sides of the needle-exchange debate agree that getting people off drugs is the best solution. But government resources have been inadequate for the task. In 1991, for example, 60 percent of New York City's estimated 200,000 injecting drug users were infected with HIV. The city had resources to provide drug treatment for only 40,000 addicts at a time. Clearly, the spread of HIV among drug users in the United States constitutes a medical and social emergency, one that we will face for years to come.

Adapted from S. Russel, "CDC Endorses Needle Swaps." *San Francisco Chronicle*, 8 March 1995; D. W. Wara, "Perinatal AIDS and HIV: Diagnosis and Treatment Update," presented at the 1992 meeting of the American Academy of Pediatrics in San Francisco; and C. Morain, "Necessary But Illegal." *American Medical News*, 12 August 1991.

- The **dose-response function** is the relationship between the amount of drug taken and the intensity or type of drug effect. This relationship is not necessarily a direct one in which increasing the dose simply increases or intensifies the effect. Rather, the effect can change with a higher dosage. A familiar example is the person who becomes friendly after one drink but belligerent and hostile after four.

- The **time-action function** is the relationship between the time elapsed since a drug was taken and the intensity of its effect. The effects of a drug are greatest when concentrations of the drug in the tissues are changing the fastest, especially if they are increasing. For example, with alcohol, intoxication is usually greater when the blood alcohol level is rising than when it is falling, even though there may actually be somewhat less alcohol in the blood when it is rising.

- The *cumulative effects* of psychoactive drugs may be different from the effects of a single dose, because over time the drugs produce physiological alterations in the body that change their effects. A given amount of alcohol, for example, will generally affect a habitual drinker less than an occasional drinker. Tolerance to some drugs, such as LSD, builds rapidly. To experience the same effect, a user has to abstain from the drug for a period of time before that dosage will again exert its original effects.

- The *method of use* has a direct effect on how strong a response a drug produces. Methods of use include ingestion, inhalation, injection, and absorption through the skin or tissue linings. Drugs are usually injected one of three ways: intravenously (IV, or mainlining), intramuscularly (IM), or subcutaneously (SQ, or "skin popping").

If a drug is taken by a method that allows the drug to enter the bloodstream and reach the brain rapidly, the effects are usually stronger and the potential for dependence is greater than when the method involves slower absorption. For example, injecting a drug generally produces stronger effects than swallowing the same drug.

Different methods of drug use are associated with different "costs," or risks. For example, injecting drugs often involves the sharing of needles, which may be contaminated with disease agents from another user's blood. For this reason, intravenous drug users are at high risk for hepatitis B and HIV infection. The surest way to prevent transmission of disease is never to share needles. Sterilizing needles using bleach may kill the HIV virus, but sterilization has to be done carefully because viruses can be transmitted in very small amounts of blood.

User Factors

The second category of factors that determine how a person will respond to a particular drug involves the person's physical characteristics. Body mass is one variable. The effects of certain drugs on a 100-pound person will be twice as great as the effect of the same amount of the drug on a 200-pound person. Other variables include general health and various subtle **biochemical** states, including genetic factors. For example, some people have an inherited ability to rapidly metabolize a cough suppressant called dextromethorphan, which also has psychoactive properties. These people must take a higher-than-normal dose to get a given cough-suppressant effect.

If a person's biochemical state is already altered by another drug, this too can make a difference. Some drugs intensify the effects of other drugs, as is the case with alcohol and barbiturates. Some drugs block the effects of other drugs, such as when a **tranquilizer** is used to relieve anxiety caused by cocaine. Interactions between drugs, including many prescription and over-the-counter drugs, can be unpredictable and dangerous.

One physical condition that requires special precautions is pregnancy. It can be risky for a woman to use any drugs at all during pregnancy, including alcohol and over-the-counter drugs like cough medicine. Risks are greatest during the first trimester of pregnancy when the fetus's body is rapidly forming and even small chemical alterations in the mother's body can have a devastating effect on development. Even later, the fetus is more susceptible than the mother to the adverse effects of drugs. The fetus may even become dependent on a drug taken by the mother and suffer withdrawal symptoms after birth.

Sometimes response to a drug is affected strongly by the user's expectations about how he or she will respond to the drug. With large doses, the chemical properties of the drug do seem to have the strongest influence on the user's response. But with small doses, psychological (and social) factors are often more important. The **set** is the user's expectations about how he or she is going to respond to the drug. When people strongly believe that a given drug will affect them a certain way, they are likely to experience those effects regardless of the drug's pharmacological properties. The **placebo** effect—when an individual receives an inert substance and yet responds as if it were an active drug—is a well-documented example of set.

Social Factors

The **setting** is the physical and social environment surrounding the drug use. If a person uses marijuana at home with trusted friends and pleasant music, the effects are likely to be different from the effects if the same dose is taken in an austere experimental laboratory with an impassive research technician. Similarly, the dose of alcohol that produces mild euphoria and stimulation at a noisy, active cocktail party might induce sleepiness and slight depression when taken at home while alone.

REPRESENTATIVE PSYCHOACTIVE DRUGS

What are the major psychoactive drugs, and how do they produce their effects? We discuss six different representative groups in this chapter: (1) opiates, (2) **central nervous system (CNS)** depressants, (3) CNS stimulants, (4) psychedelics, (5) marijuana and other cannabis products, and (6) deliriants. Some of these drugs are classified according to how they affect the body; others—the opiates and the cannabis products—are classified according to their chemical makeup. See Figure 8-1 for sources of selected psychoactive drugs.

TERMS

Dose-response function   The relationship between the amount of a drug taken and the intensity or type of drug effect.

Time-action function   The relationship between the time elapsed since a drug was taken and the intensity of a drug effect.

Biochemical   Describes the branch of chemistry that deals with the life processes of plants and animals.

Tranquilizers   Central nervous system depressants that reduce tension and anxiety.

Set   A person's expectations or preconceptions in a given situation.

Placebo   An inert or innocuous medication that is given in place of an active drug; it is often called a sugar pill.

Setting   The environment in which something is done.

Central nervous system   The brain and spinal cord.

Opiates

The opiates, also called narcotics, are natural or synthetic (laboratory-made) drugs that relieve pain, cause drowsiness, and induce **euphoria.** Opium, morphine, heroin, methadone, codeine, meperidine, and fentanyl are examples of drugs in this class. The opiates tend to reduce anxiety and to produce lethargy, apathy, and an inability to concentrate. Opiate users become less active and less responsive to frustration, hunger, and sexual stimulation. These effects are more pronounced in novice users; with repeated use, many effects diminish.

Although the euphoria associated with opiates is an important factor in their abuse, many individuals experience a feeling of vague uneasiness when they first use these drugs. They may feel nauseated, vomit, or have other unpleasant sensations. Opiates are often dependency-producing.

The various opiates have similar effects, but they do differ in dose-response and time-action characteristics. They are sometimes injected under the skin, into the muscles, or directly into the veins. They may also be taken into the body by **absorption** from the stomach and intestine, the nasal membranes, or the lungs. As mentioned earlier, how the drug is taken determines how quickly it enters body tissue. If it is injected intravenously or smoked, the tissue level will change rapidly, and more immediate behavioral changes will result.

Rates of heroin use have remained constant in recent years. A 1993 survey of college students found that less than 1 percent had used heroin within the last year.

Central Nervous System Depressants

Central nervous system **depressants,** or **sedative-hypnotics,** slow down the overall activity of the nervous system. The result can range from mild **sedation** to death, depending on the various factors involved—which drug is used, how it's taken, how tolerant the user is, and so on. CNS depressants include alcohol (discussed in Chapter 7), **barbiturates,** antianxiety agents, and various other drugs with similar effects.

Effects CNS depressants reduce anxiety and produce mood changes, muscular incoordination, slurring of speech, and drowsiness or sleep. Mental and motor functioning are also affected, but the degree varies from person to person and also depends on the kind of task the person is trying to do. Most people become drowsy with small doses, although a few become more active. When people take these drugs deliberately to alter their awareness or for social reasons, they can overcome most of the sedative effects and remain awake even with large doses, particularly if they have developed tolerance or if the environment is exciting. However, even though users may remain awake, their mental and motor functioning is affected.

Types A variety of barbiturates is available. They are similar in chemical composition and action, but they do differ in how quickly they act and how long their action lasts. Drug users call barbiturates "downers" or "downs" and refer to specific brands by names that describe the color and design of the capsules: "reds" or "red devils" for Seconal, "yellows" or "yellow jackets" for Nembutal, "blue heavens" for Amytal, and "trees" for Tuinal (a combination of secobarbital and amobarbital). People usually take barbiturates in capsules, but injecting them is also common.

Antianxiety agents, also termed tranquilizers, include the benzodiazepines such as Valium and Xanax. Other CNS depressants include methaqualone (Quaalude is the trade name of a common methaqualone compound), ethchlorvynol (Placidyl), and chloral hydrate.

Medical Uses Barbiturates, antianxiety agents, and other sedative-hypnotics are widely used to treat insomnia and anxiety disorders and to control seizures. They are also used to modify the effects of other drugs (for example, to reduce the excessive physical activity that often accompanies the use of CNS stimulants). Some CNS depressants are used for their calming properties in combination with **anesthetic agents** before operations and other medical or dental procedures.

From Use to Abuse People are usually introduced to CNS depressants either through a medical prescription or through drug-using peers. Abuse of CNS depressants for the medical patient may begin with repeated use for insomnia and progress to dependency through bigger and bigger doses at night coupled with a few capsules at stressful times during the day. The abuse of tranquilizers such as Valium often involves increasingly frequent doses during the day. If a person tries to reduce or stop the medication, feelings of anxiety may occur; the anxiety is "treated" with another dose.

Most CNS depressants, including alcohol and the barbiturates, can lead to classical physical dependence. Tolerance, sometimes for up to 15 times the usual dose, can

TERMS

Euphoria   An exaggerated feeling of well-being.

Absorption   The passage of substances through the skin, lungs, or gastrointestinal tract into the blood.

Depressant   Something that decreases nervous or muscular activity.

Sedative-hypnotics   Another term for CNS depressants. These drugs cause drowsiness or sleep.

Sedation   The induction of a calm, relaxed, often sleepy state.

Barbiturate   A common sedative-hypnotic drug.

Anesthetic agents   Drugs that produce loss of sensation with or without loss of consciousness.

Medications designed to prevent or fight disease or to alleviate symptoms are an essential part of modern medical care. But they are also powerful chemicals that have the potential for harm. Being an informed consumer can help ensure that you receive the maximum benefit from the medications you take, while minimizing your risks.

How Are Medications Classified?

Medications are classified as prescription or over-the-counter (OTC). Prescription medications are those you buy with a physician's prescription from a licensed pharmacy. OTC medications are available without a prescription and include everything from aspirin to medicated shampoo.

Generic Versus Brand-Name Medications

When a medication is first developed, it's given a patent and a generic name. The patent gives the firm that discovers it the sole right to sell the drug while the patent is in effect. When the medication comes on the market, it is usually given a brand name by the manufacturer. After the patent expires (usually in about 17 years), the drug becomes public property and other companies can make and sell the drug under its generic name or their own brand name. Generic drugs contain the same active ingredients as the original brand-name drug but may contain different inactive ingredients. Generic drugs usually cost less than their brand-name counterparts, and they can often be substituted at a substantial savings to the patient. However, for some medications it may be important that you use a particular brand; ask your physician whether a generic drug is available and suitable for you.

Side Effects

All drugs cause changes in your body's chemistry; usually these changes are helpful, but they can also harm you. Side effects can occur with all drugs. Most often side effects are mild—such as a slight headache or drowsiness—but they can also be serious. Ask your physician or pharmacist what side effects you might expect from a drug. If you suffer an unexpected or severe side effect, contact your physician.

Medication Interactions

Medications can interact with other drugs and with what you eat. If you take two or more drugs at the same time, the medications may interact and cause undesirable effects.

Food can delay or reduce the absorption of many drugs; other drugs are better absorbed or less irritating to your stomach when you take them with food. Unless otherwise directed by your physician, it's best to take medications with a full glass of water at least one hour before, or two hours after, a meal. Your physician or pharmacist will tell you if a medication should be taken with food. Alcohol and other drugs may either enhance or reduce the effect of a medication. Combining alcohol with a medication that causes sedation can result in dangerous depression of the central nervous system. Don't take medications with alcohol.

Using the same pharmacy on a continuing basis is an important health care decision. A pharmacist who knows about your medical conditions and the medications you are taking can alert you to possible interactions and answer questions about your medications.

Communicate Before You Medicate

To safely prescribe medications for you, your physician(s) must know your medical condition, what medications you are currently taking (including OTCs), whether you are allergic to any drugs, how much and how often you use alcohol, and whether you are pregnant or plan to become pregnant in the near future. Never hesitate to ask your physician or pharmacist questions about any prescription or OTC drug. You should know why you are taking it, what action you can expect it to have, what the proper dosage is, how and when you should take it, and whether there are any restrictions or side effects.

Be Informed and Act Wisely

In addition to discussing your medications with your physician and pharmacist, read all drug labels carefully—both prescription and OTC. Pay close attention to all directions, warnings, and precautions and take all your medications exactly as directed. Don't stop taking a drug unless directed to do so by your physician. Keep a list of all the prescription and OTC drugs you are taking.

Taking medications is a big responsibility. For your own health and safety, listen, read, ask questions, and understand your medications.

Source: "Medications: Know What You're Taking and Why." *Medical Essay: Supplement to Mayo Clinic Health Letter,* October 1992.

develop during a year or two of repeated use. Tranquilizers have been shown to produce physical dependence even at ordinary prescribed doses. Withdrawal symptoms are more severe than those accompanying opiate dependence and are similar to the DTs of alcoholism. They may begin as anxiety, shaking, and weakness but may turn into convulsions and possible cardiovascular collapse, which may result in death.

While intoxicated, people on depressants cannot function very well. They are mentally confused and are frequently obstinate, irritable, and abusive. After long-term use, people commonly develop poor general health and

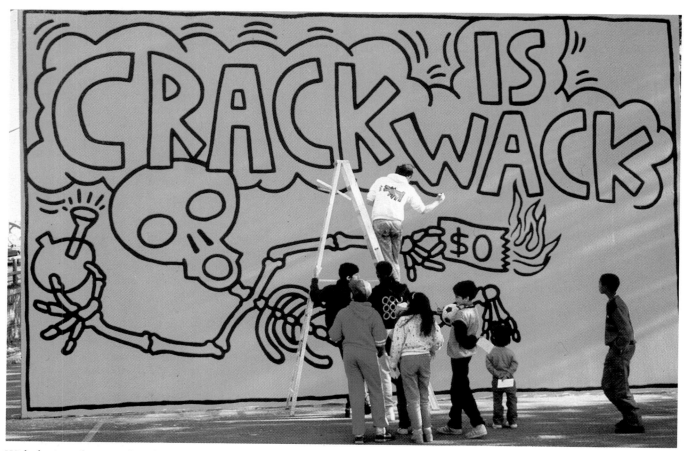

With the introduction of crack cocaine in the 1980s, the use of drugs and the incidence of associated crime rose dramatically in the United States, especially in the cities. This playground backboard, painted by the late Keith Haring, attempts to raise awareness among young people about the consequences of crack use.

may suffer from (sometimes permanent) brain damage, with impaired ability to reason and make judgments. The lack of judgment and physical coordination caused by these drugs often results in injuries and accidents.

Barbiturate dependents, like alcoholics and opiate addicts, often become preoccupied with having enough of the drug and sometimes resort to criminal activities to make sure they do. Violent behavior has also been linked with barbiturate dependence and with the use of methaqualone.

Overdosing with CNS Depressants Barbiturate overdose is one of the most frequent methods of suicide among American women. Accidental overdose can occur because the margin between a dose that produces the effects the user wants and a dose that is lethal narrows as tolerance develops. Accidental deaths can also result when people use two or more CNS depressants together, such as barbiturates and alcohol. Even if a single dose of either would not have been fatal, the combined depressant effects of both can halt breathing.

In a 1993 survey, about 2 percent of college students reported having used a CNS depressant within the past year.

Central Nervous System Stimulants

CNS **stimulants** speed up the activity of the nervous system. Under their influence, heart rate accelerates, blood pressure rises, blood vessels constrict, the pupils of the eyes and the bronchial tubes dilate, and gastric and adrenal secretions increase. There is greater muscular tension and sometimes an increase in motor activity. Small doses usually make people feel more awake and alert, less fatigued and bored. The most common CNS stimulants are cocaine, amphetamine, nicotine (discussed in Chapter 7), and caffeine.

Cocaine Usually derived from the leaves of coca shrubs that grow high in the Andes Mountains, cocaine is a potent CNS stimulant. Cocaine—also known as "coke" or "snow"—quickly produces a feeling of euphoria, which makes it a popular recreational drug. Cocaine—snorted, or inhaled—enjoyed a rapid surge in popularity during the early 1980s, when the drug's high price made it a "status" drug. Cocaine use among casual drug users began an eight-year decline in 1985. This decline ended in 1993, when, for example, an increase of 3 percent was seen in cocaine use among high school students. About 2 or 3 percent of college students use cocaine each year. The drug remains one of the country's leading public health problems. Because its price has dropped, it has entered virtually all social and economic groups in this country. Cocaine is responsible for many drug-related deaths and emergency room visits.

Methods of Use   Cocaine is usually snorted or injected intravenously, since those methods of administration provide more rapid increases of the drug's concentration in the blood and hence more intense effects. Another method of use involves heating the cocaine with ether or other chemicals and then inhaling its vapors. In "free-basing," as this practice is called, the user risks burns from sudden combustion.

A chemically similar method of processing cocaine involves baking soda and water. This yields a ready-to-smoke form of free-base cocaine, often called crack. Crack is typically available as small beads or pellets smokable in glass pipes or sprinkled on tobacco or marijuana. The tiny but potent beads can be handled more easily than cocaine powder and marketed in smaller, less expensive doses. Thus, processing cocaine into crack has increased cocaine availability to young people and others who couldn't afford to buy more expensive preparations.

Effects   The effects of cocaine are usually intense but short-lived. The euphoria lasts from 5 to 20 minutes and ends abruptly, to be replaced by irritability, anxiety, or slight depression. When cocaine is absorbed via the lungs, either by smoking or inhalation, it reaches the brain in 10 seconds or so, and the effects are particularly intense. This is part of the appeal of both free-basing and smoking crack. The effects from intravenous injections occur almost as quickly—20 seconds. Since the mucous membranes in the nose briefly slow absorption, the onset of effects from snorting takes 2 or 3 minutes. Heavy users who want to maintain the effects inject cocaine intravenously every 10 to 20 minutes.

The larger the dose of cocaine and the more rapidly it is absorbed into the bloodstream, the greater the immediate—and sometimes lethal—effects. Sudden death from cocaine is most commonly the result of excessive CNS stimulation that causes convulsions and respiratory collapse, cardiac arrhythmias (irregularities in heartbeat), excessive constriction of the arteries to the heart causing ischemia (lack of oxygen to heart muscle), and possibly heart attacks or strokes. Although rare, fatalities can occur in young people who have no underlying health problems.

Cocaine users sometimes try to alter or control their experience by using "speedball" mixtures, which combine cocaine with a depressant. However, the rapid changes thus imposed on the CNS are sometimes fatal. Comedian John Belushi died from a combination of intravenous cocaine and heroin.

Cocaine constricts the blood vessels and it acts as a local anesthetic. It is still used for minor nose surgery where bleeding is a problem. However, in the chronic cocaine snorter, repeated **vasoconstriction** produces inflammation of the nasal mucosa, which can lead to persistent bleeding and ulceration of the septum between the nostrils. Cocaine users may also become paranoid or violent.

Abuse and Dependence   When steady cocaine users stop taking the drug, they experience a sudden "crash," characterized by depression, agitation, and fatigue, followed by a period of withdrawal. Their depression can be temporarily relieved by taking more cocaine, so its continued use is reinforced. Cocaine use follows different patterns among different individuals. A binge cocaine user may go for weeks or months without using any cocaine and then take large amounts repeatedly. Although not physically dependent, a binge cocaine user who misses work or school and risks serious health consequences is clearly abusing the drug.

Cocaine Use During Pregnancy   An alarming number of babies are being exposed to cocaine before birth. Cocaine rapidly crosses the placenta and has many serious effects on the fetus. A woman who uses cocaine during pregnancy is at higher risk for miscarriage, premature labor, and stillbirth. She is more likely to deliver a low birth weight baby who has a small head circumference. Research suggests that her infant may be at increased risk for defects of the genitourinary tract, cardiovascular system, central nervous system, and extremities. It is difficult to pinpoint the effects of cocaine because many women who use cocaine also use tobacco and/or alcohol.

Infants whose mothers use cocaine may also be born intoxicated. They are typically irritable, jittery, and do not eat or sleep normally. These characteristics may affect their early social and emotional development because it may be more difficult for adults to interact with them. These effects may be related to neurological abnormalities rather than withdrawal, which may also occur.

Cocaine-affected children are at increased risk for developmental delays and learning and behavior problems

Stimulant   Something that increases nervous or muscular activity.
Vasoconstriction   A constriction of the blood vessels.

TERMS

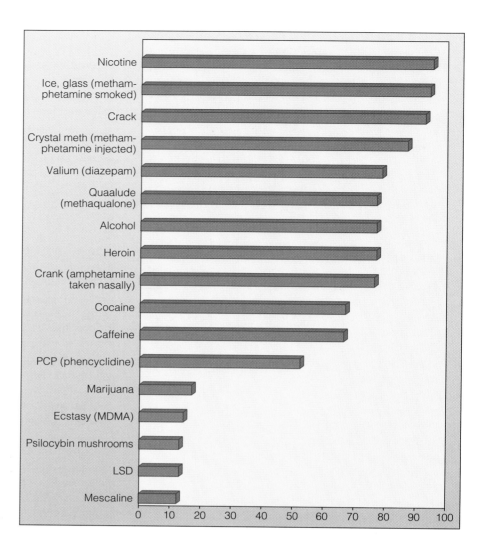

Figure 8-3 *How easy is it to get hooked on drugs?*
The numbers at the bottom of the chart are relative rankings. *Source:* L. Davis. 1990. "Why Do People Take Drugs?" *In Health,* November/December.

in their first year of life. Recent research suggests that some of these problems can disappear later in childhood if the drug-exposed infants receive adequate nutrition and skilled parenting, but it is too early to know whether effects continue into later childhood and adult life. However, children who grow up in cocaine-abusing families are at high risk for continuing problems, including accidental drug poisoning. Infants and children can also become intoxicated from the environmental smoke of freebase or crack cocaine. Cocaine passes into breast milk, as well, where it can intoxicate a breastfeeding infant.

Amphetamines Amphetamines are a group of synthetic chemicals that are potent CNS stimulants. Some common amphetamines are dextroamphetamine (Dexedrine), d-1-amphetamine (Benzedrine), and methamphetamine (Methedrine). Popular names for these drugs change often and are different in different parts of the country. Some of the more common names are "speed," "crank," "crystal," and "meth."

"Ice," a smokeable, high-potency form of methamphetamine, grew rapidly in popularity in the late 1980s and early 1990s, especially on the West Coast and in Hawaii. Easy to manufacture, ice is cheaper than crack and produces a euphoria similar to that produced by cocaine but lasting much longer. Use of ice can quickly lead to dependence (Figure 8-3). Ice is odorless, so it can't be easily detected when smoked in public. Ice has not grown in popularity as quickly as was initially feared; however, in a recent survey of high school students, about 3 percent reported having tried ice at least once.

Effects Small doses of amphetamines usually make people feel better, more alert and wide-awake, and less fatigued or bored. Small doses can produce some improvement in activities—like certain athletic contests or military maneuvers—that require extreme physical effort or endurance. Amphetamines generally increase motor activity but do not measurably alter a normal, rested person's ability to perform tasks calling for complex motor skills or high-level thinking. When amphetamines do improve performance, it's primarily by counteracting fatigue and boredom. In small doses, they also increase the heart rate and blood pressure and change sleep patterns.

Amphetamines are sometimes used to curb appetite, but after a few weeks the user develops tolerance, and higher doses are necessary. When people stop taking the drug, their appetites usually rebound, and they gain back the weight they lost unless they have made permanent changes in eating behavior. Amphetamines have other medical uses, but many physicians doubt their usefulness and consider other approaches more worthwhile and not as risky.

From Use to Abuse   Much amphetamine abuse begins as an attempt to cope with a passing situation. A student cramming for exams or an exhausted long-haul truck driver can go a little longer by "popping a benny," but the results can be disastrous. The likelihood of making bad judgments significantly increases. In addition, the stimulating effects may wear off suddenly, and the user may precipitously feel exhausted or fall asleep ("crash").

Another problem is **state dependency,** the phenomenon whereby information learned in a certain drug-induced state is difficult to recall when the person is not in that same physiological state. Test performance may deteriorate when students use drugs to study and then take tests in their normal, nondrug state.

Dependence   Repeated use of amphetamines, even in moderate doses, often leads to tolerance and the need for larger and larger doses. The result can be severe disturbances in behavior, including paranoid **psychosis** with illusions, hostility, delusions of persecution, and unprovoked violence. It is just like a nondrug psychosis except that it ends if the person stops taking the drug.

If injected in large doses, amphetamines produce a feeling of intense pleasure, followed by sensations of vigor and euphoria that last for several hours. As these feelings wear off, they are replaced by feelings of irritability and vague uneasiness. Long-term use of ice at high doses can cause paranoia, hallucinations, delusions, and incoherence. Withdrawal symptoms may include muscle aches and tremors, along with profound fatigue, deep depression, despair, and apathy. Chronic high-dose amphetamine use is often associated with pronounced psychological dependence. Chronic abusers frequently spend much of their time obsessively seeking drugs.

Women who use amphetamines during pregnancy risk premature birth, stillbirth, and early infant death. Babies born to amphetamine-using mothers have a higher incidence of cleft palate, cleft lip, and missing or deformed limbs. They may also be born dependent on amphetamines.

Other hazards of amphetamine use include malnutrition, weight loss, damage to blood vessels, strokes, and other changes in the heart and blood vessels. The use of the injection method brings an added danger, the risk of HIV infection and other blood-borne disease from contaminated needles.

Caffeine   Caffeine is probably the most popular psychoactive drug and also one of the most ancient. It is found in coffee, tea, cocoa, soft drinks, headache remedies, and over-the-counter drugs like No-Doz. In ordinary doses caffeine produces greater alertness and a sense of well-being. It also cuts down on feelings of fatigue or boredom, and using caffeine may enable a person to keep at physically exhausting or repetitive tasks longer. Such use is usually followed, however, by a sudden letdown. Caffeine does not noticeably influence a person's ability to perform complex intellectual tasks unless fatigue, boredom, alcohol, or other factors have already affected normal performance.

Caffeine mildly stimulates the heart and respiratory system, it increases muscular tremor, and it enhances gastric secretion. Higher doses may cause nervousness, anxiety, irritability, headache, disturbed sleep, and gastric irritation or peptic ulcers. In women, excessive caffeine consumption may aggravate the symptoms associated with premenstrual syndrome. Some people, especially children, are quite vulnerable to the adverse effects of caffeine. They become "wired"—hyperactive and exquisitely sensitive to any stimulation in their environment. In rare instances, the disturbance is so severe that there is misperception of their surroundings—a toxic psychosis.

Drinks containing caffeine are rarely harmful for most individuals, but some tolerance develops and withdrawal symptoms of irritability, headaches, and even mild depression do occur. Thus, although we don't usually think of caffeine as a dependency-producing drug, it is. People can usually avoid problems by simply decreasing their daily intake of caffeine (Table 8-1).

Marijuana and Other Cannabis Products

Marijuana is the most widely used illicit drug in the United States (cocaine is second). More than 30 percent of Americans—about 67 million—have tried marijuana at least once; among 18- to 25-year-olds, more than 50 percent have tried marijuana. Recent surveys of college students indicate that marijuana use is growing: about 27 percent reported using marijuana within the last year, 13 percent within the last month.

State dependency   Situation where information learned in a drug-induced state is difficult to recall when the effects of the drugs wear off.

Psychosis   A severe mental disorder in which there is a distortion of reality. Symptoms might include delusions or hallucinations.

TABLE 8-1 The Daily Dose

This chart will help you calculate your daily caffeine intake. But remember, caffeine content varies widely, depending on the product you use and how it's prepared.

Beverages	Serving Size	Caffeine (mg)
Coffee, drip	7.5 oz	115–175
Coffee, perk	7.5 oz	80–135
Coffee, instant	7.5 oz	65–100
Coffee, decaffeinated	7.5 oz	3–4
Tea, 1 minute steep	5 oz	20
Tea, 3-minute steep	5 oz	35
Tea, iced	12 oz	70
Coca-Cola	12 oz	45
Mountain Dew	12 oz	54
Dr. Pepper	12 oz	40
Pepsi Cola	12 oz	38
7 Up	12 oz	0

Foods	Serving Size	Caffeine (mg)
Milk chocolate	1 oz	1–15
Bittersweet chocolate	1 oz	5–35
Chocolate cake	1 slice	20–30

Over-the-Counter Drugs	Dose	Caffeine (mg)
Anacin, Empirin, or Midol	2	64
Excedrin	2	130
NoDoz	2	200
Aqua-Ban (diuretic)	2	200
Dexatrim (weight control aid)	1	200

Sources: Tony Chou. 1992. "Wake Up and Smell the Coffee." *Western Journal of Medicine* 157:544–53; "Caffeine Update: The News Is Mostly Good." *University of California at Berkeley Wellness Letter,* July 1988.

Marijuana is a crude preparation of various parts of the Indian hemp plant, *Cannabis sativa,* which grows in most parts of the world. THC (tetrahydrocannabinol) is the main active ingredient in marijuana. Hashish is a potent cannabis preparation derived mainly from the thick resinous materials of the flowering tops and upper leaves of the plant. THC can be synthesized, but it is an expensive process. Because of the cost, pure THC is virtually never available on the illicit market. Drugs sold as THC are almost always something else, such as methamphetamine.

Marijuana is usually smoked, but can also be ingested. Although it is usually thought of as a psychedelic, the classification of marijuana is a matter of some debate. For this reason, it is treated separately here.

Short-Term Effects and Uses As is true with most psychoactive drugs, the effects of a low dose of marijuana are strongly influenced by what the user expects and what his or her previous experience with the drug has been. At low doses, marijuana users typically experience euphoria, heightening of subjective sensory experiences, slowing down of the time sense, and a relaxed, "laid-back" attitude. These pleasant effects are the reason why this drug is so widely used. With moderate doses, these effects become stronger, and the user can also expect to have impaired memory function, disturbed thought patterns, lapses of attention, and feelings of **depersonalization,** in which the mind seems to be separated from the body. Decreased driving and workplace safety can also be expected.

The effects of marijuana with higher doses are determined mostly by the drug itself rather than by set and setting. Very high doses produce feelings of depersonalization as well as marked sensory distortion and changes in body image (such as a feeling that the body is very light). Inexperienced users sometimes think these sensations mean that they are going crazy and become anxious or even panicky. Such reactions resemble a bad trip on LSD, but they happen much less often, are less severe, and do not last as long.

Physiologically, marijuana causes increases in heart rate and dilation of certain blood vessels in the eyes, which creates the characteristic bloodshot eyes. The user also feels less inclination for physical exertion.

Cannabis preparations were once medically prescribed for a variety of human illnesses, including insomnia, migraine, depression, and epilepsy. Now, however, none of these uses can be supported. Its medical use for sedative or euphoric effects is limited because of the perceptual and cognitive changes it brings about and also because individual reactions cannot be predicted. Somewhat more promising are current investigations into the use of THC to reduce nausea and improve appetite during cancer chemotherapy. In this situation, adverse side effects are less critical. THC and related compounds are also being studied for possible use in certain forms of glaucoma, an eye disease that causes blindness.

Long-Term Effects Marijuana remains a complex, poorly understood drug; further research is needed to determine its precise physiological and psychological effects. Chronic bronchial irritation is one of the few widely agreed upon long-term effects of chronic marijuana use. Other potential adverse effects include impairment of long-term memory; gum disease; increased risk of cancers of the mouth, jaw, tongue, and lung; and impairment of the immune system. Some studies suggest that long-term marijuana use may result in decreased testosterone levels, decreased sperm counts, and increased sperm abnormalities in male users. Heavy marijuana use during pregnancy may cause impaired fetal growth and development and may act synergistically with alcohol to increase the damaging effects of alcohol on the fetus. Marijuana rapidly enters breast milk and remains there for an extended period.

Dependence   Regular users of marijuana can develop a marked tolerance to the drug, but physical dependence characterized by significant withdrawal symptoms has not been well established for marijuana use in either human or animal studies. However, as with all drugs that relieve "bad" feelings and produce "good" feelings, marijuana can become the focus of the user's life to the exclusion of other activities. The chronic marijuana user will not necessarily limit his or her drug use to cannabis. Drug uses appear to be related, and the chronic marijuana user is more likely to be a heavy user of tobacco, alcohol, and other dangerous drugs. The person who buys marijuana is in touch with the illicit drug market, and that contact may be the key to the association between marijuana use and the increased rate of subsequent use of cocaine and heroin.

Psychedelics

The term *psychedelics* refers to a group of drugs whose predominant pharmacological effect is to alter perception, feelings, and thoughts in the user. These drugs are also called hallucinogens, although at low doses hallucinations are not one of their major effects. The psychedelics include LSD (lysergic acid diethylamide), mescaline, psilocybin, STP (dimethoxy-methyl-amphetamine), DMT (dimethyl-tryptamine), and many others. These drugs are most commonly ingested or smoked. LSD ("acid") is the most widely known of the psychedelics, and we discuss it in detail here as an example of the entire group.

LSD   LSD is one of the most powerful psychoactive drugs. Tiny doses will produce noticeable effects in most people. These effects include an altered sense of time, disorders of vision, an improved sense of hearing, changes in mood, and distortions in how people perceive their bodies. There is almost always dilation of the pupils, and there may also be slight dizziness, weakness, and nausea. With larger doses, users may experience a phenomenon known as **synesthesia**, feelings of depersonalization, and other alterations in the perceived relationship between self and external reality. Many psychedelics induce biological tolerance so quickly that after a few days' use their effects are reduced greatly. The user must then stop taking the drug for several days before his or her system can be receptive to it again. These drugs cause little drug-seeking behavior and no physical dependence or withdrawal symptoms.

The immediate effects of low doses of psychedelics are largely determined by set and setting. Many effects of psychedelics are hard to describe because they involve subjective and unusual dimensions of awareness—the **altered states of consciousness** for which psychedelics are famous. A severe panic reaction ("bad trip"), which can be terrifying in the extreme, can occur at any dose of LSD. Even after the drug's chemical effects have worn off, spontaneous flashbacks and other psychological disturbances can occur. Flashbacks are perceptual distortions and bizarre thoughts that occur after the drug has been entirely eliminated from the body.

Other Psychedelics   Most other psychedelics have the same general effects that LSD has, but there are some variations. As in LSD use, the effects of small doses depend largely on psychological and social factors, the set, and the setting. A DMT **"high"** does not last as long as an LSD high; an STP trip lasts longer. Ditran and related compounds cause greater intellectual impairment and confusion than do other psychedelics.

Mescaline (peyote), the ceremonial drug of the Native North American Church, supposedly produces a trip different from that caused by LSD. Obtaining mescaline costs far more than making LSD, however, so most street mescaline is LSD that has been highly diluted. Psychedelic effects can be obtained from certain mushrooms (*Psilocybe mexicana*, or "magic mushrooms"), certain morning glory seeds, nutmeg, jimsonweed, and other botanical products, but unpleasant side effects, such as dizziness, have limited the popularity of these products.

Deliriants

Many drugs, and other substances not usually thought of as drugs, can bring on a form of abnormal behavior called **delirium,** or toxic psychosis. Delirium results from a temporary impairment of brain function. Different chemicals act on the brain in different ways, but the results are generally similar. They consist of changing levels of awareness to surrounding events, decreased ability to maintain attention to a task, and variable amounts of mental confusion. The user may also experience hallucinations, especially visual ones.

Depersonalization   A state in which a person loses the sense of his or her own reality or perceives his or her own body as unreal.

Synesthesia   A condition in which a stimulus evokes not only the sensation appropriate to it but also another sensation of a different character. An example is when a color evokes a specific smell.

Altered states of consciousness   Profound changes in mood, thinking, and perception.

"High"   The subjectively pleasing effects of a drug, usually felt quite soon after the drug is taken.

Delirium   A reversible state of mental confusion sometimes marked by emotional excitement.

TERMS

PCP Phencyclidine, also known as "angel dust," "PCP," "hog," and "peace pill," is a widely used synthetic drug that can be considered a deliriant. PCP reduces and distorts sensory input, especially **proprioception** (awareness of the position of arms and legs, joints, and so forth), and creates a state of sensory deprivation. This drug was initially used as a human anesthetic, but was unsatisfactory because of the postoperative agitation, confusion, and delirium its use caused. Since the ingredients of PCP are readily obtainable and it can be easily made, it is often available on the illicit market and is sometimes used as a cheap adulterant for other psychoactive agents.

Inhalants Inhaling certain chemicals can produce effects ranging from heightened pleasure to delirium. Inhalants fall into three major groups: (1) volatile solvents, which include adhesives and aerosols; (2) nitrites, which are found in some room odorizers and in the street drugs butyl nitrite and amyl nitrite; and (3) anesthetics, which include nitrous oxide or "laughing gas." Use of inhalants is increasing, especially among people under age 18; nearly 18 percent of all twelfth graders have used inhalants.

Inhalant use is difficult to control because users don't face the drug-procurement and use obstacles that can discourage experimentation with other drugs. Inhalants are present in a variety of seemingly harmless products, from dessert-toppings sprays to underarm deodorants, that are both inexpensive and legal. Using the drugs also requires no illegal or suspicious paraphernalia. Inhalant users get high by "sniffing," "snorting," "bagging" (inhaling fumes from a plastic bag), or "huffing" (placing an inhalant-soaked rag in the mouth).

Although different in makeup, nearly all the inhalants produce effects similar to anesthetics, which act to slow bodily functions. Low doses may cause users to feel slightly stimulated; at higher doses, users may feel less inhibited and less in control. Sniffing high concentrations of the chemicals in solvents or aerosol sprays can cause loss of conciousness, heart failure, and death. High concentrations of any inhalant can also cause death from suffocation by displacing the oxygen in the lungs and central nervous system. Deliberately inhaling from a bag or in a closed area greatly increases the chances of suffocation. Other possible effects of inhalants include damage to the nervous system (impaired perception, reasoning, memory, and muscular coordination), hearing loss, and damage to the liver, kidney, and bone marrow.

Designer Drugs

A relatively recent addition to the group of psychoactive chemicals, **"designer drugs"** are new compounds produced in clandestine laboratories. They are created by modifying existing drugs to produce **analogues.** An analogue has effects similar to those of the drug it is designed to mimic, but its origins and chemical structure are different. Use of designer drugs is increasing.

Two types of synthetic opiates have become popular designer drugs because of their heroin-like effects. Analogues of the drug meperidine (Demerol), marketed as "new heroin" or "synthetic heroin," first came to the attention of physicians because some people developed irreversible **parkinsonism** after taking the drug. Sufferers of this neurological condition experience loss of facial expression, drooling, a shuffling gait, and tremor of the hands, arms, and legs. An occasional by-product of designer heroin production caused the parkinsonism. Analogues of the drug fentanyl (Sublimaze) make up a second type of designer opiate. The best known is sold on the street as "China white." Initially touted as a safe alternative to heroin, the drug turned out to be a thousand times more potent than heroin. Numerous cases of fatal overdoses of China white have been reported since its introduction.

Methamphetamine and mescaline analogues constitute another designer drug category. MDA, known on the street as the "love drug," became a popular drug of abuse in the late 1960s. This amphetamine analogue produces a mild euphoria. Those who take it experience a desire to be with and talk to people. Like amphetamine, which it mimics, MDA can be fatal.

MDMA, known as "ecstasy" or "Adam" on the street, is chemically similar to both methamphetamine and mescaline. The drug stimulates the central nervous system and causes hallucinogenic effects. MDMA can elevate users' moods and increase feelings of intimacy with others. But it also may cause panic, anxiety, paranoid thinking, rapid heart rate, jaw clenching, involuntary eye twitching, and shaking. An overdose can cause life-threatening disturbances in heart rhythm, high blood pressure, and seizures.

DRUG USE: THE DECADES AHEAD

Drug research will undoubtedly provide new information, new treatments, and new chemical combinations in the decades ahead. New psychoactive drugs may present unexpected possibilities for therapy, social use, and abuse. Making honest and unbiased information about drugs available to everyone, however, may cut down on their abuse. Lies about the dangers of drugs—"scare tactics"—can lead some people to disbelieve any reports of drug dangers, no matter how soundly based and well documented they are.

Although the use of some drugs, both legal and illegal, has declined dramatically since the 1970s, the use of others has held steady, or increased. Mounting public concern has led to great debate and a wide range of opinions about what should be done. Efforts to combat the problem include workplace drug testing; tougher law enforce-

Codependency became a trendy term in the late 1980s, and popular authors attributed a long list of personal and social problems to what they termed "codependent behavior." However, the concept is a useful one for looking at the relationships between drug abusers (and people with other types of self-destructive habits) and those close to them. A codependent is a person who is in a continuing relationship with a drug-abusing person and whose actions help or enable that person to remain dependent. Codependency, also called enabling, removes or softens the effects of the drug use on the user. People often become enablers spontaneously and naturally. When someone they love becomes dependent on a drug, they want to help, and they assume that their good intentions will persuade the drug user to stop. Unfortunately, alcoholics and drug-dependent people have a system of denial that is strengthened rather than diminished by well-meaning attempts to help.

The habit of enabling hinders a drug-dependent person's recovery because the person never has to experience the consequences of his or her behavior. Frequently, the enabler is dependent too—on the pattern of interaction in the relationship. People who need to take care of people often marry people who need to be taken care of. Children in these families often develop the same pattern of behavior as one of their parents, either by becoming helpless or by becoming a caregiver. This is why treatment programs for drug dependency, such as Alcoholics Anonymous, Narcotics Anonymous, and Cocaine Anonymous, involve the whole family.

Have you ever been an enabler in a relationship? You may have if you have ever done any of the following:

- Given someone one more chance to stop abusing drugs, then another, and another . . .
- Made excuses or lied for someone to his or her friends, teachers, or employer
- Joined someone in drug use and blamed others for your behavior
- Lent money to someone to continue drug use
- Stayed up late waiting or gone out searching for someone who uses drugs
- Felt embarrassed or angry about the actions of someone who uses drugs
- Ignored the drug use because the person got defensive when you brought it up
- Not confronted a friend or relative who was obviously intoxicated or high on a drug

There are a number of books available in bookstores on codependency. If you come from a codependent family or see yourself developing relationships like this, consider acting now to make changes in your patterns of interaction.

---

ment and prosecution; and treatment and education. The legalization of drugs has also been proposed as a strategy to help control our nation's drug problem. With drugs entering the country on a massive scale from South America, Southeast Asia, and elsewhere and distributed through tightly controlled drug-smuggling organizations and street gangs, it remains to be seen how effective any program will be. The current federal price tag for drug control exceeds $10 billion a year, about two-thirds for law enforcement and one-third for prevention and treatment. Each year, drug abuse is linked to more than 1 million arrests, 400,000 emergency room admissions, and 8,000 deaths.

Drug Testing

One of the more controversial issues in American politics is drug testing in the workplace. It has been estimated that many workers, perhaps 1 in 10, use psychoactive drugs on the job. For some occupations, such as air traffic controllers, truck drivers, and train conductors, drug use can create significant dangers, sometimes involving hundreds of people. Some people believe that the dangers are so great that all workers should be tested and that anyone found to have traces of drugs in the blood or urine should be fired or treated. Others insist that this would violate people's right to privacy and to the freedom from unreasonable search guaranteed by the Fourth Amendment. Proponents then ask whether companies who don't test for drugs should be liable for damages if their employees cause harm to others.

Many employers now test their employees, and the U.S. armed forces test military personnel on a regular basis. However, drug testing is expensive, with costs running as high as $100 per individual test; and questions about accuracy and reliability complicate the issue. An-

TERMS

Proprioception   The sensory processes that identify the position and movement of muscles, tendons, and joints.

Designer drugs   Drugs created by altering the chemical structure of existing compounds to produce analogues with similar effects.

Analogue   A drug similar in function to the drug from which it is derived, but with a different origin.

Parkinsonism   A syndrome characterized by a masklike expression, shuffling gait, drooling, and tremor; can be drug-induced.

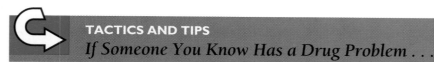

If you notice changes in behavior and mood in someone you know, they may signal a growing dependence on drugs. Signs that a person's life is beginning to center on drugs include the following:

- Sudden withdrawal or emotional distance
- Rebellious or unusually irritable behavior
- Loss of interest in usual activities or hobbies
- Decline in school performance
- Sudden change in group of friends
- Changes in sleeping or eating habits
- Frequent borrowing of money or stealing
- Secretive behavior about personal possessions, such as a backpack or the contents of a drawer
- Deterioration of physical appearance

If you believe a family member or friend has a drug problem, obtain information about resources for drug treatment available on your campus or in your community. Communicate your concern, provide him or her with information about treatment options, and offer your support during treatment. If the individual continues to deny having a problem, you may want to talk with an experienced counselor about setting up an "intervention"—a formal, structured confrontation designed to end denial by having family, friends, and other caring individuals present their concerns to the drug user. Participants in an intervention may stress the ways in which the individual is hurting others as well as himself or herself. If your friend or family member agrees to treatment, encourage him or her to attend a support group such as Narcotics Anonymous or Alcoholics Anonymous. And finally, examine your relationship with the abuser for signs of codependency. If necessary, get help for yourself; friends and family of drug users often can benefit from counseling.

other factor to be considered is that most jobs don't involve hazards, so employees who are on drugs aren't any more dangerous than employees who aren't on drugs. All these legal and practical issues mean that drug testing is likely to remain controversial throughout the 1990s.

Treatment for Drug Dependence

A variety of programs is available to help people break their drug habits. Professional treatment programs usually take the form of drug substitution programs or programs operated by rehabilitation centers. Nonprofessional self-help groups and peer counseling are also available. There is no single best method of treatment, and the relapse rate is high for all types of treatment. To be successful, a treatment program must deal with the reasons behind people's drug abuse and help them develop behaviors, attitudes, and a social support system that will help them remain drug-free.

Drug Substitution Programs   Sometimes a less debilitating drug can be substituted for one with many damaging effects, thus reducing the "costs," or risks, of the drug use. Methadone is a synthetic drug used as a substitute for heroin. When methadone is used, addicts can stop taking heroin without experiencing severe withdrawal reactions. Methadone is addictive too, but it decreases the craving for heroin and allows the individual to function normally in personal, social, and vocational activities. It also blocks the action of narcotics, so addicts don't get high even if they take heroin. Methadone treatment allows many former heroin abusers to live more useful lives.

Because they are relatively inexpensive to administer, drug substitute programs are a popular form of treatment. However, there is a significant relapse rate from methadone and other drug substitution treatment programs, as is the case with all drug dependency treatment efforts. This rate is reduced when psychological and social services are provided in addition to methadone. The fact that this type of support improves recovery rates underscores the importance of psychological factors in drug dependency.

Treatment Centers   The 1980s saw a boom in drug rehabilitation centers. Some national chains built or bought hospitals devoted solely to treating chemical dependency, and many general hospitals opened drug rehabilitation or chemical dependency units. But as the 1990s opened, skyrocketing health care costs caused the closure of many of these centers. Health insurance policies that once covered 30-day stays at drug rehabilitation centers now cover only limited outpatient visits or have no coverage for drug treatment at all. The challenge for the years ahead will be for chemical dependency centers to prove—and improve—their effectiveness and for private employers and public agencies to develop cost-effective ways to meet the needs of people in our society with drug problems.

Most treatment centers offer a variety of short- and long-term services, including hospitalization, detoxification, counseling, and other psychiatric services. A specific type of center is the therapeutic community, a residential program run in a completely drug-free atmosphere. Administered by ex-addicts, these programs use confronta-

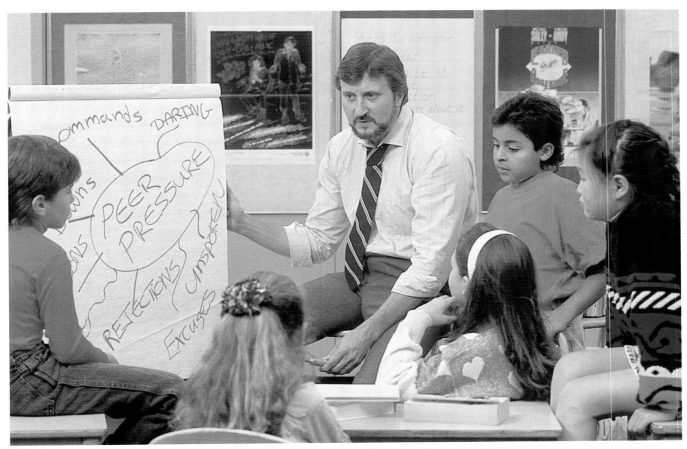

Giving young people information about the adverse effects of drugs and teaching them strategies for existing peer pressure to use drugs may help prevent future drug abuse. Young children may respond to education programs involving a respected or well-known adult.

tion, strict discipline, and unrelenting peer pressure to attempt to resocialize the addict with a different set of values. "Halfway houses," transition settings between a 24-hour-a-day program and independent living, are an important phase of treatment for some people.

Treatment centers often also offer counseling for those close to drug abusers. Drug abuse takes a toll on friends and family members, and counseling can help people work through painful feelings of guilt and powerlessness. Sometimes people close to a drug abuser develop patterns of behavior that help or enable the person to remain drug-dependent. Counseling can help people adopt realistic ideas about their role in their loved one's dependence and recovery and help them identify and change any problematic patterns of behavior.

For help in locating a treatment program in your area, call the National Drug Information and Treatment Hotline at 1-800-662-HELP (Spanish-speaking callers can phone 1-800-66-AYUDA).

Self-Help Groups and Peer Counseling Self-help groups such as Alcoholics Anonymous (AA) and Narcotics Anonymous (NA) have helped many people. Peer support is a critical ingredient of these programs. Members usually meet at least once a week. They are paired with buddies they can call for advice and support if a craving or temptation to relapse becomes overwhelming. Chapters of AA and NA meet on some college campuses; community-based chapters are listed in the phone book. Many colleges also have peer counseling programs, in which students are trained to provide confidential help for students who have drug problems. Information about peer counseling programs is usually available from the student health center.

Personal Insight What is your attitude toward drug dependency? Do you view it more as a moral violation, a criminal act, or an illness? Where do you think your ideas come from?

Prevention of Drug Abuse

Clearly, the best solution to drug abuse is prevention. Government attempts at controlling the drug problem tend to focus on stopping the production, importation,

- Bored? Go for a walk or a run; stimulate your senses at a museum or a movie; challenge your mind with a new game or book; introduce yourself to someone new.

- Stressed? Practice relaxation or visualization; try to slow down and open your senses to the natural world; get some exercise.

- Shy, lonely? Talk to a counselor; enroll in a shyness clinic; learn and practice communication techniques.

- Feeling low on self-esteem? Focus on the areas in which you are competent; give yourself credit for the things you do well. A program of regular exercise can also enhance self-esteem.

- Depressed, anxious? Talk to a friend, parent, or counselor.

- Apathetic, lethargic? Force yourself to get up and get some exercise to energize yourself; assume responsibility for someone or something outside yourself; volunteer.

- Searching for meaning? Try yoga or meditation; explore spiritual experiences through religious groups, church, prayer, or reading.

- Afraid to say no? Take a course in assertiveness training; get support from others who don't want to use drugs; remind yourself that you have the right and the responsibility to make your own decisions.

- Still feeling peer pressure? Begin to look for new friends or roommates. Take a class or join an organization that attracts other health-conscious people.

and distribution of illicit drugs. Creative effort also has to be put into stopping the demand for drugs. Developing persuasive antidrug educational programs offers the best hope for solving the drug problem in the future. Indirect approaches to prevention involve building young people's self-esteem, improving their academic skills, and increasing their recreational opportunities. Direct approaches involve giving information about the adverse effects of drugs and teaching tactics that help students resist peer pressure to use drugs in various situations. Developing strategies for resisting peer pressure is one of the more effective techniques.

Prevention in the 1990s focuses on the different motivations individuals have for using and abusing specific drugs at different ages. For example, grade school children seem receptive to programs that involve their parents or well-known adults like professional athletes. Adolescents in junior or senior high school are often more responsive to peer counselors. Many young adults tend to be influenced by efforts focusing on health education. For all ages, it is important to provide nondrug alternatives that speak to that individual's or group's specific reasons for using drugs, such as recreational facilities, counseling, or places to socialize.

The Role of Drugs in Your Life

Where do you fit into this complex picture of drug use and abuse? Chances are good that you've had experience with over-the-counter and prescription drugs, and you may or may not have had experience with one or more of the drugs described in this chapter. You probably know someone who has used or abused a psychoactive drug. Whatever your experience up to now, it's likely that you

will encounter drugs at some point in your life. To make sure you'll have the inner resources to resist peer pressure and make your own decision, cultivate a variety of activities you enjoy doing, realize that you are entitled to have your own opinion, and don't neglect your self-esteem. Like other aspects of health behavior, making responsible decisions about drug use depends on information, knowledge, and insight into yourself. Many choices are possible; making the ones that are right for you is what counts.

SUMMARY

The Drug Tradition

- Naturally occurring drugs have been used throughout history for religious, medicinal, and personal reasons. Although drug use dropped after 1900, it surged again in the 1960s; it has been declining overall since the late 1970s, although certain drugs are enjoying a revival in certain populations.

Use, Abuse, and Dependence

- People of all incomes, education levels, and ethnic backgrounds use drugs.

- Reasons for using drugs include the lure of the illicit; curiosity; rebellion; peer pressure; and the desire to alter one's mood or escape boredom, anxiety, depression, or other psychological problems.

- Drug abuse is a maladaptive pattern of drug use that persists despite adverse social, psychological, or medical consequences.

- Drug dependence involves taking a drug compulsively, which includes neglecting constructive activities because of it and continuing to use it despite experiencing adverse social effects resulting from its use. Tolerance and a withdrawal syndrome are often present.

How Drugs Affect the Body

- Drug factors include pharmacological properties, dose-response function, time-action function, cumulative effects, and method of use.
- User factors include a person's physical and psychological characteristics, such as body mass, general health, and other drugs being taken.
- The psychological set and social setting are sometimes more important in determining effects than the drug itself, if low doses are involved.

Representative Psychoactive Drugs

- Opiates relieve pain, cause drowsiness, and induce euphoria; they reduce anxiety and produce lethargy, apathy, and an inability to concentrate.
- Central nervous system depressants slow down the overall activity of the nerves; they reduce anxiety and produce mood changes, muscular incoordination, slurring of speech, and drowsiness or sleep. Physical dependency is possible with most CNS depressants, and withdrawal symptoms are severe.
- CNS stimulants speed up the activity of the nerves, causing acceleration of heart rate, rise in blood pressure, dilation of pupils and bronchial tubes, and an increase in gastric and adrenal secretions. Tolerance and physical and psychological dependence are associated with the use of CNS stimulants.
- Marijuana usually causes euphoria and a relaxed attitude at low doses; very high doses produce feelings of depersonalization and sensory distortion. Possible effects of long-term use include bronchial irritation, changes in brain function, and fertility problems.
- Psychedelics alter perception, feelings, and thought. LSD is the most widely known; its effects include an altered sense of time, disorders of vision, and changes in mood. Large doses may lead to synesthesia and depersonalization. Panic reactions and flashbacks are among the adverse effects of LSD use.
- Deliriants cause temporary impairment of brain function—changing levels of awareness to surrounding events, decreased ability to maintain attention to a task, confusion, and perhaps hallucinations.
- Inhalants are present in a variety of harmless products; they can produce delirium. Their use can lead to loss of consciousness, heart failure, suffocation, and death.
- Designer drugs are created by modifying existing drugs to produce compounds that have similar effects.

Drug Use: The Decades Ahead

- Honest and unbiased information about drugs may help cut down on their abuse; scare tactics and exaggerations are ineffective.
- Drug testing, a controversial issue in American politics, involves a basic conflict between public safety and the individual's right to privacy and freedom from unreasonable search.
- Treatment programs for drug dependence include drug substitution programs, rehabilitation centers, self-help groups, and peer counseling.
- Government attempts to control the drug problem focus on production, importation, and distribution. Persuasive antidrug educational programs are necessary; especially important is helping students develop strategies for resisting peer pressure.

TAKE ACTION

1. Find out what type of services are available on your campus or in your community to handle drug dependence. If there are none, what services are needed? Locate the school official and public health agency responsible for your campus and community and ask why these needs aren't being met.

2. Look at a recent film or television program, paying special attention to how drug use is portrayed. What messages are being conveyed? If possible, compare a recent movie with a movie made 10 or 15 years ago. Has the presentation of drug use changed? If so, how?

JOURNAL ENTRY

1. Keep track of your own drug use for a week, noting in your health journal the name of the drug, the approximate dosage, the time of day, and what you think your reasons were for taking each dose. Don't forget to include coffee, soft drinks, and over-the-counter medications. What types of drugs are you taking? Are there any patterns? Are there any signs of abuse or dependence? If you'd like to cut down, begin by making a list of alternative behaviors you could substitute for drug use.

2. *Critical Thinking:* Does a woman have an obligation to avoid alcohol and other drugs during pregnancy? What about smoking cigarettes and eating junk food? If she doesn't follow her physician's advice, should she be held legally responsible for the effects on her child? What rights do the mother and child have in this situation? In your health journal, write an essay stating your opinion; be sure to defend your position.

3. *Critical Thinking:* Do you think there is such a thing as responsible use of illegal psychoactive drugs? Are they a legitimate recreational activity? Would you change any of the current laws governing drugs? If so, how would you draw the line between legitimate and illegitimate use? Write an essay describing your position.

BEHAVIOR CHANGE STRATEGY

CHANGING YOUR DRUG HABITS

We have chosen to devote this behavior change strategy to one of the most commonly used drugs—caffeine. If there is another drug you want to cut down on or stop using, you can devise your own plan based on this one and on the steps outlined in Chapter 1.

Because caffeine supports certain behaviors that are characteristic of our culture, such as sedentary, stressful work, you may find yourself relying on coffee (or tea, chocolate, or colas) to get through a busy schedule. Such habits often begin in college. Fortunately, it's easier to break a habit before it becomes entrenched as a lifelong dependency.

Caffeine overdose can have some harmful effects on you, and knowing what they are can help motivate you to reduce your intake. You may feel increased anxiety and irritability; some people may be sensitive to caffeine and may find such exaggerated states hard to manage.

When you are studying for exams, the forced physical inactivity and the need to concentrate even when fatigued may lead you to overuse caffeine. But caffeine doesn't "help" unless you are already sleepy. And it does not relieve any underlying condition (you are just more tired when it wears off). So how can you change this pattern?

Self-Monitoring

Keep a log of how much caffeine you eat or drink. Use a measuring cup to measure coffee or tea. Using Table 8-1, convert the amounts you eat or drink into an estimate expressed in milligrams of caffeine. Be sure to include all forms, such as chocolate bars and over-the-counter medications, as well as caffeine candy, colas, cocoa or hot chocolate, chocolate cake, tea, and coffee.

Self-Assessment

At the end of the week, add up your daily totals and divide by 7 to get your daily average in milligrams. How much is too much? At more than 250 mg per day, you may well be experiencing some adverse symptoms. Are you experiencing at least five of the following? If so, you may want to cut down.

- Restlessness
- Nervousness
- Excitement
- Insomnia
- Flushed face
- Excessive sweating
- Gastrointestinal problems
- Muscle twitching
- Rambling flow of thought and speech
- Irregularities in rhythm of heartbeats
- Periods of inexhaustibility
- Excessive pacing or need to constantly move around

Set Limits

Can you restrict your caffeine intake to a daily total, and stick to this contract? If so, set a cutoff point, such as one cup of coffee. Pegging it to a specific time of day can be helpful, because then you don't confront a decision at any other point (and possibly fail). If you find you cannot stick to your limit, you may want to cut out caffeine altogether; abstinence can be easier than moderation for some people. If you experience caffeine withdrawal symptoms (headache, fatigue) when you decrease your caffeine consumption, you may want to cut your intake more gradually.

Find Other Ways to Keep Your Energy Up

If you are fatigued, it makes sense to get enough sleep or to exercise more rather than drowning the problem in coffee. Different individuals need different amounts of sleep; you may also need more sleep at different times, such as during a personal crisis or an illness. Also, exercise raises your metabolic rate for hours afterward—a handy fact to exploit when you want to feel more awake and want to avoid an irritable coffee jag. And if you've been compounding your fatigue by not eating properly, try filling up on complex carbohydrates such as whole-grain bread or potatoes instead of candy bars.

Some Tips on Cutting Out Caffeine

Here are some more ways to decrease your consumption of caffeine:

1. Keep some noncaffeine drink on hand, perhaps

decaffeinated coffee, herbal teas, hot water, or bouillon.

2. Alternate between hot and very cold liquids.

3. Fill your coffee cup only halfway.

4. Avoid the office or school lunchroom or cafeteria and the chocolate area of the grocery store. (Often people drink coffee or tea and eat chocolate simply because it's there.)

SELECTED BIBLIOGRAPHY

American Psychiatric Association. 1994. *Diagnostic and Statistical Manual of Mental Disorders,* 4th ed. (DSM-IV). Washington, D.C.: American Psychiatric Association Press.

Brook, J. S., and others. 1992. Childhood precursors of adolescent drug use: A longitudinal analysis. *Genetic, Social and General Psychology Monographs* 118(2): 195–213.

Compton, D. R., and others. 1990. Cannabis dependence and tolerance production. *Advances in Alcoholism and Substance Abuse* 9(1–2): 129–47.

Darling, M. R., and T. M. Arendorf. 1992. Review of the effects of cannabis smoking on oral health. *International Dental Journal* 42(1): 19–22.

Day, N. L., and G. A. Richardson. 1991. Prenatal marijuana use: epidemiology, methodologic issues and infant outcome. *Clinics in Perinatology* 18(1): 77–91.

Derlet, R. W., and B. Heischober. 1990. Methamphetamine: Stimulant of the '90s? *Western Journal of Medicine* 153(6): 625–28.

Duke, S. B. 1993. How legalization would cut crime. *Los Angeles Times,* 21 December.

"Forty-four Percent of College Students Are Binge Drinkers, Poll Says." 1994. *New York Times,* 7 December.

Hawkins, J. D., and others. 1992. Risk and protective factors for alcohol and other drug problems in adolescence and early adolescence: Importance for substance use prevention. *Psychological Bulletin* 112(1): 64–105.

Hecht, M. L., and others. 1992. Resistance to drug offers among college students. *International Journal of the Addictions* 27(8): 995–1017.

Imperato, P. J. 1992. Syphilis, AIDS and crack cocaine. *Journal of Community Health* 17(2): 69–71.

Kaplan, C. D., and others. 1992. Are there 'casual users' of cocaine? *CIBA Foundation Symposium* 166:57–73; 73–80.

Klonger, R. A., and others. 1992. The effects of acute and chronic cocaine use on the heart. *Circulation* 85(2): 407–19.

Nahas, G., and C. Latour. 1992. The human toxicity of marijuana. *Medical Journal of Australia* 156(7): 495–97.

National Institute on Drug Abuse. 1993. *NIDA Capsules: Designer Drugs.*

Sternbach, G. L., and J. Varon. 1992. 'Designer drugs': Recognizing and managing their toxic effects. *Postgraduate Medicine* 91(8): 169–171; 175–176.

Tobler, N. S. 1992. Drug prevention programs can work: Research findings. *Journal of Addictive Diseases* 11(3): 1–28.

U.S. Centers for Disease Control. 1992. Tobacco, alcohol and other drug use among high school students—United States. 41(37): 698–703.

U.S. Department of Health and Human Services. *National Household Survey on Drug Abuse: Main Findings 1991.* Public Health Service.

———. 1993. *Alcohol, Tobacco, and Other Drugs May Harm the Unborn.* Public Health Service. Alcohol, Drug Abuse, and Mental Health Administration: PH291.

———. 1994. *National Survey Results on Drug Use from the Monitoring the Future Study, 1975–1993.* Volume I. National Institutes of Health.

Wechsler, H., and others. 1994. Health and behavioral consequences of binge drinking in college. *Journal of the American Medical Association* 272(21): 1672–7.

Westermeyer, J. 1992. Substance abuse disorders: Predictions for the 1990s. *American Journal of Drug and Alcohol Abuse* 18(1): 1–11.

Young, S. L., and others. 1992. Cocaine: Its effects on maternal and child health. *Pharmacotherapy* 12(1): 2–17.

Zimmerman, S., and A. M. Zimmerman. 1990–91. Genetic effects of marijuana. *International Journal of the Addictions* 25(1A): 19–33.

Zuckermann, M. B. 1993. Fighting the right drug war. *U.S. News & World Report,* 26 April.

RECOMMENDED READINGS

Beattie, M. 1990. *Codependents' Guide to the Twelve Steps.* New York: HarperCollins. *A useful book for friends and loved ones of substance abusers by the writer who first popularized the now-trendy term "codependent."*

Consumer Reports Books. 1993. *The Facts About Drug Use: Coping with Drugs and Alcohol in Your Family, at Work, in Your Community.* Binghampton, N.Y.: Haworth Press. *An authoritative, unbiased book that addresses the social, psychological, and physical effects of various drugs in an easy-to-read style. It includes comprehensive information on available resources and strategies for coping with problems related to drugs and alcohol.*

Duke, S. B., and A. C. Gross. 1994. *America's Longest War: Rethinking Our Tragic Crusade Against Drugs.* New York: Tarcher/Putnam. *A Yale law professor argues for the legalization of drugs.*

Keller-Phelps, J., and A. E. Nourse. 1992. *The Hidden Addiction.* Boston: Little, Brown. *Written by two physicians, this book gives straightforward information about a range of addicting substances, from caffeine to cocaine, along with advice for avoiding or overcoming dependency problems.*

Mooney, A. J. 1992. *The Recovery Book.* New York: Workman. *Written by a physician, this helpful guide covers family relationships, support groups, work, money, and other issues involved in chemical dependency.*

U.S. Journal, Inc. 1992. *The Treatment Directory: National Directory of Alcohol, Drug Addiction and Other Addiction Treatment Programs.* Deerfield Beach, Fla.: U.S. Journal, Inc. *A helpful reference for people seeking information about treatment options for themselves or loved ones.*

9

Nutrition Facts and Fallacies

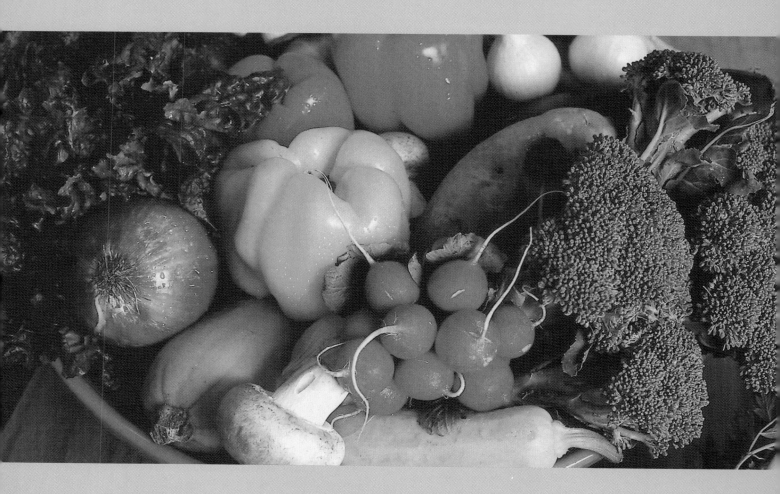

CONTENTS

In your lifetime, you'll spend about six years eating—about 70,000 meals and 60 tons of food. What you choose to eat can have profound effects on your health and well-being. Poor nutrient intake can make you more susceptible to diseases like osteoporosis and iron-deficiency anemia, while overzealous use of vitamin and mineral supplements can lead to toxicity. Your nutritional habits also affect your risk for the major chronic "killer" diseases, including heart disease, cancer, stroke, and diabetes. Choosing foods that provide adequate amounts of the nutrients you need while avoiding the substances linked to disease should be an important part of your daily life. The food choices you make will significantly influence your health both now and later in your life.

Although the science of **nutrition** is relatively young, we know what nutrients are needed for an adequate diet and what foods provide them. Understanding just the basics of a healthy diet—variety, balance, and moderation—can help you eat sensibly and protect yourself against many nutrition-related problems. For most Americans, the most likely dietary problems are overeating and an imbalance in the nutrients consumed. The *Healthy People 2000* report highlights some of the most important dietary changes that Americans can make to safeguard their health and well-being; these include reducing consumption of fat and sodium, increasing consumption of complex carbohydrates and dietary fiber, and consuming adequate amounts of iron and calcium.

NUTRITIONAL REQUIREMENTS: COMPONENTS OF A HEALTHY DIET

When you think about your diet you probably do so in terms of the foods you like to eat—a turkey sandwich and a glass of milk or a steak and a baked potato. What's important for your health, though, is the nutrients contained in those foods. Your body requires carbohydrates, proteins, fats, vitamins, minerals, and water—about 45 **essential nutrients.** The word *essential* in this context means that you must get these substances from food because your body is unable to manufacture them at all, or at least not fast enough to meet body needs. A diet containing adequate amounts of all essential nutrients is vital because nutrients provide energy, help build and maintain body tissues, and help regulate body functions.

The energy in foods is expressed as **kilocalories.** One kilocalorie represents the amount of heat it takes to raise the temperature of 1 liter of water 1° C. A person needs about 2,000 kilocalories per day to meet his or her energy needs. In common usage, people often refer to kilocalories as *calories* (a calorie is actually a very small energy unit; a kilocalorie contains 1,000 calories). We'll use the more popular term *calorie* in this chapter to stand for the larger energy unit.

Three classes of nutrients supply energy—protein, car-

bohydrates, and fats. Fats provide the most energy at 9 calories per gram; protein and carbohydrates each provide 4 calories per gram. The high caloric content of fat is one reason experts continually advise against high fat consumption—most of us don't need the extra calories. Alcohol, though it has no nutritional value, provides 7 calories per gram.

Just meeting energy needs is not enough; our bodies require adequate amounts of all the essential nutrients to grow and function properly. Many of the diet patterns followed around the world can supply these essential nutrients. Water is the major component in both foods and the human body—we are about 60 percent water—and we can live only a few days without it. Our needs for proteins, fats, carbohydrates, **vitamins,** and **minerals,** in terms of weight, are much less, but still vital. Practically all foods contain mixtures of nutrients, although foods are commonly classified according to the predominant nutrient; for example, spaghetti is thought of as a "carbohydrate" food. Let's take a closer look at the function and sources of each class of nutrients.

Proteins—The Basis of Body Structure

Proteins form important parts of the body's main structural components—muscles and bones. Proteins also form important parts of blood, enzymes, some hormones, and cell membranes. As mentioned above, proteins can provide energy for the body (4 calories per gram).

The building blocks of proteins are called **amino acids.** Twenty common amino acids are found in food; nine of these are essential parts of an adult diet: histidine, isoleucine, leucine, lysine, methionine, phenylalanine, threonine, tryptophan, and valine. The other 11 amino acids can be produced by the body, given the presence of the needed building blocks supplied by foods.

Individual protein sources are considered "complete"

Nutrition The science of food and how the body uses it in health and disease.

Essential nutrients Substances your body must get from foods because (with minor exceptions) the body cannot manufacture them at all or fast enough to meet body needs. These nutrients include vitamins, minerals, some amino acids, linoleic acid, and water.

Kilocalorie Unit of fuel potential in a diet; 1 calorie represents the amount of heat needed to raise the temperature of 1 liter of water 1° C.

Vitamins Carbon-containing substances needed in small amounts to help promote and regulate chemical reactions and processes in the body.

Minerals Inorganic compounds needed in relatively small amounts for regulation, growth, and maintenance of body tissues and functions.

Amino acids The building blocks of proteins.

TERMS

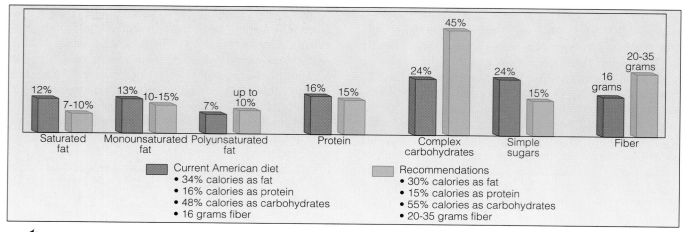

Figure 9-1   *The current American diet versus the recommended American diet.*

or "high quality" if they supply all the essential amino acids in adequate amounts and "incomplete" or "low quality" if they do not. Meat, fish, poultry, eggs, milk, cheese, and other foods from animal sources provide complete proteins. Incomplete proteins, which come from plant sources such as beans, peas, and nuts, are good sources of most essential amino acids, but are usually low in one or two.

Your concern with amino acids and complete protein in your diet should focus on what a meal supplies, rather than on what each individual food supplies. Combining two vegetable proteins, such as wheat and peanuts in a peanut butter and jelly sandwich, allows each vegetable protein to make up for the amino acids missing in the other protein. The combination yields a complete protein for the meal. By having plant proteins complement each other so that all essential amino acids are consumed in a meal, vegetarians can get the amino acids they need to synthesize the proteins their bodies require.

The leading sources of protein in the American diet are (1) beef, steaks, and roasts, (2) hamburger and meatloaf, (3) white bread, rolls, and crackers, (4) milk, and (5) pork. About two-thirds of the protein in the American diet comes from animal sources; hence, the American diet is rich in amino acids. Most Americans consume nearly twice the amount of protein they need each day. Protein consumed beyond protein needs is synthesized into fat

for energy storage or burned for energy needs. The amount of protein you eat should represent about 10–15 percent of your total calorie intake (Figure 9-1).

Fats—Essential in Small Amounts

Fats, also known as lipids, are the most concentrated source of energy at 9 calories per gram. The fats stored in your body represent usable energy and help insulate your body and support and cushion your organs. Fats in the diet help your body absorb fat-soluble vitamins, as well as add important flavor and texture to foods. Fats are the major fuel for the body during rest and light activity: Carbohydrates fuel the nervous system, brain, and red blood cells, while fats fuel most of the rest of the body's organ systems. Two fats—linoleic acid and alpha-linolenic acid—are essential components of the diet.

Most of the fats in food are in the form of triglycerides, which are composed of a glycerol molecule (an alcohol) plus three fatty acids. Fatty acids differ in the length of their carbon atom chains and in their degree of saturation (the number of double bonds contained between the carbon atoms). If no double bonds exist between the carbon atoms, the fatty acid is called **saturated.** Fatty acids with one double bond are called **monounsaturated,** and fatty acids with two or more double bonds are called **polyunsaturated.**

Food fats are often composed of both saturated and unsaturated fatty acids; the dominant type of fatty acid determines the fat's characteristics. Food fats containing large amounts of saturated fatty acids are usually solid at room temperature (these are called "fats"); they are generally found in animal products. The leading sources of saturated fat in the American diet are unprocessed animal flesh (hamburger, steak, roasts), whole milk, cheese, and hot dogs/lunch meats; other significant sources include poultry skin, ice cream, and many baked products. Food fats containing large amounts of monounsaturated and

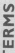

TERMS

Saturated fats   Fats with no carbon-carbon double bonds.
Monounsaturated fats   Fats with one carbon-carbon double bond.
Polyunsaturated fats   Fats containing two or more carbon-carbon double bonds.
Hydrogenation   A process by which liquid oils are turned into solid fats; used to extend the shelf life of certain foods.

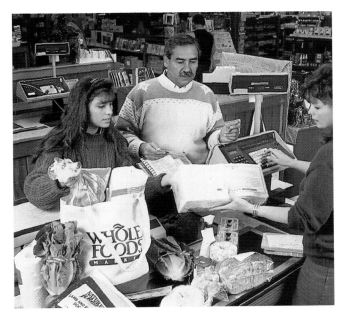

Our bodies require adequate amounts of all essential nutrients—water, proteins, carbohydrates, fats, vitamins, and minerals—in order to grow and function properly. Choosing foods to fulfill these nutritional requirements is an important part of a healthy lifestyle.

polyunsaturated fatty acids are usually from plant sources and are liquid at room temperature (these are called "oils"). Olive, canola, and peanut oils contain mostly monounsaturated fatty acids. Sunflower, corn, soybean, and safflower oils contain mostly polyunsaturated fatty acids.

Notable exceptions to these generalizations are palm oil and coconut oil, often used in processed foods; though derived from plants, these oils are highly saturated. Hydrogenated vegetable oils are also highly saturated. The process of **hydrogenation** turns many of the double bonds in unsaturated fatty acids into single bonds and produces a more solid fat from a liquid oil. Food manufacturers use this process to extend the shelf life of fats; the more double bonds a fat contains, the more likely it is to break down and turn rancid. The more solid fats that result from hydrogenation also have the texture needed to make better pastry and cake products. Hydrogenation also prevents oil from separating from the ground peanuts in peanut butter.

You need only about 1 tablespoon of vegetable oil per day incorporated into your diet to supply the essential fats. The average American diet supplies considerably more than this amount; in fact, fats make up about 34 percent of our calorie intake. Health experts recommend that we reduce our fat intake to 30 percent or less of total calories, with no more than 7 to 10 percent coming from saturated fat (see Figure 9-1). The fat content of many common foods is given in Table 9-1.

Controlling the amount of saturated fat in your diet is

TABLE 9-1 Foods and Their Fat

Percentage Fat	Food
95–100	Butter, margarine, mayonnaise, salad oil, olives, Italian dressing, heavy cream
90–95	Pecans, macadamia nuts, baking chocolate
85–90	Walnuts, egg yolk, avocado, sour cream
80–85	Almonds, cream cheese, frankfurter, pork spareribs
75–80	Peanut butter, sunflower seeds, salami, bacon, half and half
70–75	Cheddar cheese, lamb chop
65–70	American cheese, mozzarella cheese, tuna fish in oil, ground chuck
60–65	Sweet chocolate, coconut, eggs, potato chips, rich ice cream
55–60	Veal chop, milk chocolate, pie crust
50–55	Roast beef, pork chop, roast chicken with skin
45–50	Regular ice cream, whole milk, club steak, salmon
40–45	Granola, banana bread, buttered popcorn, french fries, chili, Ritz crackers
35–40	Lasagna, hamburger on a bun, chocolate chip cookies
30–35	Chicken (skinless dark meat), 2% milk
25–30	Pizza, ground round, sea bass
20–25	Chicken (skinless white meat), liver, turkey, chicken noodle soup, chocolate pudding
15–20	Halibut, oatmeal
10–15	Plain popcorn, pretzels, bread, fig bar, low-fat cottage cheese
5–10	Tortilla, brown rice, sherbet, haddock, honeydew melon, raisins
0–5	Skim milk, white rice, egg white, spaghetti, potatoes, most fruits and vegetables, beer, wine, most cereals, clear soups

How to Calculate Your Fat Intake

To calculate how much fat a food contains, you first need to know the total number of calories and grams of fat it contains. For prepared foods, food labels provide this information. Multiply the grams of fat by 9 (because there are 9 calories in a gram of fat). Then divide that number by the total calories. For example, a tablespoon of peanut butter has 8 grams of fat and 95 calories. So 8 × 9 = 72, divided by the number of calories (95) equals 0.76, or about 76 percent calories from fat.

To monitor the fat percentage in your diet, multiply the grams of fat in any individual food by 9. If the result is more than a third of the total calories, the food is relatively high in fat. You can still eat it, but make sure you limit the amount you eat—especially if it's also high in saturated fat. And make sure that you balance it with low-fat foods.

Your goal is to end up with fewer than 30 percent of your total daily calories from fat. This can be accomplished by setting a goal for fat consumption and then keeping track of the amount of fat you consume during the day. To set a goal for your daily fat consumption, first determine approximately how many calories you consume per day. Depending on your activity level, daily caloric needs range from about 2,200 to 3,500 calories for men and from about 1,700 to 2,500 for women. Multiply your chosen daily calorie intake by 30 percent (0.3) to get the maximum fat calories allowed per day. Divide this figure by 9 to get the maximum number of grams of fat you can consume per day and still stay within the 30 percent guideline at your level of caloric intake. For example, if you consume about 1,800 calories per day, your maximum fat intake would be 1,800 × 0.3 = 540 calories from fat, or 60 grams of fat. Food labels do this calculation for a 2,000 and sometimes a 2,500 calorie diet. By checking food labels you can keep a running total of the grams of fat you consume and make healthy food choices.

the most important diet-related action you can take to control your serum (blood) **cholesterol** level. An elevated serum cholesterol level is associated with an increased risk for premature heart disease. All adults, especially those who have high blood cholesterol levels (over 200 milligrams of cholesterol per 100 milliliters of blood serum), should minimize their saturated fat intake.

Certain forms of polyunsaturated fatty acids—those found in fish—may have a positive effect on cardiovascular health. Consumption of **omega-3 fatty acids** found in fish has been shown to reduce the tendency of blood to clot and to decrease inflammatory responses in the body; it even appears to lower the risk of heart disease. Because of these benefits, nutritionists now recommend that Americans increase the proportion of omega-3 polyunsaturated fats in their diet by increasing their consumption of fish. Mackerel, whitefish, herring, salmon, tuna, and lake trout are all good sources of omega-3 fatty acids.

Personal Insight Do you have emotional attachments to particular kinds of foods or meals, such as those you eat on holidays or at family gatherings? If so, do your attachments make it hard for you to evaluate those foods objectively and admit that some of them may not be good for you?

Carbohydrates—An Ideal Source of Energy

Carbohydrates are needed in the diet primarily to supply energy for body cells. Some cells, such as those found in the brain and other parts of the nervous system and in blood, use only carbohydrates for fuel. During high-intensity exercise, muscles also use primarily carbohydrates for fuel. When we don't eat enough carbohydrates to satisfy the needs of the brain and red blood cells, our bodies synthesize carbohydrates from proteins. In situations of extreme deprivation, when the diet lacks a sufficient amount of both carbohydrates and proteins, the body turns to its own proteins, causing severe muscle wasting. Crash diets and medically supervised very low carbohydrate diets used in weight reduction are the only common situations in which this would take place.

Carbohydrates can be divided into two groups: simple and complex. Table sugar, honey, fructose, glucose, and corn syrup are simple carbohydrates and contain only one or two sugar units in each molecule. Simple carbohydrates provide much of the sweetness in foods. Starches and most types of dietary fiber are complex carbohydrates; they consist of chains of many sugar units. During **digestion** in the mouth and small intestine, your body breaks down starches and double sugars into single sugar molecules, such as **glucose,** for absorption (Figure 9-2). Once glucose is in the bloodstream, cells take it up and use it for energy. The liver and muscles also take up glucose to provide carbohydrate storage in the form of the animal starch called **glycogen.**

Carbohydrates consumed beyond body needs for carbohydrate and energy are synthesized into fat and stored as such once glycogen stores are full. Any type of diet where calorie intake exceeds calorie needs can lead to fat storage and weight gain.

Carbohydrates are found primarily in plant foods, especially grains, vegetables, and fruits; milk is the only significant animal source. On average, Americans consume

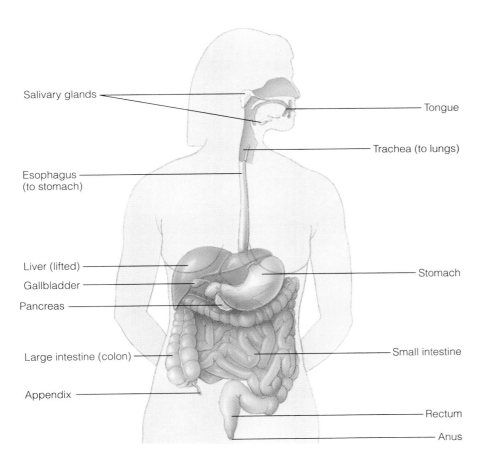

Salivary glands

Tongue

Trachea (to lungs)

Esophagus
(to stomach)

Liver (lifted)

Gallbladder

Pancreas

Stomach

Large intestine (colon)

Small intestine

Appendix

Rectum

Anus

Figure 9-2 *The digestive tract.*
Digestion of carbohydrates begins in the
mouth, but most digestion takes place in
the small intestine and stomach.

over 200 grams of carbohydrates per day (about 48 percent of total calorie intake), well above the minimum of 50 to 100 grams of essential carbohydrate required by the body. However, health experts recommend that Americans increase their consumption of carbohydrates—particularly complex carbohydrates—to 55 percent of total calories. This increase in carbohydrate consumption should take place at the expense of fat intake. Potatoes, rice, pasta, bread, vegetables, and beans are all good sources of complex carbohydrates.

Dietary Fiber—A Closer Look

Dietary fiber (also known as "bulk" or "roughage") includes plant substances that are difficult or impossible for humans to digest. Fiber passes through your intestinal tract and provides bulk for feces (stool) in the large intestine; this facilitates elimination. Some types of fiber are metabolized by bacteria in the large intestine into products such as acids and gases; too much fiber intake can therefore lead to intestinal gas.

Nutritionists classify fibers as soluble or insoluble; each group has important physiological effects on your body. **Soluble fiber** binds cholesterol-containing compounds in the intestine, thereby lowering your blood cholesterol level. Soluble fiber also slows your body's absorption of glucose. Therefore, under medical supervi-

sion, a diet high in soluble fiber has a place in the treatment of diabetes and high serum cholesterol levels. Chapter 15 will discuss the latest research findings on the effect of fiber on blood cholesterol in more detail.

Insoluble fiber primarily binds water, making feces bulkier and softer so they pass more quickly and easily through the intestines. A diet high in insoluble fiber can help prevent a variety of health problems, including constipation, hemorrhoids, and diverticulitis (a painful condition in which abnormal pouches in the wall of the large intestine are produced and then become inflamed). Stud-

Cholesterol A waxy substance found in the blood and cells and implicated in heart disease.

Omega-3 fatty acid A polyunsaturated fatty acid in which the double bonds begin after the third carbon atom on the chain.

Digestion Process of breaking down foods in the gastrointestinal tract into compounds your body can absorb.

Glucose A simple sugar that is your body's basic fuel.

Glycogen An animal starch stored in the liver and muscles.

Soluble fiber Fiber that dissolves in water or is broken down by bacteria in the large intestine.

Insoluble fiber Fiber that does not dissolve in water and is not broken down by bacteria in the large intestine.

TERMS

TABLE 9-2 *Vitamins: Their Functions and Food Sources*

Vitamin	Function	Food Sources
Thiamin	Conversion of carbohydrates into usable forms of energy	Yeast, mushrooms, whole-grain and enriched breads and cereals, liver, pork, lean meats, poultry, eggs, fish, beans, nuts
Riboflavin	Energy release; maintenance of skin, mucous membranes, and nervous structures	Dairy products, liver, whole-grain and enriched breads and cereals, lean meats, poultry, leafy vegetables
Niacin	Conversion of carbohydrates, fats, and protein into usable forms of energy; essential for growth, synthesis of hormones	Eggs, chicken, turkey, fish, milk, grains, nuts, enriched breads and cereals, lean meats
B-6 (pyridoxine, pyridoxal, pyridoxamine)	More than 60 enzyme reactions, mostly involving proteins	Liver, lean meats, fish, poultry, whole grains, legumes
B-12	Synthesis of red and white blood cells; other metabolic reactions	Liver, meat, eggs, milk
Folate	Blood cell production, maintenance of nervous system	Liver, leafy vegetables, oranges, whole grains
Biotin	Metabolism of fats, carbohydrates, and proteins	Cauliflower, egg yolks, nuts, cheese
Pantothenic acid	Metabolism of carbohydrates, fats, and proteins	Widely distributed in all foods
A (retinol)	Maintenance of eyes, vision, skin, linings of the nose, mouth, digestive and urinary tracts, immune function	Liver, milk, butter, cheese, fortified margarine, carrots, spinach, most other vegetables and fruits that are dark green, yellow, or orange
C (ascorbic acid)	Maintenance and repair of connective tissue, bones, teeth, cartilage; promotes wound healing	Peppers, broccoli, brussels sprouts, citrus fruits, tomatoes, potatoes, cabbage
D (cholecalciferol)	Aids in calcium and phosphorus metabolism; promotion of calcium absorption; development and maintenance of bones and teeth	Fortified milk, fish liver oils; sunlight on skin produces vitamin D
E (tocopherol)	Protection and maintenance of cellular membranes	Vegetable oils, whole grains, leafy vegetables, asparagus, peaches; smaller amounts widespread in foods
K	Production of prothrombin and other factors essential for blood clotting	Green leafy vegetables, other vegetables, liver, milk; widespread in other foods

ies have linked high levels of insoluble fiber in the diet with lower incidences of colon cancer; conversely, a low-fiber diet can increase the risk for colon cancer. There is even some evidence that high levels of insoluble fiber can suppress and reverse precancerous changes that can lead to colon and rectal cancer.

All plant foods contain some dietary fiber. Fruits, **legumes,** oats (especially oat bran), barley, and psyllium (found in some laxatives) are rich in soluble fiber. Wheat (especially wheat bran), cereals, grains, and vegetables are good sources of insoluble fiber. Processing can remove

fiber from foods, so fresh fruits and vegetables and foods made from whole grains are the richest sources of fiber.

Although it's not yet clear exactly how much and what types of fiber would be ideal to consume, most experts feel that the average American would benefit from an increase in daily fiber intake. We currently consume about 16 grams a day; a better goal would be 20–35 grams a day. Emphasizing fruits, vegetables, cereals, legumes, and whole grains in the diet makes this fiber goal easy to obtain and gives a nice mixture of both soluble and insoluble fibers.

1. Consume or process vegetables immediately after purchasing (or harvesting).

   The longer vegetables are kept before they are eaten or processed, the more vitamins are lost, especially vitamin C and folate.

2. Store vegetables and fruits properly.

   If you can't eat fruits and vegetables immediately after purchasing (or harvesting) but plan to do so within a few days, keep them in the refrigerator. Place them in covered containers or plastic bags to lessen moisture loss.

   The best method for longer-term preservation is to freeze fruits and vegetables when possible. Canning fruits and vegetables preserves them, but it's a lot of work and causes a greater nutrient loss.

3. Reduce preparation and cooking of vegetables and other foods.

   The more preparation and cooking of foods that is done before eating, the greater the nutrient loss. To reduce the losses:

- Avoid soaking vegetables in water.
- When possible, cook vegetables, like potatoes, in their skins.
- Don't soak and rinse rice before cooking; you'll wash off the B vitamins.
- Cook in as little water as possible.
- Bake, steam, or broil vegetables. Microwave cooking retains vitamins. If you stew meats, consume the broth too.
- When boiling, use tight-fitting lids to diminish evaporation of water.
- Cook vegetables in as short a time as possible. Develop a taste for a more crunchy texture.
- Don't thaw frozen vegetables before cooking.
- Prepare lettuce salads right before eating.

Vitamins—Organic Micronutrients

Vitamins are organic (carbon-containing) substances required in very small amounts to promote specific chemical reactions within living cells (Table 9-2). Humans need 13 vitamins. Four are fat-soluble (A, D, E, and K), while nine are water-soluble (C, and the eight "B-complex" vitamins: thiamin, riboflavin, niacin, vitamin B-6, folate, vitamin B-12, biotin, and pantothenic acid). Because patients can survive for many years without becoming ill on intravenous feeding formulated with just these substances and the other essential nutrients, it appears that no vitamins remain to be discovered.

Many vitamins act with catalysts to initiate or speed up chemical reactions. Vitamins provide no energy to the body directly but instead are used to unleash the energy stored in carbohydrates, proteins, and fats. Some vitamins form substances that act as **antioxidants.** These are compounds that can decrease the breakdown of foodstuffs, such as when the vitamin C in orange juice is used to stop sliced bananas from turning brown. Antioxidants also aid in the preservation of healthy cells in the body. When the body uses oxygen or breaks down certain fats, it gives rise to substances called "free radicals." In their search for electrons, free radicals react with fats, proteins, and DNA, damaging cell membranes and mutating genes. Antioxidants react with free radicals and donate electrons, rendering them harmless. Key vitamin antioxidants in our diet are vitamin E, vitamin C, and the vitamin A derivative beta-carotene. Obtaining a regular intake of these nutrients is vital for maintaining the health of the body.

If your diet lacks a particular vitamin, or if you don't consume enough of it, characteristic symptoms of deficiency develop. Vitamin A deficiency can cause blindness, niacin deficiency can lead to mental illness, vitamin B-6 deficiency can cause seizures, vitamin B-12 deficiency can cause a severe type of anemia, and vitamin D deficiency can cause growth retardation. The best known deficiency disease is probably **scurvy,** caused by vitamin C deficiency; it killed many sailors on long ocean voyages until people realized in the eighteenth century that eating oranges and lemons could prevent it. Even today people develop scurvy; its presence suggests a very poor intake of fruits and vegetables, which are often rich sources of vitamin C.

Vitamin deficiency diseases are most often seen in developing countries. They are rare in the United States because vitamins are readily available from our food supply.

Legumes Vegetables such as peas and beans that are high in fiber and are also important sources of protein in a vegetarian diet.

Antioxidants Substances that can lessen the breakdown of foodstuffs or body constituents. Their actions include binding oxygen and donating electrons to free radicals.

Scurvy A disease caused by lack of vitamin C in which wounds fail to heal, the gums bleed, and teeth are loosened.

TERMS

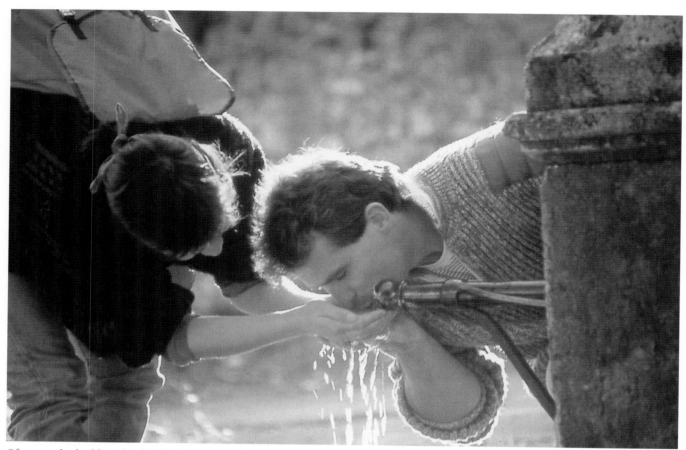

Often overlooked but absolutely crucial to life, water is an essential part of our diet.

People suffering from alcoholism currently run the greatest risk of vitamin deficiencies, especially from the water-soluble vitamins thiamin, vitamin B-6, and folate.

Extra vitamins in the diet can be harmful, especially when taken as supplements. Some vitamins can produce toxic results when regularly consumed in high quantities; as always, the dose determines the effect—health or ill health.

Water—Vital but Often Ignored

Water is the major component in both foods and the human body—you are about 60 percent water. Your need for other nutrients, in terms of weight, is much less than your need for water. You can live up to 50 days without food, but only a few days without water.

Water is distributed all over the body—among lean and other tissues and in urine and other body fluids. Water is used in the digestion and absorption of food and is the medium in which most of the chemical reactions take place within the body. Some water-based fluids like blood transport substances around the body, while other fluids serve as lubricants or cushions. Water also helps regulate body temperature.

Water is contained in almost all foods, particularly in liquids, fruits, and vegetables. The foods and fluids you consume provide 80 to 90 percent of your daily water intake; the remainder is generated through the metabolism of energy nutrients. You lose water each day in urine, feces, and sweat and through evaporation in your lungs. To maintain a balance between water consumed and water lost, you need to take in about 1 milliliter of water for each calorie you burn—that's about 2 liters or 8 cups of fluid per day—more if you live in a hot climate or engage in vigorous exercise.

Thirst is the body's first sign of dehydration, a signal that it needs more water. If this thirst mechanism is faulty, as it may be during illness or vigorous exercise, hormonal mechanisms can help conserve water by reducing the output of urine. Severe dehydration causes weakness and can lead to death.

Minerals—Inorganic Micronutrients

Minerals are inorganic (non-carbon-containing) compounds you need in relatively small amounts to help regulate body functions, aid in growth and maintenance of body tissues, and act with catalysts in the release of energy (Table 9-3). There are about 17 essential minerals. The major minerals—those that the body needs in

TABLE 9-3 Selected Minerals: Their Functions and Food Sources

Mineral	Function	Food Sources
Calcium	Maintenance of bones and teeth; blood clotting; maintenance of cell membranes; control of nerve impulses	Milk and milk products, tofu, fortified orange juice and bread, sardines, leafy vegetables
Phosphorus	Bone growth and maintenance (teams with calcium); energy transfer in cells	Present in nearly all foods, especially milk, cheese, bakery products, and meats
Magnesium	Transmission of nerve impulses; energy transfer; composition of many enzyme systems	Widespread in foods and water (except soft water) and especially found in wheat bran, milk products, beans, nuts, and leafy vegetables
Iron	Component of hemoglobin (carries oxygen to tissues) and myoglobin (in muscle fibers) and enzymes	Liver, lean meats, legumes, enriched flour; absorption enhanced by presence of vitamin C
Iodide	Essential part of thyroid hormones; regulation of body metabolism	Iodized salt, seafood
Zinc	More than 70 enzyme reactions including synthesis of proteins, RNA, and DNA	Meat, eggs, liver, and seafood (especially oysters), milk, whole grains
Copper	Iron metabolism and red blood cell formation	Liver, shellfish, nuts, dried beans

amounts exceeding 100 milligrams—include calcium, phosphorus, magnesium, sodium, potassium, and chloride. The essential trace minerals—those that you need in minute amounts—include copper, fluoride, iodide, iron, selenium, and zinc.

Characteristic symptoms develop if an essential mineral is consumed in a quantity too small or too large for good health. The minerals most commonly lacking in our diets are iron and calcium—and possibly zinc and magnesium. We should focus on good food choices for these nutrients. Lean meats are rich in iron and zinc, while low-fat or nonfat milk is an excellent choice for calcium. Plant foods are good sources of magnesium. Iron-deficiency **anemia** is a problem in many age groups and researchers fear poor calcium intakes are sowing the seeds for future **osteoporosis**, especially in women.

NUTRITIONAL GUIDELINES: PLANNING YOUR DIET

Various scientific and governmental groups have established nutrition guidelines to help you plan a healthy diet. The **Recommended Dietary Allowances (RDAs)**, Estimated Safe and Adequate Daily Intakes (ESADDIs), and Estimated Minimum Requirements are standards for nutrient intake designed to prevent nutrient deficiencies. The **Food Guide Pyramid** then translates these nutrient recommendations into a food-group plan that, when followed, ensures a balanced intake of the essential nutri-

ents. To provide further guidance in choosing foods, **Dietary Guidelines for Americans** have been established to address the prevention of certain diet-related chronic diseases.

Personal Insight How have your eating habits changed since you've entered college? Do you feel more comfortable with your current habits or less? Why?

Recommended Dietary Allowances (RDAs)

The Food and Nutrition Board of the National Academy of Sciences meets approximately every five years to set

Anemia A deficiency in the oxygen-carrying material in the red blood cells.

Osteoporosis A condition, mostly affecting women, in which the bones become extremely thin and brittle and break easily.

Recommended Dietary Allowances (RDAs) Amounts of certain nutrients considered adequate to meet the needs of most healthy people.

Food Guide Pyramid Food-group plan that provides practical advice to ensure balanced intake of the essential nutrients.

Dietary Guidelines for Americans Seven general principles of good nutrition intended to help prevent certain diet-related diseases.

TERMS

TABLE 9-4 Recommended Dietary Allowances, Revised 1989[a,b,c]

Category	Age (years) or Condition	Weight[d] (kg)	(lb)	Height[d] (cm)	(in)	Protein (g)	Fat-Soluble Vitamins — Vitamin A (µg RE)	Vitamin D (µg)	Vitamin E (mg α-TE)	Vitamin K (µg)
Infants	0.0–0.5	6	13	60	24	13	375	7.5	3	5
	0.5–1.0	9	20	71	28	14	375	10	4	10
Children	1–3	13	29	90	35	16	400	10	6	15
	4–6	20	44	112	44	24	500	10	7	20
	7–10	28	62	132	52	28	700	10	7	30
Males	11–14	45	99	157	62	45	1,000	10	10	45
	15–18	66	145	176	69	59	1,000	10	10	65
	19–24	72	160	177	70	58	1,000	10	10	70
	25–50	79	174	176	70	63	1,000	5	10	80
	51 +	77	170	173	68	63	1,000	5	10	80
Females	11–14	46	101	157	62	46	800	10	8	45
	15–18	55	120	163	64	44	800	10	8	55
	19–24	58	128	164	65	46	800	10	8	60
	25–50	63	138	163	64	50	800	5	8	65
	51 +	65	143	160	63	50	800	5	8	65
Pregnant						60	800	10	10	65
Lactating	1st 6 Months					65	1,300	10	12	65
	2nd 6 Months					62	1,200	10	11	65

[a] The allowances, expressed as average daily intakes over time, are intended to provide for individual variations among most normal people as they live in the United States under usual environmental stresses. Diets should be based on a variety of common foods in order to provide other nutrients for which human requirements have been less well defined.

[b] Estimated Safe and Adequate Daily Dietary Intakes (ESADDIs) for adults: 30–100 µg biotin; 4.0–7.0 mg pantothenic acid; 1.5–3.0 mg copper; 2.0–5.0 mg manganese; 1.0–4.0 mg fluoride; 50–200 µg chromium; 75–250 mg molybdenum. (See *Recommended Dietary Allowances*, 10th edition, for information on other age groups.)

[c] Estimated Minimum Requirements of healthy adults: 500 mg sodium; 750 mg chloride; 2,000 mg potassium. (See *Recommended Dietary Allowances*, 10th edition, for information on other age groups.)

[d] Weights and heights of reference adults are actual medians for the U.S. population of the designated age. The use of these figures does not imply that the height-to-weight ratios are ideal.

RDAs and related guidelines; the most recent version was published in 1989 (Table 9-4). The RDA for a vitamin or mineral is set by estimating the range for normal human needs, selecting the number at the high end of the range, and then adding amounts to account for needed body storage and losses during food preparation.

The aim of the RDAs is to guide you in meeting your nutrition needs with food, rather than with vitamin and mineral supplements. This aim is important because recommendations have not yet been set for some essential nutrients; not enough is known about these nutrients for the Food and Nutrition Board to actually set a recommended level of intake. Because many supplements contain only nutrients with established RDAs, using them to meet nutrient needs can leave you deficient in other nutrients. Meeting these recommendations with food ensures a balanced intake of all essential nutrients.

No nutrient is absolutely needed daily. You can survive for a few days on a diet without water and about one year on a diet without vitamin A. But diets meeting only half the recommended intake levels are likely to be insufficient to replace daily losses of nutrients and thus over the long run can lead to a deficiency. Signs and symptoms of nutritional deficiency may be subtle and develop slowly. Decreased effectiveness of the immune system, reduced organ function, decreased ability to carry oxygen in the bloodstream, and general ongoing cell damage may not be apparent for a long period of time. You may become ill more often and not really know why. Though your diet may be inadequate, you still may show no telltale signs. So it's best to eat a diet that meets your projected nutrient needs on a daily basis.

A variant of the RDA is the **Daily Values**, which have been set by the FDA as a means of expressing nutrient

		Water-Soluble Vitamins							Minerals				
Vitamin C (mg)	Thiamin (mg)	Riboflavin (mg)	Niacin (mg)	Vitamin B-6 (mg)	Folate (µg)	Vitamin B-12 (µg)	Calcium (mg)	Phosphorus (mg)	Magnesium (mg)	Iron (mg)	Zinc (mg)	Iodine (µg)	Selenium (µg)
30	0.3	0.4	5	0.3	25	0.3	400	300	40	6	5	40	10
35	0.4	0.5	6	0.6	35	0.5	600	500	60	10	5	50	15
40	0.7	0.8	9	1.0	50	0.7	800	800	80	10	10	70	20
45	0.9	1.1	12	1.1	75	1.0	800	800	120	10	10	90	20
45	1.0	1.2	13	1.4	100	1.4	800	800	170	10	10	120	30
50	1.3	1.5	17	1.7	150	2.0	1,200	1,200	270	12	15	150	40
60	1.5	1.8	20	2.0	200	2.0	1,200	1,200	400	12	15	150	50
60	1.5	1.7	19	2.0	200	2.0	1,200	1,200	350	10	15	150	70
60	1.5	1.7	19	2.0	200	2.0	800	800	350	10	15	150	70
60	1.2	1.4	15	2.0	200	2.0	800	800	350	10	15	150	70
50	1.1	1.3	15	1.4	150	2.0	1,200	1,200	280	15	12	150	45
60	1.1	1.3	15	1.5	180	2.0	1,200	1,200	300	15	12	150	50
60	1.1	1.3	15	1.6	180	2.0	1,200	1,200	280	15	12	150	55
60	1.1	1.3	15	1.6	180	2.0	800	800	280	15	12	150	55
60	1.0	1.2	13	1.6	180	2.0	800	800	280	10	12	150	55
70	1.5	1.6	17	2.2	400	2.2	1,200	1,200	320	30	15	175	65
95	1.6	1.8	20	2.1	280	2.6	1,200	1,200	355	15	19	200	75
90	1.6	1.7	20	2.1	260	2.6	1,200	1,200	340	15	16	200	75

content on food labels. The Daily Values are based on two dietary standards—the RDAs, used for vitamins and minerals, and current scientific consensus, used for nutrients for which there is no RDA per se, such as protein, saturated fat, and dietary fiber. Nutrient content is expressed as a percentage of the Daily Values.

Many countries publish their own nutrient guides, as does the World Health Organization (WHO). These guidelines differ slightly from one another because there is disagreement among scientists about requirements and because different diets can lead to slightly different vitamin and mineral needs.

Food Guide Pyramid

Most of us learned about food groups in grade school. We learned that by choosing foods from each group, we could have a healthy diet. The fundamental principles of this food guide are moderation, variety, and balance—a theme echoed throughout this chapter. A diet is balanced if it contains appropriate amounts of each nutrient; choosing foods from each of the food groups helps insure that. The latest version of the food-group plan is the U.S. Department of Agriculture's Food Guide Pyramid (Figure 9-3). It is based on a recommended number of servings from six food groups: (1) a milk, yogurt, and cheese group; (2) a meat, poultry, fish, dry beans, eggs, and nut group; (3) a fruit group; (4) a vegetables group; (5) a breads, cereals, rice and pasta group; and (6) a fats, oils, and sweets group. Caution is advised when choosing from the last group, although foods within that group can supply the essential fats for our diet (Table 9-5).

If you're worried about maintaining a healthy weight or want to lose weight, the Food Guide Pyramid can help you create food plans with as few as 1,600–1,800 calories and meet the adult RDAs of all essential nutrients, except possibly for iron in some women who have heavy menstrual flow. For those women, foods fortified in iron, such as breakfast cereals, can supply the deficit. If 1,600 calories is too many calories for you, first try to become more active; it's hard to design an adequate diet for young adults that supplies fewer than 1,600 calories. If you can't increase your energy output, you can include some nutrient-fortified foods.

Daily Values   A simplified version of the RDAs used in food-product labels; also included are values for nutrients with no RDA per se.

TERMS

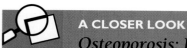
Osteoporosis is a condition in which the bones become dangerously thin and fragile over time. As the disease progresses, losses in bone density lead first to poor bone strength and then to an increased risk of fractures, back pain, height loss, and a curving of the spine. Osteoporosis develops gradually over the years. After age 35, we all lose more bone mass than our bodies replace, but many of us retain enough throughout our lives to avoid serious problems.

Who Is at Risk?

Osteoporosis afflicts four times as many women as men. Women are more susceptible because they generally have less bone mass to begin with. More importantly, women commonly experience rapid bone loss in the first few years following menopause. There is also an important genetic factor—Caucasian and Asian women get osteoporosis more often than do black women, and the risk is even greater for small-boned women and those with a family history of osteoporosis.

Other factors can increase the likelihood of osteoporosis: abnormal menstrual periods, early menopause or surgical removal of the ovaries, a history of anorexia nervosa, the use of certain drugs, smoking, and the habitual consumption of alcohol.

What Can You Do?

Childhood, adolescence, and the first years of adulthood are the times to build bones strong enough to cover bone loss in later years. However, lifestyle factors at any point during the lifespan can decrease the loss of bone density over time.

Exercise can help prevent osteoporosis by strengthening the bones that are most likely to be affected. Many experts recommend a regular routine of weight-bearing exercise, such as walking, running, or aerobic dancing. But any benefit derived from exercise may be lost within a year after the exercising stops. Therefore, exercising is just as important for a woman in her forties and fifties who is trying to prevent bone loss as it is for a younger woman who is trying to increase her bone mass. Recent research indicates that weight training exercises can increase bone density, even when taken up later in life.

Exercise alone is not a sufficient defense against the kind of bone loss that can lead to osteoporosis. Sufficient calcium and adequate vitamin D are both important in preventing the condition. Calcium is necessary for healthy bones, especially during childhood and adolescence, when bones are growing. The recommended dietary allowance of calcium for people between 11 and 24 is 1,200 mg per day, approximately as much as in a quart of milk. After age 25, the recommended amount drops down to 800 mg daily, although pregnant and nursing women need more. However, a recent NIH Consensus Conference recommended up to a total of 1,500 mg per day through age 24, 1,000 mg per day through age 50, and 1,500 mg per day after age 50 for men and women not taking estrogen.

Getting enough calcium in the diet takes some careful planning, especially since foods traditionally recognized as high in calcium are also high in fat. Low-fat and nonfat dairy products, tofu, canned salmon, and sardines eaten with the bones are all calcium-rich foods. Other good sources are dark-green vegetables such as collard or turnip greens, bok choy, kale, and broccoli and calcium-fortified orange juice, fruit drinks, and bread.

Vitamin D is necessary for the body to absorb calcium. The body makes its own vitamin D when it is exposed to the sun, and the vitamin is also available in such foods as milk.

The Menopause Connection

Menopause is a natural accelerator of bone loss. The presence of estrogen inhibits bone loss, but after menopause a woman's body stops producing estrogen, and bone loss increases rapidly. Whether osteoporosis develops is determined by the specific constellation of interacting factors such as heredity, diet, and the individual's bone density.

Estrogen replacement at menopause significantly reduces further bone loss, but there is a question about the extent to which long-term use increases cancer risk. It is therefore recommended that estrogen-replacement therapy be considered on an individual basis by women and their physicians. Overall, for most women at high risk for osteoporosis, a combination of estrogen and calcium is one of the most effective treatments.

Dietary Guidelines for Americans

To provide further guidance for choosing a healthy diet, the U.S. Department of Agriculture and the Department of Health and Human Services have issued Dietary Guidelines for Americans, most recently in 1990. What follows is a summary of the advice provided by the Dietary Guidelines, with additional comments from various health-related organizations, including the Surgeon General, the American Heart Association, the National Cancer Institute, and the National Academy of Sciences.

1. *Eat a variety of foods.* Focus on the Food Guide Pyramid we just discussed, choosing an appropriate number of servings from each group. Choose a variety of foods from within each group to take advantage of the fact that certain foods are better sources of some nutrients than other foods are. Everyone, especially adolescent girls and women, should take special care to meet their RDA for calcium and iron. Limit your

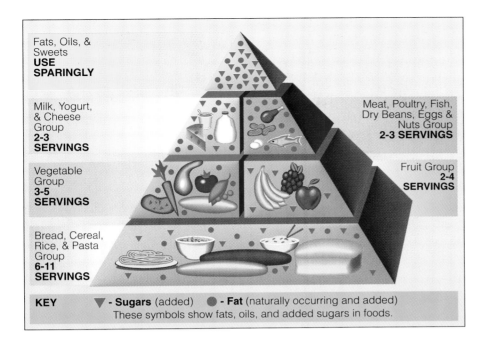

Fats, Oils, & Sweets
USE SPARINGLY

Milk, Yogurt, & Cheese Group
2-3 SERVINGS

Meat, Poultry, Fish, Dry Beans, Eggs & Nuts Group
2-3 SERVINGS

Vegetable Group
3-5 SERVINGS

Fruit Group
2-4 SERVINGS

Bread, Cereal, Rice, & Pasta Group
6-11 SERVINGS

KEY   ▼ - **Sugars** (added)   ● - **Fat** (naturally occurring and added)
These symbols show fats, oils, and added sugars in foods.

Figure 9-3   *The Food Guide Pyramid: a guide to daily food choices.*
The Pyramid is an outline of what to eat each day. It's not a rigid prescription, but a general guide that lets you choose a healthful diet that's right for you. The Pyramid calls for eating a variety of foods to get the nutrients you need and at the same time the right amount of calories to maintain a healthy weight. The Pyramid also focuses on fat because many Americans eat too much fat, especially saturated fat. *Source:* U.S. Department of Agriculture, Human Nutrition Information Service. 1992. *Food Guide Pyramid.* Home and Garden Bulletin No. 249.

protein intake to no more than twice the RDA and don't take a nutrient supplement in quantities greater than 150 percent of the Daily Value.

2. *Maintain healthy weight.* Emphasize balancing food intake with regular physical activity to avoid creeping overweight and eventual obesity. Excess body fat increases the risk for diabetes, heart disease, cancer, and other diseases. Those who are overweight shouldn't try to lose more than ½ to 1 pound per week. Weight loss should be accomplished by increasing physical activity and eating low-calorie, nutrient-rich foods—grains, vegetables, and fruits— not fat and fatty foods, sugar and sweets, and alcoholic beverages. Diets with fewer than 800–1,000 calories per day can be hazardous and should be followed only under medical supervision.

3. *Choose a diet low in fat, saturated fat, and cholesterol.* Limit your fat intake to 30 percent or less of total calories. Limit your intake of saturated fat to one-third of your total fat intake (10 percent of total calories) and dietary cholesterol to 300 milligrams per day. The average American consumes 12 percent of total calories as saturated fat and about 230 (for women) to 370 (for men) milligrams of dietary cholesterol per day. Experts recommend choosing lean meat, fish, poultry, and dry beans and peas as protein sources; using nonfat or low-fat milk and milk products; limiting your intake of fat-rich foods and oils high in saturated fat; trimming fat off meats; broiling, baking, or boiling instead of frying; and moderate use of fat-containing foods such as deep-fried foods.

4. *Choose a diet with plenty of vegetables, fruits, and grain products.* Emphasize complex, rather than simple carbohydrates. Five or more servings of vegetables or fruits daily and six or more servings of breads, cereals, and legumes daily is a good goal and will help you reach a daily dietary fiber consumption of 20–35 grams.

5. *Use sugars only in moderation.* Moderation here means less than 15 percent of total calories—about 75 grams of simple sugars per day, or about 15 teaspoons. Reducing sugar consumption means cutting back on items with added sugar, such as baked goods, sweetened beverages, and presweetened breakfast cereals.

6. *Use salt and sodium only in moderation.* Sodium is an essential nutrient, but you need only about 500 milligrams per day—that translates into only about ¼ teaspoon of salt. Most Americans consume 8 to 12 times this amount. It's recommended that you limit your sodium intake to no more than 2.4 to 3 grams per day, or about 1¼ to 1½ teaspoons of salt. A restriction of this magnitude does require a change in food habits for many people, such as eliminating processed (lunch) meats, salted snack foods, most canned and prepared soups, regular cheese, and many tomato-based products. You can begin to make this change by learning to enjoy the flavors of unsalted foods, adding little or no salt during cooking or at the table, and flavoring foods with herbs, spices, or lemon juice.

7. *If you drink alcoholic beverages, do so in moderation.* Men should consume no more than two drinks daily. Women should drink no more than one drink daily, and alcohol should not be consumed during pregnancy. One drink is the equivalent of 5 ounces of

TABLE 9-5 Food Guide Pyramid

This guide lets you easily turn the RDA into food choices. You can get all essential nutrients by eating a balanced variety of foods each day from the food groups listed here. Eat a variety of foods in each food group and adjust serving sizes appropriately to reach and maintain a desirable weight. This pattern will yield only about 1,600–1,800 calories.

Choosing some plant proteins and following the other suggestions listed should provide a diet adequate in all nutrients, except possibly iron for women who experience a heavy menstrual flow.

Food Group	Serving	Major Contributions	Foods and Serving Sizes*
Milk, yogurt, and cheese	2 (adult[ll]) 3 (children, teens, young adults, and pregnant or lactating women)	Calcium Riboflavin Protein Potassium Zinc	1 cup milk 1$^1/_2$ oz cheese 2 oz processed cheese 1 cup yogurt 2 cups cottage cheese 1 cup custard/pudding 1$^1/_2$ cups ice cream
Meat, poultry, fish, dry beans, eggs, and nuts	2–3	Protein Niacin Iron Vitamin B-6 Zinc Thiamin Vitamin B-12[†]	2–3 oz cooked meat, poultry, fish 1–1$^1/_2$ cups cooked dry beans 4 T peanut butter 2 eggs $^1/_2$–1 cup nuts
Fruits	2–4	Vitamin C Carbohydrates Fiber	$^1/_4$ cup dried fruit $^1/_2$ cup cooked fruit $^3/_4$ cup juice 1 whole piece of fruit 1 melon wedge
Vegetables	3–5	Vitamin A Vitamin C Folate Magnesium Carbohydrates Fiber	$^1/_2$ cup raw or cooked vegetables 1 cup raw leafy vegetables
Bread, cereals, rice, and pasta	6–11	Starch Thiamin Riboflavin[§] Iron Niacin Folate Magnesium[‡] Carbohydrates Fiber[‡] Zinc[‡]	1 slice of bread 1 oz ready-to-eat cereal $^1/_2$–$^3/_4$ cup cooked cereal, rice, or pasta
Fats, oils, and sweets			Foods from this group should not replace any from the other groups. Amounts consumed should be determined by individual energy needs.

*May be reduced for child servings
†Only in animal food choices
‡Whole grains especially
§If enriched
ll25 years of age or older

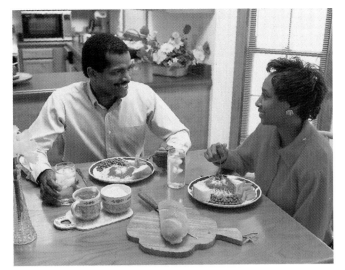

This couple's dinner of spaghetti with marinara sauce, carrots, peas, and bread is high in complex carbohydrates, vitamin A, vitamin C, folate, and dietary fiber.

TACTICS AND TIPS
Reducing the Fat in Your Diet

- Steam, boil, or bake vegetables, or stir fry them in a small amount of vegetable oil.
- Season vegetables with herbs and spices rather than with sauces, butter, or margarine.
- Try lemon juice on salad or use a yogurt-based salad dressing instead of mayonnaise or sour cream dressings.
- To reduce saturated fat, use vegetable oil instead of butter or margarine. Use tub margarine instead of stick margarine in baked products.
- Replace whole milk with skim or low-fat milk in puddings, soups, and baked products. Substitute plain low-fat yogurt, blender-whipped cottage cheese, or buttermilk in recipes that call for sour cream.
- Choose lean cuts of meat, and trim any visible fat from meat before and after cooking. Remove skin from poultry before or after cooking.
- Roast, bake, or broil meat, poultry, or fish so that fat drains away as the food cooks.
- Use a nonstick pan for cooking so added fat will be unnecessary; use a vegetable spray for frying.
- Chill broths from meat or poultry until the fat becomes solid. Spoon off the fat before using the broth.
- Eat a low-fat vegetarian main dish at least once a week.

wine, 12 ounces of beer, or 1½ ounces of distilled spirits. Remember, alcoholic beverages are high in calories and low in nutrients.

These guidelines do not apply equally to everyone. We vary in our susceptibility to developing high serum cholesterol levels, high blood pressure, obesity, cancer, and the other health problems these guidelines seek to counteract. You should consider your own health status and apply these guidelines appropriately to address current or potential health problems.

Personal Insight Do you feel good after you eat a healthy meal? Are your good feelings physical or emotional or both?

The Vegetarian Alternative

Some people choose a diet with one essential difference from the diets we've already described—foods of animal origin (meat, poultry, fish, eggs, milk) are eliminated or restricted. Today, about 12 million Americans follow a vegetarian diet. Most do so because they think foods of plant origin are a more natural way to nourish the body. Some do so for religious, health, ethical, or philosophical reasons. If you choose to be a vegetarian, you can be confident you can meet your nutritional needs by following a few basic rules. (Vegetarian diets for children and pregnant women warrant individual professional guidance.)

There is a variety of vegetarian styles; the wider the variety of the diet eaten, the easier it is to meet nutritional needs. **Vegans** eat only plant foods. **Lacto-vegetarians** eat plant foods and dairy products. **Lacto-ovo-vegetari-** ans eat plant foods, dairy products, and eggs. Finally, **partial** or **semivegetarians** eat plant foods, dairy products, eggs, and usually a small selection of poultry, fish, and other seafood. Including some animal protein in a diet makes planning much easier.

A food-group plan has been developed for lacto-vegetarians; it includes 6–11 servings from grains and 2–4 servings from legumes, nuts, and seeds. Add to this 3–5 servings from a vegetable group, 2–4 servings from a fruit group, and two or more servings from the milk, yogurt, and cheese group to complete the plan. By following this

Vegans Vegetarians who eat no animal products at all.
Lacto-vegetarians Vegetarians who include milk and cheese products in their diet.
Lacto-ovo-vegetarians Vegetarians who eat no meat, poultry, or fish, but do eat eggs and milk products.
Partial or semivegetarians Vegetarians who include eggs, dairy products, and small amounts of poultry and seafood in their diet.

TERMS

plan, the lacto-vegetarian should have no problem obtaining an adequate diet. Consuming fruits with most meals is especially helpful, because any vitamin C present will improve iron absorption (the iron in plants is more difficult to absorb than is that in animal sources).

In contrast to those who eat dairy products, the vegan has to do much more special diet planning to obtain all essential nutrients. A vegan must take special care to consume adequate amounts of protein, riboflavin, vitamin D, vitamin B-12, calcium, iron, and zinc.

It takes a little planning and common sense to put together a good vegetarian diet. If you are a vegetarian or are considering becoming one, devote some extra time and thought to your diet. It's especially important that you eat as wide a variety of foods as possible to ensure that all of your nutritional needs are filled.

A PERSONAL PLAN: MAKING INTELLIGENT CHOICES ABOUT FOOD

Now that you understand the basis of good nutrition and a healthy diet, you can put together a diet that works for you. There probably is an ideal diet for you based on your particular nutrition and health status, but there is no single type of diet that provides optimal health for everyone. Many cultural dietary patterns encompass the practices recommended by nutrition experts: eating a variety of foods, maintaining a healthy body weight, and maintaining a physically active lifestyle.

Reading Food Labels to Learn More About What You Eat

To make intelligent choices about food, you should learn to read and understand food labels. In December 1992, the federal government enacted new and dramatically different guidelines for food labels. Almost all food packages are now required to have the new labels.

Food labels are designed to help consumers make food choices based on the nutrients of most concern to health. The labels show how much fat, saturated fat, cholesterol, protein, dietary fiber, and sodium the food contains. In addition to listing nutrient content by weight, the labels put the information in the context of a daily diet of 2,000 calories that includes no more than 65 grams of fat (approximately 30 percent of total calories). For example, if a serving of a particular product has 260 calories and 13 grams of fat, the label will tell you that that amount of fat is 20 percent of what you should eat each day.

The labels require uniform serving sizes. This means that consumers looking at different brands of salad dressing, for example, can compare calories and fat content based on the same serving amount. The regulations also require that foods meet strict definitions if their packaging includes the terms "light," "low-fat," or "high-fiber." A

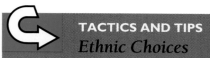

TACTICS AND TIPS
Ethnic Choices

	Choose Often	Choose Less Often
Chinese	Chinese greens Rice, brown or white Steamed beef with pea pods Stir-fry dishes Wonton soup	Crispy duck Egg rolls Fried rice Kung pao (fried chicken) Pork spare ribs
Japanese	Chiri nabe (fish stew) Sushi, sashimi (raw fish) Yakitori (grilled chicken)	Age tofu (fried tofu) Tonkatsu (fried pork) Tempura (fried chicken, shrimp, or vegetables)
Thai	Forest salad Larb (minty chicken salad) Po tak (seafood soup) Yum neua (broiled beef with onions)	Fried fish, duck, or chicken Curries with coconut milk Yum koon chaing (sausage with peppers)
Italian	Cioppino (seafood stew) Minestrone soup (vegetarian) Pasta with marinara sauce Pasta primavera (pasta with vegetables)	Antipasto Cannelloni, ravioli Fettucini alfredo Garlic bread White clam sauce
Mexican	Beans and rice Black bean/vegetable soup Burritos, bean Enchiladas, bean Gazpacho Tortillas, steamed Tostadas, bean or chicken	Chiles rellenos Chimichangas Enchiladas, beef or cheese Flautas Guacamole Nachos or fried tortillas Quesadillas
Indian	Chapati (tortilla-like bread) Dal (lentils) Karhi (chick-pea soup) Khur (milk/rice dessert) Tandoori, chicken or fish	Bhatura (fried bread) Coconut milk Ghee (clarified butter) Korma (rich meat dish) Samosa (fried meat and vegetables in dough)

Source: *Runner's World*, January 1990, p. 25.

footnote on the label gives suggested intakes of fat, saturated fat, cholesterol, sodium, carbohydrate, and fiber for both a 2,000-calorie diet and a 2,500-calorie diet, as space on the label permits. A sample label is shown in Figure 9-4.

Who Should Take Vitamin or Mineral Supplements?

You may wonder whether or not to take vitamin or min-

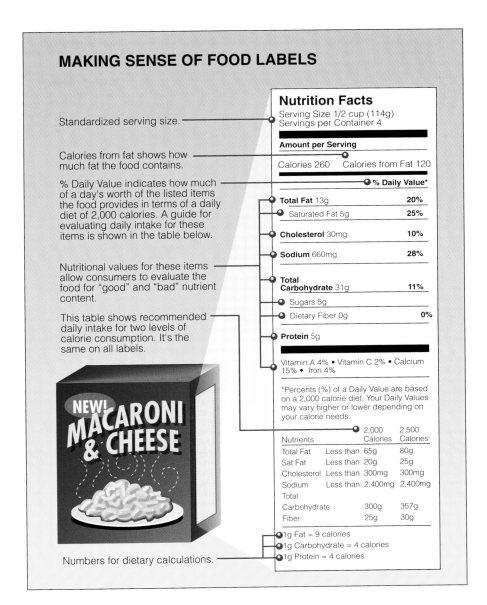

MAKING SENSE OF FOOD LABELS

Standardized serving size.

Calories from fat shows how much fat the food contains.

% Daily Value indicates how much of a day's worth of the listed items the food provides in terms of a daily diet of 2,000 calories. A guide for evaluating daily intake for these items is shown in the table below.

Nutritional values for these items allow consumers to evaluate the food for "good" and "bad" nutrient content.

This table shows recommended daily intake for two levels of calorie consumption. It's the same on all labels.

Numbers for dietary calculations.

Nutrition Facts
Serving Size 1/2 cup (114g)
Servings per Container 4

Amount per Serving

Calories 260   Calories from Fat 120

% Daily Value*

Total Fat 13g	**20%**
Saturated Fat 5g	**25%**
Cholesterol 30mg	**10%**
Sodium 660mg	**28%**
Total Carbohydrate 31g	**11%**
Sugars 5g	
Dietary Fiber 0g	**0%**
Protein 5g	

Vitamin A 4% • Vitamin C 2% • Calcium 15% • Iron 4%

*Percents (%) of a Daily Value are based on a 2,000 calorie diet. Your Daily Values may vary higher or lower depending on your calorie needs:

Nutrients		2,000 Calories	2,500 Calories
Total Fat	Less than	65g	80g
Sat Fat	Less than	20g	25g
Cholesterol	Less than	300mg	300mg
Sodium	Less than	2,400mg	2,400mg
Total Carbohydrate		300g	357g
Fiber		25g	30g

1g Fat = 9 calories
1g Carbohydrate = 4 calories
1g Protein = 4 calories

Figure 9-4   *The current food label.*
A sample label for macaroni and cheese is shown here.

eral supplements. To answer this question, first look closely at your diet. Does it follow the Food Guide Pyramid, especially emphasizing whole grains, low-fat and nonfat dairy products, leafy and dark-green vegetables, foods containing vitamin C, and a serving of vegetable oils? If so, men are probably meeting their nutrient needs; some women (those with heavy menstrual flows) may still need more iron to compensate for that lost. Secondly, do you regularly consume a fortified breakfast cereal? Most breakfast cereals have extra vitamins and minerals added, some even matching 100% of the adult Daily Values.

Nutrition scientists generally agree that most people can obtain needed vitamins and minerals from a healthy diet. Improve your diet where needed. After that, consider whether you need a supplement. Talk to a registered dietitian and your physician.

Recently a panel of nutrition scientists suggested certain cases when vitamin and mineral supplements should be considered.

- Women with excessive bleeding during menses may need iron.
- Women who are pregnant or breastfeeding may need extra iron, folate, and calcium.
- People with very low calorie intakes need the range of vitamins and minerals covered by the RDA.
- Some vegetarians may need extra calcium, iron, zinc, and vitamin B-12.
- Newborns, under the direction of a physician, need a single dose of vitamin K.
- People with certain illnesses or diseases, and those on certain medications, may need supplementation of specific vitamins and minerals at the direction of a physician.

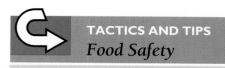
- Thoroughly wash hands with hot soapy water before and after handling food, especially raw meat, fish, poultry, or eggs, which may contain *Salmonella* bacteria.

- Don't let groceries sit in a warm car; bacteria will grow in warm temperatures. Get them home to the refrigerator or freezer promptly.

- Don't buy food in containers that leak, bulge, or are severely dented—the deadly botulism toxin may be present.

- Make sure counters, cutting boards, dishes, and other equipment are thoroughly cleaned before and after use, especially if they have come in contact with raw meat, fish, poultry, or eggs.

- Thoroughly rinse and scrub fruits and vegetables, with a brush, if possible. Peel them, if appropriate, even though you'll peel away some of the nutrients. Remove outer leaves of leafy vegetables, such as lettuce and cabbage.

- If possible, use separate cutting boards for meat and for foods that will be eaten raw, such as fruits or vegetables.

- Cook foods thoroughly, especially beef, poultry, fish, pork, and eggs. This is of the utmost importance. Cooking

kills most microbes. Don't eat raw animal products.

- Trim fat from meat, poultry, and fish and remove skin (which contains most of the fat) from poultry and fish. Discard fats and oils found in broths and pan drippings. (Pesticide residues concentrate in the animals' fat.)

- Cook stuffing separately from poultry; or wash poultry thoroughly, stuff immediately before cooking, and then transfer the stuffing to a clean bowl immediately after cooking.

- Store foods below 40° or above 140° F. Do not leave cooked or refrigerated foods, such as meats or salads, at room temperature for more than two hours.

- Avoid coughing or sneezing over foods, even when you are healthy, and cover any cuts on your hands.

- Use only pasteurized milk.

- Throw back the big fish—the little ones have less time to take up and concentrate pesticides and other harmful residues.

Adapted from Food-borne Illness. 1995. *Mayo Clinic Health Letter,* March; and Food and Drug Administration. 1988. "Safety First: Protecting America's Food Supply." *FDA Consumer,* November, p. 26.

If you decide to take a vitamin and mineral supplement, the Council on Scientific Affairs of the American Medical Association recommends a supplement containing between 50 and 150 percent of the adult Daily Values for vitamins. We suggest the same guidelines for minerals.

In sum, most of us can rely on a healthy diet for our nutrient needs. Few people need to resort to regular use of a nutrient supplement, and those who do should do so under professional guidance.

Getting Reliable Nutrition Advice

Americans face an avalanche of conflicting nutrition advice from newspapers, magazines, books, and television programs—advice that can have profound effects on food choices. In order to choose a healthy diet, you must learn to sift through this information and find reliable resources to answer your questions.

Nutrition labels can be an important source of information. However, not all materials provided by the food industry promote healthy food choices. If you have a question about nutrition, it's probably most convenient to ask a faculty member in the nutrition department on your campus. Local registered dietitians and home economists are also helpful resources, as is your family physician.

Most large communities contain a service called "Dial a Dietitian" where you can phone a registered dietitian and receive nutrition information free of charge.

You should look for the credential "Registered Dietitian" (R.D.) when seeking a nutrition counselor because these individuals are specially trained to translate nutritional needs into healthful, tasty diets. An R.D. credential guarantees that the person has a good nutrition background.

Whenever people need detailed nutrition advice, they usually also require a physician's consultation. The presence of one health problem often indicates the presence of still another, and a physician needs to evaluate the total health of a person to make a proper diagnosis. A complete and accurate diagnosis then allows the registered dietitian to design the proper diet.

The Food Supply: Is It Safe?

Many people worry about additives or pesticide residues in their food. However, the greatest threat to the safety of the food supply comes from microorganisms that cause food-borne illness. Raw or undercooked animal products, such as chicken, hamburger, and oysters, pose the greatest risk for contamination. About one-third to one-half of all diarrhea cases in America—more than 20 million each year—are caused by food-borne organisms. Your last bout of "flu" may very well have been food-borne illness. The symptoms of both are often the same: diarrhea, vomiting, fever, and weakness. Although the effects of food-borne illness are usually not serious, some groups, such as children and the elderly, are more at risk for severe complications like rheumatic diseases, seizures, blood poisoning, and other ailments.

Environmental contaminants are also present in the food-growing environment, but few of them ever enter the food and water supply in amounts sufficient to cause health problems. Environmental contaminants include various minerals, antibiotics, hormones, pesticides, PCBs, and naturally occurring substances such as cyanogenic glycosides (found in lima beans and the pits of some fruits) and certain molds. Their effects depend on many factors, including concentration, length of exposure, and the age and health status of the person involved. Safety regulations attempt to keep our exposure to environmental contaminants at safe levels, but monitoring is difficult and many substances (such as pesticides) persist in the environment long after being banned from use.

Adequate nutrition from a varied diet provides a key part of your defense against small doses of contaminants, since a healthy body has much greater resistance to their effects. If you consume a variety of foods in moderation, you will have less chance of suffering negative health consequences from contaminants.

Additives in Food: Are They Dangerous?

Today, some 2,800 substances are intentionally added to foods for one or more of the following reasons: (1) to maintain or improve nutritional quality, (2) to maintain freshness, (3) to help in processing or preparation, or (4) to alter taste or appearance. The most widely used are sugar, salt, and corn syrup; these three, plus citric acid, baking soda, vegetable colors, mustard, and pepper account for 98 percent by weight of all food additives used in the United States.

The amount of an additive that can be used in food processing must be kept to the lowest amount needed to do the job and is also limited to 0.01 to 0.001 of the dose that is found safe to administer to animals. If the additive is known to cause cancer in animals, then it generally cannot be intentionally used in foods at all. If you consume a variety of foods in moderation, the chance of suffering negative health consequences from food additives is minimal.

Overall, the American food supply is outstandingly safe, whether you're concerned with additives, pesticides, or bacteria. With reasonable precautions in preparing food and avoiding substances to which you seem to be sensitive, you can be confident that the food supply is not causing you harm. By far the greatest dietary risks to your long-term health come from overconsumption of calories, fat, and sodium.

SUMMARY

- Choosing foods that provide needed nutrients is an important part of daily life. Food choices made in youth can significantly affect health in later years.

Nutritional Requirements: Components of a Healthy Diet

- The fuel potential in our diet is expressed in calories.
- To function at its best, the human body requires about 45 essential nutrients in specific proportions. People get the nutrients needed to fuel their bodies and maintain tissues and organ systems through the foods they eat.
- Proteins, made up of amino acids, form muscles and bones and help make up blood, enzymes, hormones, and cell membranes. Foods from animal sources provide complete proteins; plants provide incomplete proteins, but combinations of plant proteins yield complete proteins.
- Fats, a concentrated source of energy, also help insulate the body and cushion the organs; 1 tablespoon of vegetable oil per day supplies the essential fats. Dietary fat intake should be limited to 30 percent of total calories.
- Carbohydrates supply energy to the brain and other parts of the nervous system as well as to red blood cells. The body needs 50–100 grams of carbohydrates a day; much more is usually consumed.
- Dietary fiber includes plant substances difficult or impossible for humans to digest. Insoluble fibers like wheat bran hold water and increase bulk in the stool; soluble fibers like oat bran bind cholesterol-containing compounds in the intestine and slow glucose absorption.
- The 13 vitamins needed in the diet are organic substances that promote specific chemical and cell processes within living tissue. Deficiencies can cause serious illnesses and even death.
- Water is used to digest and absorb food, to transport substances around the body, to lubricate joints and organs, and to regulate body temperature. Lack of water can cause death within a few days.
- The approximately 17 minerals needed in the diet are inorganic substances that regulate body functions, aid in growth and maintenance of body tissues, and help in the release of energy from foods. The minerals most commonly lacking are iron and calcium.

Nutritional Guidelines: Planning Your Diet

- Recommended Dietary Allowances (RDAs) are recommended intakes for essential nutrients that meet the needs of healthy persons.

- The Food Guide Pyramid contains six food groups; choosing foods from each every day helps insure appropriate amounts of necessary nutrients. The fundamental principles of the Food Guide Pyramid are moderation, variety, and balance.

- The Dietary Guidelines for Americans address prevention of diet-related diseases like cardiovascular disease, cancer, and diabetes. The guidelines advise: (1) eat a variety of foods, (2) maintain a healthy weight, (3) choose a diet low in fat, (4) choose a diet with plenty of fruits, vegetables, and grain products, (5) use sugars only in moderation, (6) use sodium only in moderation, and (7) drink alcohol in moderation, if at all.

- A vegetarian diet can meet human nutritional needs. Although including dairy products makes diet planning easier, a vegan can meet all needs through careful planning and a wide variety of foods.

A Personal Plan: Making Intelligent Choices About Food

- Almost all foods have labels that show how much fat, cholesterol, protein, fiber, and sodium they contain. Serving sizes are standardized, and health claims are carefully regulated.

- Most people don't need vitamin and mineral supplements. Those who may include pregnant and breastfeeding women, vegetarians, and people who are ill or taking certain medications.

- Reliable nutritional advice can be obtained from registered dietitians; some people will also need consultation with a physician.

- Food-borne illness is a greater threat to health than are additives and environmental contaminants.

- Food additives maintain or improve nutritional quality, maintain freshness, help in processing, and alter taste or appearance.

TAKE ACTION

1. Read the list of ingredients on three or four canned or packaged foods that you enjoy eating. If any ingredients are unfamiliar to you, find out what they are and why they have been used. A nutrition textbook from the library may be a helpful resource.

2. Investigate the nutritional and dietary guidelines that are used to prepare the food served in your school. Are they consistent with what you've learned in this chapter? If not, try to find out more about the guidelines that have been used and why they were chosen.

3. Prepare a flavorful low-fat vegetarian and/or ethnic meal. (Check your local library for appropriate cookbooks.) How do the foods included in the meal and the preparation methods differ from what you're used to?

JOURNAL ENTRY

1. In your health journal, keep track of everything you eat and drink for three or four days. Calculate the average number of servings of each food group you consume per day. Then see how well your average daily intake meets the guidelines in the Food Guide Pyramid.

2. Put together three sample daily menus that follow the Food Guide Pyramid. Keep the dietary guidelines in mind as you make your food selections from each group. Also be sure to base your menus around foods you enjoy eating.

3. *Critical Thinking:* Analyze patterns of food advertising on television by recording the number and types of ads that appear each hour. If possible, compare the number and types of products advertised during an hour of cartoons or other children's programs, an hour of daytime programs, and an hour of prime-time programs. What patterns do you see? What types of information do the ads present? Are they geared toward different segments of the population? Do they encourage healthy eating?

BEHAVIOR CHANGE STRATEGY

IMPROVING YOUR DIET

If you want to alter your diet, some of the major health behavior change strategies we have already examined can help you. Here are some suggestions for behavior management that you can use to lower your fat consumption, raise your fiber intake, or make other changes in your diet.

Establishing a Baseline

Let's say that you want to do two things to your diet: (1) cut out all candy while walking between classes or while on errands in town and (2) eat more fresh fruits and raw vegetables.

Begin by keeping track of your candy consumption. In a journal jot down the time of day and what occurred be-

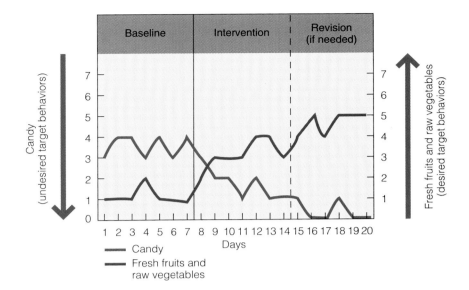

Candy (undesired target behaviors)

Fresh fruits and raw vegetables (desired target behaviors)

Baseline | Intervention | Revision (if needed)

— Candy
— Fresh fruits and raw vegetables

Days

fore and after you ate the candy. On a chart such as the one shown here, keep track of the number of times each day you eat candy. Because you also want to add more fruits and vegetables to your diet, also keep notes on the kinds of foods you have been eating at meals. You can include this information on the same chart or you can keep two graphs.

Intervention

Once you have established your baseline levels, begin to make some changes in those routines that seem to precede your eating candy. For example, you might find that you have been eating candy from a vending machine that you walk by every day after class. If this is the case, try another route that allows you to avoid the machine. If you find that you usually are hungry at one particular time of day and that you rarely have lunch or a healthful snack with you, try to keep a healthful snack on hand so that you won't be caught off guard and be pushed toward eating candy (which always seems to be available). Putting fresh or dried fruit in a backpack or pocket every morning can help. You can use the same sort of strategy to increase the number of fruits and vegetables in your diet: Specifically, you will need to shop for these food items in *advance* and prepare them *ahead of time* so that they are readily available.

Revision (If Needed)

You may discover that your initial plan works perfectly or that it works well for three weeks but then loses its effectiveness. Watch out for programs that become stale and lose their strength, and, of course, revise an ineffective program entirely once you have given it a real try. The critical data from your journal can help you to decide how to revise your program. Plotting the data on a prominently displayed chart can encourage you to continue.

Social Eating Events

Avoiding an attractive candy vending machine may be a lot easier than cutting back on late-night pizza binges; the former involves only you while the latter involves you and your friends. It's harder to make adjustments in social eating patterns, but there are some strategies that you can try. First, tell your friends that you would prefer to try something new to eat instead of pizza, such as popcorn. Being assertive in such matters can be very helpful; you may discover some allies who share your views about the type of food you want to eat. Second, try to cut down on these group activities without eliminating them entirely. Of course, you can try to change or limit the kinds of food you eat at these times, but it's generally very difficult to refrain from joining in once you're actually in the social situation.

Systematic Changes in Other Habits

Many people begin an exercise program or begin to increase their routine activity levels (walks after meals, and so on) at the same time that they try to adjust their diet. While it isn't a good idea to try to make too many significant changes at one time, you may want to experiment with other changes while you're making adjustments in your diet.

SELECTED BIBLIOGRAPHY

Achterberg, C., and others. 1994. How to put the Food Guide Pyramid into practice. *Journal of the American Dietetic Association* 94:1030.

ADA Reports: Position of the American Dietetic Association: Use of nutritive and nonnutritive sweeteners. 1993. *Journal of the American Dietetic Association* 93:816.

ADA Reports: Position of the American Dietetic Association: Vegetarian diets. 1993. *Journal of the American Dietetic Association* 93:1317.

Alaimo, K., and others. 1994. Dietary intake of vitamins, minerals, and fiber of persons ages 2 months and over in the United States. *Third National Health and Nutrition Examination Survey*, Phase 1, 1988–91, Advance Data 258:1, November 14.

Anderson, J. W., and others. 1994. Health benefits and practical aspects of high-fiber diets. *American Journal of Clinical Nutrition* 59:1242S.

———. 1991. Lipid responses of hypercholesterolemic men to oat-bran and wheat-bran intakes. *American Journal of Clinical Nutrition* 54:678.

Blackburn, H. 1994. Strategies for reducing dietary risk factors: the high risk individual versus population-wide interventions. *Nutrition* 10:636.

Bray, G. A. 1992. Pathophysiology of obesity. *American Journal of Clinical Nutrition* 55:488S.

Clark, N. 1991. How to pack a meatless diet full of nutrients. *The Physician and Sports Medicine* 19:31.

Cutler, R. G. 1991. Antioxidants and aging. *American Journal of Clinical Nutrition* 53:3735.

Diet, nutrition and the prevention of chronic diseases—A report of the WHO study group on diet, nutrition and prevention of noncommunicable diseases. 1991. *Nutrition Reviews* 49:291.

Dwyer, J. T. 1991. Dietary change: Convergence of prevention and treatment measures. *Topics of Clinical Nutrition* 6:42.

———. 1991. Nutritional consequences of vegetarianism. *Annual Reviews of Nutrition* 11:61.

Filer, L. J. 1991. Recommended dietary allowances: How did we get where we are? *Nutrition Today*, September/October.

Food and Nutrition Board. 1989. *Recommended Dietary Allowances*. Revised. Washington, D.C.: National Academy of Sciences—National Research Council.

Glore, S. R., and others. 1994. Soluble fiber and serum lipids: A literature review. *Journal of the American Dietetic Association* 94:425.

Haddad, E. H. 1994. Development of a vegetarian food guide. *American Journal of Clinical Nutrition* 59:1248S.

Halliwell, B. 1994. Free radicals and antioxidants: A personal view. *Nutrition Reviews* 52:253.

Hecht, A. 1991. Preventing food-borne illness. *FDA Consumer*, January/February, 18.

Herbert, V., and T. S. Kasdan. 1994. Misleading nutrition claims and their gurus. *Nutrition Today*, May/June, 28.

Holick, M. F. 1994. McCollum Award Lecture: Vitamin D—new horizons for the 21st century. *American Journal of Clinical Nutrition* 60:619.

Kurtzwell, P. 1994. Food label close-up. *FDA Consumer*, April, 15.

Lachance, P., and L. Langseth. 1994. The RDA concept: Time for a change? *Nutrition Reviews* 52:266.

Lofgren, P. A., and others. 1994. Eating in America today: A dietary pattern and intake report. *Food and Nutrition News* 66:9.

Mayes, P. A. 1993. Nutrition, digestion, and absorption. In Murray, R. K., and others, eds. *Harper's Biochemistry*. East Norwalk, Conn.: Appleton & Lange.

Mayfield, E. 1994. A consumer's guide to fats. *FDA Consumer*, May, 15.

McDowell, M. A., and others. 1994. Energy and macronutrient intakes of persons ages 2 months and over in the United States. *Third National Health and Nutrition Examination Survey*. Advanced Data No. 255, October 24.

NIH Consensus Development Panel on Optimal Calcium Intake. 1994. Optimal calcium intake. *Journal of the American Medical Association* 272:1942.

Papazian, R. 1991. Osteoporosis treatment advances. *FDA Consumer*, April, 29–32.

Perkin, B. B. 1990. Dietary guidelines for Americans, 1990 edition. *Journal of the American Dietetic Association* 90:1725.

Saling, J. 1992. Staying ahead of osteoporosis. *Take Care*, Winter, 8–10.

Saltos, E., and others. 1994. The new food label as a tool for healthy eating. *Nutrition Today*, May/June, 18.

Slavin, J. L. 1990. Dietary fiber: Mechanism or magic on disease prevention. *Nutrition Today*, November/December, 6.

Woteki, C. E., and P. R. Thomas. 1991. *Improving America's Diet and Health*. Washington, D.C.: National Academy Press.

RECOMMENDED READINGS

Barrett, S., and W. Jarvis. 1993. *The Health Robbers: A Close Look at Quackery in America*. New York: Prometheus Books. *A careful look at nutrition quackery written by two noted "quackbusters."*

Finn, S. C., and L. Stern. 1992. *The Real Life Nutrition Book*. New York: Penguin. *A nice review of nutrition for the consumer, written by a past president of the American Dietetic Association.*

Herbert, V., and G. J. Subak-Sharpe, eds. 1994. *Total Nutrition: The Only Guide You Will Ever Need—From the Mount Sinai School of Medicine*. New York: St. Martins Press. *An excellent review of current nutrition topics written by a noted physician, scientist, and nutrition expert.*

Wardlaw, G. M., and P. M. Insel. 1996. *Perspectives in Nutrition*. 3rd ed. St. Louis: Mosby-Yearbook. *An easy-to-understand review of major concepts in nutrition—from infancy to elderly years.*

Woteki, C. E., and P. R. Thomas. 1992. *Eat for Life*. Washington, D.C.: National Academy Press. *A summary of* Improving America's Diet and Health *(listed above) designed for the lay public. This volume is packed with up-to-date and useful information on the relationship between diet and health status.*

The Facts About Fast Food

Burger King

	Serving size	Calories	Protein	Carbohydrates	Fat: Total	Polyunsaturated fat	Monounsaturated fat	Saturated fat	Cholesterol	Sodium	Potassium	Phosphorus	Vitamin A	Vitamin C	Thiamine	Riboflavin	Niacin	Calcium	Iron	Zinc	% cal from fat
	gm		gm	gm	gm	gm	gm	gm	mg	mg	mg				% Daily Value						
Whopper	270	614	27	45	36	13	11	12	91	865	N/A	N/A	11	20	24	24	34	8	27	N/A	53
Whopper with cheese	294	706	32	47	44	13	13	16	116	1177	N/A	N/A	19	20	24	28	34	22	27	N/A	56
Hamburger	108	272	15	28	11	1	5	4	37	505	N/A	N/A	3	5	15	15	19	4	15	N/A	36
Bacon double cheeseburger	160	507	33	26	30	2	13	14	108	809	N/A	N/A	8	*	23	29	36	18	21	N/A	53
Burger buddies (pair)	129	349	18	31	17	1	8	7	52	717	N/A	N/A	9	8	32	24	23	11	19	N/A	44
BK Broiler chicken sandwich	154	267	22	28	8	3	3	2	45	728	N/A	N/A	4	6	45	45	60	4	15	N/A	27
Ocean Catch fish fillet sandwich	165	479	16	31	33	12	13	8	45	736	N/A	N/A	*	*	48	25	48	5	13	N/A	62
Chicken tenders (6 piece)	90	236	16	14	13	2	8	3	38	541	N/A	N/A	2	*	7	5	40	*	2	N/A	50
Chunky chicken salad	258	142	20	8	4	1	1	1	49	443	N/A	N/A	92	34	10	10	47	4	7	N/A	25
Garden salad	223	95	6	8	5	0	1	3	15	125	N/A	N/A	100	58	5	6	4	15	6	N/A	47
French fries (medium, salted)	116	372	5	43	20	2	12	5	0	238	N/A	N/A	*	5	5	*	12	*	7	N/A	48
Onion rings	97	339	5	38	19	2	12	5	0	628	N/A	N/A	15	*	10	6	12	11	3	N/A	50
Chocolate shake	284	326	9	49	10	0	4	6	31	198	N/A	N/A	7	4	6	28	*	31	4	N/A	28
Croissan'wich w/bacon, egg, & cheese	118	353	16	19	23	2	12	8	230	780	N/A	N/A	10	*	23	27	15	14	10	N/A	59
Breakfast Buddy	84	255	11	15	16	8	6	16	127	492	N/A	N/A	5	*	19	17	13	8	10	N/A	56

* Contains less than 2% of the Daily Value of these nutrients.
N/A—not available

Domino's Pizza

(1 serving = 2 slices)

	Serving size (gm)	Calories	Protein (gm)	Carbohydrates (gm)	Fat: Total (gm)	Polyunsaturated fat (gm)	Monounsaturated fat (gm)	Saturated fat (gm)	Cholesterol (mg)	Sodium (mg)	Potassium (mg)	Phosphorus	Vitamin A	Vitamin C	Thiamine	Riboflavin	Niacin	Calcium	Iron	Zinc	% cal from fat
															% Daily Value						
Cheese (2 slices)		376	22	56	10	1	3	6	19	483	N/A	N/A	7	<4	33	25	17	17	13	N/A	24
Pepperoni (2 slices)		460	24	56	18	2	7	9	28	825	N/A	N/A	7	<4	37	24	28	19	15	N/A	35
Sausage/mushroom (2 slices)		430	24	55	16	2	6	8	28	552	N/A	N/A	8	<4	40	30	30	20	17	N/A	33
Veggie (2 slices)		498	31	60	19	2	7	10	36	1035	N/A	N/A	10	<6	39	52	25	39	26	N/A	34
Deluxe (2 slices)		498	27	59	20	2	9	9	40	954	N/A	N/A	9	<5	35	23	35	23	23	N/A	36
Ham (2 slices)		417	23	58	11	1	4	6	26	805	N/A	N/A	4	<4	37	19	28	19	19	N/A	24

N/A—not available

KFC
(Kentucky Fried Chicken)

	Serving size (gm)	Calories	Protein (gm)	Carbohydrates (gm)	Fat: Total (gm)	Polyunsaturated fat (gm)	Monounsaturated fat (gm)	Saturated fat (gm)	Cholesterol (mg)	Sodium (mg)	Potassium (mg)	Phosphorus	Vitamin A	Vitamin C	Thiamine	Riboflavin	Niacin	Calcium	Iron	Zinc	% cal from fat
															% Daily Value						
Original Recipe—wing	53	172	12	5	11	2	6	3	59	383	N/A	N/A	*	*	2	4	15	3	3	N/A	58
center breast	103	260	25	8	14	2	8	4	92	609	N/A	N/A	*	*	5	8	49	3	4	N/A	48
drumstick	57	152	14	3	9	2	5	2	75	269	N/A	N/A	*	*	3	7	13	*	4	N/A	53
Extra Tasty Crispy—wing	57	231	11	8	17	2	10	4	63	319	N/A	N/A	*	*	2	4	15	2	3	N/A	66
center breast	110	344	23	15	21	2	12	5	80	636	N/A	N/A	*	*	5	8	47	2	5	N/A	55
drumstick	68	205	14	7	14	2	8	3	72	292	N/A	N/A	*	*	4	8	17	*	6	N/A	61
Hot & Spicy—wing	62	244	12	9	18	2	10	4	65	459	N/A	N/A	*	*	2	4	16	2	3	N/A	66
center breast	122	382	24	16	25	3	14	6	84	905	N/A	N/A	*	*	7	8	46	2	6	N/A	59
drumstick	70	207	11	10	14	1	8	3	75	406	N/A	N/A	*	*	4	9	16	*	46	N/A	61
Lite 'N Crispy—center breast	86	220	N/A	N/A	12	N/A	N/A	3	57	416	N/A	N/A	N/A	N/A	N/A	N/A	N/A	N/A	N/A	N/A	49
drumstick	47	121	N/A	N/A	7	N/A	N/A	2	51	196	N/A	N/A	N/A	N/A	N/A	N/A	N/A	N/A	N/A	N/A	52
Kentucky nuggets (6)	95	284	16	15	18	2	10	4	66	865	N/A	N/A	*	*	6	7	28	2	4	N/A	57
Buttermilk biscuit (1)	65	235	5	28	12	2	5	3	1	655	N/A	N/A	*	*	16	11	13	10	9	N/A	46
Mashed potatoes & gravy	98	71	2	12	2	—	1	—	<1	339	N/A	N/A	*	*	*	2	6	2	2	N/A	25
Corn-on-the-cob	73	90	3	16	2	1	0	1	<1	11	N/A	N/A	3	2	5	4	5	*	2	N/A	20
Coleslaw	90	114	1	13	6	3	2	1	4	177	N/A	N/A	*	47	2	2	*	3	2	N/A	47

* Contains less than 2% of the Daily Value of these nutrients.
N/A—not available

Jack in the Box

	Serving size (gm)	Calories	Protein (gm)	Carbohydrates (gm)	Fat: Total (gm)	Polyunsaturated fat (gm)	Monounsaturated fat (gm)	Saturated fat (gm)	Cholesterol (mg)	Sodium (mg)	Potassium (mg)	Phosphorus	Vitamin A	Vitamin C	Thiamine	Riboflavin	nNiacin	Calcium	Iron	Zinc	% cal from fat
												% Daily Value									
Breakfast Jack	126	307	18	30	13	2.5	5	5.2	203	871	N/A	N/A	9	*	31	24	15	17	17	N/A	38
Supreme crescent	146	547	20	27	40	7.8	18.9	13.2	178	1053	N/A	N/A	11	*	43	32	21	15	15	N/A	66
Hamburger	96	267	13	28	11	2.0	4.9	4.1	26	556	N/A	N/A	*	*	10	15	10	15	10	N/A	37
Double cheeseburger	149	467	21	33	27	3.1	11.6	12.3	72	842	N/A	N/A	8	*	10	20	30	40	15	N/A	52
Jumbo Jack	222	584	26	42	34	8	13	11	73	733	N/A	N/A	*	*	24	17	9	14	17	N/A	52
Bacon bacon cheeseburger	242	705	35	41	45	8.7	15.7	14.9	113	1240	N/A	N/A	7	13	16	28	44	25	28	N/A	57
Chicken Fajita Pita (1)	189	292	24	29	8	1.4	3.6	2.9	34	703	N/A	N/A	10	*	50	10	30	25	15	N/A	25
Chicken supreme	245	641	27	47	39	11.4	14.8	10	85	1470	N/A	N/A	8	10	26	19	55	24	16	N/A	55
Fish supreme	218	510	24	44	27	7.7	11.4	6.1	55	1040	N/A	N/A	*	9	26	14	21	16	15	N/A	48
Taco salad	402	503	34	28	31	1.6	11.9	13.4	92	1600	N/A	N/A	27	15	19	31	29	41	21	N/A	55
Egg rolls—3 piece	165	437	3	54	24	2.6	12.5	6.8	29	957	N/A	N/A	*	6	39	19	30	8	20	N/A	49
Chicken strips—4 piece	112	285	25	18	13	.7	7.9	3.1	52	695	N/A	N/A	*	*	7	7	56	*	4	N/A	41
Taquitos—5 piece	134	362	15	42	15	1.8	8.4	3.3	24	462	N/A	N/A	*	3	6	7	11	15	15	N/A	37
Seasoned curly fries	109	358	5	3	20	.5	13.3	4.7	0	1030	N/A	N/A	*	9	11	6	15	3	9	N/A	50
Onion rings	103	380	5	38	23	.9	15.2	5.5	0	451	N/A	N/A	*	5	19	10	13	3	12	N/A	54
Chocolate milkshake	322	330	11	55	7	<1	2.1	4.3	25	270	N/A	N/A	*	*	10	35	2	35	4	N/A	19

* Contains less than 2% of the Daily Value of these nutrients.
N/A—not available

McDonald's

	Serving size (gm)	Calories	Protein (gm)	Carbohydrates (gm)	Fat: Total (gm)	Polyunsaturated fat (gm)	Monounsaturated fat (gm)	Saturated fat (gm)	Cholesterol (mg)	Sodium (mg)	Potassium (mg)	Phosphorus	Vitamin A	Vitamin C	Thiamine	Riboflavin	Niacin	Calcium	Iron	Zinc	% cal from fat
												% Daily Value									
Cheeseburger	116	305	15	30	13	1	7	5	50	725	N/A	N/A	8	4	20	15	20	20	15	N/A	38
QuarterPounder®	166	410	23	34	20	1	11	8	85	645	N/A	N/A	4	6	25	15	35	15	20	N/A	44
McLean Deluxe™	206	320	22	35	10	1	5	4	60	670	N/A	N/A	10	10	25	20	35	15	20	N/A	28
Big Mac®	215	500	25	42	26	1	16	9	100	890	N/A	N/A	6	2	30	25	35	25	20	N/A	47
Filet-O-Fish®	141	370	14	38	18	6	8	4	50	730	N/A	N/A	2	*	20	8	45	15	10	N/A	44
McChicken®	187	415	19	39	20	7	9	4	50	830	N/A	N/A	2	4	60	10	45	15	15	N/A	43
Chicken fajitas	82	185	11	20	8	3	3	2	35	310	N/A	N/A	2	8	10	10	20	8	4	N/A	39
Medium french fries	97	320	4	36	17	1.5	12	3.5	0	150	N/A	N/A	*	20	15	*	15	*	4	N/A	48
Chicken McNuggets® 6 pce		270	20	17	15	1.5	10	3.5	55	580	N/A	N/A	*	*	8	8	40	*	6	N/A	50
Chef salad	265	170	17	8	9	1	4	4	111	400	N/A	N/A	100	35	20	15	20	15	8	N/A	48
Chunky chicken salad	255	150	25	7	4	1	2	1	78	230	N/A	N/A	170	45	15	10	45	4	6	N/A	24
Egg McMuffin	135	280	18	28	11	1	6	4	235	710	N/A	N/A	10	*	30	20	20	25	15	N/A	35
Bacon, egg & cheese biscuit	153	440	15	33	26	2	16	8	240	1215	N/A	N/A	10	*	25	20	10	20	15	N/A	53
Breakfast burrito	105	280	12	21	17	7	6	4	135	580	N/A	N/A	10	10	20	15	10	10	8	N/A	55
Chocolate lowfat milkshake	323	320	11	66	1.7	0.1	0.9	0.7	10	240	N/A	N/A	6	*	8	30	2	35	*	N/A	5

* Contains less than 2% of the Daily Value of these nutrients.
N/A—not available

Taco Bell

N/A—not available

	Serving size (gm)	Calories	Protein (gm)	Carbohydrates (gm)	Fat: Total (gm)	Polyunsaturated fat (gm)	Monounsaturated fat (gm)	Saturated fat (gm)	Cholesterol (mg)	Sodium (mg)	Potassium (mg)	Phosphorus	Vitamin A	Vitamin C	Thiamine	Riboflavin	Niacin	Calcium	Iron	Zinc	% cal from fat
												(% Daily Value)									
Taco	78	183	10	11	11	1	N/A	5	32	276	159	N/A	7	2	3	8	6	8	6	N/A	54
Soft taco	92	225	12	18	12	1	N/A	5	32	554	196	N/A	4	2	26	13	14	12	13	N/A	48
Tostada w/red sauce	156	243	9	27	11	1	N/A	4	16	596	401	N/A	13	75	4	10	3	18	9	N/A	41
Chicken soft taco	107	213	14	19	10	2	N/A	4	52	615	233	N/A	4	4	13	13	17	8	35	N/A	42
Taco supreme	92	230	11	12	15	1	N/A	8	32	276	205	N/A	11	5	4	10	6	11	6	N/A	59
Bean burrito w/red sauce	206	357	15	63	14	2	N/A	4	9	1148	495	N/A	7	88	27	117	14	19	21	N/A	35
Burrito supreme w/red sauce	255	503	20	55	22	2	N/A	8	33	1181	501	N/A	18	43	29	123	18	19	22	N/A	39
Fiesta bean burrito	114	226	8	29	9	1	N/A	3	9	652	307	N/A	5	57	12	13	11	15	15	N/A	35
Nachos Bell Grande	287	649	22	61	35	3	N/A	12	36	997	674	N/A	23	96	7	20	11	30	19	N/A	48
Chicken MexiMelt	107	257	14	19	15	2	N/A	7	48	779	150	N/A	10	4	12	14	7	22	20	N/A	53
Mexican pizza	223	575	21	40	37	10	N/A	11	52	1031	408	N/A	20	51	21	19	19	26	21	N/A	58
Taco salad	575	905	34	55	61	12	N/A	19	80	910	673	N/A	33	125	33	33	24	32	33	N/A	61
Light taco	78	140	12	11	5	N/A	N/A	1.5	20	290	N/A	N/A	6	0	N/A	N/A	N/A	8	0	N/A	36
Light soft taco	99	180	13	19	5	N/A	N/A	2.5	25	550	N/A	N/A	4	0	N/A	N/A	N/A	4	6	N/A	28
Light taco supreme	106	160	13	14	5	N/A	N/A	1.5	20	340	N/A	N/A	10	4	N/A	N/A	N/A	8	0	N/A	31
Light soft taco supreme	128	200	14	23	5	N/A	N/A	2.5	25	610	N/A	N/A	10	4	N/A	N/A	N/A	4	6	N/A	25

N/A—not available

Wendy's

	Serving size (gm)	Calories	Protein (gm)	Carbohydrates (gm)	Fat: Total (gm)	Polyunsaturated fat (gm)	Monounsaturated fat (gm)	Saturated fat (gm)	Cholesterol (mg)	Sodium (mg)	Potassium (mg)	Phosphorus	Vitamin A	Vitamin C	Thiamine	Riboflavin	Niacin	Calcium	Iron	Zinc	% cal from fat
												(% Daily Value)									
Single with everything	210	420	25	35	21	2.1	7.3	5.5	70	890	430	N/A	5	15	25	10	35	10	30	N/A	45
Wendy's Big Classic	260	570	27	47	33	2.5	7.4	5.6	80	1085	525	N/A	10	20	30	15	35	15	35	N/A	52
Jr. hamburger	111	260	15	33	9.0	1.9	4.0	3.0	35	570	215	N/A	2	4	25	10	20	10	20	N/A	31
Jr. bacon cheeseburger	155	430	22	33	25	2.7	6.9	5.2	50	840	290	N/A	2	15	30	50	25	10	20	N/A	52
Grilled chicken sandwich	175	320	24	37	9	6.9	3.0	2.2	60	815	340	N/A	2	8	30	15	50	10	25	N/A	25
Fish fillet sandwich	170	460	18	42	25	10	9.6	4.7	50	780	320	N/A	2	2	40	25	20	10	15	N/A	49
Country fried steak sandwich	145	440	14	45	25	4.3	7.6	5.7	35	870	215	N/A	2	2	30	15	25	10	20	N/A	51
French fries (small)	91	240	3	33	12	.77	7.98	2.5	0	145	510	N/A	*	10	10	2	10	*	4	N/A	45
Crispy chicken nuggets (6)	93	280	14	12	20	3.8	9.6	4.5	50	600	200	N/A	*	*	6	6	30	*	4	N/A	64
Chili and cheese	403	500	15	71	18	3.3	3.30	4.0	25	630	1270	N/A	15	60	20	100	25	8	28	N/A	32
Salad Dressing — Blue Cheese (2oz. packet)	54	324	<1	<1	36	22.14	N/A	6.84	36	378	36	N/A	*	*	*	*	*	*		N/A	100
Garden salad	231	70	4	9	2	.23	0	0	0	60	500	N/A	110	70	10	10	6	10	8	N/A	26
Taco salad	490	530	27	55	23	.27	.03	.07	35	825	800	N/A	30	40	20	35	15	40	30	N/A	39
Frosty dairy dessert (small)	243	340	9	57	10	.39	2.58	5	40	200	625	N/A	8	*	8	50	2	30	6	N/A	26

* Contains less than 2% of the Daily Value of these nutrients.
N/A—not available

10

Weight Management

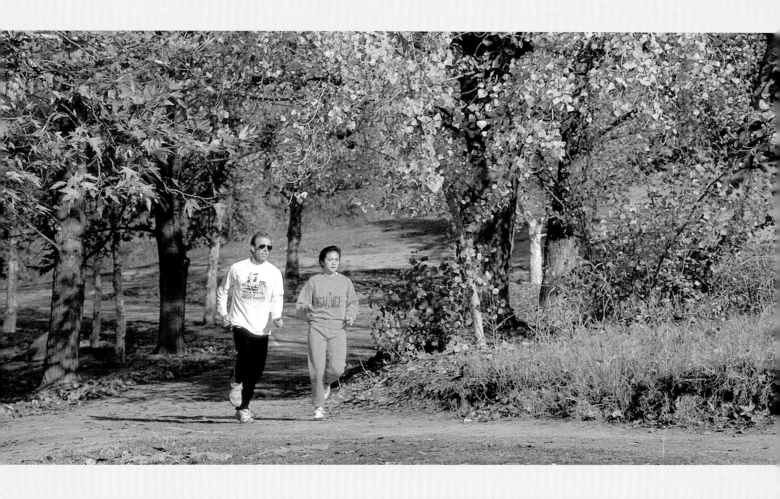

CONTENTS

There is a "secret" to weight management: Maintain a moderate level of total calories, minimize fat calories, and get lots of exercise. Unfortunately, this simple formula is not as exciting as the latest fad diet or the "scientific breakthrough" that promises slimness without effort. If only calories didn't count, or exercising just a few minutes a day could produce a beautifully proportioned body, then the continuing stream of diet books, special programs, dietary supplements, and medical procedures for weight loss that assault the American public year after year might disappear. **Obesity** would not be the public health problem or the personal agony that it is for so many. Fad diets and promises of being able to get something for nothing are the fool's gold of weight control.

Yet more and more Americans are going on diets. At any given time, more than one-third of the American public is engaged in dieting behavior. Research shows that many girls start dieting during adolescence and that the rate of dieting reaches 60 percent or more during the college years. Males too are getting caught up in the dieting craze. Furthermore, this bad habit is taking hold at younger and younger ages; many have started dieting in high school or even grade school. Twenty-two percent of tenth-grade girls reported frequent dieting, and another 10 percent engaged in fasts. There have even been reports of failure to thrive—a syndrome involving undernourishment and retarded growth—in infants whose affluent parents put their babies on a diet, mistakenly thinking this would reduce their child's risk of later obesity! Yet, despite all the concern about body weight, the prevalence of obesity is increasing.

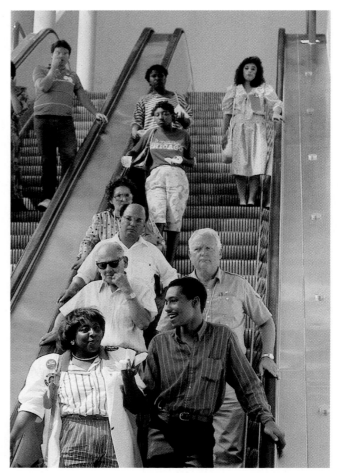

The typical American lifestyle does not lead naturally to healthy weight management. Labor-saving devices such as escalators help reinforce our sedentary habits.

LIFESTYLE AND WEIGHT

At the turn of the century, Americans consumed a diet very different from that of the 1990s, and they got much more exercise. Americans today actually eat somewhat fewer calories overall (down about 3 percent), but they eat more fat and more refined sugars and fewer complex carbohydrates. Since 1910, the percentage of calories consumed from fat increased from 32 percent to 34 percent, while that from complex carbohydrates—vegetables, grains, rice, legumes, and pasta—declined from 38 percent to 24 percent. Eating foods high in fat and refined sugar, usually in the form of candy, ice cream, cookies, and pastries, is a favorite modern way of coping with stress. Fats and simple sugars make up nearly 60 percent of all calories consumed in the 1990s. In large part, these changes reflect the trend toward more processed foods and away from fresh, unprocessed foods and complex carbohydrates.

Despite the increased interest in fitness during recent years, Americans today get far less exercise than did their great-grandparents. In earlier times, people walked or rode bicycles more often than they drove. Most worked on farms or did manual labor. They were able to eat more and weigh less because they didn't have the dubious benefits of labor-saving devices. Daily energy expenditure has decreased over the past 200 years as our nation has changed from an agricultural, to an industrial, and now to an information economy. Fewer and fewer people have jobs that require strenuous physical labor. From 1965 to 1977 alone, daily energy expenditure was thought to have dropped by 200 calories a day—due largely to automobiles, remote control devices for television and garage doors, and a host of electrical appliances that do our work for us.

People from other countries often deplore the prevalence of obesity in this country. Financially, most Americans can afford to eat more meat than can people in the rest of the world, who still consume mostly complex carbohydrates. Gasoline here is cheap in comparison to its cost elsewhere, and most Americans view automobiles as a necessity. American cities are not particularly safe for walking or riding bicycles, which are still the primary means of transportation for most people in the world. The

It's easier to incorporate small switches and substitutions in your eating habits than to initiate radical changes. These simple suggestions for a more healthful diet can reduce your fat and calorie intake considerably while still satisfying your appetite. To put these numbers in perspective, if you consume 2,000 calories a day, you should eat no more than about 66 grams of fat—that way fat will contribute less than 30% of your daily calories.

Instead of Eating	Substitute	To Save*
1 croissant	1 plain bagel	35 calories, 10 grams fat
1 whole egg	1 egg white	65 calories, 6 grams fat
1 oz. cheddar cheese	1 oz. part-skim mozzarella	35 calories, 4 grams fat
1 oz. cream cheese	1 oz. cottage cheese (1% fat)	74 calories, 9 grams fat
1 T whipping cream	1 T evaporated skim milk, whipped	32 calories, 5 grams fat
3.5 oz. lamb chop, untrimmed, broiled	3.5 oz. lean leg of lamb, trimmed, broiled	219 calories, 28 grams fat
3.5 oz. pork spare ribs, cooked	3.5 oz. lean pork loin, trimmed, broiled	157 calories, 17 grams fat
1 oz. regular bacon, cooked	1 oz. Canadian bacon, cooked	111 calories, 12 grams fat
1 oz. hard salami	1 oz. extra-lean roasted ham	75 calories, 8 grams fat
1 beef frankfurter	1 chicken frankfurter	67 calories, 8 grams fat
3 oz. oil-packed tuna, light	3 oz. water-packed tuna, light	60 calories, 6 grams fat
1 regular-size serving fast-food French fries	1 medium-sized baked potato	125 calories, 11 grams fat
1 oz. potato chips	1 oz. thin pretzels	40 calories, 9 grams fat
1 oz. corn chips	1 oz. plain air-popped popcorn	125 calories, 9 grams fat
1 T sour-cream dip	1 T bottled salsa	20 calories, 3 grams fat
1 glazed doughnut	1 slice angel-food cake	110 calories, 13 grams fat
3 chocolate sandwich cookies	3 fig bar cookies	4 grams fat
1 cup ice cream (premium)	1 cup sorbet	320 calories, 34 grams fat

*The values listed are the most significant savings; smaller differences are not shown. Weights given for meats are edible portions.
Reprinted permission of *University of California at Berkeley Wellness Letter*, P.O. Box 10922, Des Moines, IA 50340.

typical American lifestyle does not naturally promote healthy eating or adequate exercise. And the results of our lifestyle are clear from recent national surveys, which indicate that about 26 percent of Americans are overweight. More women than men are affected, especially African American women. Overweight is also more common among people who have low incomes and people of low educational attainment. The percentage of the American population that is overweight continues to rise. It's no wonder that dieting has practically become an American institution.

More children and adolescents are developing weight problems than ever before. Even so, nearly 80 percent of adolescents arrive at early adulthood with "normal" body weight (that is, neither too fat nor too lean). In fact, many young adults get away with terrible eating and exercise habits and don't develop a weight problem. But as the rapid growth period of adolescence slows, it becomes necessary to adopt a healthy lifestyle in order to maintain normal weight without undue effort. As family and career obligations increase and less time and perhaps motivation

Obesity A serious, prevalent, and chronic health problem affecting 26 percent of the population of the United States. Technically the term means "overfat" and is defined as 20 percent above ideal body weight.

TERMS

are available for other things, living a healthy lifestyle becomes a greater and greater challenge. A good time to develop such a lifestyle is early in adulthood, when healthy habits and behavior patterns have a better chance of taking a firm hold.

ADOPTING A HEALTHY LIFESTYLE

Four factors are crucial to the kind of lifestyle that will naturally yield a healthy body weight: what goes into your mouth, what you do with your body, what goes on in your head, and how you cope with life. In other words, nutrition, physical activity, thinking and emotions, and habits and behavior patterns are the keys to successful maintenance of normal weight. These four factors are discussed in detail in this section.

Nutrition

Too often nutrition is a topic studied in a class on health, and too seldom does it become personally relevant to most people's lives. Knowing about nutrients and a balanced diet may help, but actually making healthy food choices day to day is what really counts. What goes into your mouth directly affects health and body weight. In particular, too much dietary fat and refined sugar can undermine good health in the long run, whereas eating more complex carbohydrates and keeping total calories at a moderate level produces a healthy body weight with little effort.

Fat Most experts agree that the real problem in the American diet is overconsumption of dietary fats. Although no more than 30 percent of total calories (and preferably less) should come from fat, Americans get about 34 percent of their calories from fat sources. (See Chapter 9 for the correct method of calculating the percentage of calories from fat.) Oils, margarine, butter, cream, and lard are almost pure fat. Meat and processed foods such as pastries contain a great deal of "hidden" fat, while nuts, seeds, and avocados are plant sources of fat. Most fat in the American diet comes from fatty red meats, dairy products, and processed foods, including snack foods like potato and corn chips. You can substantially decrease your fat consumption by moving closer to a vegetarian (complex carbohydrate) diet: Eating more fruits, vegetables, grains, and legumes and decreasing overall meat consumption. Learn to substitute leaner choices (fish or poultry without the skin) for high-fat choices such as bacon, sausage, and ribs.

Sugar Some people equate sugar with fatness, even though there is no evidence that fat people consume more sugar than thin people. Sugar is a health problem primarily because it causes tooth decay. Still, for some who are

trying to maintain a reasonable body weight, sugar can be a problem. Sugar is a major component of many favorite foods in the American diet, which are often also high in fat. Ice cream, for example, is 63 percent sugar, 27 percent fat, and only 10 percent protein. An ounce of milk chocolate is 59 percent sugar, 33 percent fat, and 8 percent protein. Under such names as corn syrup, corn sweetener, honey, molasses, fructose, sucrose, and dextrose, sugar is added to processed foods such as breads, crackers, cereals, sauces, salad dressings, fruit-flavored yogurt, soft drinks, and bacon and cured meats.

Protein Americans worry far too much about the protein content of their diet. The typical American eats an average of 70–100 grams of protein every day. An adult male needs only 60 grams of protein a day and an adult female only 45 grams. Special dietary supplements that provide extra protein are totally unnecessary for most people; and, in fact, protein not needed by the body for growth and tissue repair will be stored as body fat. Foods high in protein are often also high in fat.

Complex Carbohydrates People concerned about their weight often eliminate bread, pasta, and potatoes—the starches or "carbs" in the diet—in the mistaken belief that cutting these calories will help control weight. In fact, complex carbohydrates from these sources as well as from fresh vegetables, legumes, and whole grains help maintain proper weight. In contrast to fat calories, which the body can easily convert to body fat, calories from complex carbohydrates actually cost the body calories to digest. Furthermore, eating a large amount of complex carbohydrates makes you feel full. In fact, eating a high-carbohydrate/low-fat diet can even result in weight loss without conscious restriction of calories and without exercise! The real problem in terms of obesity is not eating too many complex carbohydrates, but adding high-fat sauces and toppings to them. Changing the composition of your diet in favor of a higher carbohydrate-to-fat ratio may require retraining your taste buds so that you get used to bread without butter, potatoes without sour cream, and pasta with a vegetable sauce instead of a cream sauce or cheese.

Hunger and Satiety What you put in your mouth also affects your experience of hunger and satiety. One theory says that the brain senses hunger when the blood sugar gets too low and that this sensation triggers eating. The resulting increase in blood sugar presumably produces **satiety**—feelings of fullness. However, blood sugar level varies under normal conditions, and it's not clear exactly how variations in blood sugar affect hunger. Another theory says that low levels of **serotonin** (a neurotransmitter) in the brain are associated with feelings of hunger and high levels with satiety. People who eat a diet high in fat and low in complex carbohydrates tend to have lower than normal levels of serotonin in their brains. Theoretically, eating a diet low in fat and high in complex carbohydrates should help us avoid feelings of hunger.

Most people infer that they're hungry when their stomach growls or when they get the "shakes" from not eating. However, research suggests that many people are unable to recognize stomach contractions as a signal of their hunger. They might confuse anxiety or physiological arousal with feeling hungry. Telling such people to "eat only when hungry" is poor advice. It's better to say, "stop eating when full," since people are much better at knowing when they feel full than when they feel hungry. Unfortunately, many people who know they're full keep eating because the food tastes good. We all need to mentally monitor feelings of fullness and be guided by adequate portion control in order to maintain normal weight.

Eating Habits Equally important to weight control is eating small, frequent meals—three a day or more, plus planned, appropriate snacks if desired. Some people—especially young people on the go—skip breakfast and even lunch, thinking they're saving calories. When they do finally eat, they're often so hungry they can't stop eating for the rest of the night. Gradually their eating pattern gets shifted to later and later in the day, until finally they "can't" eat breakfast in the morning. They're still full from the night before! In addition, waiting to eat until late in the day often results in shopping for a meal on an empty stomach and feeling stressed and fatigued from a day without sufficient body fuel. Insufficient energy contributes to poor performance. Failure to do a job well then leads to feelings of stress. This stress can result in making poor food choices, overeating, and possibly drinking too much alcohol. Eating eventually seems to be an effective means of self-soothing and distraction from problems. This cyclical pattern sets the stage for future problems with food.

A healthier approach is to develop a *structure* to guide eating. This structure involves having a more-or-less regular time for meals. (Weekends and vacations may differ from weekdays.) It also means establishing a set of *decision rules* that guide food choices. These rules indicate what choices are "allowed" for breakfast, lunch, and dinner, when high-fat or high-sugar choices may be indulged in, what are the preferred substitutions for the less healthy choices, and so forth. For example, the rule governing breakfast choices might be, "Choose a sugar-free, high-fiber cereal with nonfat milk most of the time. Once in a while (no more than once a week) a poached or soft-boiled egg is okay. Save pancakes and waffles for special occasions." The decision rule governing dinner entrees might be, "Choose chicken or fish most of the time. Avoid cream sauces. Once in a while if a steak is desired, make it a small fillet or flank steak."

Decreeing some food "off limits" is generally not a good idea. Doing so sets up a struggle to be vigilant and resist the urge to eat that food, but almost everyone eventually succumbs to the forbidden food rather than feel deprived. The guiding principle should be "everything in moderation." If a particular food becomes troublesome, it could be placed off limits temporarily until control over it is regained.

Exercise and Physical Activity

Regular endurance exercise strengthens the heart and cardiovascular system, creates greater endurance and energy, provides a means of managing stress, and helps prevent osteoporosis. Exercise also burns calories and keeps the **metabolism** geared to using food for energy instead of storing calories. And perhaps most importantly, exercise builds lean body mass, which in turn can increase metabolism. People with low metabolic rates are more likely to become overweight than are those with normal or elevated metabolic rates. The greater the amount of fat-free body mass—muscle—the higher the metabolism. Your body burns more calories when your metabolism is more active, meaning you can eat more without necessarily gaining weight.

Research has established that obese people are clearly less physically active than their nonobese peers, and there is universal agreement that increased physical activity plays a critical role in long-term weight management success. Those who say that exercise isn't worthwhile for weight loss because "you have to play volleyball for 32 hours to burn enough calories to lose just one pound of fat" overlook the metabolic boost that results from exercise—and that lasts even beyond the period of exercise.

A well-rounded exercise program that includes endurance exercise, weight training, and activities to promote flexibility, relaxation, and enjoyment is best for wellness and weight management. Moderate endurance exercise, sustained for 45 minutes to an hour, can help you lose body fat and keep it off. The longer the duration of a session of endurance exercise, the more fat you'll burn as fuel. Weight training helps increase or maintain lean body mass during diet-induced weight loss. Because of the important role of lean body mass in metabolism, its maintenance means you'll burn more calories even when you're not exercising. (Women need not fear that weight training will result in weight gain and bulky muscles because females lack the necessary hormones to add muscle bulk easily.)

Satiety Feelings of fullness after eating, perhaps associated with blood sugar levels or with serotonin levels in the brain.

Serotonin A neurotransmitter in the brain that has a calming effect; carbohydrate deprivation causes serotonin depletion.

Metabolism Refers to the sum of all of the vital processes in which energy and nutrients from foods are made available to and utilized by the body.

TERMS

You need to adopt a weight management plan that will last a lifetime. Look through the following list of strategies and adopt those that will be most useful for you.

- When shopping for food, make a list and stick to it. Don't shop when you're hungry. Avoid aisles that contain problem foods.

- When serving food, use a small food scale to measure out portions before putting them on your plate. Serve meals on small plates and in small bowls to help you eat smaller portions without feeling deprived.

- Eat three meals a day; replace impulse snacking with planned, healthy snacks. Drink plenty of water to help fill you up.

- Eat only in specifically designated spots. Remove food from other areas of your house or apartment. When you eat, just eat—don't do anything else, such as read or watch TV.

- Eat more slowly. Pay attention to every bite and enjoy your food. Try putting your fork or spoon down between bites.

- For problem foods, try eating small amounts under controlled conditions. Go out for a scoop of ice cream, for example, rather than buying half a gallon for your freezer.

- If you cook a large meal for friends, send leftovers home with your guests.

- When you eat out, choose a restaurant where you can make healthy food choices. Ask the waiter or waitress not to put bread and butter on the table before the meal; request that sauces and salad dressings be served on the side.

- If you're eating at a friend's, eat a little and leave the rest. Don't eat to be polite; if someone offers you food you don't want, thank the person and decline firmly. To turn down dessert or second helpings, try "No thank you, I've had enough" or "It's delicious, but I'm full."

- Develop strategies for handling stress—go for a walk or use a relaxation technique. Practice positive self-talk.

- Incorporate more physical activity into your life. Begin a fitness program that includes endurance exercise and resistance weight training, ride your bike or walk instead of driving, take the stairs instead of the elevator, and so on.

- Tell family and friends that you're making some changes in your eating and exercise habits. Ask them to be supportive.

Adapted from J. D. Nash. 1986. *Maximize Your Body Potential*. (Menlo Park, Calif.: Bull Publishing).

Living a healthy lifestyle also means taking advantage of routine opportunities to get exercise. Try taking the stairs instead of the elevator, walking or biking instead of driving, and so forth. In the long term, even a small increase in activity level can result in weight loss.

The message about exercise is that regular exercise, maintained throughout life, makes weight management easier. The sooner you establish good habits, the better. The key to success is to make exercise an integral part of the lifestyle you enjoy now and will enjoy in the future. Chapter 11 contains many suggestions for becoming a more active, physically fit person.

Thinking and Emotions

What goes on in your head is the third component of a healthy lifestyle and successful weight management. Research on people who have a weight problem indicates that low self-esteem and the negative emotions that accompany it are significant problems. This low self-esteem often results in part from mentally comparing the actual self to an internally held picture of the "ideal self." The greater the discrepancy, the larger the impact on self-es-

teem and the more likely the presence of negative emotions.

Often our internalized "ideal self" is the result of having adopted perfectionistic goals and beliefs about how we and others "should" be. Examples of such beliefs include, "If I don't do things perfectly, I'm a failure" and "It's terrible if I'm not thin." These irrational beliefs may actually cause stress and emotional disturbance. The remedy is to challenge such beliefs and replace them with more realistic ones.

The beliefs and attitudes you hold give rise to self-talk, an internal dialogue you carry on with yourself about events that happen to and around you. Positive self-talk includes leading yourself through the steps of a job and then praising yourself when it's successfully completed. Negative self-talk takes the form of self-deprecating remarks, self-blame, and angry and guilt-producing comments. Negative self-talk can undermine efforts at self-control and lead to feelings of anxiety and depression.

Your beliefs and self-talk influence how you interpret what happens to you and what you can expect in the future, as well as how you feel and react. A healthy lifestyle is supported by having realistic beliefs and goals and by engaging in positive self-talk and problem-solving efforts.

Coping Strategies

The fourth component of a healthy lifestyle is adequate and appropriate coping strategies for dealing with the stresses and challenges of life. One strategy that some people adopt for coping is eating. (Others use drugs, alcohol, smoking, spending, gambling, and so on, to cope.) So, when boredom presents itself, eating can provide entertainment. Food may be used to alleviate loneliness or as a pickup for fatigue. Eating provides distraction from difficult problems and is a means of punishing the self or others for real or imagined transgressions.

People who lead healthy lifestyles have learned more effective ways to get their needs met. They have learned to communicate assertively and to manage interpersonal conflict effectively and don't shrink from problems or overreact. The person with a healthy lifestyle knows how to create and maintain relationships with others and has a solid network of friends and loved ones. Food is used appropriately—to fuel life's activities and growth and for personal satisfaction, not to manage stress.

Personal Insight Do you sometimes overeat? If so, are you more likely to overeat in certain situations, at certain times of the day, or with particular people? Do you overeat when you're in a particular frame of mind?

A CLOSER LOOK AT BODY WEIGHT

How many times have you or one of your friends said "I'm overweight"? Probably quite a few. But how do you decide whether you or someone else is overweight? At what point does being overweight affect your health? And how much should you weigh?

The answers to these questions are complex. Total body weight—expressed in pounds or kilograms—is the most commonly used measure of overweight. Total body weight can be an indicator of health risks, but a more important measure of the health effects of body weight is the composition of this weight. The human body is composed of lean body mass (bones and teeth, water, muscles, connective and organ tissues) and body fat. The percentage of body fat is of primary concern because too much or too little body fat can have negative effects on health. The location of stored body fat also has health implications.

These three factors—body weight, body composition, and the distribution of body fat—can be measured and evaluated by a variety of means. The results of these assessments can help determine whether people face any increased risks due to their weight or percentage of body fat. Although in common usage we tend to use the terms *overweight* and *obese* very loosely, they actually refer to specific ranges of body weight or body fatness. People who meet the criteria for severe overweight or obesity face additional health risks.

In this section, we review some of the techniques for assessing weight and body composition and then look at the health implications of obesity.

Assessing Your Weight and Body Composition

Several different approaches can be used to assess body weight, body composition, and body fat distribution. Each has advantages and disadvantages that need to be considered.

Height-Weight Tables The most common way to assess total body weight is to refer to a height-weight table. These tables are usually based on mortality statistics from life insurance companies. They give ranges of "ideal," "recommended," or "desirable" weights, adjusted for sex, height, and sometimes frame size.

Most experts agree that these tables have inherent problems. They are based on data that is not representative of the American population; they don't take age into account; and they typically use arbitrary frame size categories. In addition, the ranges of weights recommended in height-weight tables as "healthy" (that is, associated with minimum mortality) are too narrow.

Despite these limitations, the U.S. Food and Drug Administration and the Health and Human Services Department have recently published a new height-weight table (Table 10-1). The table gives a range of suggested weights based on height and age. Both sexes are included in one table; the higher weights in each range generally apply to men, the lower to women.

Underwater Weighing One of the most accurate methods for assessing body composition is *hydrostatic weighing,* or weighing under water. Since the density of fat is different from that of lean tissue, these masses can be estimated by either measuring the amount of water displaced or by comparing the difference between the underwater and the dry weighings.

The range of "normal," healthy values for body fat content in young adults is about 10 to 18 percent for men and 18 to 25 percent for women. The values for women are higher because women need more body fat for certain reproductive functions, including regular menstruation. Individuals who engage in vigorous, regular exercise may have much less body fat. However, too little body fat—less than 8 percent for women or 5 percent for men—can cause health problems, including muscle wasting and fatigue. For women, a very low percentage of body fat is also associated with **amenorrhea** and loss of bone mass.

TABLE 10-1 Guidelines for "Healthy" Weights*

	Suggested Weight (Without Clothes or Shoes)	
Height (ft-in)	19 to 34 Years	35 Years and Over
5-0	97–128	108–138
5-1	101–132	111–143
5-2	104–137	115–148
5-3	107–141	119–152
5-4	111–146	122–157
5-5	114–150	126–162
5-6	118–155	130–167
5-7	121–160	134–172
5-8	125–164	138–178
5-9	129–169	142–183
5-10	132–174	146–188
5-11	136–179	151–194
6-0	140–184	155–199
6-1	144–189	159–205
6-2	148–195	164–210
6-3	152–200	168–216
6-4	156–205	173–222

*Both sexes are combined in one table; the higher weights generally apply to men, the lower to women.

Source: U.S. Department of Health and Human Services. 1990. *Nutrition and Your Health: Dietary Guidelines for Americans* (Washington, D.C.: U.S. Government Printing Office, Home and Garden Bulletin 232).

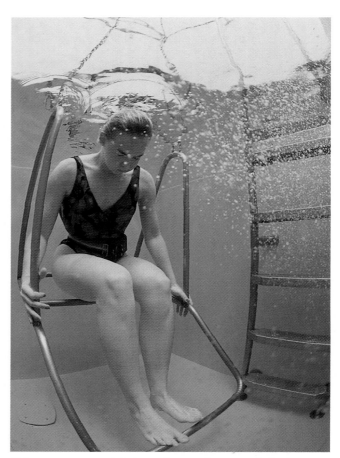

This young woman is being submerged as part of a hydrostatic weighing procedure, one of several methods for measuring the percentage of body weight that is fat. A very high or very low percentage of body fat is associated with health problems.

Skinfold Measurements A more convenient method for determining percentage of body fat is the skinfold thickness technique, which measures the thickness of fat under the skin. A technician grasps a fold of skin at a predetermined location and measures it using an instrument called a caliper. Repeated measurements are taken from several areas of the body, and the results are computed from formulas that predict body fatness from skinfold thickness.

Electrical Impedance Analysis Body fat can also be assessed by the newly popular technique of electrical impedance analysis. Electrodes are attached to the body in several areas, and a harmless electrical current is trans-mitted from electrode to electrode. The electrical conduction through the body favors the path of the lean tissues over the fat tissues. A computer can calculate fat percentage from these current measurements.

Body Mass Index Another approach to determining whether a person is overweight is **body mass index (BMI)**, defined as body weight (in kilograms) divided by the square of height (in meters) or BMI = kg/m^2 (Figure 10-1). BMI correlates highly with direct measures of body fat.

The National Academy of Sciences (NAS) recommends that people between the ages of 19 and 24 maintain a BMI between 19 and 24, with an increase of 1 for each succeeding decade. These lower suggested values for young people reflect the fact that even a small degree of overweight at younger ages is associated with serious health problems and lower life expectancy. For all ages and sexes, a BMI below 19 is considered underweight and unhealthy.

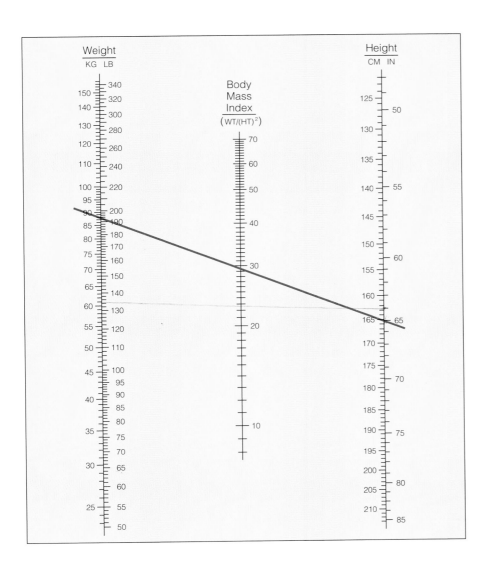

Figure 10-1 *Body mass index (BMI).* To determine your BMI, place a ruler or other straight edge so that it intersects your body weight under the weight column on the left and your height in the height column on the right. Read your BMI where the ruler intersects the center column. For example, the red line shows that a person who weighs 190 pounds and is 65 inches tall has a BMI of 29.5.

Waist-to-Hip Ratio Another approach to assessing overweight and its associated health risks focuses on the distribution of body fat. Fat located in the waist and abdomen is more metabolically active and associated with greater risk of disease and premature death than is fat in the thighs, hips, and buttocks. The higher the ratio of waist to hip measurement, the greater the risk. To determine your ratio, simply measure your waist and hips and then divide the waist measurement by the hip measurement. Ratios of more than 1.0 for men or 0.8 for women suggest elevated risk.

Defining Overweight and Obesity The term **overweight** is usually used in reference to total body weight or body mass index. In terms of height-weight tables—the least accurate approach to body weight assessment—anyone with a body weight above the "healthy" range is considered overweight. In terms of BMI, anyone with a BMI between 27 and 30 is considered overweight, and anyone with a BMI over 30 is considered severely overweight. About 12 percent of Americans have BMI over 30.

Using the body composition approach, researchers have defined obesity as a body-fat content greater than 25 percent of total body weight for males and greater than 30 percent for females. This condition is also termed **overfat**. Using height-weight tables, researchers define obesity as being 20 percent or more above a person's upper limit for weight, adjusted for sex and height (some researchers use 30 percent).

Amenorrhea Absence of menstruation.

Body mass index (BMI) A measure of relative body weight nearly independent of height and correlating highly with more direct measures of body fat. It is calculated by dividing total body weight in kilograms by the square of body height in meters.

Overweight Body weight or body mass index that falls above the range associated with minimum mortality.

Overfat A condition in which a person has more body fat than is considered to be healthy. The amount differs according to gender (females naturally have more body fat than males), race, and ethnicity.

TERMS

Anyone who meets the criteria for overweight or obesity or who has an elevated waist-to-hip ratio faces increased health risks.

A Radical Answer   For most of us, our body weight and percentage of body fat fall somewhere under the levels associated with significant health risks. For us, these assessment tests don't really answer the question, "How much should I weigh?" Height-weight tables, body composition analyses, and BMI and waist-to-hip ratio measurements can best serve as general guides or estimates for body weight. They can't account for individual genetic, racial, or ethnic differences that cause variations from "average" population weights but that may still be healthy. Perhaps it's time for a radical idea: To answer the question of what you "should" weigh, let your lifestyle be your guide. Don't focus on a particular weight as your goal. Focus on living a lifestyle that includes eating moderate amounts of healthful foods, getting plenty of exercise, thinking positively, and learning to cope with stress. Then let the pounds fall where they may. For most people, the result will be close to the recommended weight ranges discussed earlier. For some, their weight will be somewhat higher than societal standards—but right for them. By letting a healthy lifestyle determine your weight, you can avoid the dieting hysteria and fixation on body weight that grips this country.

Health Implications of Obesity

In general, the health risks of obesity increase with its severity, reaching significance when BMI exceeds 27. These risks include higher rates of cardiovascular disease, hypertension, gallbladder disease, and diabetes. Obesity may be associated with a more dangerous blood lipid profile: high levels of triglycerides, total cholesterol, and low-density lipoproteins and low levels of high-density lipoproteins. Obesity is also associated with certain types of cancer, including cancer of the colon, prostate, gallbladder, ovary, endometrium, breast, and cervix. Women who are obese are more likely to suffer from menstrual abnormalities and complications during pregnancy. With more severe obesity, respiratory problems and degenerative joint disease are common.

How dangerous obesity is depends to some extent on where excess fat is located in the body. As mentioned earlier, people who carry their body fat in their trunk and abdomen are at greater risk for health problems than are people who carry fat in their hips, thighs, and buttocks. The risks associated with body fat stored primarily in the midsection include higher rates of heart disease, hypertension, stroke, and diabetes. Men are more likely than women to store excess fat in the midsection and to develop a "beer belly," whether or not they drink alcohol. Women typically store fat in the lower body, but women who exhibit the male pattern of fat distribution face the increased health risks associated with it.

Considerable controversy exists over whether there is a threshold at which the health risks of obesity increase sharply or whether risks from obesity increase in a linear fashion as weight increases. Some argue that being as little as 5 percent overweight elevates risk, but 20 to 30 percent overweight is more commonly seen as the point at which health risks increase significantly.

OVERCOMING A WEIGHT PROBLEM

Why do some people become obese and others remain thin? A variety of factors work together to determine body weight and body fatness, including genetics, metabolism, and lifestyle. But for whatever reasons it occurs, obesity is a problem that requires action.

What Contributes to a Weight Problem?

Although the picture is far from complete, we know that physical factors, as well as psychological, cultural, and social factors, play a significant role in determining body weight. In particular, heredity and metabolism have been linked to a tendency toward obesity.

Genetic Factors and the Environment   Both genetic and environmental factors influence the development of obesity. Genes influence body fat distribution, metabolic rate, and the ease with which weight is gained after overeating. Between 25 and 70 percent of the variance in body mass index among people is estimated to be due to genetics and associated biological factors. In a study of identical twins reared apart, the weights of each pair of twins were found to be very similar. In another study that compared adoptees and their biological parents, the weights of the adoptees were found to be more like those of the biological parents than the adoptive parents. Other research has shown that if both parents are overweight, their children are twice as likely to be overweight as children who have only one overweight parent. All of these studies point to a genetic component in the determination of body weight.

Balanced against the contribution of genetic factors are environmental influences. For example, in a study comparing men born and raised in Ireland with their biological brothers who lived in the United States, the American men were found to weigh on average 6 percent more than their Irish brothers. Presumably, environmental factors like diet and exercise are responsible for this difference in weight. Thus, the tendency to develop obesity may be inherited, but the expression of this tendency is affected by environmental influences.

The message you should take from this research is that genes are not destiny. With increased exercise and decreased food consumption, even those with a genetic ten-

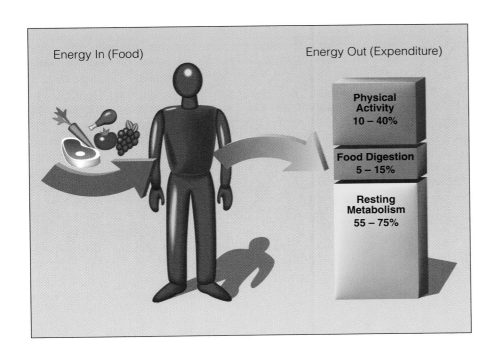

Figure 10-2 *Energy balance equation.* Total energy expenditure in humans is composed of physical activity, digestion, and resting metabolism.

dency toward obesity can maintain a healthy body weight.

Set Point Theory Set point theory holds that body weight, or, more precisely, body fat, is automatically regulated at a relatively constant level, in much the same manner as body temperature and blood pressure. The body "defends" this set point and defeats attempts to change levels of body fat with a variety of compensatory responses, such as increasing or decreasing metabolic rate or feelings of hunger. Proponents of this theory claim that the only way to lower set point is through increased exercise. So far, the operation of a set point has been demonstrated conclusively only in animals. Recent research suggests that if a set point for humans exists, it is probably a range rather than a specific point, and it is probably greatly affected by diet and exercise.

Fat Cell Theory According to fat cell theory, the quantity of fat stored in the body is the result of the number of fat cells that a person has and their size. People with an above-average number of fat cells may have been born with them or may have developed them at certain critical times because of overfeeding. Childhood-onset obesity, or hyperplasia, is thought to be the result of developing too many fat cells. Adult-onset obesity, or hypertrophy, is the result of developing bigger, rather than more, fat cells. Some very obese people are thought to have a combination of both too many fat cells and extraordinarily large fat cells. As the theory goes, having extra fat cells creates a biological pressure to keep these fat cells full. New fat cells

are most likely to develop in response to prolonged overeating when existing fat cells reach the limit of their fat storage capacity. It is unclear whether the number of fat cells can be decreased if weight is kept off for an extended period. More research is needed to determine the actual relevance of fat cell theory to the development and maintenance of obesity in humans.

Metabolism and Energy Balance Metabolism is the sum of all the vital processes in which energy and nutrients from foods are made available to and utilized by the body. The largest component of metabolism, measured as **resting metabolic rate (RMR)**, is the energy required to maintain vital bodily functions, including respiration, temperature regulation, and blood pressure, while the body is at rest. As shown in Figure 10-2, this component of metabolism accounts for 55 to 75 percent of energy used. The energy required to digest food accounts for an additional 5 to 15 percent of daily energy expenditure. The remaining 10 to 40 percent of energy is expended during physical activity; this represents the biggest variable in energy use among people.

Metabolic rate differs from person to person, depending on a variety of genetic and behavioral factors. A higher

Resting metabolic rate (RMR) The energy required to maintain vital bodily functions, including respiration, heart rate, and blood pressure.

percentage of body fat is associated with a lower metabolic rate. Thus, obese people have relatively lower metabolic rates than thin people, partly because thin people dissipate more calories through heat loss. And women, with their larger percentage of body fat, have lower metabolic rates than men.

Recent evidence also suggests that people with a history of weight loss have lower metabolic rates. For example, a man who formerly weighed 165 pounds but who now weighs 150 pounds must eat about 15 percent fewer calories to maintain his new, lower weight than a man who has weighed 150 pounds throughout adult life. Researchers found that among individuals who had lost weight, both RMR and the energy required to perform physical tasks were lowered. The message from this research is that although weight loss can be achieved and maintained, it requires ongoing attention to diet and exercise.

Exercise affects metabolic rate in several ways. When people exercise, they increase their RMR (the number of calories their bodies burn at rest), and they also increase their lean body mass, which is associated with a higher metabolic rate. The exercise itself also burns calories, raising total energy expenditure. The higher a person's energy expenditure, the more the person can eat without gaining weight.

Two factors in the energy balance equation illustrated in Figure 10-2 are under individual control—the amount of energy taken in as food and the number of calories expended through physical activity. Exercise is thus an important part of weight management. Studies have shown that obese adults are less physically active than their average-weight peers. However, this doesn't prove that inactivity causes obesity; it may be that obesity causes inactivity. There is universal agreement, however, that increased physical activity is a critical component of long-term success in weight management.

Weight Cycling

Repeated dieting resulting in cycles of weight loss and weight gain ("yo-yo dieting") has been implicated as being harmful—both to weight management and to overall health. The hypothesis is that cycling increases the body's efficiency at extracting and storing calories from food, making weight loss progressively more difficult with each successive diet. Although some studies have found support for this phenomenon, most have not; and current thinking is that weight cycling probably does not result in increased food efficiency. Some studies have shown a link between weight variability and cardiovascular disease mortality, although it is not clear whether this is actually the result of repeated dieting. Similarly, there is some evidence that weight cycling is associated with altered body fat distribution and increased preference for dietary fat. More research is needed to clarify the effects of weight cycling on weight management and disease mortality.

Eating Habits and Psychological Problems

Although "common sense" suggests that obesity results from overeating, this is a matter of controversy. Studies in the 1970s using self-reports of food intake found no apparent difference between the caloric intakes of obese and nonobese people. More recent studies using different methods have raised serious questions about the accuracy of self-reported caloric intakes and about the findings of the earlier studies. More recent research indicates that approximately 25 to 45 percent of obese people treated in professional hospital and university-based weight control programs report problems with binge eating. Obese binge eaters generally do not compensate for their overeating by purging or exercising. Consuming large amounts of food during binges may be an important factor in the development of obesity for some people.

An important qualification to this finding is that very few obese people seek treatment in such programs, and those that do tend to also report elevated levels of depression and more psychological problems in general. The prevalence of binge eating among obese people who do not participate in such weight control programs is not known. Studies have shown that in general, obese and nonobese individuals do not differ significantly in psychological functioning.

Externality Theory

Externality theory proposes that the obese might be more sensitive to external cues to eat. Researchers looked for evidence that time of day, elapsed time between eating episodes, sight of food, and association of eating with particular cues might account for differences between lean and obese people. Environmental cues *are* intimately linked to eating behavior, but this was found to be true for people in every weight category. Overweight people on the average are more responsive than lean people to food cues in the environment, but many people of normal weight are too.

Lifestyle and Weight

Most weight problems are in fact lifestyle problems. Researchers have found a strong relationship between socioeconomic status (SES) and obesity, with the prevalence of obesity going down as SES level goes up. One major study found that the rate of obesity in women was 30 percent for the lower SES group, 16 percent for the middle group, and only 5 percent for the higher group. More women are obese at lower SES levels than are men, but men are somewhat more obese at the higher SES levels than are women. These differences may reflect the greater sensitivity and concern for a slim physical appearance among upper SES women. It may also reflect the greater acceptance of obesity among low-income and certain ethnic groups, as well as different cultural values related to food choices.

In addition to poor nutrition and lack of adequate exercise, an unhealthy lifestyle is characterized by too many obligations and too few rewards. Sometimes the seeds of an unhealthy lifestyle are planted early, in the family of origin. When a family advocates setting high goals for accomplishment, being a perfectionist, putting work first, and not balancing obligations with personal rewards, it establishes the basis for a lifestyle that may support a weight problem.

Social and cultural influences further complicate the picture. Food is used to show friendship and caring; it is part of the social fabric and is involved in celebrations and social gatherings. In our society, eating well and sharing food with friends are highly valued activities. Food is a symbol of love and caring.

> *Personal Insight*   What do you recall about your family's eating habits as you were growing up? Were certain foods given as a reward or withheld as a punishment? Were you encouraged to always "clean your plate"? How have these family eating habits affected your attitudes toward food and your current eating behavior?

Do Diets Work?

The 1990s are taking shape as the anti-dieting decade. Popular books proclaim that diets don't work, and anti-dieting books are outselling the latest diet books. Feminist writers argue that the beauty ideal advocated by society, and dietary efforts that try to attain this ideal, constitute the continued oppression of women. Advocates of self-acceptance are critical of attempts to treat obesity. And commercial weight loss programs have come under unprecedented scrutiny by government regulators. The central issue is, do diets work?

The popular press states that 95 percent of all diets fail. In fact, this frequently cited figure is based on descriptive data from a 30-year-old study of overweight people who enrolled in a hospital nutrition clinic. A recent survey of more than 20,000 readers of *Consumer Reports* found that of those who reported losing a significant amount of weight and maintaining the loss, 72 percent had done so on their own and only 5 percent had ever enrolled in a hospital-based program. (Most used a diet of their own invention, a diet from a book or magazine, or joined an exercise program or a commercial diet or self-help program.) Clearly, data from hospital-based programs should not be used as a basis for concluding that diets don't work for most people.

In fact, not all diets fail. Several programs that combine very low calorie diets with intensive education and behavior modification have reported good long-term results. Significant weight losses have also been reported in population and community studies and in studies of professional programs. The programs most likely to produce good results involved comprehensive behavioral treatment including a combination of behavior modification, a special diet, and an exercise program.

If diets do work, at least sometimes, for whom do they work? Little is known about people who diet on their own. Even less is known about those who are not obese but who diet in order to maintain normal weight. Two recent surveys found that nonobese individuals who had dieted reported losses of 8–12 pounds for their most recent effort. Does such "preventive dieting" actually prevent or delay weight gain, or does it set up conditions for an eventual eating disturbance? Dieting often precedes the development of **eating disorders,** but many individuals diet and don't develop a problem. The general conclusion is that dieting alone is not sufficient to cause an eating disturbance.

It is possible that dieting may be helpful for some people. Clearly, adopting a healthy diet with a moderate intake of calories, especially fat calories, and engaging in regular exercise can be beneficial for everyone. Whether more stringent dieting should be undertaken is a question of balancing risks and benefits. The prevailing wisdom is that those with marked obesity can reduce health risks by losing weight—provided that effective treatment programs that also address issues such as binge eating and depression are available and utilized.

For people of normal weight, excessive concern about dieting can set the stage for future problems. Dieting is a complex issue in children and adolescents, in whom growth, physical maturation, self-concept, body image, and peer relationships change rapidly. Young people who are overweight may need assistance and treatment in order to prevent obesity as well as future health problems. Normal weight or underweight young people should avoid overconcern about weight or preoccupation with shape. Accepting one's body, rather than undertaking a relentless pursuit of an unrealistic ideal, is important for the health and well-being of all people.

Hazards and Rewards in the Search for the "Perfect" Body

The American focus on attaining a perfect body has prompted a flood of weight loss programs, fad diets, health clubs, exercise equipment, appetite-reducing medicines, and books on diet, nutrition, and fitness. Presumably, with the right combination of programs, exercise, and eating plans, one can attain the promised rewards of a healthier, slimmer, fitter, more aesthetically appealing body.

Eating disorder   Any of a number of disorders characterized by gross disturbances in eating or eating-related behaviors.

TERMS

Despite the recent growth of an anti-dieting movement, dieting is part of the American way of life. Data from two large national surveys indicate that about 24 percent of men and 40 percent of women are currently dieting. The rates are even higher among young people. Chronic dieting among teenagers can lead to retardation of physical growth, menstrual irregularities, and possibly to the development of eating disorders.

During adolescence, both boys and girls become sensitive about their size and physical appearance. Studies have consistently shown a high prevalence of dissatisfaction with body weight or shape among male and female adolescents. The cultural pressure to be thin, especially for female adolescents, coupled with the social stigma of obesity, may well predispose weight-conscious youth to dieting, abnormal eating patterns, and eating disorders.

Setting large weight loss goals in response to cultural ideals of attractiveness can set people up for failure and psychological distress. Dieters may suffer from depression, persistent irritability, inability to concentrate, sleep difficulties, and preoccupation with food and weight. When they fail to attain their goal of thinness, they may feel they're weak or suffer from a character flaw. Such ideas can undermine their chances of developing a truly healthy lifestyle, one that will allow them to maintain a reasonable body weight easily and naturally.

Smaller weight loss goals are much more realistic and can have very beneficial effects. For an obese person, losing as little as 10 pounds can reduce blood pressure as much as antihypertensive medication. People participating in behavioral weight loss programs tend to experience improvement in mood.

Obesity *is* a serious health risk, but weight management needs to take place in a positive and realistic atmosphere. The hazards of excessive dieting and overconcern about body weight need to be countered by a change in attitude about what constitutes the perfect body and a reasonable body weight. The current ideals of ultra-thin and ultra-fit need to change. A reasonable body weight must take into account an individual's weight history, social circumstances, metabolic profile, and psychological well-being.

Personal Insight How do you feel about your body weight, shape, and size? Do you have strong feelings about what an ideal male and female body should look like? Where do you think you've learned these ideals?

Resources for Getting Help

What should you do if you are overweight? Several approaches are possible.

Doing It Yourself Research indicates that people are far more successful than was previously thought at losing

weight and keeping it off. One study found that about 64 percent of the people achieved long-term success without joining a formal program or getting special help. Other researchers investigated the characteristics that distinguished those who lost at least 20 percent of body weight and maintained this loss for two years or more. Virtually all maintained their success by making exercise a permanent part of their lifestyle. They also kept tabs on their weight and habits. In addition, they learned to develop their own diet, exercise, and maintenance plans, and they became more involved in and excited by activities other than eating—such as careers, projects, and special interests.

If you need to lose weight, focus on adopting the healthy lifestyle we've described. The "right" weight for you will naturally evolve, and you won't have to diet. However, if you must diet, do so in combination with exercise, and avoid very-low-calorie diets. Realize that most low-calorie diets cause a rapid loss of body water at first. When this phase passes, weight loss declines. As a result, dieters are often misled into believing that their efforts are not working. They then give up, not realizing that smaller losses later in the diet are actually better than the initial big losses, because later loss is mostly fat loss, whereas initial loss was primarily fluid.

Diet Books Many people who try to lose weight by themselves fall prey to one or more of the dozens of diet books on the market. Although a very few of these do contain useful advice and tips for motivation, most make promises they can't fulfill. Some guidelines for evaluating and choosing a diet book can be offered:

1. Reject books that advocate an unbalanced way of eating. These include books advocating a high-carbohydrate-only diet or those advocating low-carbohydrate/high-protein diets.

2. Reject books that claim to be based on a "scientific breakthrough" or to have the "secret" to success.

3. Reject books that use gimmicks, like combining foods in special ways to achieve weight loss, rotating levels of calories, or purporting that a weight problem is due to food allergies, food sensitivities, or yeast infections.

4. Reject books that promise quick weight loss or limit the selection of foods.

5. Accept books that advocate a balanced approach to diet plus exercise and sound nutrition advice.

Dangerous Do-It-Yourself Options: Dietary Supplements Using commercially available supplements for modified fasting can be a dangerous option, especially if they are the sole source of nutrition, because there is no medical monitoring by a physician. Such approaches include powders used to make shakes that substitute for some or all of the daily food intake, as well as food bars. Many provide fewer than 800 calories a day. Although the

Getting Started on a Sensible Weight Loss Program

Would you like to lose weight on your own? Here are some tips for getting started on a program of weight management that will last a lifetime.

Motivation and Commitment

Make sure you are motivated and committed before you begin. Failure at weight loss is a frustrating experience that can make it more difficult to lose weight in the future. Think about the reasons you want to lose weight. Self-focused reasons, such as to feel good about yourself or to have a greater sense of well-being, are often associated with success. Trying to lose weight for others or out of concern for how others view you is a poor foundation for a weight loss program. Make a list of your reasons for wanting to lose weight and post it in a prominent place.

Creating a Negative Energy Balance

When your weight is constant, you are burning approximately the same number of calories as you are taking in. To tip the energy balance toward weight loss, you must either consume fewer calories or burn more calories through physical activity, or both. One pound of body fat represents 3,500 calories. To lose weight at the recommended rate of one-half to one pound per week, you must create a negative energy balance of 1,750 to 3,500 calories per week or 250 to 500 calories per day. To generate your negative energy balance, it's usually best to begin by increasing your activity level rather than decreasing your calorie consumption.

Increasing Your Level of Physical Activity

Exercise is a crucial component of weight management. You can increase your activity level both by beginning a program of regular exercise and by incorporating more physical activity into your daily routine. Just 30 minutes of moderate walking or cycling can provide a significant contribution—150 calories—toward your daily negative calorie balance; an hour of cycling or slow jogging burns about 500 calories. Chapter 11 has more information about putting together a successful program of regular exercise.

Don't try to use exercise to "spot reduce." Leg lifts, for example, contribute to fat loss only to the extent that they burn calories; they don't burn fat just from your legs. You can make parts of your body appear more fit by exercising them, but the only way you can reduce fat in any specific part of your body is to create an overall negative energy balance.

Making Changes in Your Diet and Eating Habits

If you can't generate a large enough negative calorie balance solely by increasing physical activity, you may want to supplement exercise with small cuts in your calorie intake. Don't think of this as "going on a diet"—your goal is to make small changes in your diet that you can maintain for a lifetime. Focus on cutting your fat intake (refer back to the box on "Eating Smart") and on eating a variety of nutritious foods in moderation. Don't try skipping meals, fasting, or very-low-calorie diets. These strategies seldom work, and they can have negative effects on your ability to manage your weight and on your overall health.

Making changes in eating habits is another important strategy for weight management. If your program centers on conscious restriction of certain food items, you're likely to spend all your time thinking about the forbidden foods. Focus on *how* to eat rather than *what* to eat. Try adopting some of the behaviors listed in the box "Strategies for Managing Your Weight"—you may find that your new eating habits make it much easier for you to achieve and maintain a healthy weight.

---

products available today are much improved over the liquid-protein supplements that contributed to many dieters' deaths in the 1970s, only careful medical evaluation and monitoring can significantly reduce the risk of such an approach. Furthermore, dietary supplements teach reliance on patented products, not on sound, lifelong eating habits. And although weight loss can be rapid, muscle tends to be lost too, and weight is often regained when the supplements are discontinued.

Over-the-Counter Diet Aids   A large number of over-the-counter diet aids are available to those seeking a magic pill to do away with extra pounds. Many of these tout gimmicks, such as exotic-sounding herbs, grapefruit juice extract, and amino acids (L-glutamine, L-arginine), none of which has been proven to affect appetite or weight loss. So far, over 111 ineffective ingredients have been identified as components of various diet aids.

The most common ingredient in diet aids sold in drugstores is *phenylpropanolamine hydrochloride (PPA)*. The Food and Drug Administration (FDA) has declared that PPA is a safe and effective appetite suppressant for weight loss. Though less potent, PPA is similar to amphetamines, a class of drugs available legally only by prescription. It acts as a mild stimulant and suppresses the desire to eat.

Studies on the effectiveness of PPA are contradictory. A recent study found that while PPA was effective in suppressing appetite, the average weight loss of people taking it over a six-week period was only two pounds greater than for those receiving a placebo. Without a conscious effort to reduce calorie intake, increase activity, and change eating behavior, such weight loss is unlikely to be

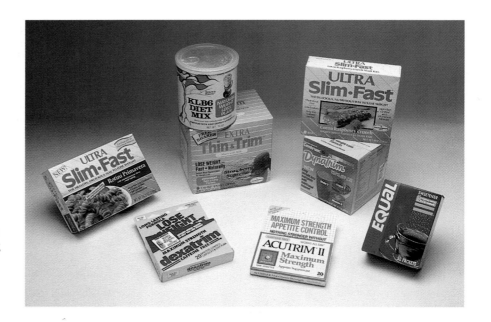

Over-the-counter diet aids such as those shown here can be helpful in controlling hunger and weight in the short term, but they are not a miracle cure. Long-term weight management requires life-long healthy diet and exercise habits.

maintained. Furthermore, there is concern over the safety of PPA because it can cause dizziness, headaches, rapid pulse, palpitations, sleeplessness, and hypertension. Use of PPA is not approved by the FDA for periods longer than 12 weeks.

The second most common ingredient of diet aids sold in drugstores is *fiber.* Oat bran, guar gum, hemicellulose, cellulose, corn bran, pectin, psyllium seed, apple fiber, and lignin have all been promoted as weight-loss aids. Manufacturers claim these work by "swelling in the stomach and absorbing liquids" to provide a feeling of fullness. In fact, dietary fiber acts as a bulking agent in the large intestine, not in the stomach. The FDA has found no data to warrant classifying any type of fiber as an aid in weight control or as an appetite suppressant. Furthermore, most of these products provide a mere 1 to 3 grams of fiber per day, which doesn't contribute much toward the recommended daily intake of 20 to 35 grams. In 1992 the FDA banned guar gum and 110 other ingredients from use in nonprescription diet aids because they had not been proven safe and effective.

The bottom line on over-the-counter diet aids is *caveat emptor*—buyer beware. There is no quick and easy way to lose weight. The most effective answer is to develop healthy diet and exercise habits and to make these part of your lifestyle.

Commercial, Group, and Medical Programs

A variety of options is available if you want help, support, or advice for your weight management program. Different types of programs may work for different individuals, but a little research can help you locate a program that suits your needs and preferences. Many commercial weight

loss programs include counseling sessions, nutrition education, exercise planning, and behavior modification training; they can be expensive, though, and some require purchase of special foods or supplements.

Self-help groups that focus on weight management can offer support and encouragement. Your physician or a registered dietitian can also help you put together a successful weight management program. Many registered dietitians can be found in private practice or conducting weight management programs through hospitals or clinics. For cases of severe obesity, a physician's advice is probably indicated.

Selecting a Weight Reduction Approach

No single approach to weight reduction is appropriate for all individuals, and no one type of program stands above all others. After eliminating those approaches that are dangerous or fraudulent, you will have a number of options. The challenge is to find the one that's best for you.

The first step is to decide how serious your weight problem is. If you are less than 20 percent overweight, you might consider a self-directed approach—cutting back on fat calories and increasing exercise on your own—or reconsidering whether in fact you need to lose weight. Be sure you are pursuing a reasonable weight, given your family history and lifestyle.

If you are 20 to 40 percent overweight, you might consider joining a self-help group, one of the commercial weight loss programs, a behavioral program led by a health professional, or a work site program. More serious degrees of overweight, 40 to 100 percent, may require a more aggressive approach. Consider getting private counseling, joining a hospital-based program, participating in a medically supervised very-low-calorie diet (VLCD) with a maintenance program, or going to a residential program such as Pritikin.

If you are 100 percent or more overweight, or have 100 pounds or more to lose, a medically supervised VLCD should be your first choice. With appropriate pretreatment assessment, open-ended treatment that includes a maintenance program, and the help of a professional staff that includes dietitians, physicians, and psychologists, this approach is effective for about 65 percent of those who participate. Should this approach fail, the most drastic (but often successful) treatment is surgery. Discuss this alternative with your physician.

Once you narrow your options, take into consideration your own needs and preferences. You may prefer a group program to individual care. You may need supervised exercise, while others may be able to exercise on their own. Choosing a program that fits your lifestyle will increase your chances of success.

EATING DISORDERS

Problems with body weight and weight control are not limited to excessive body fat. A growing number of people, especially adolescent girls and young women, experience what are called "eating disorders," characterized by severe disturbances in eating and eating-related behaviors. The major eating disorders are **anorexia nervosa, bulimia nervosa,** and **binge eating disorder.** The essential feature of anorexia and bulimia is a disturbance in the perception of body shape and weight. Anorexia nervosa is characterized by a refusal to maintain a minimally normal body weight. Bulimia nervosa is characterized by re-

peated episodes of binge eating followed by inappropriate compensatory behaviors such as self-induced vomiting, misuse of laxatives or diuretics, fasting, or excessive exercise. Binge eating disorder is characterized by binge eating without any compensatory behaviors. Eating disorders are associated with depression, anxiety, low self-esteem, and increased health risks, including, in some cases, increased risk of premature death.

Western society's emphasis on extreme thinness as the ideal for females places many young women in conflict about their weight. Although the typical woman under the age of 30 has become heavier by 5 or 6 pounds since the 1960s, the "ideal" body—as reflected by winners of the Miss America Pageant and models—has become thinner. This widening gap between reality and ideal is reflected in high rates of body dissatisfaction.

Eating disorders are far more prevalent in industrialized countries than in developing ones. In the United States, eating disorders affect more women than men, more whites than nonwhites, and more younger people (under age 30) than older people. Some studies suggest

TERMS

Anorexia nervosa   An eating disorder characterized by a refusal to eat enough food to maintain normal, healthy body weight and/or the use of measures to produce severe weight loss. Anorexics do experience hunger and appetite but resist the impulse to eat.

Bulimia nervosa   An eating disorder characterized by alternating binging and purging by means of vomiting, laxatives or diuretics, or excessive exercise. Bulimics can be normal weight or overweight.

Binge eating disorder   An eating disorder characterized by uncontrollable urges to eat. People suffering from binge eating disorder are often overweight.

Human bodies come in a tremendous range of sizes and shapes, and people don't have to fit any particular standard to be healthy. Unfortunately, over the last few decades our society has tended to embrace a single ideal, especially for women—slim but fit. The media expose us to this single "right" look relentlessly, and the beauty and fitness industries promise to help us attain it.

As a result, Americans have become preoccupied with their appearance and ever more dissatisfied with their bodies. In 1972, 15 percent of men and 25 percent of women surveyed said that they were dissatisfied with their bodies. In 1987, 34 percent of men and 38 percent of women surveyed expressed dissatisfaction. In a recent survey, only 30 percent of eighth grade girls were content with their bodies, compared to 70 percent of their male classmates. The higher levels of dissatisfaction among women reflect the cultural belief that women's value is largely a function of their physical appearance and that they should strive to be beautiful, slim, and fit. Men are also concerned about appearance, but they are taught that their success doesn't depend solely on their looks.

Research indicates that such detailed attention to physical appearance has a negative effect on self-esteem. We become increasingly critical of ourselves for not attaining the right weight and look. Some people (usually women) who are dissatisfied with their appearance also develop a distorted body image. They look in the mirror and see only "flaws"—areas in which they fail to match the culture's physical ideal. They focus critically on these perceived flaws and then generalize from them to their whole body. They may conclude that their bodies are totally unacceptable and even disgusting, when the truth is that they simply don't conform to the cultural ideal.

These distorted ideas about the body may extend to ideas about the self in general. Our bodies shape our sense of identity because they represent how we appear to the rest of the world. When our body image is distorted, it interferes with a healthy sense of self-worth and can lead to feelings of anxiety and depression, as well as to chronic dieting. It also puts people at risk for developing eating disorders.

Research has shown that people can turn dissatisfaction into satisfaction by learning to perceive their bodies differently. One study attempted to correct body image distortions among young women who were of appropriate weight for their height but thought they were overweight. These women tended to think "globally," applying negative thoughts to their entire body. As part of a six-week therapy program, they learned to view themselves more realistically, replacing negative thoughts with positive ones while looking in the mirror. They also learned to put their supposed flaws in perspective. By the end of the program they had become more confident and comfortable with themselves.

A more sensible approach in the long run is to change our attitudes about our bodies, replacing faultfinding with respect. What our bodies need is moderate exercise, healthy foods, adequate sleep, and opportunities for relaxation. When we treat our bodies better, we feel better about ourselves. Another thing we can do is add interests to our lives besides counting calories and watching the scale. By broadening our roles and activities, we make it clear to ourselves and others that how we look is not the sum of what we are.

How accurate is your own body image? Do you like your body the way it is, or are you caught up in a quest for "the perfect body"? To assess the health of your attitudes toward your body, answer the questions on the questionnaire that follows. If your score indicates that you have a negative body image, you can take steps to change it. Look in the mirror and notice the features you like. "Forgive" those features you're worried about, and view them realistically as only a part of your entire body. When you see idealized standards presented by the beauty and fitness industries, realize that one of their goals is to increase your dissatisfaction with yourself. Most of all, put your concerns about your physical appearance in perspective. Remember, your worth as a human being is not a function of how you look.

---

that eating disorders are more prevalent among people of middle and upper-middle socioeconomic status. Certain occupations also appear to be associated with a higher prevalence of eating disorders; these include modeling, ballet, and some sports, in which professional advancement requires maintenance of very low body weight.

Anorexia Nervosa

A person suffering from anorexia nervosa doesn't eat enough food to maintain a reasonable body weight. Anorexics have an intense fear of gaining weight or becoming fat. Their body image is distorted, so that even when they're emaciated they think they're fat. When confronted about being dangerously thin, anorexics often respond with disbelief. Their entire sense of self-worth is tied up in their evaluation of their body shape and weight.

Anorexics may engage in compulsive behaviors or rituals that help keep them from eating, though some anorexics also binge eat. They commonly use vigorous and prolonged physical activity to reduce body weight as well. Anorexics are often introverted, emotionally reserved, and socially insecure. They tend to favor health foods, be obsessive about health issues, and prepare meals for others without eating them themselves.

Anorexia affects between 1 and 3 million Americans, mostly women. It's been estimated that 1 percent of pre-college girls have some form of anorexia nervosa.

Assessing Your Body Image

		Never	Some-times	Often	Always
1.	I dislike seeing myself in mirrors.	0	1	(2)	3
2.	When I shop for clothing, I am more aware of my weight problem, and consequently I find shopping for clothes somewhat unpleasant.	0	(1)	2	3
3.	I'm ashamed to be seen in public.	(0)	1	2	3
4.	I prefer to avoid engaging in sports or public exercise because of my appearance.	0	(1)	2	3
5.	I feel somewhat embarrassed about my body in the presence of someone of the opposite sex.	0	(1)	2	3
6.	I think my body is ugly.	0	1	(2)	3
7.	I feel that other people must think my body is unattractive.	0	1	(2)	3
8.	I feel that my family or friends may be embarrassed to be seen with me.	(0)	1	2	3
9.	I find myself comparing myself with other people to see if they are heavier than I am.	0	1	2	(3)
10.	I find it difficult to enjoy activities because I am self-conscious about my physical appearance.	0	(1)	2	3
11.	Feeling guilty about my weight problem preoccupies most of my thinking.	0	1	(2)	3
12.	My thoughts about my body and physical appearance are negative and self-critical.	0	1	(2)	3

Now, add up the number of points you have circled in each column: _____   0 + _4_ + _10_ + _3_

= 17

Score Interpretation

The lowest possible score is 0, and this indicates a positive body image. The highest possible score is 36, and this indicates an unhealthy body image. A score higher than 14 suggests a need to develop a healthier body image.

Adapted from "Emancipation from Emaciation." 1994. *Harvard Women's Health Watch,* August; J. Rodin. 1992. "Body mania." *Psychology Today,* January/February; and C. Sacra. 1990. "Mirror images." *Health,* March. Questionnaire used with permission. J. D. Nash. 1986. *Maximize Your Body Potential* (Palo Alto, Calif.: Bull Publishing).

Health Risks of Anorexia Nervosa   Because of extreme weight loss, the anorexic is likely to stop menstruating, become intolerant of cold, and develop low blood pressure and heart rate. Anorexics develop dry skin that is often covered by fine, neonatal-like body hair called lanugo. Their hands and feet may swell and take on a blue color.

Anorexia nervosa has been linked to a variety of medical complications, including dental problems and disorders of the cardiovascular, gastrointestinal, and endocrine systems. When body fat is virtually gone and muscles are severely wasted, the body turns to its own organs in a desperate search for protein. Death can occur from heart failure caused by electrolyte imbalances. As many as 18 percent of patients with anorexia nervosa die of complications related to the disorder. Depression is also a serious risk, and about half the fatalities due to anorexia are from suicide.

Treatment of Anorexia Nervosa   The physical and psychological aspects of anorexia must be addressed in treatment. The crucial first step is to restore body weight as much as possible. This usually has to be done in a specialized inpatient setting because anorexics tend to cling to their unrealistic beliefs and resist treatment. While controversial, drugs may be included as part of the treatment.

Psychotherapy for anorexia includes education, behavior modification, and changing maladaptive patterns of thinking. Anorexics need to learn about the physical risks of self-starvation and the importance of healthy eating habits. They have to adopt habits that will allow them to regain and sustain a healthy weight. They have to change their irrational thinking, learn to tolerate imperfection in themselves, and gain some perspective on the arbitrary cultural standard of thinness.

Bulimia Nervosa

Bulimia nervosa is characterized by recurring episodes of binge eating (consuming a huge amount of food in a discrete period of time) followed by purging. During a binge, bulimics feel that they can't stop eating or control what or how much they eat. To compensate for the binge, bulimics induce vomiting and/or use laxatives or diuretics. They may also use strict dieting, fasting, or vigorous exercise to maintain normal weight. Bulimics may binge up to 20 to 30 times per day, consuming over 6,000 calories in 24 hours. Bulimia can be difficult to recognize because bulimics conceal their eating habits and usually maintain normal weight.

Like anorexics, bulimics have a morbid fear of becoming fat, and they base their sense of self-worth on their body shape and weight. Bulimics are typically more socially outgoing than anorexics—and more socially deviant. Bulimics are more likely to smoke and to abuse alcohol and other drugs. They tend to prefer junk food to health food. Bulimics also tend to have fluctuating moods that vary from persistent fatigue and depression to feelings of agitation accompanied by impulsive behaviors. They often have a strong need for social approval. Bulimics place high demands on themselves but have few strategies for coping with stress.

Restrictive eating and purging are attempts made by bulimics to control their bodies and, by extension, their surroundings. Many bulimics have been in relationships (family and interpersonal) that were unpredictable, where they didn't feel safe. The binge-purge cycle has the quality of a ritual: Bulimics are able to plan, follow through, and predict how they will feel during and after the bulimic episode. The sense of security and control the bingeing and purging brings is what reinforces and perpetuates the behavior.

Among college women, the incidence of bulimia has variously been reported to range from 2 to 19 percent. In a sample of 18- to 30-year-olds in the general population, 3 to 4 percent of women were reported to have bulimia. The number of women who occasionally engage in bulimic behaviors, but don't develop the disorder, may be as high as 14 percent.

Health Risks of Bulimia Nervosa   The binge-purge cycle of bulimia places a tremendous strain on the body and can have serious health effects. Contact with vomited stomach acids erodes tooth enamel. Bulimics often develop dental caries because they binge on foods that contain large amounts of simple sugars. Repeated vomiting or the use of laxatives, in combination with deficient calorie intake, can damage the liver and kidneys and cause cardiac arrhythmia. Chronic hoarseness and esophageal tearing with bleeding may also result from vomiting. More rarely, binge eating can lead to rupture of the stomach. Although many bulimics maintain normal weight, even small amounts of weight loss to a lower-than-normal weight can cause menstrual problems. And although less often associated with suicide or premature death than is anorexia, bulimia is associated with increased depression, excessive preoccupation with food and body image, and sometimes disturbances in intellectual functioning.

Treatment of Bulimia Nervosa   The symptom that usually brings bulimics into treatment is vomiting, which they often find shameful and distressing. The treatment for bulimia is similar to that of anorexia. Bulimics need to learn about nutrition, the physiology of body weight, and the dangers of their method of weight control. They need to adopt a regular pattern of eating meals and snacks and learn to use moderation rather than restriction in choosing foods. Cognitive techniques for combating bulimia include substituting coping thoughts for anxiety-producing ones and challenging dysfunctional attitudes about food and weight. Antidepressant drugs can be used in cases of depression.

Binge Eating Disorder

Binge eating disorder is a newly recognized eating disorder. The symptoms of this disorder are the same as those of bulimia nervosa, except that the purging behavior does not occur. In addition, loss of control is indicated by the presence of at least three of the following symptoms:

- Eating more rapidly than normal
- Eating until feeling uncomfortably full
- Eating large amounts of food when not feeling physically hungry
- Eating large amounts of food throughout the day with no planned mealtimes
- Eating alone because of being embarrassed by how much one is eating
- Feeling disgusted with oneself, depressed, or very guilty after overeating

A person with binge eating disorder is often overweight; dieters seem to be most susceptible to the disorder. There is evidence that between 25 and 45 percent of obese dieters, most of whom are women, may have binge eating disorder. Whether overweight or normal weight, bingers report more negative moods and emotional disturbances than nonbingers. The binge eater is likely to engage in obsessive thinking and frequently experience anxiety, self-doubt, and guilt.

Health Risks of Binge Eating Disorder The health risks of compulsive binge eating without purging are not as well documented as those associated with anorexia or bulimia. Since most people with the disorder are obese, they face all the health risks associated with obesity. In addition, obese bingers are more likely than nonbingers to experience negative moods and emotional distress, especially depression.

Treatment of Binge Eating Disorder Treatments are just beginning to be developed for binge eating disorders. Obese bingers are more likely to drop out of any kind of obesity treatment than are nonbinging dieters. Thus a primary objective for successful treatment is to find ways to keep bingers in treatment. Bingers need to develop more effective ways to cope with their emotions and to recover from relapses in their weight management programs. Another useful strategy is to develop patterns of positive self-talk directed at reaching goals.

When You or Someone You Know Needs Help . . .

How can you tell if you or someone you know needs help? Begin by taking the self-test in the box "In Quest of the Perfect Body." A score of 14 or above indicates that you have a level of body dissatisfaction that may place you at risk for an eating disorder. If you think you may have an eating disorder or be at risk for developing one, contact a psychologist or other licensed therapist who specializes in this kind of problem. For further information, contact the National Association of Anorexia Nervosa and Associated Disorders (708-831-3438). You can help others by learning to recognize the symptoms that suggest the existence of an eating disorder:

- Looking underweight or wearing baggy clothes all of the time
- Not eating in front of others or toying with food
- Disappearing for a while after eating
- Smelling like he or she has vomited
- Exhibiting hyperactivity with no apparent fatigue
- Showing agitated behavior or disorganized thinking
- Complaining of abdominal discomfort
- Complaining of feeling fat but looking normal or even underweight

If more than a few of these signs are present, try talking to your friend about your concerns. Remember that anorexics tend to deny their symptoms and refuse treatment. Bulimics are often more cooperative. Suggest that your friend seek professional help immediately. She could talk with the school counselor or nurse. If she refuses and you feel sure that she is anorexic, you may need to take stronger measures, such as contacting her family or letting a teacher or counselor at school know. Whatever you do, be sure to let your friend know that you care and want to help. Admitting to having an eating disorder can be quite painful. Reaching out for help is an act of courage.

Today's Challenge

Eating disorders can be seen as the logical extension of the concern with weight that pervades American society. Most people don't succumb to irrational or distorted ideas about their bodies, but many do become obsessed with dieting. The challenge facing Americans today is achieving a healthy body weight without excessive dieting—by adopting and maintaining sensible eating habits, an active lifestyle, realistic and positive attitudes and emotions, and creative ways to handle stress.

SUMMARY

Lifestyle and Weight Control

- The overweight problem that plagues American society can be traced to a sedentary, high-stress lifestyle and a diet based on overly refined and processed foods.

Adopting a Healthy Lifestyle

- The four key factors in maintaining normal weight are nutrition, physical activity, thinking and emotions, and coping strategies.
- Although sugar causes tooth decay, the real problem in the American diet is too much fat.
- Protein is amply supplied in the typical American diet. Excess dietary protein is stored as body fat.
- Eating more complex carbohydrates is a key component in maintaining a healthy body weight. The body has to expend energy to digest complex carbohydrates, and eating starchy foods makes you feel full.
- Eating small, frequent meals and having a structure to guide eating and decision rules to guide food choices are helpful weight management strategies.
- Physical activity is an important part of weight management because it burns calories, increases lean body mass, and keeps the metabolism geared up to active levels.
- Many people have an internalized "idealized self," based on perfectionistic irrational beliefs, with which they frequently compare themselves. Such comparisons can lead to low self-esteem and other emotional problems and to negative "self-talk."
- Maintaining a healthy body weight also depends on having a repertoire of appropriate techniques for coping with stress and other challenges.

A Closer Look at Body Weight

- Height-weight tables are a popular, though often inaccurate, means of assessing body weight. Body mass index measures body weight but correlates highly with direct measures of body fat. Techniques for analyzing body composition include hydrostatic weighing, skinfold measurements, and electrical impedance analysis.

- The ratio of waist and hip measurements can be used to assess the health risks of body fat distribution.

- Rather than concerning themselves with elaborate measurements, individuals should focus on the four factors that go into maintaining normal weight.

- Obesity increases a person's risk for a variety of health problems, including cardiovascular disease, gallbladder disease, diabetes, and certain cancers. People who tend to carry their body fat in their trunk and abdomen are at greater risk than people who carry body fat in their hips, thighs, and buttocks.

Overcoming a Weight Problem

- Genetic factors influence many physical characteristics, but people can control whether they actually become obese by modifying their behavior and adopting a healthy lifestyle.

- Set point theory suggests that the body has a certain natural weight and resists moving away from it by very much.

- Fat cell theory suggests that obese people were born with more or larger fat cells than normal-weight people or developed them during childhood.

- Resting metabolism is the single largest determinant of energy expenditure. Physical activity is the only component of energy expenditure over which we have much control.

- It is not clear whether, in general, obese people eat more than do people of normal weight. Binge eating is a serious problem for many dieters.

- No particular personality characteristics are consistently found among the obese, nor do they have a higher rate of psychological problems.

- There is a strong association between weight problems and socioeconomic status, overweight being more common among people of lower SES.

- The high rate of dieting in the United States is due in part to unrealistic cultural ideals of thinness. Modest weight loss can benefit health.

- People can be successful at losing weight and maintaining a healthy body weight on their own, usually through a combination of diet and exercise.

- Diet books should be carefully evaluated because many advocate useless or dangerous steps. Some over-the-counter diet aids can be helpful, but none is effective without individual effort. Supplements for modified fasting can be dangerous.

- Different approaches to weight reduction are appropriate for different individuals. The best choice depends on how severely overweight a person is and his or her lifestyle and preferences.

Eating Disorders

- Dissatisfaction with body weight and shape are common to all eating disorders. Serious physical and psychological health risks are associated with eating disorders.

- Anorexia nervosa is characterized by self-starvation, increased physical activity, distorted body image, intense fear of gaining weight, and amenorrhea. It is potentially fatal. Treatment involves restoring body weight, addressing underlying psychological problems, and changing eating habits.

- Bulimia nervosa is characterized by intense concern with body weight, recurrent episodes of uncontrolled binge eating, and frequent purging, either by self-induced vomiting or the use of laxatives or diuretics. Treatment usually involves behavior modification and cognitive therapy.

- Binge eating disorder involves binging without compensatory purging. It is most common among obese dieters.

- Although eating disorders are extreme conditions, many Americans are obsessed with dieting. The challenge is to maintain normal body weight by balancing diet and exercise.

TAKE ACTION

1. Interview some people who have successfully lost weight and kept it off. What were their strategies and techniques? Do you think their approach would work for others?

2. Find out what percentage of your body weight is fat by taking one of the tests described in this chapter at your campus health clinic, sports medicine clinic, or health club. If you have too high a proportion of body fat, consider taking steps to reduce it.

JOURNAL ENTRY

1. Monitor your diet for a week to see exactly how much fat and sugar you consume. If these amounts are excessive, make a list of specific steps you can take to reduce them, such as those suggested in the boxes in this chapter.

2. Make a list of at least five things you could do each day to become more physically active. Your list might include things such as riding your bike to class instead of driving and walking up stairs instead of taking the elevator. For each item on your list, describe the lifestyle adjustments you'd need to make—for example, leaving for class five minutes earlier to allow for cycling time.

3. *Critical Thinking:* Evaluate some of the weight loss resources in your community. First, investigate a commercial weight management program that operates in your community. Write an evaluation of it in terms of the 11 criteria listed in the box in this chapter. How does the program measure up? Next, look at the frozen diet dinners in your supermarket, such as Weight Watchers and Lean Cuisine. How do they compare in terms of calories, fat content, and nutritional value?

BEHAVIOR CHANGE STRATEGY

A WEIGHT MANAGEMENT PLAN

The behavior management plan described in Chapter 1 provides an excellent framework for a weight management program. Following are some suggestions about specific ways you can adapt that general plan to controlling your weight.

Goal-setting

Choose a reasonable weight you think you would like to reach over the long term, and be willing to renegotiate it as you get further along. Break your long-term goal into a series of short-term goals. Focus on reaching each short-term goal until you get close to your long-term goal. Likewise, when setting behavioral goals, break them down into small, reasonable steps—big enough to be a challenge but not so big that you can't accomplish each step. Don't try to convert to a new behavior pattern all at once. Shape your new way of behaving by designing small, manageable steps that will get you to where you want to go.

Self-monitoring

Keep a chart, journal, or record of your weight and behavior change progress. Try keeping a record of everything you eat. Write down what you plan to eat, the quantity, and the caloric content as well. Do this *before* you eat it. You'll find that just having to record something that is "not okay" to eat is likely to stop you from eating it. If you also note what seems to be triggering your urges to eat

(for example, you feel bored, it's lunchtime, someone offered you something, it was there so you ate it), you'll become more aware of your weak spots and be better able to take corrective action.

Stimulus Control

Figure out what makes you want to eat. Then engineer your environment so that these cues are eliminated (or avoid them if you can't get rid of them). Go through your pantry and refrigerator and throw out or give away "trouble" food—ice cream, candy, cookies, etc. Avoid driving past the doughnut shop that always beckons you to stop. Ask your friends or fellow students not to offer you snack food. Anticipate problem situations and plan ways to handle them more effectively.

Exercise

Evaluate your energy expenditure. Keep a daily log of both routine daily activity and planned exercise. Consider how you can find ways to increase your energy output simply by increasing routine physical activity, such as walking or taking the stairs. If you are not already involved in a regular exercise routine aimed at increasing endurance and building or maintaining lean body mass, seek help from someone who is competent to help you plan and start an appropriate exercise routine. If you are already doing regular physical exercise, evaluate your program according to the guidelines in Chapter 11.

Social Support

Get others to help. Get someone to join your efforts to adopt a healthy lifestyle. Make an appointment with someone to exercise together. Talk to friends and family about what they can do to support your efforts. Give them lots of praise for helping.

Reward Yourself Appropriately

Use lots of self-praise; avoid self-criticism, even when you slip. Plan special nonfood treats for yourself—a walk, a movie, an afternoon's reprieve from studying—when you accomplish a small step or short-term goal. Don't wait for the long-term goal to reward yourself. Reward yourself often and for anything that counts toward success.

Cognitive Strategies

Give yourself credit for even the smallest successes. Don't discount anything you can possibly count as progress. Tell yourself what you need to do next to stay on track. Think about your accomplishments and achievements. Congratulate yourself. Avoid demanding too much of yourself. Don't be a perfectionist; let yourself be human. Above all, don't criticize yourself!

Learn to Recover from Slips

When you have a slip (and you will, because you are human), learn from it. Decide what you might do to reduce the risk of its happening again. Identify the "high-risk" situations that set you up to backslide. Figure out how you can avoid such situations or change your response so that you win.

SELECTED BIBLIOGRAPHY

Bray, G. A. 1989. Obesity: Basic aspects and clinical applications. *The Medical Clinics of North America* 78(1).

Brownell, K. D. 1991. Dieting and the search for the perfect body: Where physiology and culture collide. *Behavior Therapy* 22:1–12.

———. 1993. Whether obesity should be treated. *Health Psychology* 12:339–341.

Brownell, K. D., and J. Rodin. 1994. The dieting maelstrom: Is it possible and advisable to lose weight? *American Psychologist* 49:781–791.

Brownell, K. D., and T. A. Wadden. 1991. The heterogeneity of obesity: Fitting treatments to individuals. *Behavior Therapy* 22:153–77.

———. 1992. Etiology and treatment of obesity: Understanding a serious, prevalent, and refractory disorder. *Journal of Consulting and Clinical Psychology* 60:505–17.

Fairburn, C. G., and G. T. Wilson. 1993. *Binge Eating: Nature, Assessment, and Treatment.* New York: The Guilford Press.

Fitzgibbon, M. L., M. R. Stolley, and D. S. Kirschenbaum. 1993. Obese people who seek treatment have different characteristics than those who do not seek treatment. *Health Psychology* 12:342–345.

Gortmaker, S. L., W. H. Dietz, Jr., L. W. Y. Cheung. 1990. Inactivity, diet, and the fattening of America. *Journal of the American Dietetic Association* 90:1247–52.

Haddock, C. K., W. R. Shadish, R. C. Klesges, and R. J. Stein. 1994. Treatments for childhood and adolescent obesity: Meta-analysis. *Annals of Behavioral Medicine* 16:235–244.

Jeffery, R. W., R. R. Wing, and S. A. French. 1992. Weight cycling and cardiovascular risk factors in obese men and women. *American Journal of Clinical Nutrition* 55:641–44.

Kuczmarski, R. J. 1992. Prevalence of overweight and weight gain in the United States. *American Journal of Clinical Nutrition* 55:495S–502S.

Pi-Sunyer, F. X. 1991. Health implications of obesity. *American Journal of Clinical Nutrition* 53:1595S–1603S.

Rand, C. S. W., and J. M. Kuldau. 1992. Epidemiology of bulimia and symptoms in a general population: Sex, age, race, and socioeconomic status. *International Journal of Eating Disorders* 11:37–44.

Sichieri, R., J. E. Everhart, and V. S. Hubbard. 1992. Relative weight classifications in the assessment of underweight and overweight in the United States. *International Journal of Obesity* 16:303–12.

Stallone, D. D., and A. J. Stunkard. 1991. The regulation of body weight: Evidence and clinical implications. *Annals of Behavioral Medicine* 13:220–30.

Steiger, H., F. Y. K. Leung, G. Puentes-Neuman, and N. Gottheil. 1992. *International Journal of Eating Disorders* 11:121–31.

"Why Lost Weight Finds Its Way Back." 1995. *San Francisco Chronicle,* 9 March, pp. A1, A13.

Wilson, G. T., and B. T. Walsh. 1991. Eating disorders in the DSM-IV. *Journal of Abnormal Psychology* 100:362–65.

Wing, R. R. 1993. Obesity and related eating and exercise behaviors in women. *Annals of Behavioral Medicine* 15:124–134.

Wooley, S. C., and D. M. Garner. 1991. Obesity treatment: The high cost of false hope. *Journal of the American Dietetic Association* 91:1248–51.

RECOMMENDED READINGS

Bailey, C. 1991 (Revised edition). *The New Fit or Fat.* Boston: Houghton Mifflin. *Originally published in 1977, this entertaining book describes ways to become healthy by developing better diet and exercise habits.*

Finn, S., and L. S. Kass. 1992. *The Real Life Nutrition Book.* New York: Penguin Books. *The philosophy behind this book, which covers the nutrition basics, is that your lifestyle should dictate your nutrition and fitness regimen.*

Goldberg, L. 1991. *The New Controlled ChEATing Weight-Loss and Fitness Program.* Kansas City: Andrews and McMeel. *Entertaining and motivating, this diet book tells how to eat your favorite foods without guilt. Even so, it gives responsible diet advice and advocates that exercise accompany dieting.*

Nash, J. D. 1986. *Maximize Your Body Potential.* Palo Alto, Calif.: Bull Publishing. *Called "the most helpful book on lifetime weight management" by the* Journal of Nutrition Education, *this comprehensive book on nutrition, exercise, behavior, and the psychological aspects of weight management helps the reader assess his or her situation and plan effective action.*

———. 1992. *Now That You've Lost It: How to Maintain Your Best Weight.* Palo Alto, Calif.: Bull Publishing. *Keeping the weight off once one gets to goal weight is often the toughest part of a weight management effort, and this book addresses the psychological and motivational factors that can produce long-lasting success.*

Roth, G. 1991. *When Food Is Love.* New York: Dutton. *This book explores the relation between eating disorders and close relationships, including early family experiences.*

Exercise for Health and Fitness

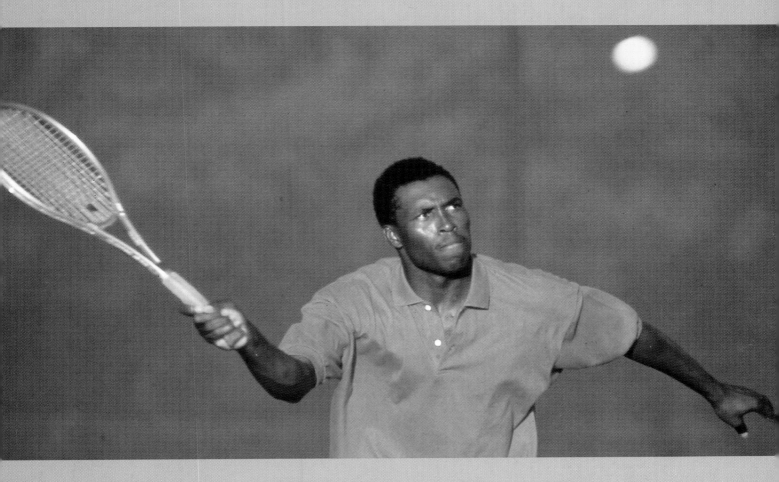

CONTENTS

Exercise is part of the lives of millions of Americans. People are walking, jogging, and working out in gyms and fitness centers. They're talking about weight training, aerobic exercise, cardiorespiratory capacity, and body composition. Colleges are stressing regular exercise programs, and businesses are providing recreational and fitness facilities for their employees.

But the "fitness boom" is not without its casualties. Some people start an exercise program without enough thought and drop it a few months later because it's too time-consuming, inconvenient, or boring. Some rush into sports or activities without proper training or knowledge, only to get benched with a sprained ankle or sore knee a week or two later. Many "weekend warriors" suffer overuse injuries from trying to squeeze all their activities into a 48-hour period.

Most of these difficulties arise because people don't have the basic knowledge and understanding they need to exercise properly and get the most from it. Many choose inappropriate activities or do too much too soon. When their program doesn't work out, they become frustrated and discouraged about exercise in general. At the same time, some people remain on the sidelines because they simply don't know where to begin. If you have ever been confused about the best way to get in shape and stay in shape, this chapter will help you understand the basics of exercise so you can put together a physical fitness plan that will work for you. If approached correctly, exercise and sports can contribute immeasurably to health and well-being, add fun and joy to life, and provide the foundation for a lifetime of fitness.

WHAT IS PHYSICAL FITNESS AND WHY IS IT IMPORTANT?

Physical fitness is the ability to adapt to the demands and stresses of physical effort. It has many components, some related to general health and others related more specifically to particular sports or activities. The components most important for health include the following:

- Cardiorespiratory endurance
- Flexibility
- Muscular strength, power, and endurance
- Body composition (proportion of fat to lean body mass)

In addition to some or all of these, physical fitness for a particular sport or activity might include the following:

- Coordination
- Speed
- Agility
- Balance
- Skill

Although some components may overlap, each is largely independent and requires specific types of exercise to develop it. Your body has the ability to adapt to physical stress and improve its function; that is, through specific physical activities, you can increase your heart and lung capacity, develop stronger muscles, become more flexible, improve your performance in particular sports, and so on. In general, your level of physical fitness is directly related to the amount and intensity of your physical activity.

Why is physical fitness so important? Part of the answer to this question lies in your genetic inheritance. Your body is a wonderful moving machine, designed to be active. Your bones, joints, and ligaments provide a support system for movement; your muscles perform the motions of work and play; your heart and lungs nourish your cells as you move through your daily life. Millions of years of evolution have made your body a precision tool capable of astonishing feats of speed, strength, endurance, and skill, all in the service of survival. But your body is made to work best when it is active. Left unchallenged, bones lose their density, joints stiffen, muscles become weak, and cellular energy systems begin to degenerate. To be truly well, you must be active.

Unfortunately, modern life for most Americans provides few built-in occasions for vigorous activity—people don't have to hunt, fight, or work strenuously all day for their dinner, as human beings did in the past. Technological advances have made our lives increasingly inactive and sedentary; we drive cars, ride escalators, watch television, and push papers around at school or work. Growing evidence points to lack of physical activity as a prime contributing factor to the array of perplexing degenerative diseases we now see in our society—heart disease, cancer, stroke, obesity, diabetes, and hypertension, among others. Overall, sedentary people have been found to have up to 50 percent more health problems than people with active lifestyles.

A major physical fitness study that followed 13,000 men and women for eight years found that inactive men were almost $3\frac{1}{2}$ times more likely to die over the course of the eight years than active men, and inactive women were over $4\frac{1}{2}$ times more likely to die than active women. Being sedentary was found to be as risky as having hypertension, high cholesterol, high blood-sugar levels, or obesity. An encouraging finding is that even mild exercise, such as a brisk walk for 30 to 60 minutes a day, every other day, was enough to make a substantial difference in an individual's risk of death. The conclusion is obvious: Exercise and physical activity are good for your health.

There is another basic reason to be physically fit, of course: It's fun and it feels good. Some people are active not because they're thinking about health benefits but simply because they enjoy it, whether they're skiing, swimming, hiking, playing basketball, or engaging in any of innumerable other activities. Sports provide the oppor-

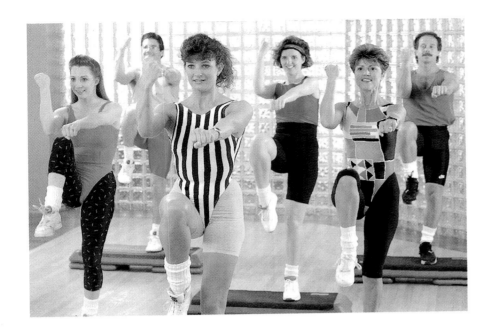

Endurance exercise conditions the heart, improves the function of the entire cardiorespiratory system, and has many other health benefits as well. An effective personal fitness program should be built around an activity like running, walking, biking, swimming, or aerobic dance.

tunity to be active, to develop strength and skills, to improve and excel, to challenge yourself or an opponent, to share victory and defeat with fellow team members, to compete. Many people who play sports feel that physical performance is an integral part of an active and exciting lifestyle.

As one of the most important—and most controllable—factors in a person's general health, exercise is mentioned in many other contexts in this book. It can help you to manage stress, to maintain your emotional well-being, to control your weight, to boost your immune system, and to protect yourself against serious diseases later in life. It does all this by improving the overall functioning of your body in ways detailed more fully in the rest of this chapter.

Personal Insight Was exercise part of your family life when you were growing up? How much do your parents exercise? Do you think you're influenced by their attitudes and habits? How will you motivate your own children to exercise?

WHY IS EXERCISE SO GOOD FOR YOU?

The health benefits of exercise can be divided into five general categories—improved cardiorespiratory efficiency and health, more efficient metabolism and better control of body fat, improved psychological and emotional well-being, improved muscular strength and flexibility, and improved health over the whole life span.

Improved Cardiorespiratory Efficiency

The most important kind of exercise is **cardiorespiratory endurance** (or **aerobic**) **exercise.** It improves heart and lung functioning. As fitness pioneer Kenneth Cooper remarked, "You can live without big muscles or a nice figure, but you can't live without a healthy heart." This type of exercise helps your body become a more efficient machine, better equipped to cope with physical challenges. *Aerobic* means "requiring oxygen." In very-high-intensity exercise, such as sprinting, the body relies on an energy system that doesn't require much oxygen, but that can operate only for short periods of time. For these reasons, very-high-intensity exercise doesn't develop the cardiorespiratory system to the same extent as does aerobic exercise.

The primary effect of endurance exercise is to improve the ability of the heart, lungs, and circulatory system to carry oxygen to the body's tissues. The heart pumps more blood per beat, resting heart rate slows down, the number of red blood cells increases, blood supply to the tissues improves, and resting blood pressure decreases. A fit cardiorespiratory system doesn't have to work as hard at rest and at low levels of exercise, because it functions more efficiently. A healthy heart can better withstand the stresses and strains of daily life and meet the occasional emergen-

Physical fitness   The extent to which the body can respond to the demands of physical effort.

Cardiorespiratory endurance exercise (or aerobic)
Rhythmical, large-muscle exercise for a prolonged period of time. Partially dependent on the ability of the cardiovascular system to deliver oxygen to tissues.

TERMS

The Power of Exercise: How It Affects the Mind

If you've ever gone for a long, brisk walk after a hard day's work, you know how refreshing exercise can be. Exercise can improve mood, stimulate creativity, clarify thinking, relieve anxiety, and provide an outlet for anger or aggression. But why does exercise make you feel good? Does it simply take your mind off your problems, or does it cause a physical reaction that affects your mental state?

Until recently, scientists were unable to learn whether the mood-altering effects of physical activity were based on some sort of physical or chemical reaction or whether these effects were merely "in the mind." Current research indicates that exercise triggers many physical changes in the body that can alter mood. Scientists are now trying to explain how and why exercise affects the mind.

Some researchers are looking at the physical structure of the brain. They think the effect of exercise on the mind may be due to the close proximity of two specific areas of the brain—the motor cortex, which is responsible for the movement of muscles in the body, and a nearby area that is responsible for thought and emotion. As muscles work more vigorously, nerve cells transmit signals with much greater frequency, stimulating the motor cortex. This increased brain activity may also stimulate the nearby areas of the brain.

Other researchers suggest that exercise stimulates the release of endorphins, substances that can suppress fatigue, produce euphoria, and decrease pain. Endorphins affect the human body much as the opium-based drug morphine does. The pituitary gland, located in the base of the brain, produces greater amounts of endorphins during vigorous exercise. If you are a long-distance runner, you have probably experienced a sense of euphoria, called a "runner's high," after running several miles. This euphoria, which contributes to an athlete's endurance, may be due to increased production of endorphins.

In theory, endorphins flow through the bloodstream and find their way into the area of the brain that controls mood. So far, no evidence has been found indicating that they actually reach this part of the brain. The theory remains promising, but further research is needed to determine the exact role of endorphins in our sense of well-being.

A third area of research focuses on changes in brain activity during and after exercise. Currently, researchers recognize that two changes occur. The first is an increase in alpha wave activity. Alpha brain waves indicate a highly relaxed state; meditation also induces alpha wave activity. The increase in alpha waves starts some time after exercise is begun and continues well beyond the end of the exercise period.

The second change is an alteration in the levels of the **neurotransmitters** norepinephrine, dopamine, and serotonin—chemicals that increase alertness and reduce stress. Higher levels of these neurotransmitters can also improve state of mind in people who suffer from depression. Not only does exercise trigger a change in these neurotransmitters, but some effects of exercise, such as an increase in body temperature, also further alter their levels.

You might wonder how much exercise is needed to improve your overall mood. Some studies have compared a sedentary lifestyle with a lifestyle that included walking a few times a week. After several weeks, the inactive individuals showed no change in before-and-after tests of psychological well-being, but the moderately active individuals showed significant improvement. So no matter what the exact explanation for this mind-body connection turns out to be, it makes sense to take advantage of it today.

Adapted from D. C. Nieman. 1995. *Fitness and Sports Medicine* (Menlo Park, Calif.: Bull Publishing); D. C. Nieman. 1989. "Exercise and the Mind." *Women's Sports and Fitness* 11(17): 54–57; "Fitness Update." *Consumer Reports on Health,* August 1992.

---

cies that make extraordinary demands on the body's cardiorespiratory resources.

Endurance exercise also has a positive effect on the balance of lipids, or fatlike substances such as cholesterol and triglycerides, that are circulating in the blood. Lipids are involved in the formation of plaques, or fatty deposits, on the inner lining of the coronary arteries. Cholesterol is carried in the blood by **lipoproteins,** which are classified according to size and density. Cholesterol carried by low-density lipoproteins (LDL) tends to stick to the walls of coronary arteries, and high-density lipoproteins (HDL) tend to pick up excess cholesterol in the bloodstream and carry it back to the liver for excretion from the body. The total amount of HDL and the relative amounts of HDL and LDL in the blood are very important factors involved in the development of coronary heart disease. Recent studies have shown that people with low levels of HDL have an increased risk of coronary heart disease even if their total cholesterol is low. The good news is that one excellent way to increase your HDL and lower your LDL is to exercise.

Endurance exercise also protects the cardiorespiratory system from the effects of stress. Many studies have shown that excessive stress and anxiety are associated with poor cardiorespiratory health. Psychological stress prompts increased secretion of **epinephrine** and **norepinephrine,** the so-called fight-or-flight hormones, which are thought to speed the development of atherosclerosis, or hardening of the arteries. Excessive hostility has also been found to be associated with an increased risk of heart disease. Exercise decreases the secretion of hormones triggered by emotional stress, and it can diffuse

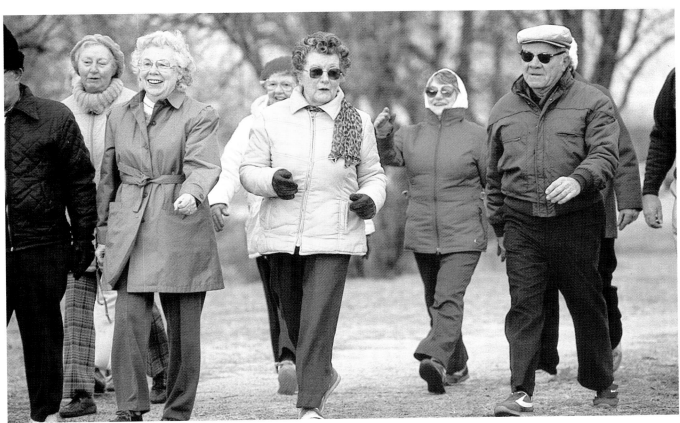

It makes sense to choose activities that will add enjoyment to your life for years to come. In this group of older people we can see the rewards of a lifetime of fitness and smart exercise habits.

hostility by providing an emotional outlet for pent-up anger.

More Efficient Metabolism and Better Control of Body Fat

A second major effect of endurance exercise is to improve the efficiency of the body's metabolism, the complicated process by which the body converts chemical or food energy into mechanical or work energy. This process involves hormones, oxygen, fuels, and enzymes. A physically fit person is better able to generate useful energy, to use fats for energy, and to regulate hormones. One theory holds that the bodies of physically active people process food faster and get rid of cancer-causing agents before they can create a problem. This may explain the lower rates of colon cancer among fit people.

A related effect of endurance exercise, of course, is simply to expend calories and thus help regulate energy balance and body weight. Without exercise, it is extremely difficult to eat a nutritious diet and maintain an ideal body weight. Sedentary people may gain weight on a good diet simply because they are taking in more calories than they are using. Weight training can also help with weight control by increasing or maintaining muscle mass.

Improved Psychological and Emotional Well-Being

Most people who participate in sports or vigorous exercise have noted a number of social, psychological, and emotional benefits of being active. The joy of a well-hit cross-court backhand, the euphoria of a run through the park, or the rush of a downhill schuss through deep snow powder provides pleasure that transcends health benefits alone. Competent performance of a physical activity serves as proof that you can master skills and control your efforts, which in turn enhances your self-image. Exercise improves the appearance of your body, which also tends

Neurotransmitters Substances that transmit nerve impulses.

Lipoproteins (*low-density lipoproteins, LDL; high-density lipoproteins, HDL*) Substances in blood, classified according to size, density, and chemical composition, that transport fats.

Epinephrine A hormone secreted principally by the adrenal medulla with a wide variety of functions, such as stimulating the heart, making carbohydrates available in the liver and muscles, and releasing fat from fat cells.

Norepinephrine A hormone released from the adrenal medulla and nerve endings of the autonomic nervous system. Has many of the same effects as epinephrine.

TERMS

to make you feel better about yourself. Exercise can offer an arena for harmonious interaction with other people as well as opportunities to strive and excel. Since physically fit people develop greater physical efficiency, they have plenty of energy and lead lives that are full and varied.

Beyond these personal and interpersonal benefits, positive feelings associated with exercise have a physiological basis in hormones and body chemicals. Exercise decreases the secretion of stress-related hormones, as noted earlier, and it alleviates depression and anxiety by providing an emotional outlet. Additionally, researchers are studying the effect of **endorphins** and other hormonelike substances whose production increases during vigorous exercise.

Improved Strength and Flexibility

Most of the benefits already discussed are benefits of cardiorespiratory endurance exercise, but exercises designed to improve muscular strength and endurance, joint flexibility, and posture are also crucial to your physical well-being. Back pain, for example, plagues a large percentage of the population. In most cases, it can be directly traced to weak abdominal and spinal muscles with poor muscular endurance; inadequate flexibility in the spine, hips, and legs; and chronically poor posture.

A basic principle in physical training is "Use it or lose it!" If muscles aren't used, they degenerate. If joints aren't moved, they become stiff. But if you do specific exercises for strength and flexibility, your functioning both in sports and in everyday life is improved. Muscular strength, for example, is an advantage whether you're hitting a baseball, unscrewing the lid of a jar, or moving your furniture into a new apartment. Stronger muscles make it easier to move the body, and they're also less susceptible to injury and disability, especially in the long term. Similarly, flexible joints that are pain-free and capable of normal movement are less likely to impede your activities, whether you're sprinting to class or running a marathon. Good posture helps to keep your spine properly aligned, which helps keep your back and neck pain-free. And an attractive, fit, healthy-looking body helps you feel good about yourself and project self-confidence and radiant well-being.

Improved Health over the Life Span

Exercising regularly may be the single most important thing you can do in your twenties to improve the quality of your life in your forties, fifties, sixties, and beyond. Physically fit individuals are less likely to develop the diseases and disabilities now associated with middle age in our society, including heart disease, stroke, diabetes, and high blood pressure. They may be able to avoid fatigue, weight gain, memory loss, and other problems associated with aging. Their cardiorespiratory systems tend to resemble those of people 10 or more years younger than themselves. With flexible spines, strong hearts and muscles, lean bodies, and a repertoire of physical skills they can call on for exercise and enjoyment, these people have the potential to maintain their physical and mental well-being throughout their entire lives.

A specific benefit of exercise, especially for women, is protection against **osteoporosis,** a disease that results in loss of bone density and poor bone strength (see Chapter 9). Weight-bearing exercise, which includes almost everything except swimming, helps build bone during the teens and twenties, when bones are still growing. Older people with denser bones can endure the bone loss that comes with osteoporosis better than can people whose bones are not as dense. Strength training can increase bone density throughout life. With stronger bones, stronger muscles, and better balance, fit people are less likely to suffer the bone fractures that debilitate so many older people.

DESIGNING YOUR EXERCISE AND FITNESS PROGRAM

The best exercise and fitness program has two primary characteristics: It promotes your health and it's fun for you to do. Exercise doesn't have to be a chore. On the contrary, it can provide some of the most pleasurable moments of your day, once you make it a habit. A little thought and planning will help you achieve these goals.

If you are over 35 or have questions about your health, get a medical examination before beginning an exercise program. Diabetes, asthma, heart disease, or extreme obesity are conditions that may call for a modified program. If you have an increased risk of heart disease because of smoking, high blood pressure, or obesity, have an exercise **electrocardiogram (ECG)** before beginning a program. This checkup can help ensure that your program is a benefit to your health rather than a potential hazard.

Cardiorespiratory Endurance Exercises

Exercises that condition your heart and lungs should have a central role in your fitness program. The best exercises for developing **cardiorespiratory endurance** are those that stress a large portion of the body's muscle mass for a

TERMS

Endorphins Substances resembling opium that are secreted by the brain. They seem to be involved in modulating pain.

Osteoporosis A bone disease characterized by the loss of bone mineral. It is particularly prevalent in postmenopausal women.

Electrocardiogram (EKG or ECG) A recording of the changes in electrical activity of the heart.

Cardiorespiratory endurance The extent to which the heart and lungs can respond to physical exercise.

If you're someone who doesn't like jogging or swimming, who never learned to ski or play tennis, or who refuses to spend money on a health club, don't despair. You can still get into great shape—by walking!

Many people aren't aware that the physical conditioning value and aerobic effects of walking approach those of more strenuous exercise. If done briskly or long enough, walking can be as beneficial as jogging or any other endurance exercise for developing cardiorespiratory fitness. Walking promotes increased lung action, stimulates blood circulation, lowers elevated blood pressure, activates many large muscle groups, and even strengthens bones, perhaps lowering the risk of osteoporosis. Walking also tones the body and promotes weight loss, especially when combined with a low-fat diet. And like many other forms of exercise, walking helps reduce the effects of stress.

Perhaps the best news is that these benefits come with very little cost. Compared with other forms of exercise, walking has a very low injury rate, and the potential for pleasure is high. Also encouraging is the fact that even a modest program of 15 minutes of walking three times a week produces health benefits, as long as the pace puts your heart rate in the target range (see the box on determining your target heart rate).

You can vary the intensity of your workouts by walking briskly on level ground, taking to the hills, and then finishing on the flats. When walking uphill, try leaning forward slightly—it's easier on your leg muscles. Surprisingly, walking downhill can be harder on your body than walking uphill; it can jar the joints, especially the knees, and cause muscle soreness.

Walking uphill burns more calories than walking on flat land. If you weigh 150 pounds, walking at 3.5 miles an hour on flat terrain burns about 300 calories per hour. On a gentle incline (a 4 percent grade), the same pace burns almost 400 calories an hour. On a slightly steeper incline (an 8 percent grade), nearly 500 calories per hour are consumed.

To increase the physical benefits of your walking program and to avoid boredom, try these variations:

- Choose diverse terrains. Walking on grass or gravel burns more calories than walking on a dirt track. Walking on sand increases calorie consumption dramatically.

- Walk up and down stairs every day; skip all escalators and elevators.

- Swing or pump your arms for an upper body workout.

- Use hand weights while you walk to boost your heart rate and calorie consumption (but not if you have high blood pressure or heart disease). Begin with 1-pound weights and increase gradually, if you wish, but the weights shouldn't add up to more than 10 percent of your body weight. Don't use ankle weights; they increase the risk of injury.

- Stride-walk—lengthen your stride, swing your arms more, and pick up your pace.

- Retrowalk—walk backwards to work your back, abdominal, and thigh muscles. (Be sure to choose a smooth, unobstructed surface, such as a track.)

- Walk in water. The deeper the water and the faster the pace, the higher the calorie-burning value. Waist-high water is ideal, but you can achieve the same benefits in shallow water by walking faster and longer.

- Learn racewalking, a sport that involves moving your body forward as quickly as possible without breaking into a run. It eliminates the up-down motions of regular walking. Racewalking takes study, practice, and, at competitive levels, intensive training.

As a form of regular exercise, walking offers many advantages over other activities. It's comfortable, convenient, affordable, and safe. It also lends itself to socializing, sharing, and enjoying nature. And because it's so easy and pleasurable, you're likely to continue walking long after you've dropped more exotic or strenuous sports.

Adapted from E. E. Esckilsen. 1992. "The Short Walk to Health." *Take Care.* Summer, pp. 1–3; "Better Walking Workouts," *University of California at Berkeley Wellness Letter,* September 1992, pp. 4–5.

---

prolonged period of time. These include walking, jogging, running, swimming, bicycling, and aerobic dancing. Games such as racquetball, tennis, basketball, and soccer are also good if the skill level and intensity of the game are sufficient to provide a vigorous workout.

Specific recommendations have been made by the American College of Sports Medicine for the kind and amount of exercise that provide the optimal workout for your heart and lungs. They have defined three dimensions of training that should be taken into consideration: frequency, intensity, and duration of exercise. Frequency refers to the number of times per week you exercise; intensity refers to how hard you work; and duration refers to the length of your exercise session. Basic recommendations for quantity and quality of exercise are outlined in Table 11-1.

Frequency of Training The optimal workout schedule for endurance training is three to five days per week. Beginners should start with three and work up to five days. Training more than five days a week often leads to injury for recreational athletes. While recent evidence suggests

TABLE 11-1 Recommended Quantity and Quality of Exercise for Healthy Adults

Mode of activity	Cardiorespiratory endurance exercises such as running-jogging, walking-hiking, swimming, skating, bicycling, rowing, cross-country skiing, rope skipping, and various game activities; resistance training; flexibility exercises
Frequency of training	3 to 5 days per week
Intensity of training	55 to 90 percent of maximum heart rate or 40 to 85 percent of maximum oxygen uptake
Duration of training	15 to 60 minutes of continuous aerobic activity; duration dependent on the intensity of the activity
Resistance training	At least one set of 8 to 12 repetitions of 8 to 10 exercises that condition the major muscle groups; recommended minimum frequency—at least two days per week
Flexibility training	Statically stretch the major muscle groups for 5 repetitions of 10 to 30 seconds, at least 3 times per week. Use caution when performing exercises that require substantial skill or flexibility, particularly if you are older, less flexible, or less experienced.

Sources: American College of Sports Medicine. 1991. *Guidelines for Exercise Training and Prescription.* Philadelphia: Lea & Febiger; American College of Sports Medicine. 1990. *ACSM Position Stand. The Recommended Quantity and Quality of Exercise for Developing and Maintaining Cardiorespiratory and Muscular Fitness in Healthy Adults.*

that you get some health benefits from exercising from only one or two days per week, you risk injury because your body never gets a chance to adapt fully to regular exercise training.

Intensity of Training The most misunderstood aspect of conditioning, even among experienced athletes, is training intensity. Intensity is the crucial factor in attaining a training effect—that is, in increasing the body's cardiorespiratory capacity. A primary purpose of endurance training is to increase **maximal oxygen consumption (MOC).** MOC represents the maximum ability of the cells to use oxygen and is considered the best measure of cardiorespiratory capacity. Intensity of training is the crucial factor in attaining a training effect—that is, in increasing the body's cardiorespiratory capacity—and in improving MOC. The ideal intensity for increasing MOC is 55 to 90 percent of maximum heart rate or 40 to 85 percent of MOC.

However, it's not true that the harder you work, the better it is for you. Working too hard can cause injury, just as not working hard enough provides little benefit. One of the easiest ways to determine exactly how intensely you should work involves measuring your heart rate. It is not necessary or desirable to exercise at your maximum heart rate—the fastest heart rate possible before exhaustion sets in—in order to improve your cardiorespiratory capacity. Beneficial effects occur at lower heart rates with a much lower risk of injury.

After you begin your fitness program, you may improve quickly, because the body adapts readily to new ex-

ercises at first but slows after the first month or so. The more fit you become, the harder you will have to work to improve. By monitoring your heart rate, you will always know if you are working hard enough to improve, not hard enough, or too hard. For most people, a fitness program involves attaining an acceptable level of fitness and then maintaining that level. There is no need to keep working indefinitely to improve; doing so only increases the chance of injury. After you have reached the level you want, you can maintain fitness by exercising at the same intensity approximately three times per week, 20 minutes per session.

Many people work out using a technique known as **periodization of training,** or *cycle training.* This technique involves varying the intensity of the workout from one session to the next so that you're rested on the days you exercise the hardest. For example, the intensity schedule of a week-long series of workouts might be (1) hard, (2) easy, (3) moderate, (4) easy, (5) moderate, (6) rest, and (7) rest. A hard workout might be practiced at the high end of the target heart rate range, a moderate workout in the middle of the range, and an easy workout at the low end of the range. Cycle training allows your body to adapt rapidly to intense workouts by giving it time to recover between strenuous sessions. Competitive athletes also use yearly cycles—varying workouts during different times of the year and competitive season.

Duration of Training The length of time you should spend on a workout depends on its intensity. If you are walking, swimming slowly, or playing a stop-and-start

Determining Your Target Heart Rate

Your *target heart rate* is the rate at which you should exercise to experience cardiorespiratory benefits. Your target heart rate is based on your maximum heart rate, which can be estimated from your age. (If you are a serious athlete or face possible cardiovascular risks from exercise, you may want to have your maximum heart rate determined more accurately through a treadmill test in a physician's office, hospital, or sports medicine laboratory.) Your target heart rate is actually a range—the lower value corresponds to moderately intense exercise while the higher value is associated with high-intensity activities. Target heart rates for people in the age groups between 20 and 60 are shown in the accompanying table.

You can monitor the intensity of your workouts by measuring your pulse either at your wrist or at one of your carotid arteries, located on either side of your Adam's apple. Your pulse rate drops rapidly after exercise, so begin counting immediately after you have finished exercising. You will obtain the most accurate results by counting beats for 15 seconds and then multiplying by 4 to get your heart rate in beats per minute. To build cardiorespiratory endurance, you must exercise at your target heart rate for a minimum of 15 minutes, at least three times per week.

Maximum and Target Heart Rates Predicted from Age

Age (in years)	Predicted Maximum Heart Rate (in beats per minute)	Target Heart Rate Range (in beats per minute)
20–24	200	149–174
25–29	200	149–174
30–34	194	145–170
35–39	188	142–165
40–44	182	138–160
45–49	176	134–155
50–54	171	131–151
55–59	165	128–146
60–64	159	124–142
65+	153	121–137

Adapted from Metropolitan Life Insurance Company charts and Karvonen formula (target heart rate = 0.6 or 0.8 × [HR_{max} − HR_{rest}] + HR_{rest}).

game like tennis, you should participate for 45 to 60 minutes. High-intensity exercises such as running that keep your heart rate in the target zone for at least 15 minutes can be practiced for a shorter period of time. The recreational athlete should start off with less vigorous activities and only gradually increase intensity. For most people, continuous endurance exercise should last from 15 minutes (high-intensity activities) to 60 minutes (low-intensity activities).

You can use these three dimensions of cardiorespiratory endurance training—frequency, intensity, and duration—to construct a fitness program that strengthens your heart and lungs and provides all the benefits described earlier in this chapter. Build your program around at least 15 minutes of continuous aerobic activity at your target heart rate three to five times a week. Then add exercises that develop the other components of fitness.

Flexibility Exercises

Flexibility, or stretching, exercises are perhaps the most neglected part of fitness programs, but they are extremely

Maximal oxygen consumption (MOC) The body's maximum ability to transport and use oxygen.

Periodization of training A training technique that systematically varies the volume and intensity of the workouts.

1. **Shoulder blade scratch** (shoulders, arms)
Reach back with one arm as if to scratch your shoulder blade. Use your other hand to extend the stretch. Alternate arms.

2. **Towel stretch** (arms, shoulders, chest)
Grasp a rolled towel at both ends and slowly bring it back over your head as far down as possible. Keep your arms straight. (The closer your hands are, the greater the stretch.)

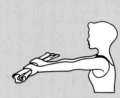

3. **Alternate knee-to-chest** (lower back)
With hands behind your knees, bring one knee up to your chest. Curl your head toward your knee. Keep the other leg on the floor. Alternate knees.

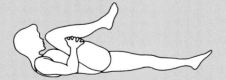

4. **Double knee-to-chest** (buttocks, lower back)
Same as alternate knee-to-chest (3), except bring both knees up to your chest.

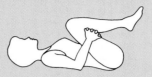
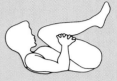

5. **Sole stretch** (groin)
With the soles of your feet pressed together, pull your feet toward you while pressing your knees down with your elbows.

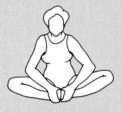

6. **Seated toe touch** (hamstrings)
Sit with your legs straight. Fold one leg in front and gradually reach for the toes of your other foot. Eventually you will be able to grasp your feet at the instep. Keep your head down. Alternate legs.

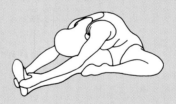

7. **Seated foot-over-knee twist** (hips)
Seated as depicted, turn at the hips to face the rear. Hold your ankle to keep your foot on the floor. Alternate legs.

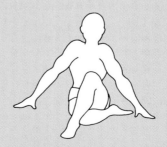
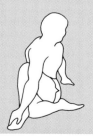

8. **Prone knee flexion** (quadriceps)
Lying on your side with one arm tucked behind your head, use the other arm to slowly pull one foot up toward your buttocks. Flex the leg up until you feel the stretch in your quadriceps. Alternate legs.

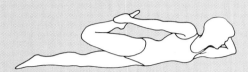

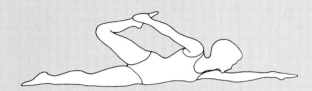

9. **Wall lean** (lower legs)
Lean against the wall with one leg bent and the other straight. Keep your back straight and your heels on the floor. Bend the knee of the straight leg—this changes the stretch from the calf muscle to the Achilles tendon. Alternate legs.

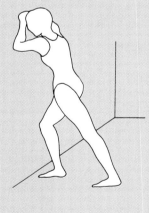

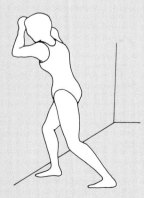

10. **Stride stretch** (hips, hamstring)
Assume the racer's starting position and stretch one leg backward. Keep your head down. Alternate legs.

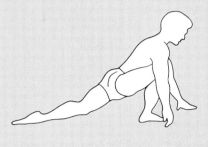

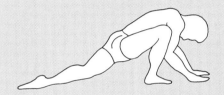

Source: I. Kusinitz and M. Fine. 1995. *Your Guide to Getting Fit.* 3rd ed. (Mountain View, Calif.: Mayfield).

The Dangers of Anabolic Steroids

Anabolic steroids are drugs that resemble male hormones such as testosterone and are widely used by athletes in sports like track and field, weight lifting, and football. Athletes take them in the hope of gaining weight, strength, power, speed, endurance, and aggressiveness. Recently young people who are not athletes have begun taking these drugs to improve their appearance. Studies indicate that as many as 400,000 American teens may have experimented with steroids. Steroid use is costly both to athletic careers and to health.

Steroids work by enhancing the anabolic (tissue-building) properties of male hormones. These include accelerated growth of muscle, bone, and red blood cells and enhanced neural conduction. Most experts feel that anabolic steroids are effective in improving some types of athletic performance—but only at a cost to health, because they have dangerous side effects.

The physiological side effects of steroid use include reduced testosterone production, testicular function, and sperm cell production, which in turn can lead to atrophy of the testes. These changes may reverse themselves after use stops, but prolonged use may permanently disturb the delicate hormone regulatory system. Anabolic steroids also increase fluid retention and may harm the immune system. Libido (sex drive) may increase or decrease.

Steroid use by women and children may have masculinizing effects, including hair growth on face and body, deepening of the voice, oily skin, increased sweat gland activity, acne, and baldness. In women, some of these changes are irreversible. Women may also experience clitoral enlargement and menstrual irregularity. Children initially experience accelerated maturation followed by premature closure of growth centers in the long bones.

Taken orally, anabolic steroids also present a risk of toxicity, particularly to the liver. Prolonged use has been linked to severe liver disorders such as blood-filled cysts, liver cancer, and bile duct obstruction.

Several factors associated with steroid use are linked to increased risk of coronary heart disease: high levels of blood cholesterol and triglycerides, high blood pressure, and low levels of high-density lipoproteins (HDLs). Many athletes use steroids for long periods of time (10 to 20 years), risking premature death from atherosclerosis. High blood pressure is also common, probably due to fluid retention.

A variety of other side effects has been reported, including psychological disorders, muscle cramps, gastrointestinal distress, headache, dizziness, sore nipples, and abnormal thyroid function. Some of these side effects even show up in people who have taken only low doses for short periods of time.

---

important. They are necessary to maintain the normal range of motion in the major joints of the body. Some exercises, such as running, actually decrease flexibility because the movements they entail require only a partial range of motion. It's important to do stretching exercises at least three to five times a week.

Stretching should be performed statically. "Bouncing" (ballistic stretching) is dangerous and counterproductive. Stretch to the point of tightness in the muscle and hold the position 10 to 30 seconds. Do five repetitions of exercises for the major muscle groups and joints of the body—neck, shoulders, back, hips, thighs, hamstrings, and calves. You should feel a pleasant, mild stretch as you let the muscles relax; stretching shouldn't be painful. There are large individual differences in flexibility, so don't feel you have to compete with others during stretching workouts. Flexibility increases gradually over a period of time. You can set apart a special time for these exercises or do them before or after your aerobic exercise. You may develop more flexibility if you do them after exercise, because your muscles are warmer then and can be stretched farther.

Muscle Strengthening Exercises

Exercises that develop muscular strength and muscular endurance should also be included in any program designed to promote health. Your ability to maintain correct posture and to move efficiently depends in part on adequate muscle fitness. Strengthening exercises also increase muscle tone, which improves the appearance of your body. A lean, healthy-looking body is certainly one of the goals and one of the benefits of an overall fitness program.

Muscular strength and endurance can be developed in many ways, from weight training to calisthenics. (Taking **anabolic steroids** is *not* a safe or healthy way to increase muscle strength or endurance; in fact, it runs counter to all the practices that promote good health discussed in this chapter.) Common exercises such as sit-ups, push-ups, pull-ups, and wall-sitting (leaning against a wall in a seated position and supporting yourself with your leg muscles) maintain the muscular strength of most people if they practice them three to five days a week. To condition and tone your whole body, choose exercises that

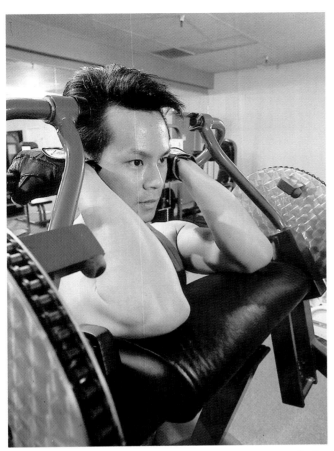

Building muscular strength is an important component of a fitness program. Weight training is just one way to increase strength, improve muscle tone, and enhance the overall appearance of the body.

work the major muscles of the shoulders, chest, back, arms, abdomen, and legs.

To increase strength, you must do **resistive exercise**—exercises in which your muscles must exert force against a significant resistance. Resistance can be provided by weights, exercise machines, or your own body weight. Your muscles become stronger when you subject them to **overload,** an exercise stress that is more severe than what they are used to. By pushing your muscles to temporary fatigue and by gradually increasing the amount of resistance or the number of times they must resist, you force them to adapt to greater physical stress. If you use heavy resistance with few repetitions (1 to 10), you build muscle strength and size. If you use lighter resistance and do more repetitions, you improve muscular endurance (the ability to exert force over a longer period of time). Strength training improves performance in most sports and has become a prominent part of the training program of many athletes. In general, you have to train at least twice a week for an hour to experience significant results. You also have to allow recovery time between work-outs—two to four days—to train properly and avoid injury.

There are three different kinds of strengthening exercises. **Isometric exercises** involve applying force without movement, such as when you contract your abdominal muscles. This static type of exercise is valuable for toning and strengthening muscles. Isometrics can be practiced anywhere and don't require any equipment. Try holding your stomach in for 10 to 30 seconds several times during the day (but don't hold your breath—that can restrict blood flow to your heart and brain). Within a few weeks, you'll notice the effect of this isometric exercise. Isometrics are particularly useful when recovering from an injury.

Isokinetic exercises involve exerting force at a constant speed against an equal force exerted by a specialized strength training machine. Proponents of this type of exercise claim that training at faster speeds produces a training effect more specific to the rapid movements used in sports. Isokinetic machines are considerably more expensive than traditional weight training equipment and so are not as widely available.

Isotonic exercises involve applying force with movement, as, for example, in weight training exercises such as the bench press. These are the most popular type of exercises for increasing muscle strength and seem to be most valuable for developing strength that can be transferred to other forms of physical activity. They include exercises using barbells, dumbbells, weight machines, and the body's own weight, as in push-ups or sit-ups.

Examples of isotonic exercises for various muscle groups include the bench press for the chest; the overhead press, the behind-the-neck press, and upright rowing for the shoulders; barbell and dumbbell curls for the arms; pull-ups and chin-ups for the upper back; sit-ups and crunches for the abdominals; and squats and leg presses for the legs. Exercises are repeated until the muscles are fatigued, and muscle contraction—the lifting or pushing part of the exercise—is always accompanied by an exhalation. Begin with a weight that you can lift fairly easily for 10 repetitions, and do three sets (groups) of 10 repetitions of each exercise. Increase your level of exertion gradually over a period of weeks. To learn how to do these exercises properly so they increase your muscle strength and don't cause injury, you should receive instruction from a trainer in a gym, a health club, a physical education class, or a Y or community recreation department.

Training in Specific Skills

The fourth element in your fitness program is learning the skills required in the sports or activities in which you choose to participate. Taking the time and effort to acquire competence means that instead of feeling ridiculous, becoming frustrated, and giving up in despair, you achieve a sense of mastery and add a new physical activity to your repertoire.

The first step in learning a new skill is to get help. Sports like tennis, golf, sailing, and skiing require mastery of basic movements and techniques, so instruction from a qualified teacher can save you hours of frustration and increase your enjoyment of the sport.

Skill is also important in conditioning activities such as jogging, swimming, and cycling. Some instruction on technique from a coach or fellow participant can often help you to train more efficiently. Even if you learned a sport as a child, additional instruction now can help you refine your technique, get over stumbling blocks, and relearn skills that you may have learned incorrectly.

Putting It All Together

Now that you know the basic components of a fitness program, you can put them all together in a program that works for you. Remember to include the following:

- Cardiorespiratory endurance exercise—do at least 20 minutes of aerobic exercise at your target heart rate three to five times a week
- Muscle strengthening exercise—work the major muscle groups two to three times a week
- Flexibility exercise—do stretches three to five times a week
- Skill training—incorporate some or all of your aerobic or strengthening exercise into an enjoyable sport or physical activity

In any program, it's important to *warm up* before you exercise and *cool down* afterwards. Warming up enhances your performance and decreases your chances of injury. Your muscles work better when their temperature is elevated slightly above resting level. Warming up helps your body's physiology gradually progress from rest to exercise. Blood needs to be redirected to active muscles, and your heart needs time to adapt to the increased demands of exercise. Warm-up helps spread **synovial fluid** throughout joints, which helps protect surfaces from wear and tear.

A warm-up session should include low-intensity movements similar to those in the activity that will follow. Low-intensity movements include hitting forehands and backhands before a tennis game and running a 12-minute mile before progressing to an 8-minute one. Some experts also recommend warm-up stretching exercises for flexibility after the warm-up and before intense activity.

Cooling down after exercise is important to restore circulation to its normal resting condition. When you are at rest, a relatively small percentage of your total blood volume is directed to muscles, but during exercise as much as 85 percent of the heart's output is directed to them. During recovery from exercise, it is important to continue exercising at a low level to provide a smooth transition to the resting state. Cooling down helps maintain the return of blood to your heart.

Personal Insight In our society, boys and men tend to be more active in sports and physical activities than do girls and women. Why do you think that is? How do you feel about it?

GETTING STARTED AND KEEPING ON TRACK

Once you have a program that fulfills your basic fitness needs and suits your personal tastes, adhering to a few basic principles will help you improve at the fastest rate, have more fun, and minimize the risk of injury. These principles include buying appropriate equipment, eating and drinking properly, and managing your program so it becomes an integral part of your life.

Selecting Equipment

When you're sure of the activities you're going to do, buy the best equipment you can afford. Good equipment will enhance your enjoyment and decrease your risk of injury. Part of the "fitness fad" has been a wave of new equipment and clothing. Some of it is truly revolutionary: New skis allow you to go faster with better control, new tennis racquets make it easier to hit the ball over the net, and new materials make sports clothing more comfortable and fashionable. Unfortunately, some new products are either overpriced or of poor quality. A flashy but overweight tennis racquet can produce an elbow injury, and a shoe that can't absorb shock can cause leg pains.

Before you invest in a new piece of equipment, investigate it. Is it worth the money? Does it produce the results its proponents claim for it? Is it safe? Does it fit properly and is it in good working order? Look for equipment that provides a genuine workout, such as stationary bicycles, cross-country skiing machines, or stair-climbers, not passive devices such as massage machines and rubberized

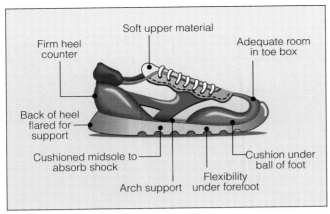

Figure 11-1 *What to look for in a running shoe.*

suits. Ask the experts (coaches, physical educators, and sports instructors) for their opinion. Better yet, educate yourself. Every sport, from running to volleyball, has its own magazine. A little effort to educate yourself will be well rewarded.

Footwear is perhaps the most important piece of equipment for almost any sport. Buy shoes that fit properly and that are appropriate for the activity. Running shoes, court shoes (for tennis, racquetball, basketball, and so on), and shoes for aerobic dance and exercise have different characteristics. Figure 11-1 shows the characteristics of an ideal running shoe.

Eating and Drinking for Exercise

Most people do not need to change their eating habits when they begin a fitness program. Many athletes and other physically active people are lured into buying aggressively advertised vitamins, minerals, and protein supplements. The truth is that in almost every case a well-balanced diet (see Chapter 9) contains all the energy and nutrients needed to sustain an exercise program.

A balanced diet is also the key to improving your body composition when you begin to exercise more. One of the promises of a fitness program is a decrease in body fat and an increase in lean, muscular body mass. As mentioned earlier, the control of body fat is determined by the balance of energy in the body. If more calories are consumed than are expended through metabolism and exercise, then fat increases. If the reverse is true, fat is lost. The best way to control body fat is to follow a diet containing adequate but not excessive calories and to exercise.

The one change in diet that some long-distance runners and other athletes make is to increase the proportion of carbohydrates they consume. Diets that are higher than average in carbohydrates can benefit athletes because carbohydrates increase the amount of **glycogen** present in the body. Glycogen, a carbohydrate stored in muscles and the liver, is vitally important for sustaining physical activity over long periods of time. When levels of this substance are low, the athlete feels sluggish, weak, and tired. One exciting discovery in sports medicine in recent years has been that consuming carbohydrate drinks during exercise can improve performance and that drinking them immediately after exercise rapidly replenishes glycogen.

One of the most important principles to follow when you're exercising is to drink enough water. Your body depends on water to sustain many chemical reactions and to maintain correct body temperature. Sweating during exercise depletes your body's water supply and can lead to dehydration if fluids aren't replaced. Serious dehydration can cause reduced blood volume, increased heart rate, raised body temperature, muscle cramps, heat stroke, and other serious problems. Drinking water before and during exercise is important to prevent dehydration and enhance athletic performance.

Thirst alone is not a good indication of how much you need to drink, because thirst is quickly depressed by drinking even small amounts of water. Most of your weight loss immediately after exercise is from loss of fluids. If you rely on thirst, it can take 24 hours or more to replace these fluids. Ideally, you should restore your body fluids before you exercise vigorously again. As a rule of thumb, try to drink about 8 ounces of water (more in hot weather) for every 30 minutes of heavy exercise. Bring a water bottle with you when you exercise so you can replace your fluids while they're being depleted. Water—preferably cold—or diluted carbohydrate drinks such as Cytomax or Gatorade are the best fluid replacements. Carbohydrate drinks are good because they also supply energy and electrolytes, such as sodium and potassium. You don't need to take salt pills—your body is very efficient at sparing electrolytes during exercise.

Managing Your Fitness Program

How can you tell when you're in shape? When do you stop improving and start maintaining? How can you stay motivated? These are important questions if your program is going to become an integral part of your life and if the principles behind it are going to serve you well in the years ahead.

Consistency: The Key to Physical Improvement It's important to be able to recognize when you have achieved the level of fitness that is adequate for you. This level will vary, of course, depending on your goals, the intensity of your program, and your natural ability. Your

Synovial fluid Fluid found within many joints that provides lubrication and nutrition to the cells of the joint surface.

Glycogen A complex carbohydrate, found largely in the liver and skeletal muscle, that serves as a carbohydrate storage depot.

TERMS

body gets into shape by adapting to increasing levels of physical stress. If you don't push yourself by increasing the intensity of your workout—by adding weight or running a little faster or a little longer—no change will occur in your body.

But if you subject your body to overly severe stress, it will break down and become distressed, or injured. Overdoing exercise is just as bad as not exercising hard enough. No one can become fit overnight. Your body needs time to adapt to increasingly higher levels of stress. The process of improving fitness, of training, involves a countless number of stresses and adaptations. If you feel extremely sore and tired the day after exercising, then you have worked too hard. Injury will slow you down just as much as a missed workout.

Consistency is the key to getting into shape without injury. Steady fitness improvement comes when you overload your body consistently over a long period of time. The best way to ensure consistency is by keeping a training journal in which you record the details of your workouts—how far you ran, how much weight you lifted, how many laps you swam, and so on. This record will help you evaluate your progress and plan your workout sessions intelligently. Don't increase your exercise volume by more than 5 to 10 percent per week.

Assessing Your Fitness

When are you "in shape"? It depends. One person may be out of shape running a mile in 5 minutes; another may be in shape running a mile in 12 minutes. As mentioned earlier, your ultimate level of fitness depends on your goals, your program, and your natural ability. The important thing is to set goals that make sense for you.

If you are interested in finding out exactly how fit you are before you begin a program, the best approach is to get an assessment from a modern sports medicine laboratory. Such laboratories can be found in university physical education departments and medical centers. Here you will receive an accurate profile of your capacity to exercise. Typically, your endurance will be measured on a treadmill or bicycle, your body fat will be estimated, and your strength and flexibility will be tested. This evaluation will reveal whether your physical condition is consistent with good health, and the personnel at the laboratory can suggest an exercise program that will be appropriate for your level of fitness.

Assessing your own fitness is more difficult, but a very rough estimate of your cardiorespiratory fitness can be obtained by checking your time in the 1.5-mile run or walk. Use the table in Wellness Worksheet 11-1 (located in the study guide in the back of the book) to find out in general terms whether your level of fitness is consistent with good health.

Staying with Your Program

Once you have attained your desired level of fitness, you can maintain it by exercising on a regular basis at a consistent intensity, three to five times a week. You must work at the intensity that brought you to your desired fitness level. If you don't, your body will become less fit because less is expected of it. In general, if you exercise at the same intensity over a long period, your fitness will level out and can be maintained easily. Sometimes it's easiest to stay with a program if you spend money to take a class or join a club. Exercising with a friend is also a good motivator.

What if you run out of steam? A variety of specific suggestions for staying with your program are given in the Behavior Change Strategy at the end of this chapter. It's also a good idea to have a goal, anything from fitting into the same size jeans you used to wear to successfully skiing down a new slope. Remember, you can have goals without striving to improve your fitness.

Varying your program is another way to stay interested. Some people alternate two or more activities—swimming and jogging, for example—to improve a particular component of fitness. The practice, called **cross-training**, can help prevent boredom and overuse injuries. It's a good idea to explore many exercise options. Consider competitive sports at the recreational level—swimming, running, racquetball, volleyball, golf, and so on. Find out how you can participate in an activity you've never done before—canoeing, hang gliding, windsurfing, backpacking. Try new activities, especially ones that you will be able to do for the rest of your life. Get maps of the park, recreational, or wilderness areas near you and go exploring. Fill a canteen, pack a good lunch, and take along a wildflower or bird book. Every step you take will bring you closer to your ultimate goal—fitness and health that last a lifetime.

> **Personal Insight** Do you exercise because you like it or because you think you should? Is there any form of exercise that you do just for the love of it?

SUMMARY

What Is Physical Fitness and Why Is It Important?

- The components of overall *physical fitness* include cardiorespiratory endurance; flexibility; muscular strength, power, and endurance; and body composition. Components of fitness for a specific activity might include coordination, speed, agility, balance, and skill.

- The body works best when it *is* active. By improving the overall functioning of the body, exercise can help in managing stress, maintaining emotional well-being, controlling weight, boosting the immune system, and protecting against serious diseases.

Why Is Exercise So Good for You?

- Cardiorespiratory endurance (or aerobic) exercise improves the ability of the heart, lungs, and circulatory system to carry oxygen to the body's tissues. This efficiency means that the heart does not have to work as hard in daily life and can meet emergency needs.
- Exercise has a positive effect on the balance of lipids in the blood; exercise increases HDLs and lowers LDLs. Exercise also decreases the secretion of hormones triggered by emotional stress and helps diffuse hostility.
- Endurance exercise improves the efficiency of the body's metabolism, helping to regulate energy balance and body weight.
- Exercise has social, psychological, and emotional benefits. Positive feelings associated with exercise have a physiological basis in hormones and body chemicals.
- Exercises designed to improve muscular strength and endurance, joint flexibility, and posture are also essential to fitness.
- Beginning to exercise regularly can improve health over the life span. Physical fitness helps prevent heart disease, stroke, diabetes, and high blood pressure; it may help prevent fatigue, weight gain, memory loss, and other problems associated with aging. Exercise is especially helpful in preventing osteoporosis.

Designing Your Exercise and Fitness Program

- The best exercise and fitness programs develop all fitness components, promote health, and are fun to do.
- Cardiorespiratory endurance exercises stress a large portion of the body's muscle mass for a prolonged period of time.
- To be effective, endurance exercise should be undertaken three to five days a week and last from 15 minutes (high-intensity activities) to 60 minutes (low-intensity activities).
- Intensity of training is crucial to increasing the body's maximal oxygen capacity; monitoring the heart rate helps ensure that a workout is done at the appropriate intensity.

- Flexibility, or stretching, exercises are necessary to maintain the normal range of motion in the major joints of the body.
- Exercises to develop muscular strength and endurance are necessary for correct posture, efficient movement, and muscle tone. Resistive exercises are necessary to increase muscle strength.
- Learning the skills required for specific sports or activities helps people achieve a sense of mastery and adds new physical activities to their exercise programs.
- Warming up exercises decrease chances of injury by helping the body gradually progress from rest to exercise as blood is redirected to active muscles.
- Cooling down after exercise involves continuing to exercise at a low level to provide a smooth transition to the resting state.

Getting Started and Keeping on Track

- Good equipment enhances enjoyment and decreases risk of injury. Footwear is especially important; it should fit properly and be appropriate for the activity.
- A well-balanced diet contains all the energy and nutrients needed to sustain a fitness program. Increasing the proportion of carbohydrates can benefit some athletes.
- When exercising, it's important to drink enough water, which is necessary to prevent dehydration and maintain correct body temperature.
- The ultimate level of fitness depends on the goals, the program, and natural ability. Fitness levels can be evaluated at sports medicine laboratories.
- A desired level of fitness can be maintained by exercising three to five times a week at a consistent intensity. Ways to stay motivated include having specific goals, enjoying the activity, working out with a friend or group, and maintaining interest by varying the program.

TAKE ACTION

1. Go to your school's physical education office and ask for a comprehensive listing of all the exercise and fitness facilities available on your campus. Visit the facilities you haven't yet seen and investigate the activities that are done there. If there are sports or activities you'd like to try, consider doing so.

2. Habit helps us conserve energy as we go through our daily lives, but it also blinds us to areas we could change. Identify 10 ways you can incorporate more physical activity into your life by changing a habit, such as walking instead of riding the bus, taking the

stairs in a certain building instead of the elevator, and so on. Try several of these new habits this week.

JOURNAL ENTRY

1. In your health journal, list the positive behaviors and attitudes that help you avoid a sedentary lifestyle and stay fit. How can you strengthen these behaviors and attitudes? Then list the negative behaviors and attitudes that block a physically active lifestyle. Which ones can you change? How can you change them?

2. *Critical Thinking:* Study the ads for fitness products and clubs on television, in popular magazines, and in your local newspaper. What markets are they targeting? How do they try to appeal to their audience? What other messages are they sending? Write a short essay describing your findings.

BEHAVIOR CHANGE STRATEGY

PLANNING A PERSONAL EXERCISE PROGRAM

Although most people recognize the importance of incorporating exercise into their lives, many find it difficult to do. No single strategy will work for everyone, but the general steps outlined here should help you create an exercise program that fits your goals, preferences, and lifestyle. A carefully designed contract and program plan can help you convert your vague wishes into a detailed plan of action. And the strategies for program compliance outlined here and in Chapter 1 can help you enjoy and stick with your program for the rest of your life.

Step 1: Set Goals

Setting specific goals to accomplish by exercising is an important first step in a successful fitness program because it establishes the direction you want to go. Your goals might be specifically related to health, such as lowering your blood pressure and risk for heart disease, or they might relate to other aspects of your life, such as improving your tennis game or the fit of your clothes. If you can decide why you're starting to exercise, it can help you to keep going.

Think carefully about your reasons for incorporating exercise into your life, and then fill in the goals portion of the Personal Fitness Contract.

Step 2: Select a Sport or Activity

As discussed in the chapter, the success of your fitness program depends upon the consistency of your involvement. You should select activities that encourage your

commitment: The right program will be its own incentive to continue; poor activity choices provide obstacles and can turn exercise into a chore.

When choosing activities for your fitness program, you should consider the following:

- Is this activity fun? Will it hold my interest over time?
- Will this activity help me reach the goals I have set for myself?
- Will my current fitness and skill level allow me to participate fully in this activity?
- Can I easily fit this activity into my daily schedule? Are there any special requirements (facilities, partners, equipment, etc.) that I must plan for?
- Can I afford any special costs required for equipment or facilities?
- (If you have special exercise needs due to a particular health problem.) Does this activity conform to my special health needs? Will it enhance my ability to cope with my specific health problem?

Using the guidelines listed above, select a number of sports and activities and fill in the "Program Plan" portion of the Fitness Contract. Does your program meet the criteria of a complete fitness program discussed in the chapter?

Step 3: Make a Commitment

Complete your Fitness Contract and Program Plan by signing your contract and having it witnessed and signed by someone who can help make you accountable for your progress. By completing a written contract you will make a firm commitment and will be more likely to follow through until you meet your goals.

Step 4: Begin and Maintain Your Program

Start out slowly to allow your body time to adjust. Be realistic and patient—meeting your goals will take time. The following guidelines may help you to start and stick with your program:

- Set aside regular periods for exercise. Choose times that fit in best with your schedule and stick to them. Allow an adequate amount of time for warm-up, cool-down, and a shower.
- Take advantage of any opportunity for exercise that presents itself (for example, walk to class, take the stairs instead of the elevator).
- Do what you can to avoid boredom. Do calisthenics to music or watch the evening news while riding your stationary bicycle.
- Exercise with a group that shares your goals and general level of competence.
- Vary the program. Change your activities periodically. Alter your route or distance if biking or jogging.

Personal Fitness Contract

I, _____ , am contracting with myself to follow an exercise program to work at the following goals.

Fitness Goals

(Note as many as appropriate)

1. _____
2. _____
3. _____
4. _____
5. _____

Program Plan

Activities	Components (Check ✓)					Intensity	Duration	Frequency (Check ✓)						
	CRE	BC	MS	ME	F			M.	Tu.	W.	Th.	F.	Sa.	Su.
1.														
2.														
3.														
4.														
5.														
6.														
7.														
8.														
9.														
10.														

I will begin my program on _____ .

I agree to maintain a record of my activity, assess my progress periodically, and, if necessary, revise my goals.

Signed _____   Date _____

Witness _____

Note: You should conduct activities for achieving CRE goals at your target heart rate.

Adapted from Ivan Kusinitz and Morton Fine. 1995. *Your Guide to Getting Fit*, 3rd ed. Mountain View, Calif.: Mayfield.

Change racquetball partners or find a new volleyball court.

- Establish minigoals or a point system and work rewards into your program. Until you reach your main goals, a system of self-rewards will help you stick with your program. Rewards should be things you enjoy and that are easily obtainable.

Step 5: Record and Assess Your Progress

Keeping a record that notes the daily results of your program will help remind you of your ongoing commitment to your program and give you a sense of accomplishment. Create daily and weekly program logs that you can use to track your progress. You should record the activity type, frequency, and duration. Keep your log handy and fill it in immediately after each exercise session. Post it in a visible place to both remind you of your activity schedule and offer incentive for improvement.

Here are some additional tips to help make your program a success:

- If in the first few weeks you find that your program is unrealistic, revise the goals and activity information on your contract. Expect to make many adjustments in your program along the way.

- Don't expect your progress to be even and regular. You will notice fluctuations: On some days your progress will be excellent, while on others you will barely be able to drag yourself through the scheduled activities.

- Don't rush yourself. Overzealous exercising can result in discouraging discomforts and injuries. Your program is meant to last a lifetime, so begin slowly and increase your activity level gradually.

- If you notice that you are slacking off, try to list the negative thoughts and behaviors that are causing noncompliance. Devise a strategy to decrease the frequency of negative thoughts and behaviors. Adjust your program plan and reward system to help renew your enthusiasm and commitment to your program.

- Review your goals. Visualize what it will be like to reach them, and keep these pictures in your mind as an incentive to stick to your program.

SELECTED BIBLIOGRAPHY

American College of Sports Medicine. 1991. *Guidelines for Exercise Testing and Prescription.* Philadelphia: Lea and Feibiger.

Berlin, J. A., and G. A. Colditz. 1990. A meta-analysis of physical activity in the prevention of coronary heart disease. *American Journal of Epidemiology* 132:612–628.

Bijnen, F. C., C. J. Caspersen, and W. L. Mosterd. 1994. Physical inactivity as a risk factor for coronary heart disease: A WHO and International Society and Federation of Cardiology position statement. *Bulletin of the World Health Organization* 72(1): 1–4.

Blair, S. N., and H. W. Kohl. 1988. Physical activity or physical fitness: Which is more important for health? *Medical Science Sports Exercise* 20:S8.

Blair, S. N., H. W. Kohl, R. S. Paffenbarger, D. G. Clark, K. H. Cooper, and L. W. Gibbons. 1989. Physical fitness and all-cause mortality: A prospective study of healthy men and women. *Journal of the American Medical Association* 262:2395–2401.

Brooks, G. A., and T. D. Fahey. 1987. *Fundamentals of Human Performance.* New York: Macmillan.

Fahey, T. D., ed. 1986. *Athletic Training: Principles and Practice.* Mountain View, Calif.: Mayfield.

Haskell, W. L., and others. 1992. Cardiovascular benefits and assessment of physical activity and physical fitness in adults. *Medicine and Science in Sports and Exercise* 24:S201–20.

———. 1994. Effects of intensive multiple risk factor reduction on coronary atherosclerosis and clinical cardiac events in men and women with coronary artery disease. The Stanford Coronary Risk Intervention Project (SCRIP). *Circulation* 89:975–990.

Hickson, R. C., K. Hidaka, and C. Foster. 1994. Skeletal muscle fiber type, resistance training, and strength-related performance. *Medicine and Science in Sports and Exercise* 26:593–8.

Hickson, J. F., and I. Wolinsky. 1989. *Nutrition in Exercise and Sport.* Boca Raton, Fla.: CRC Press.

Israel, R. G., and others. 1994. Relationship between cardiorespiratory fitness and lipoprotein(a) in men and women. *Medicine and Science in Sports and Exercise* 26:425–431.

Komi, P. V., ed. 1992. *Strength and Power in Sports.* London: Blackwell Scientific Publications.

LaFontaine, T., and others. 1994. The effect of physical activity on all cause mortality compared to cardiovascular mortality: A review of research and recommendations. *Mo. Med.* 91:188–94.

McAuley, D. 1994. Exercise, cardiovascular disease and lipids. *British Journal of Clinical Practice* 47:323–7.

Nieman, D. C. 1995. *Fitness and Sports Medicine.* 3rd ed. Menlo Park, Calif.: Bull Publishing.

Porcari, J. P., C. B. Ebbeling, A. Ward, P. S. Freedson, and J. M. Rippe. 1989. Walking for exercise testing and training. *Sports Medicine* 8:189–200.

Rodriguez, B. L., and others. 1994. Physical activity and 23-year incidence of coronary heart disease morbidity and mortality among middle-aged men. The Honolulu Heart Program. *Circulation* 89:2540–44.

Safran, M. R., A. V. Seaber, and W. E. Garrett. 1989. Warm-up and muscular injury prevention. *Sports Medicine* 8:239–49.

Yeager, K. K., and C. A. Macera. 1994. Physical activity and health profiles of United States women. *Clin. Sports. Med.* 13:329–35.

RECOMMENDED READINGS

Anderson, B. 1980. *Stretching.* Bolinas, Calif.: Shelter Publications. *A complete guide to stretching that includes stretching programs for general fitness, for many sports and activities, and for care of the back.*

Cooper, K. 1983. *The Aerobics Program for Total Well-Being.* New York: Bantam Books. *A comprehensive guide to shaping up your heart and lungs.*

Fahey, T. 1994. *Basic Weight Training for Men and Women,* 2nd ed. Mountain View, Calif.: Mayfield. *A practical guide to developing training programs tailored to individual needs.*

Fahey, T. D., and G. Hutchinson. 1992. *Weight Training for Women.* Mountain View, Calif.: Mayfield. *A practical guide to developing a healthier, stronger body, it contains complete coverage of topics of special interest to women.*

Kusinitz, I., and M. Fine. 1995. *Your Guide to Getting Fit.* 3rd ed. Mountain View, Calif.: Mayfield. *A step-by-step guide to developing a personalized fitness program.*

Maglischo, E. W., and C. F. Brennan. 1984. *Swim for the Health of It.* Mountain View, Calif.: Mayfield. *Includes discussions of conditioning and stroke techniques for people who want to use swimming to improve their health and physical fitness.*

Meyers, C. 1992. *Walking: A Complete Guide to the Complete Exercise.* New York: Random House. *Offers strategies for putting together individualized walking programs for weight control and cardiovascular fitness.*

Nokes, T. D. 1991. *Lore of Running.* 3rd ed. Champaign, Ill.: Human Kinetics. *A comprehensive guide that includes discussions of the physiology of running; training for running; and recognizing, avoiding, and treating running injuries.*

Pryor, E., and M. Kraines. 1996. *Keep Moving! It's Aerobic Dance.* 3rd ed. Mountain View, Calif.: Mayfield. *Discusses the fitness principles and techniques every aerobic dancer should know.*

Van der Plas, R. 1990. *The Bicycle Fitness Book: Riding Your Bike for Health and Fitness.* Rev. ed. Mill Valley, Calif.: Bicycle Books. *Includes practical advice on choosing equipment, riding safely, and putting together a personal training program.*

12

Cardiovascular Disease and Cancer

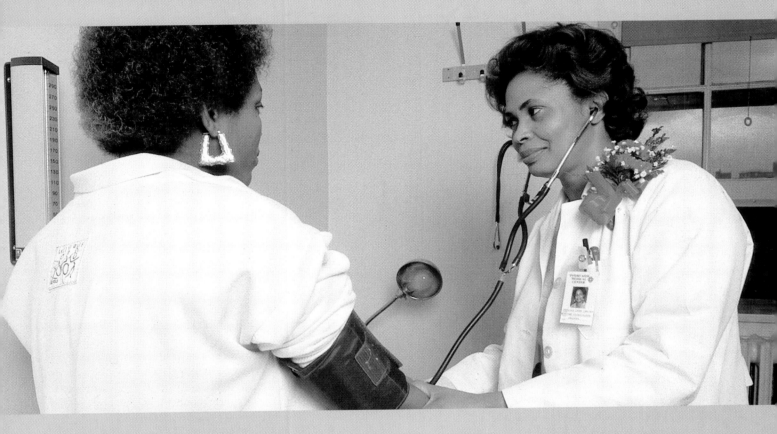

CONTENTS

The breakthroughs in medical science that have eradicated some diseases (such as smallpox and polio) and reduced the impact of others (such as streptococcal infections) have left **cardiovascular disease** and cancer high on the list of threats to human life. Both are lifestyle diseases, although genetics and the physical environment also play a role. This chapter discusses both the causes of these diseases and ways to reduce your risk of developing them.

THE CARDIOVASCULAR SYSTEM

The **cardiovascular system** consists of the heart and blood vessels (veins, arteries, and capillaries); together they pump and circulate blood throughout the body. Blood travels through two separate circulatory systems, the right and left sides of the heart. The right side pumps blood to and from the lungs; this is called the **pulmonary circulation.** The left side pumps blood through the rest of the body; this is called the **systemic circulation** (Figure 12-1). A person weighing 150 pounds has about 5 quarts of blood, which is circulated about once every minute.

The heart is a four-chambered muscle, shaped like a cone and about the size of a fist (Figure 12-2). It is located just beneath the ribs, under the left breast. Its role is to pump oxygen-depleted blood to the lungs and to pump oxygenated blood to the rest of the body. Used, oxygen-depleted blood enters the right upper chamber, or **atrium,** of the heart through the **vena cava,** the largest vein in the body. Valves prevent it from flowing the wrong way. As it fills, the right atrium contracts and pumps blood into the right lower chamber, or **ventricle,** which, when it contracts, pumps blood through the **pulmonary artery** into the lungs. There blood picks up oxygen and discards carbon dioxide. Cleaned, oxygenated blood then flows through the pulmonary veins into the left atrium. As this chamber fills, it contracts and pumps blood into the powerful left ventricle. When the left ventricle contracts, blood is pumped through the **aorta,** the body's largest artery, which feeds into the rest of the blood vessels in the body. The period of contraction of the heart is called **systole;** the period of relaxation between contractions is called **diastole.**

Blood vessels are classified by size and function. Veins carry blood *to* the heart, arteries carry it *away* from the heart. Arteries have thick elastic walls that enable them to expand and relax as blood is pumped into them under pressure from the heart. Veins have thinner walls. After leaving the heart, the aorta branches into smaller and smaller arteries. Two vital arteries branch off the aorta to carry blood back to the tissues of the heart itself; these are the **coronary arteries.** The smallest arteries, called **arterioles,** branch still further into **capillaries,** tiny vessels only one cell thick.

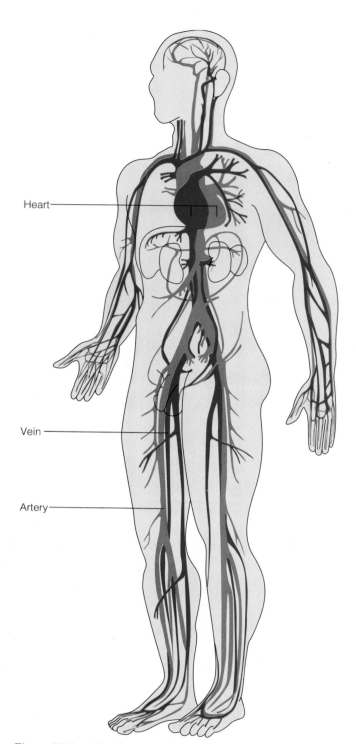

Heart

Vein

Artery

Figure 12-1 *Circulation in the body.*

TERMS

Cardiovascular disease (CVD) Diseases of the heart and blood vessels.

Cardiovascular system The heart and blood vessels.

Pulmonary circulation The portion of the circulatory system governed by the right side of the heart; the circulation of blood between the heart and the lungs.

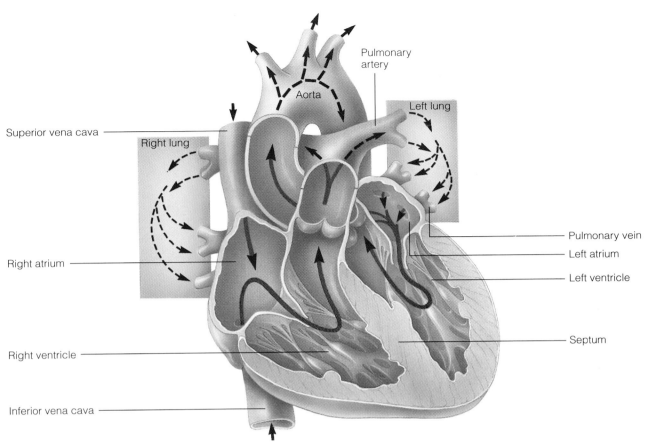

Figure 12-2 *Circulation in the heart.*

An exchange of nutrients and waste products takes place between the capillaries and the tissues, so that the oxygen- and nutrient-rich blood becomes oxygen-poor, waste-carrying blood. This blood empties out of the capillaries into small veins called **venules**, then into the larger veins that return it to the heart. From there the cycle is repeated.

RISK FACTORS FOR CARDIOVASCULAR DISEASE

Researchers have identified a variety of factors associated with increased risk for cardiovascular disease. They are grouped into two categories: major risk factors and contributing risk factors. Some major risk factors are linked to controllable lifestyle factors such as diet, exercise habits, and ways of dealing with stress and can therefore be changed. Others are beyond the individual's control and cannot be changed.

Major Risk Factors That Can Be Changed

The American Heart Association has identified four major risk factors for CVD that can be changed. These are to-

TERMS

Systemic circulation   The portion of the circulatory system governed by the left side of the heart; the circulation of blood between the heart and the rest of the body.

Atria   The two upper chambers of the heart in which blood collects before passing to the ventricles; also called auricles (*sing.* atrium).

Vena cava   Large vein through which blood is returned to the right atrium of the heart.

Ventricles   The two lower chambers of the heart from which blood flows through arteries to the lungs and other parts of the body.

Pulmonary artery   The artery that receives blood from the right ventricle and carries it to the lungs.

Aorta   The large artery that receives blood from the left ventricle and distributes it to the body.

Systole   Contraction of the heart.

Diastole   Relaxation of the heart.

Coronary arteries   Two arteries branching from the aorta that provide blood to the heart muscle.

Arterioles   The smallest arteries that end in capillaries.

Capillaries   Very small blood vessels that distribute blood to all parts of the body.

Venules   Small veins.

TABLE 12-1 Cholesterol Guidelines

Total blood cholesterol

Less than 200 mg/dl	Desirable*
200–239 mg/dl	Borderline high
240 mg/dl or more	High

LDL cholesterol

Less than 130 mg/dl	Desirable*
130–159 mg/dl	Borderline high
160 mg/dl or more	High

HDL cholesterol

More than 45 mg/dl	Desirable*
35–45 mg/dl	Borderline low
Less than 35 mg/dl	Low

*For adults without known heart disease.

Source: The American Heart Association; the National Cholesterol Education Program.

TACTICS AND TIPS
Controlling Cholesterol Through Diet

A diet that improves cholesterol levels is high in dietary fiber and low in fat, saturated fat, and cholesterol. To lower your risk for CVD, try some of these dietary changes.

Decrease Intake	Increase Intake
Whole milk	Nonfat and low-fat milk
Hard cheeses, cream cheese	Low-fat cottage cheese, nonfat yogurt
Beef, pork, sausage, bacon	Fish, skinless chicken, turkey
Butter, high-fat mayonnaise	Vegetable oil, mustard
Ice cream	Sherbet, frozen yogurt
Palm and coconut oils	Olive and vegetable oils
Many luncheon meats	Turkey, chicken meats
Many prepared baked goods	Fruits, vegetables
Egg yolks (egg whites are OK)	Beans, cereals, pasta, bread

bacco use, high blood pressure, unhealthy blood cholesterol levels, and physical inactivity.

Tobacco Use People who smoke a pack of cigarettes a day have twice the risk of heart attack that nonsmokers have; smoking two or more packs a day triples the risk. And when smokers do have heart attacks, they are two to four times more likely than nonsmokers to die from them. And you don't have to smoke to be affected. Environmental tobacco smoke (ETS) in high concentrations has been linked to the development of CVD.

Smoking harms the cardiovascular system in several ways. Smoking can reduce levels of **high-density lipoproteins (HDL),** the so-called "good cholesterol," in the bloodstream. The psychoactive drug in tobacco, nicotine, is a central nervous system stimulant, causing increased blood pressure and heart rate. The carbon monoxide in cigarette smoke displaces oxygen in the blood, reducing the amount of oxygen available to the heart and other parts of the body. Cigarette smoking also causes the **platelets** in blood to become sticky and cluster, shortens platelet survival, decreases clotting time, and increases blood thickness. All these effects increase a person's risk of heart attack and other cardiovascular disease.

Smokers' risk for CVD drops rapidly after quitting, regardless of how long or how much they've smoked. Three years after quitting, a person who smoked a pack a day or less has about the same risk of death from CVD as a person who has never smoked.

High Blood Pressure High blood pressure (**hypertension**) is a risk factor for many types of cardiovascular disease but is also considered a form of disease itself. High blood pressure occurs when too much force or pressure is exerted against the walls of the arteries. If your blood pressure is high, your heart has to work harder to push the blood forward. Over time, a strained heart weakens and tends to enlarge, which weakens it further. Increased blood pressure also scars and hardens arteries and arterioles, making them less elastic. Heart attacks, strokes, **atherosclerosis,** and kidney failure can result. High blood pressure usually has no early warning signs, so it's important to have your blood pressure tested at least once a year. If yours is high, your physician can help you lower it through diet, weight management, exercise, and, if necessary, medication. (High blood pressure and atherosclerosis are discussed in greater detail later in the chapter.)

Cholesterol Cholesterol is a fatty, waxlike substance, or lipid, that circulates through the bloodstream. Adequate cholesterol is essential for the proper functioning of the body. However, excess cholesterol can clog arteries and increase the risk of cardiovascular disease.

Our bodies obtain cholesterol in two ways: from the liver, which manufactures it, and from the foods we eat. If our blood contains more of the "bad" type of cholesterol than we can use or dispose of, the excess is deposited on artery walls.

Cholesterol Testing   The first step in controlling cholesterol is to have your total blood cholesterol level tested. The National Cholesterol Education Program (NCEP) recommends testing for all adults at least once every five years, beginning at age 20, or at least every three years if there is a family history of heart disease. "Desirable" total cholesterol readings for middle-aged adults are 200 milligrams per deciliter of blood (mg/dl) or lower. Readings of 240 mg/dl or above are considered "high"; readings between 200 and 240 mg/dl are "borderline high" (Table 12-1). For those aged 19 and under, the "desirable" level is below 170 mg/dl. An estimated 94.6 million American adults—over half the adult population—have total cholesterol levels of 200 mg/dl or higher.

The American Heart Association recommends that cholesterol testing measure both total cholesterol level and the level of high-density lipoproteins, or HDL (discussed below). If total cholesterol measures over 200 and HDL measures under 35, a more extensive lipid analysis test is in order.

Good Versus Bad Cholesterol   Cholesterol is carried in the blood in protein-lipid packages called lipoproteins. Lipoproteins can be thought of as one-way shuttles that transport cholesterol to and from the liver through the circulatory system. **Low-density lipoproteins (LDLs)** are known as "bad" cholesterol because they shuttle cholesterol from the liver to the organs and tissues that require it. If the LDLs transport more cholesterol than the body can use, the excess is deposited in the blood vessels. When it accumulates, it can block arteries and cause heart attacks and strokes. High-density lipoproteins (HDLs), or "good" cholesterol, shuttle unused cholesterol back to the liver for recycling. High LDL levels and low HDL levels are associated with high risk for CVD; low levels of LDL and high levels of HDL are associated with lower risk (see Table 12-1).

Can Cholesterol Be Too Low?   Some recent evidence suggests that very low levels of cholesterol may be unhealthy. Studies have found that the death rate for people with total cholesterol levels below 160 mg/dl is equivalent to the death rate for people with very high cholesterol levels. For example, very low cholesterol is associated with an increased risk of certain strokes. People with very low cholesterol levels also have an increased risk of certain cancers, liver disease, and lung disease. It's possible that lack of adequate cholesterol interferes with the production of crucial materials such as sex hormones and **lung surfactant.** The findings about very low cholesterol levels are still preliminary, and no guidelines regarding low cholesterol have been established. However, some cardiovascular disease experts suggest that cholesterol levels between 180 and 200 mg/dl may be optimal.

A Dietary Plan for Controlling Cholesterol   For most Americans, changing their diets to lower their total cholesterol level means cutting total fat intake and substituting unsaturated fats for saturated fats. The NCEP recommends that all Americans over the age of 2 adopt a diet in which total fat consumption is no more than 30 percent of total daily caloric intake. No more than one-third of those fat calories should come from saturated fat, which is found in animal products, palm and coconut oil, and hydrogenated vegetable oils. Saturated fat influences the production and excretion of cholesterol by the liver, so decreasing your saturated fat intake is the most important dietary change you can make to control your cholesterol.

One-third or more of your fat calories should come from monounsaturated fats, such as olive or canola oil; intake of these oils may raise HDL levels. And up to one-third of your fat calories should come from polyunsaturated fats, which may help you lower your total cholesterol level without reducing HDL.

Animal products contain cholesterol as well as saturated fat. The NCEP recommends limiting dietary cholesterol to 300 mg or less per day, slightly more than the amount in one egg. (Vegetable products do not contain cholesterol.)

Research has linked other dietary factors to improving cholesterol levels. Dietary fiber can help reduce cholesterol by trapping the bile acids the liver needs to manufacture cholesterol and carrying them to the large intestine, where they are excreted. Good sources of fiber include wheat bran, oatmeal, psyllium, barley, legumes, apples, pears, figs, and the pulp of citrus fruits. Omega-3 fatty acids, found in fish and shellfish, may also be helpful in lowering cholesterol. Some experts recommend eating fish or seafood two or three times a week; fish-oil capsules are not recommended, however, because they have not been proven effective and they add calories and fat to

---

High-density lipoproteins (HDLs)   Blood fats that help transport cholesterol out of the arteries and thus protect against heart diseases.

Platelets   Microscopic disk-shaped cell fragments in the blood. These disintegrate on contact with foreign objects and release chemicals that are necessary for the formation of blood clots.

Hypertension   Sustained abnormally high blood pressure.

Atherosclerosis   The principal form of arteriosclerosis; in atherosclerosis, the inner layers of artery walls are made thick and irregular by deposits of a fatty substance. The internal channel of arteries becomes narrowed, and blood supply is reduced.

Low-density lipoproteins (LDLs)   Blood fats that transport cholesterol from the liver to organs and tissues; excess is deposited on artery walls, where it can eventually block the flow of blood to the heart and brain.

Lung surfactant   Chemical fluid coating the surface of the lungs that lowers surface tension, aids in gas exchange, and helps keep the lungs from collapsing.

TERMS

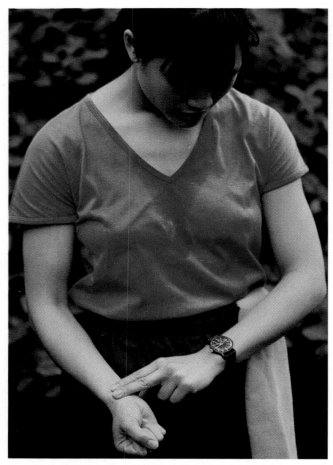

One of the primary benefits of endurance exercise is its conditioning effect on the heart and lungs. A lifetime of sensible exercise habits offers protection against cardiovascular disease later in life.

the diet. Alcohol, particularly certain components of red wine, has been shown to increase HDL cholesterol levels. However, experts don't recommend alcohol consumption as a strategy for preventing CVD either. The other risks of alcohol, including automobile crashes and alcoholism, outweigh any potential benefits.

Two other steps in cholesterol control are regular exercise and smoking cessation. Smoking lowers your HDL. Exercise, which is the closest thing to a "magic bullet" against disease, raises HDL.

Physical Inactivity   In 1992, the American Heart Association elevated a sedentary lifestyle to the ranks of major risk factors for CVD, putting it on a par with smoking, unhealthy cholesterol levels, and high blood pressure. Lack of exercise had previously been considered only a contributing factor. Exercise lowers CVD risk by helping to decrease blood pressure, increase HDL levels, maintain desirable weight, and prevent or control diabetes.

An estimated 35 to 50 million Americans are so sedentary that they are at high risk for developing CVD. They can reduce their risk significantly with as little as 90 minutes a week of mild exercise like walking, gardening, or bowling. Moving from a mild exercise program to a moderate one—say 30 minutes to an hour of brisk walking or cycling, four or more times a week—reduces risk even more. Moving from a moderate to an intense program provides little added benefit in terms of CVD prevention, although intense exercise can improve your strength, endurance, and athletic performance. See Chapter 11 for information on developing a complete, personalized exercise program.

Personal Insight   What sort of health habits did your family have when you were growing up? Did members of your family exercise? Smoke? What kind of diet did they eat? How do your current habits compare? In what ways have your family's habits affected your current lifestyle?

Contributing Risk Factors That Can Be Changed

Various other factors that can be changed have been identified as contributing to risk for cardiovascular disease, including overweight, diabetes, responses to stress, and psychological and social factors.

Overweight   A person whose body weight is more than 30 percent above the recommended level is at higher risk for heart disease and stroke even if no other risk factors are present. Excess weight increases the strain on the heart by contributing to high blood pressure and high cholesterol. It can also lead to diabetes, another CVD risk factor (see below). As discussed in Chapter 10, the distribution of body fat is also significant: Fat that collects in the torso is more dangerous than fat that collects around the hips. A prudent diet and regular exercise are the best ways to achieve and maintain a healthy body weight. Avoid yo-yo dieting—evidence suggests that repeatedly losing and regaining weight may be more harmful to the cardiovascular system than living with some excess weight.

Diabetes   In a person with **diabetes,** the pancreas produces insufficient insulin to metabolize glucose. People with diabetes are at increased risk for CVD because the disease affects the levels of cholesterol in the blood. Diabetes appears to have both a genetic component and a behavioral component. The best way to avoid diabetes is to exercise regularly and control body weight.

Stress   Excessive stress may contribute to CVD over time. If the alarm reaction (the "fight-or-flight" response) is triggered repeatedly, it can put a strain on the heart and blood vessels. In addition, people sometimes adopt un-

Current research indicates that individuals who have a persistently hostile outlook, a quick temper, and a mistrusting, cynical attitude toward life are more likely to develop heart disease than are individuals with a calmer, more trusting attitude. Why should this be the case? What is the link between chronic hostility and the heart?

The connection is most likely to be found in the physiological mechanism of the stress response (see Chapter 2). Studies show that people who are prone to chronic hostility experience the stress response more intensely and frequently than do more relaxed individuals. When they encounter the irritations of daily life, their blood pressure increases much more than is the case for less hostile people. They also seem to have trouble shutting down the stress response. Less hostile people tend to calm down much more quickly, taking the stress off their bodies—especially their hearts.

Are You Hostile?

How hostile do you think you are? To get an idea, read the following questions and respond to each with *never, sometimes, often,* or *always.*

- When people do things (or fail to do things) that prevent you from doing what you want to do, do you begin to think that they are selfish, mean, inconsiderate, incompetent, or stupid?

- When people do things that strike you as messy, selfish, inconsiderate, incompetent, or stupid, do you quickly experience feelings of frustration, irritation, anger, or rage?

- When you experience the feelings mentioned above, are they accompanied by physical sensations like increases in heart rate, breathing rate, perspiration, and so on?

- When you have these experiences, are you likely to express your feelings, whether in words, body language, facial expression, or action, to the person you see as responsible?

If you answer *often* or *always* to two or more of these questions, it's likely that your level of hostility is creating a health risk for you.

Developing a "Trusting Heart"

According to Redford Williams, noted researcher and author of *The Trusting Heart* and *Anger Kills,* hostile people can learn to change their attitudes and, in doing so, reduce their risk of heart disease. Just as hostility increases the risk of heart disease, having a trusting heart—being slow to anger, ex-

pecting the best of others, and spending minimal time feeling resentful, irritable, and angry—appears to prevent heart disease. Williams has created a 17-point behavior modification plan for developing a more trusting—and healthier—heart:

1. Reason with yourself. Try to talk yourself out of being upset. Then drop the matter.

2. Stop hostile thoughts, feelings, and urges. Silently shout "Stop!" at them.

3. Distract yourself. Look at a magazine when waiting in line. Sing along with a tape when stuck in traffic.

4. Meditate. Practice emptying your mind of thoughts 15 minutes a day. Use these skills when you become angry.

5. Avoid overstimulation. Cut back on nicotine, caffeine, and sweets. Exercise regularly.

6. Assert yourself. Learn to calmly and respectfully ask others to change a specific behavior.

7. Care for a pet.

8. Listen. Learning to listen to others will reduce misunderstandings and improve your relationships.

9. Practice trusting others. Begin with simple situations, such as letting a friend choose a restaurant.

10. Take on community service to reinforce your sense of connectedness with other people.

11. Increase your empathy. Learn to understand other people's needs and motivations.

12. Be tolerant. Intolerance is accompanied by anger.

13. Forgive. When you cannot change what was done, release your anger by forgiving the person who hurt you.

14. Have a confidant. Cultivate at least one relationship intimate enough that you can rely on each other for emotional and physical support.

15. Learn to laugh at yourself when you're getting hostile.

16. Become more religious. Being an active participant in a religious community can help you achieve a more positive outlook.

17. Pretend this is the last day of your life. Does this argument matter in the long run?

For a full discussion of these points, see Williams' book *Anger Kills.*

- *CVD* in all its forms kills about 860,000 Americans per year. Nearly one in two Americans dies of CVD. More than one-sixth of the victims are under age 65.
- *High blood pressure* afflicts about 50 million Americans. About 36,000 die from it each year.
- *Coronary heart disease* afflicts 7.2 percent of Americans aged 20 and older. 1.5 million will have a heart attack this year. About one-third of them will die.
- *Stroke* strikes about 500,000 Americans each year. It kills 150,000 a year.
- *Rheumatic heart disease* afflicts 1.3 million Americans. It kills about 6,000 every year.

- *CVD* has a greater impact on African Americans. The death rate for African American men is 46.8 percent higher than for white men. The death rate for African American women is 68.9 percent higher than for white women.
- *CVD* will cost the nation about $137.7 billion in 1995 for medical services and lost productivity.
- If all forms of CVD were eliminated, total life expectancy in the U.S. would rise by 9.8 years.

Source: The American Heart Association. 1995. *Heart and Stroke Facts: 1995 Statistical Supplement.*

---

healthy habits as a means of dealing with severe stress; they may start smoking, overeating, or skipping meals. (See Chapter 2 for information on effective strategies for managing stress.)

Psychological and Social Factors   In the 1970s, two astute cardiologists noticed that people with hard-driving, aggressive personalities had a high incidence of heart disease. They dubbed this heart-attack-prone personality "Type A"; its laid-back, healthier counterpart was termed "Type B." In the 1980s, further research found that only certain traits in the Type A personality—hostility, cynicism, and anger—increase the risk for heart disease.

Other links between personality and CVD are the subject of ongoing research. Several recent studies suggest that people who hide psychological distress—even from themselves—have a higher rate of heart disease than people who experience similar distress but share it with others. Lack of social support has also been linked with an increased risk for CVD. Low socioeconomic status and low educational attainment are other risk factors. These associations are probably due to a variety of factors, including lifestyle and access to health care.

Personal Insight   Would you characterize yourself as a hostile or cynical person? If not, do you know anyone you would characterize that way? What do you think causes a person to have this type of personality?

Major Risk Factors That Can't Be Changed

A number of major risk factors for CVD can't be changed: heredity, aging, being male, and racial and ethnic factors.

- *Heredity.* The tendency to develop CVD seems to be inherited. If your father or mother has had heart or blood vessel disease, you are at greater risk of developing CVD yourself. High cholesterol levels, abnormal blood clotting problems, diabetes, and obesity are other CVD risk factors that have genetic links. It's important to remember that people who inherit a tendency for CVD aren't destined to develop it. They may, however, have to work harder than other people to prevent cardiovascular problems.
- *Aging.* The risk of heart attack increases dramatically after age 65. About 55 percent of all heart attack victims are age 65 or older, and almost four out of five who suffer fatal heart attacks are over 65. For people over 55, the incidence of stroke more than doubles in each successive decade. However, many people in their thirties and forties, especially men, have heart attacks.
- *Being Male.* Although CVD is the leading killer of both men and women in the United States, men face a greater risk of heart attack than women, especially earlier in life. Until age 55, men also have a greater risk of high blood pressure than women. The incidence of stroke is about 19 percent higher for males than females. Estrogen production, which is highest in the childbearing years, may offer premenopausal women some protection against CVD. However, when heart attacks occur, they are more deadly for women than for men: 39 percent of women who have heart attacks die within a year compared to 31 percent of men.
- *Racial and Ethnic Factors.* African American men and women have moderate high blood pressure twice as often as do whites and severe high blood pressure three times as often, putting blacks of both sexes at greater risk of heart disease and stroke. Puerto Ricans,

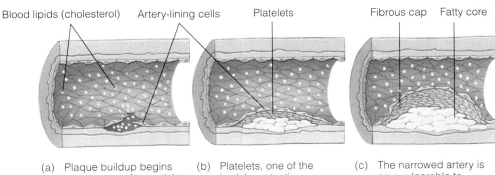

Blood lipids (cholesterol)   Artery-lining cells   Platelets   Fibrous cap   Fatty core

(a) Plaque buildup begins when excess fat particles, called lipids, collect beneath cells lining the artery that have been damaged by smoking, high blood pressure, or other causes.

(b) Platelets, one of the body's protective mechanisms, collect at the damaged area and cause a cap of cells to form, isolating the plaque within the artery wall.

(c) The narrowed artery is now vulnerable to blockage by clots that can form if the cap breaks and the fatty core of the lesion combines with the clot-producing factors in the blood.

Figure 12-3 *Stages of plaque development.*

Cuban Americans, and Mexican Americans are also more likely to suffer from high blood pressure and angina (a warning sign of heart disease) than are non-Hispanic white Americans. These differences may be due in part to differences in education, income, and other socioeconomic factors. Asian Americans historically have had far lower rates of CVD than white Americans. However, recent studies indicate that cholesterol levels among Asian Americans are rising, presumably because of the adoption of a high-fat American diet.

MAJOR FORMS OF CARDIOVASCULAR DISEASE

Cardiovascular disease is the leading cause of death in the United States, claiming one life every 34 seconds. More Americans die from diseases of the heart and blood vessels than from the next five leading causes of death combined. In fact, almost half of all Americans who die this year will die from CVD. Though we typically think of CVD as primarily affecting men and the elderly, heart attack is the number one killer of American women. And 45 percent of heart attacks and 28 percent of strokes occur in people younger than 65 years of age.

The chief forms of CVD are atherosclerosis, high blood pressure, stroke, congestive heart failure, congenital heart disease, and rheumatic heart disease. Most forms have elements in common; we treat them separately here for the sake of clarity.

Atherosclerosis

One of the most common cardiovascular diseases is atherosclerosis, the principal form of arteriosclerosis, or hardening of the arteries. Atherosclerosis is a slow, pro-

gressive process that often begins in childhood. Arteries become narrowed by deposits of fat, cholesterol, and other substances. As these deposits, called **plaques,** accumulate on the walls of the arteries, the arteries lose their elasticity and are unable to expand and contract (Figure 12-3). The flow of blood through the narrowed arteries is restricted. Platelets in the blood may get stuck on a plaque and form a blood clot (**thrombus**), which further restricts the flow of blood, blocking the artery and depriving the heart, brain, or other organ of the vital oxygen carried by the blood. When a coronary artery is blocked, the result is a *coronary thrombosis,* which is one type of heart attack. When a cerebral artery (leading to the brain) is blocked, the result is a *cerebral thrombosis,* a type of stroke.

What causes atherosclerosis? Although there are many possible contributing factors, four of the main factors are cigarette smoking, high levels of blood cholesterol, hypertension (high blood pressure), and physical inactivity. Of these, the most important is smoking.

Hypertension

Every time the heart contracts, or beats (systole), blood pressure increases. When the heart relaxes between beats (diastole), the pressure decreases. Blood pressure can fluctuate considerably, depending on different factors. For example, when you're excited or when you're exercis-

Diabetes A disorder characterized by high blood sugar levels and the inability of the body to take up and use glucose; it is caused by an insufficient supply of the hormone insulin.

Plaque A deposit of fatty (and other) substances on the inner wall of the arteries.

Thrombus A blood clot that forms in a blood vessel and remains attached there.

TERMS

TABLE 12-2 Blood Pressure Classification

Classification	*Systolic	*Diastolic	What to do
Normal	Below 130	Below 85	Recheck in 2 years
High normal	130–139	85–89	Recheck in 1 year
Mild hypertension	140–159	90–99	Confirm within 2 months
Moderate hypertension	160–179	100–109	See physician within a month
Severe hypertension	180 or above	110 or above	See physician immediately

Examples

120/80	Normal
135/85	High normal
145/95	Mild hypertension
160/105	Moderate hypertension
180/115	Severe hypertension

Adapted from The National High Blood Pressure Education Program and the fifth report of the Joint National Committee on Detection, Evaluation, and Treatment of High Blood Pressure, *Archives of Internal Medicine,* 25 January 1993.

*Based on an average of two or more readings on two or more occasions.

ing, the heart pumps more blood into your arteries and your blood pressure rises. But when blood pressure exceeds normal limits most of the time, a person is considered to have high blood pressure, or hypertension. It can result from either increased output of blood by the heart due to overweight or increased resistance to blood flow in the arteries due to narrowing and hardening. Either way, the heart is working harder than normal and the arteries are under greater strain.

High blood pressure is often called a "silent killer" because it usually has no early warning signs. It's possible to have high blood pressure for years without realizing it. During those years, it may be causing damage to vital organs and blood vessels, including the heart and coronary arteries. Blood vessels in the kidneys, for example, may rupture from constant pressure, causing kidney damage or failure. In the eyes, pressure on capillaries in the retina may cause tiny hemorrhages, resulting in blindness.

An estimated 50 million Americans have high blood pressure, and only a small percentage have it under control. There is no cure. Having your blood pressure checked at least once a year is the key to avoiding the complications of hypertension.

Measuring Your Blood Pressure
Blood pressure is measured with a stethoscope and an instrument called a **sphygmomanometer.** Blood pressure is expressed as two numbers—for example, 120/80. The first is systolic pres-

sure, the pressure when the ventricular heart contraction is occurring; the second is diastolic pressure, the pressure when the heart is relaxed. The unit of measurement is millimeters of mercury (mm Hg).

Blood pressure readings can be quite variable, depending on such factors as anxiety, excitement, and setting. For this reason, it's best to compute an average based on at least three measurements on different days. Average blood pressure readings for young adults in good physical condition are 110 to 120 mm Hg systolic over 70 to 80 mm Hg diastolic. Elevated blood pressure in adults is defined as a systolic pressure of 140 mm Hg or more and/or a diastolic pressure of 90 mm Hg or more (Table 12-2).

What Causes Hypertension?
In up to 95 percent of the cases of hypertension, the cause is unknown. High blood pressure of unknown cause is called **essential hypertension,** which most likely involves many factors, including diet, obesity, alcohol abuse, physical and emotional stress, and psychological and genetic factors. Environmental factors alone probably do not produce hypertension in someone without a genetic predisposition to it.

In the remaining cases, the condition is a symptom of another problem, such as a defect in a kidney or other organ. In these cases, referred to as **secondary hypertension,** blood pressure usually returns to normal when the underlying problem is corrected surgically.

Treating Hypertension Cases of mild hypertension (see Table 12-2) can frequently be treated by changes in diet alone, such as restricted salt intake in salt-sensitive people, reduced caloric intake, or both. In people who are overweight, weight loss may also help lower blood pressure. Treatment of more severe hypertension often also involves the use of **antihypertensive drugs.**

Heart Attacks

Every year about 1.5 million Americans have a heart attack. Although a heart attack may come without warning, it is the end result of a long-term disease process. The most common form of heart disease is coronary artery disease caused by atherosclerosis. When one of the coronary arteries—the arteries that branch off the aorta and supply blood directly to the heart muscle—becomes blocked by a blood clot, a heart attack results. A heart attack caused by a clot is called a **coronary thrombosis,** a **coronary occlusion,** or a **myocardial infarction.** In myocardial infarction, part of the heart muscle (myocardium) may die from lack of oxygen.

If the heart attack is not fatal—that is, if enough of the muscle is undamaged to permit life to continue—the muscle begins to repair itself. It does so through a process called **collateral circulation,** in which small blood vessels open to take over the functions of the blocked artery and to move more blood through the damaged area. As healing takes place, scar tissue replaces part of the injured muscle.

Angina Arteries narrowed by disease may still be open enough to deliver blood to the heart. At times, however—chiefly during emotional excitement, stress, or physical exertion—the heart requires more oxygen than narrowed arteries can accommodate. Chest pain, called **angina pectoris,** is a signal that the heart is not getting enough blood to supply the oxygen it needs. Angina pain is felt as an extreme tightness in the chest and heavy pressure behind the breastbone or in the shoulder, neck, arm, hand, or back. This pain, although not actually a heart attack, is a warning that the load on the heart must be reduced. Angina may be controlled in a number of ways (with diet and drugs), but its course is unpredictable. Over a period of months or years, the narrowing often goes on to full blockage and a heart attack.

Arrhythmias Of the roughly 500,000 heart attack deaths each year, about half happen within the first hour from an abnormal heartbeat called an arrhythmia, which usually results from damaged heart muscle. Sudden death can be caused by failure of the heart's natural pacemaker, which normally sends electrical impulses through the heart at a rate of 60 to 100 times per minute. A normal heart rhythm can often be restored using a defibrillator, which gives an electrical shock to the heart. This must be done within three to four minutes unless blood flow is restored through **cardiopulmonary resuscitation (CPR).**

Helping a Heart Attack Victim Most people who suffer a fatal heart attack do so within two hours from the time they experience the first signals. Therefore, recognizing the signals and responding immediately by getting to the nearest hospital or clinic with 24-hour emergency cardiac facilities is critical. If the person loses consciousness, emergency cardiopulmonary resuscitation (CPR) should be initiated by a qualified person. Damage to the heart muscle increases with time. If the victim gets to the emergency room quickly enough, a clot-dissolving agent can be injected to dissolve a clot in the coronary artery.

Detecting and Treating Heart Disease Physicians have a variety of diagnostic tools to evaluate the condition of the heart and the arteries. To determine whether a person is at risk of a heart attack, physicians order a stress or exercise test, in which the patient runs on a treadmill while being monitored for heart rhythm abnormalities with an **electrocardiogram (ECG).** Certain characteristic changes in the heart's electrical activity while under stress can reveal particular heart problems, such as restricted blood flow to the heart muscle.

Sphygmomanometer An instrument for measuring blood pressure.

Essential hypertension Persistent elevated blood pressure without known or specific cause.

Secondary hypertension High blood pressure caused by disease such as kidney dysfunctioning or tumor.

Antihypertensive drugs Prescribed drugs that lower blood pressure.

Coronary thrombosis A clot in a coronary artery, often causing sudden death.

Coronary occlusion Partial or total obstruction of a coronary artery, as by a clot; usually resulting in myocardial infarction.

Myocardial infarction A heart attack in which the heart muscle is damaged through lack of blood supply.

Collateral circulation The movement of blood by a system of smaller blood vessels when a main vessel is blocked.

Angina pectoris A condition in which the heart muscle does not receive enough blood, causing severe pain in the chest and often in the left arm and shoulder.

Cardiopulmonary resuscitation (CPR) A technique involving mouth-to-mouth breathing and chest compression to keep oxygen flowing to the brain.

Electrocardiogram (ECG) A test to detect abnormalities by measuring the electrical activity in the heart.

Magnetic resonance imaging (MRI) (also **nuclear magnetic resonance imaging**) A computerized imaging technique that uses a strong magnetic field and radio frequency signals to examine a thin cross section of the body; no x-rays are involved.

Other tools allow the physician to visualize the patient's heart and arteries. **Magnetic resonance imaging (MRI)**, also called **nuclear magnetic resonance imaging (NMR)**, uses powerful magnets to look inside the heart. **Radionuclide imaging** involves injecting radioactive markers into the bloodstream and then using sensitive cameras to determine if the heart is well-supplied with blood and its chambers are functioning properly. Other tests involve threading a catheter through arteries and into the heart. Dye is injected through the catheter; x-rays are used to trace the liquid's flow. The resulting pictures, called **angiograms** or **arteriograms**, reveal the presence of any obstructions.

A variety of treatments, ranging from changes in diet to major surgery, is available if a problem is detected. Along with a low-fat diet, regular exercise, and smoking cessation, one frequent nonsurgical recommendation for people at high risk of CVD is for them to take one-half an aspirin tablet a day. Aspirin has an anticlotting effect; it discourages platelets in the blood from sticking to arterial plaque and forming clots. Too much aspirin, however, may increase risks of certain types of stroke and cause ulcers or gastrointestinal bleeding.

The most common surgical procedure performed today for coronary disease is **balloon angioplasty**, or **percutaneous transluminal angioplasty (PCTA)**. This technique involves threading a catheter with an inflatable balloon tip through the artery until it reaches the area of blockage. The balloon is then inflated, flattening the fatty plaque and widening the arterial opening.

Coronary bypass surgery is performed on nearly 400,000 men and women a year. Surgeons remove a healthy blood vessel, usually a vein from one of the patient's legs, and graft it to one or more coronary arteries to bypass a blockage. A heart-lung machine must be used to maintain the patient's circulation while the operation is taking place.

Whatever treatment is used, the person with heart disease is also advised to make behavior and lifestyle changes, such as changing the diet to improve blood cholesterol levels and quitting smoking. Otherwise, the arteries simply become clogged again, and the same problems recur a few years later.

Stroke

For brain cells to function as they should, they must have a continuous and ample supply of oxygen-rich blood. If brain cells are deprived of blood for more than a few minutes, they die. A **stroke**, also called a *cerebrovascular accident* (CVA), occurs when the blood supply to the brain is cut off. Stroke can be particularly serious because injured brain cells, unlike those of other organs, cannot regenerate. Hypertension and atherosclerosis are primary risk factors for stroke.

Types of Strokes　There are three major types of stroke. The most common is the *thrombotic stroke,* caused by a blood clot, or *thrombus,* that forms in one of the cerebral arteries (Figure 12-4). This condition, called **cerebral**

thrombosis, is likely to occur when the cerebral arteries become narrowed or damaged by atherosclerosis.

A second type of stroke, the *embolic stroke,* occurs when a wandering blood clot, or **embolus,** is carried in the bloodstream and becomes wedged in one of the cerebral arteries. This event is called a **cerebral embolism.**

The third type of stroke, the *hemorrhagic stroke,* is the least common but most severe type of stroke. It occurs when a blood vessel in the brain bursts, spilling blood into the surrounding tissue and causing damage to it. When a **cerebral hemorrhage** occurs, cells normally nourished by the artery are deprived of blood and cannot function.

Bleeding of an artery in the brain may also be caused by a head injury or by the bursting of an **aneurysm.** An aneurysm is a blood-filled pocket that bulges out from a weak spot in an artery wall. Aneurysms in the brain may remain stable and never break. But when they do, the result is a stroke.

Effects of a Stroke

The interruption of the blood supply to any area of the brain prevents the nerve cells there from functioning, in some cases causing death. Of the 500,000 Americans who have strokes each year, approximately one-third die within a year. Those who survive usually have some lasting disability. Which parts of the body are affected depends on the area of the brain affected. Nerve cells control sensation and most of our bodily movements, so a stroke may cause paralysis, walking disability, speech impairment, or memory loss. The severity of the stroke and its long-term effects depend on which brain cells have been injured, how widespread the damage is, how effectively the body can restore the blood supply, and how rapidly other areas of the brain can take over.

Detecting and Treating Stroke

Strokes can be treated, but effective treatment requires prompt recognition of symptoms and correct diagnosis of the type of stroke that has occurred. Warning signs of a stroke include the following:

- Sudden numbness or weakness of the face, arm, and leg on one side of the body
- Loss of speech or difficulty speaking or understanding speech
- Dimming or loss of vision, especially in only one eye
- Unexplained dizziness, particularly if other symptoms are present

Some stroke victims have a **transient ischemic attack (TIA),** or ministroke, days, weeks, or months before they have a full-blown stroke. TIAs produce temporary stroke-like symptoms, such as weakness or numbness in an arm or leg, speech difficulty, or dizziness, but these symptoms are brief and don't seem to cause permanent damage.

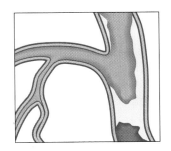
(a) Thrombus

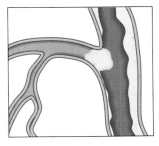
(b) Embolism

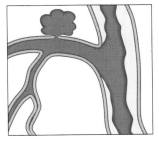
(c) Hemorrhage

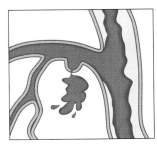
(d) Aneurysm (ruptured)

Figure 12-4 *Causes of stroke.*
Five out of six strokes are caused by blood clots, either a thrombus (a) or an embolism (b). A hemorrhagic stroke (c), is more serious and occurs when a blood vessel in the brain bursts. When an aneurysm ruptures (d), a stroke results.

TERMS

Radionuclide imaging An imaging technique that uses radioisotopes and a scanning camera to produce a pictorial representation of the radioisotope markers taken up in a particular organ, such as the heart.

Angiogram (also **arteriogram**) A picture of the arterial system taken after injection of a dye that is opaque to x-rays.

Balloon angioplasty (also **Percutaneous transluminal angioplasty, or PCTA**) A technique in which a catheter with a balloon on the tip is inserted into an artery; the balloon is then inflated at the point of obstruction in the artery, pressing the plaque against the artery wall to improve blood supply.

Coronary bypass surgery Surgery in which a vein is grafted from a point above to a point below an obstruction in a coronary artery, improving the blood supply to the heart.

Stroke An impeded blood supply to some part of the brain resulting in the destruction of brain cells (also called *cerebrovascular accident*).

Cerebral thrombosis A clot in a vessel that supplies blood to the brain.

Embolus A blood clot that breaks off from its place of origin in a blood vessel and travels through the bloodstream.

Cerebral embolism Blockage of a blood vessel in the brain, caused by blood clots or other material carried in the blood from other parts of the body.

Cerebral hemorrhage Bleeding in or near the brain.

Aneurysm A sac formed by a distention or dilation of the artery wall.

Transient ischemic attack (TIA) A small stroke; usually a temporary interruption of blood supply to the brain, causing numbness or difficulty with speech.

TIAs should be taken as warning signs of a stroke and reported to a physician.

A person who has had or is having a stroke should be rushed to the hospital for diagnosis and treatment. Tests may include an electrocardiogram (which measures the electrical activity of the heart), an **electroencephalogram** (which measures nerve cell activity in the brain), and a **computerized tomography (CT)** scan (a painless technique that can assess brain damage). The CT scan uses a computer to construct a picture of the brain from x-rays beamed through the head.

If the tests reveal that the stroke was caused by a blood clot, the person can be treated with the same kind of clot-dissolving drugs that are being used to treat coronary artery blockages. If tests reveal that the stroke was caused by a cerebral hemorrhage, drugs may be prescribed to lower the blood pressure, which is usually high. If detection and treatment of stroke come too late, rehabilitation is the only treatment. Although damaged or destroyed brain tissue cannot regenerate, the brain can find new pathways, and some functions can be taken over by other parts of the brain. Some spontaneous recovery starts immediately after a stroke and continues for a few months.

Rehabilitation consists of various types of therapy: physical therapy, which helps strengthen muscles and improve balance and coordination; speech and language therapy, which helps those whose speech has been damaged; and occupational therapy, which helps improve hand-eye coordination and everyday living skills. Progress varies from person to person and can be unpredictable. Some people recover completely in a matter of days or weeks, but most stroke victims who survive struggle with disability for the rest of their lives.

Congestive Heart Failure

A number of conditions, including high blood pressure, heart attack, atherosclerosis, rheumatic fever, and birth defects, can damage the heart's pumping efficiency. When the heart cannot maintain its regular pumping rate and force, fluids begin to back up. When this extra fluid seeps through capillary walls, edema (swelling) results, most commonly in the legs and ankles, but sometimes in other parts of the body as well. Fluid can collect in the lungs and interfere with breathing, particularly when a person is lying down. This condition is called **pulmonary edema;** the entire process is **congestive heart failure.**

Congestive heart failure can be controlled. Treatment includes reducing the workload on the heart, modifying salt intake, and using drugs that help the body eliminate excess fluid. Drugs used to treat congestive heart failure include digitalis, which increases the pumping action of the heart; diuretics, which help the body eliminate excess salt and water; and vasodilators, which expand the blood vessels, decrease the pressure, and allow blood to flow more easily, which in turn makes the heart's work easier.

Heart Disease in Children

Although most cardiovascular disease occurs in adults—and usually in middle-aged or older adults at that—it can occur in children, usually as congenital heart disease or as a result of rheumatic fever.

Congenital Heart Disease   About 32,000 children born each year in the United States have a defect or malformation of the heart or major blood vessels. These conditions are referred to collectively as **congenital heart disease.** They cause 5,600 deaths a year.

The most common congenital defects are holes in the wall that divides the lower chambers of the heart. Holes may also occur in the wall between the upper chambers. With these defects the heart produces a distinctive sound, making diagnosis relatively simple. Another defect is **coarctation of the aorta,** which is a narrowing, or constriction, of the aorta. Heart failure may result unless the constricted area is repaired by surgery.

Most of the common congenital defects can now be accurately diagnosed and treated with medication or surgery. Important in saving lives is the early recognition that the newborn infant who shows blue appearance, respiratory difficulty, or failure to thrive may be suffering from congenital heart disease.

Rheumatic Heart Disease   A leading cause of heart trouble in children is **rheumatic fever,** a consequence of untreated strep throat. Rheumatic fever can damage the heart muscle and heart valves. Symptoms of strep throat are the sudden onset of a sore throat, painful swallowing, fever, swollen glands, headache, nausea, and vomiting. Strep infections can be diagnosed by rapid laboratory detection tests. The symptoms of rheumatic fever are generally vague, making diagnosis difficult. Symptoms in children include loss of weight or failure to gain weight; a low

TERMS

Electroencephalogram (EEG)   A test that measures nerve cell activity in the brain.

Computerized tomography (CT) scan   A test using computerized x-ray images to create a cross-sectional depiction of tissue density.

Pulmonary edema   Accumulation of water in the lungs.

Congestive heart failure   A condition resulting from the heart's inability to pump out all the blood that returns to it. Blood backs up in the veins leading to the heart, causing an accumulation of fluid in various parts of the body.

Congenital heart disease   Disease present at birth due to malformation of the heart or its major blood vessels.

Coarctation of the aorta   A congenital defect in which the aorta is narrowed or constricted.

Rheumatic fever   A disease, mainly of children, characterized by fever, inflammation, and pain in the joints; often damages the heart muscle.

but persistent fever; poor appetite; repeated nose-bleeds without apparent cause; jerky body movements; pain in the arms, legs, or abdomen; fatigue; and weakness. Rheumatic fever can usually be prevented by treating strep throat, when it occurs, with antibiotics.

PROTECTING YOURSELF FROM CARDIOVASCULAR DISEASE

What can you do now, while you're still young, to improve your chances of avoiding CVD? Here are a number of important steps you can take:

- Have your blood pressure measured by a physician or other health care provider at least once a year, even if your blood pressure has been normal in the past. Self-administered blood pressure tests in pharmacies and other public places may be misleading and are no substitute for a test performed by a trained professional. If your blood pressure is high, follow your physician's advice on how to lower it.

- Have your blood cholesterol measured if you've never had it done. Finger-prick tests at health fairs and other public places are generally fairly accurate, especially if they're offered by a hospital or other reputable health group. When you know your "number," follow these guidelines from the National Cholesterol Education Program:

    If your cholesterol is under 200 mg/dl, maintain a healthy lifestyle—including eating a low-fat diet, getting regular exercise, maintaining a healthy body weight, and not smoking—and get another test within five years.

    If your cholesterol is between 200 and 239 mg/dl, have a second test performed and average the results. If that number falls in the same range, and if you do not have any form of CVD or two other risk factors for CVD, change your diet to improve your cholesterol. In addition, eliminate any other risk factors you have and get tested again in about one year. If you have CVD or other risk factors for CVD, your physician should order a more detailed cholesterol analysis, including measurement of HDL and LDL. You should begin a cholesterol-improving diet and follow any other therapy recommended by your physician.

    If your cholesterol is 240 mg/dl or more, your physician should order a detailed cholesterol analysis and suggest therapy based on the results. You should begin a cholesterol-improving diet immediately.

- Get regular exercise. Sedentary people can significantly reduce their risk of premature death from CVD just by walking a dog every day, taking up gardening, playing golf on weekends, enrolling in a weekly dance class, or joining a bowling league. People who have already built mild exercise into their weekly routines can reduce their CVD risk even further by exercising a little harder, a little more often, or both. Exercise programs needn't be rigid or strenuous to provide protection from CVD. The American Medical Association recommends exercising a total of between 90 minutes and four hours each week.

- If you smoke, quit. If you live or work with people who smoke, encourage them to quit—for their sake and yours (see Chapter 7).

- Bring your diet into line with the guidelines of the National Cholesterol Education Program. Consume fewer than 30 percent of your total daily calories as fat; fewer than 10 percent should come from saturated fat. Eat fewer than 300 milligrams of dietary cholesterol a day. Choose foods high in fiber and complex carbohydrates. And adjust your caloric intake to achieve or maintain a healthy body weight.

- Develop effective ways to handle stress and anger. Refer to Chapter 2 for suggestions about how to manage stress and avoid its negative consequences.

- Follow your physician's advice about any medical problems you may have, such as diabetes.

In a sense, some of us choose our diseases when we choose the way we live. On the other hand, sometimes it's difficult to see that other choices are possible. Our competitive society fosters certain values and behaviors. When there's still work to do, it's not always easy to leave the desk or computer terminal and take the time to exercise and eat a healthy meal instead of fast food. But if we can see that we have choices, if we can learn to mediate the negative effects of the "fast track," we can perhaps make cardiovascular disease less inevitable in our lives.

WHAT IS CANCER?

Cancer is a group of diseases characterized by uncontrolled growth of abnormal cells. If the spread of these abnormal cells is not controlled, cancer can cause death. Most cancers take the form of tumors, although not all tumors are cancers. A tumor is simply a mass of new tissue that serves no physiological purpose. It can be benign, like a wart, or malignant, like most lung cancers; the terms **malignant tumor** and **malignant neoplasm** are synonymous with *cancer.* **Benign tumors** are made up of

---

Malignant tumor   A tumor that is cancerous and capable of spreading.

Malignant neoplasm   A cancerous growth. A new growth of abnormal cells.

Benign tumor   A tumor that is not malignant or cancerous.

TERMS

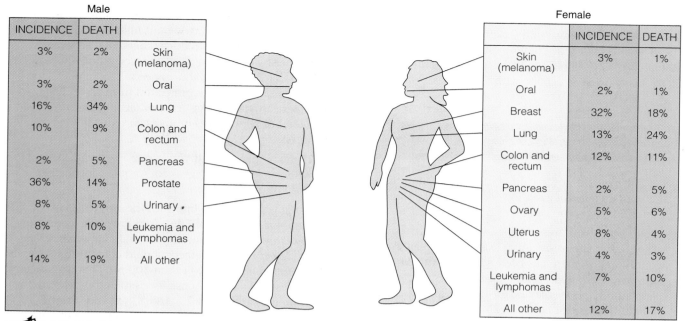

Male

INCIDENCE	DEATH	
3%	2%	Skin (melanoma)
3%	2%	Oral
16%	34%	Lung
10%	9%	Colon and rectum
2%	5%	Pancreas
36%	14%	Prostate
8%	5%	Urinary
8%	10%	Leukemia and lymphomas
14%	19%	All other

Female

	INCIDENCE	DEATH
Skin (melanoma)	3%	1%
Oral	2%	1%
Breast	32%	18%
Lung	13%	24%
Colon and rectum	12%	11%
Pancreas	2%	5%
Ovary	5%	6%
Uterus	8%	4%
Urinary	4%	3%
Leukemia and lymphomas	7%	10%
All other	12%	17%

VITAL STATISTICS

Figure 12-5 *Cancer incidence by site and sex, and cancer deaths by site and sex.*
Percentages shown are estimates for 1995, excluding nonmelanoma skin cancer. The "incidence" column indicates what percentage of all cancers occurred in each site; the "death" column indicates what percentage of all cancer deaths were attributed to each type. Note: Columns do not all total 100 percent due to rounding. *Source:* American Cancer Society, 1995. *Cancer Facts and Figures, 1995.*

cells similar to the surrounding normal cells and are enclosed in a membrane that prevents them from penetrating neighboring tissues. They are dangerous only if their physical presence interferes with bodily functions. A benign brain tumor, for example, can cause death if it blocks the blood supply to the brain. A malignant tumor, or cancer, is capable of invading surrounding structures, including blood vessels, the **lymph system,** and nerves. It can also spread, or *metastasize,* to distant sites via the blood and lymphatic circulation and so can produce invasive tumors in almost any part of the body. A few cancers, like the **leukemias,** or cancers of the blood, don't produce a mass and so aren't properly called tumors. But since the leukemic cells do have the fundamental property of rapid, uncontrolled growth, they are still malignant and therefore cancers.

Metastasis occurs because cancer cells do not stick to each other as strongly as normal cells do and so may not remain at the site of the original or *primary tumor.* They break away and can pass through the lining of lymph or blood vessels to invade nearby tissue. They can also drift to distant parts of the body, where they establish new colonies of cancer cells. This traveling and seeding process is called metastasizing, and the new tumors are called *secondary tumors,* or *metastases.*

Traveling cancer cells can follow two courses. They can produce secondary tumors in the lymph nodes and be carried through the lymph system to form secondary sites elsewhere, or they can invade blood vessels and circulate through the vessels to colonize other organs. This ability of cancer cells to metastasize makes early cancer detection critical. To control the cancer and prevent death, every cancerous cell must be removed. Once cancer cells enter either the lymph or the blood system, it is extremely difficult to stop their spread to other organs of the body.

Every case of cancer begins as a change in a cell that allows it to grow and divide when it should not. Normally (in adults), cells divide and grow at a rate just sufficient to replace dying cells. When you cut your finger, for example, the cells around the wound divide more rapidly to heal the wound. When the wound is healed, the rate of cell growth and division returns to normal. In contrast, a malignant cell divides without regard for normal control mechanisms and gradually produces a mass of abnormal cells, or a tumor. It takes about a billion cells to make a mass the size of a pea, so a single tumor cell must go through many divisions, often taking years, before the tumor grows to a noticeable size. Eventually it produces a sign or symptom that is determined by its location in the body. In the breast, for example, a tumor may be felt as a lump and diagnosed as cancer by x-ray or **biopsy.** In less accessible locations, like the lung, ovary, or bowel, a tumor may be noticed only after considerable growth has taken place and may then be detected only by an indirect symptom—for instance, a persistent cough or unexplained bleeding or pain. In the case of leukemia, there is no lump, but the changes in the blood will eventually be noticed as increasing fatigue, infection, or abnormal bleeding.

Types of Cancer

The behavior of tumors arising in different body organs is characteristic of the tissue of origin. (Figure 12-5 shows the major cancer sites and the incidence of each type.) Since each cancer begins as a single (altered) cell with a specific function in the body, the cancer will retain some of the properties of the normal cell for a time. So, for instance, a cancer of the thyroid gland may produce too much thyroid hormone and cause hyperthyroidism as well as cancer. Usually, however, a cancer loses its resemblance to normal tissue as it continues to divide, and it becomes a group of rogue cells with increasingly unpredictable behavior.

Malignant tumors are classified according to the types of cells that give rise to them. The most common cancers are carcinomas, sarcomas, lymphomas, and leukemias (the suffix -oma means "tumor"). **Carcinomas,** the most common form of cancer, arise from the **epithelial layers** (outside layers) of cells, which are usually the most actively growing cells in the adult body. Important epithelial layers include the skin, the epithelium of glandular organs (breast, uterus, prostate), and cells lining the respiratory tract (lungs, bronchial tubes), gastrointestinal tract (mouth, stomach, colon, rectum), and urinary tract. Carcinomas metastasize primarily via the lymph vessels. In breast cancer, cells that break away from the tumor metastasize to the nearby lymph nodes. In fact, counting the number of lymph nodes that contain cancer cells is one of the principal methods of predicting the outcome of the disease; the probability of a cure is much greater when the lymph nodes do not contain cancer cells.

Sarcomas occur less often than carcinomas. They arise from connective and fibrous tissue like muscle, bone, cartilage, and the membranes covering muscles and fat. Sarcomas have the reputation of metastasizing primarily by way of the blood vessels. **Lymphomas** are cancers of the lymph nodes, part of the body's infection-fighting system. They are closely related to leukemias, and like leukemias, they arise from changes in the white blood cells.

Leukemias are cancers of the blood-forming cells, which reside chiefly in the bone marrow; these cancers are due to an abundance of abnormal white cells. Rapid growth of these cells displaces the red blood cell precursors from the bone marrow and can lead to anemia. Because malignant white cells no longer fight infection, the immune system also loses its ability to defend against bacteria, viruses, and other infectious organisms.

There is a great deal of variation in how easily different cancers can be detected and how well they respond to treatment. For instance, basal cell skin cancer (one type of skin cancer) is easily detected, grows slowly, and is very accessible. Although there are over 800,000 cases per year in the United States, virtually all are cured. On the other hand, cancer of the pancreas, fortunately far less frequent, is difficult to detect and only rarely approachable surgically. Only about 3 percent of patients are alive 5 years after diagnosis. In general, the ability of the **oncologist** to predict how a specific tumor will behave is imperfect; since every tumor arises from a unique set of changes in a single cell, predicting the course of the disease is always uncertain.

Incidence of Cancer

In 1995, about 1,252,000 people in the United States were diagnosed as having cancer. More than half will be cured, but about 44 percent will eventually die as a result of their cancer. These grim statistics exclude more than 800,000 cases of the curable types of skin cancer. About 85 million Americans now living will eventually develop cancer, or about one in three, according to present rates. Cancer is second only to heart disease as a cause of death in the United States.

Is the incidence of cancer increasing or decreasing? The question must be answered carefully, because the American population is aging and cancer strikes more frequently with advancing age. As the nation improves its cardiovascular health through better eating and exercise habits, people are living longer and so are increasingly likely to die of cancer rather than of heart attack or stroke. When cancer death rates are adjusted for the effects of an older population, death rates from major types of cancer appear to be leveling off or decreasing. The only major exception to this trend is lung cancer, which is increasing rapidly in women. The rate of death from lung cancer in women today parallels the increased rate of smoking in women about twenty years ago.

COMMON CANCERS

A discussion of all types of cancer would be beyond the scope of this book, but in this section we look at some of the most common cancers and their causes, prevention, and treatment.

Lung Cancer

Lung cancer is the most common cause of cancer death in the United States and is responsible for over 157,000 deaths each year. For over 40 years breast cancer was the major cause of cancer death in women, but since 1987, lung cancer has surpassed breast cancer as a killer of women. The chief risk factor in lung cancer is tobacco smoke, which accounts for 87 percent of cancers. When smoking is combined with exposure to other environmental carcinogens, such as radioactive radon gas present in some residences or asbestos particles from insulation installed prior to 1970, the risk of cancer can be multiplied by a factor of 10 or more.

The smoker is not the only one at risk. In early 1993, the Environmental Protection Agency classified environmental tobacco smoke (ETS) as a human **carcinogen**— that is, a substance that causes cancer in humans. Long-term exposure to ETS increases risk for lung cancer. The smoke from the burning end of the cigarette, called secondhand or sidestream smoke, has significantly higher concentrations of the toxic and carcinogenic compounds found in mainstream smoke, including nitrosamines, ammonia, and nicotine. It's estimated that ETS causes about 3,000 lung cancer deaths each year.

Lung cancer is difficult to detect at an early stage, and it is difficult to cure even when detected early. Symptoms of lung cancer don't usually appear until the disease has advanced to the invasive stage. Signals such as a persistent cough, chest pain, or recurring bronchitis may be the first indication of the tumor's presence. Lung cancer is most often treated by surgery; if all the tumor cells can be removed, a cure is possible. Unfortunately, lung cancer is usually detected only after it has begun to spread, and most lung cancer cells are resistant to almost all forms of **chemotherapy.** It isn't surprising that only about 13 per-

cent of lung cancer patients are alive 5 years after diagnosis. The rate of survival has improved only slightly during the past 10 years.

Colon and Rectal Cancer

Another common cancer in the United States is colon and rectal cancer (also called colorectal cancer). It is the second leading cause of cancer death, after lung cancer. This cancer is clearly linked both to diet and to genetic susceptibility (discussed in the next section). In countries where diets are low in fat and high in fiber, the incidence of this cancer may be only 10 or 20 percent of that seen in the United States. Many people are uniquely susceptible to colon cancer because of heredity, but even for those of us most susceptible, attention to diet can make a significant difference. Decreasing the amount of fat and increasing the amount of insoluble fiber (found in fruits, vegetables, and whole grains) in your diet can minimize your risks of colon cancer. Just as cessation of smoking can reverse precancerous changes in the lung, a high-fiber diet can slow or even reverse precancerous changes in colon cells.

Colon cancer rarely occurs before the age of 40, but to have the best chance of preventing it, you should begin to make dietary changes now. Most colon cancers arise from preexisting **polyps,** small growths on the wall of the colon that may gradually drift toward malignancy over a period of years. The tendency of an individual to form colon polyps appears to be determined by specific genes, so you should be particularly vigilant if colon cancer has occurred among your close relatives. A polyp may be directly visualized using a **sigmoidoscope,** a flexible fiber-optic device inserted through the rectum. The sigmoidoscope and related instruments allow both visualization and biopsy of the polyp, or even its removal, without the need for major surgery.

The standard warning signs of colon cancer are bleeding from the rectum or a change in bowel habits. A rectal examination can detect some rectal tumors, and a stool occult blood test, done during a routine physical exam, can detect small amounts of blood in stool long before obvious bleeding would be noticed. The American Cancer Society recommends that this examination be performed annually after age 40. Colon and rectal cancer is more curable than lung cancer, particularly if it is caught before it spreads beyond the bowel to other parts of the body. The 5-year survival rate is 58 percent overall—about 89 percent if the tumor is localized, but only 40 percent if it has spread.

Breast Cancer

Breast cancer is the most common cancer in women and causes almost as many deaths in women as lung cancer. In men, breast cancer occurs only rarely. In the United States, about one woman in nine will develop breast cancer during her lifetime. In 1995, breast cancer was diagnosed in approximately 182,000 American women, and about 46,000 died from the disease. About 79 percent of patients survive at least 5 years after the diagnosis is made, and most of these achieve a complete cure.

Only a small percentage of breast cancer cases occurs before the age of 30, but a woman's risk doubles every five years between the ages of 30 and 45 and then increases more slowly, by 10 to 15 percent every five years after age 45. The majority of breast cancers are diagnosed in women over 50. When breast cancer does occur, a cure is most likely if the tumor is detected when it is still small. Since this is an increasingly common cancer, attention to screening is a good investment even for younger women.

Risk Factors for Breast Cancer   Breast cancer has been called a "disease of civilization," because incidence is high in industrialized Western countries but remains low in less developed non-Western countries. This pattern has led some researchers to point to a link between breast cancer and the Western lifestyle, which is sedentary and includes a diet high in calories and fat and low in fiber. There is also a strong genetic factor in breast cancer. A woman who has two close relatives with breast cancer is four to six times more likely to develop the disease than is a woman who has no close relatives with breast cancer. However, even though genetic factors do increase the risk of breast cancer, only about 20 percent of cancers occur in women with a family history of the disease.

Other risk factors include alcohol use, certain kinds of benign breast disease, obesity, use of oral contraceptives, early first menstruation, late menopause, and late first childbirth. The unifying factor for many of these risk factors may be the female sex hormone estrogen. Estrogen circulates in a woman's body in high concentrations during the years between puberty and menopause, and it promotes the growth of responsive cells in a variety of sites. Fat cells also produce estrogen, and estrogen levels are higher in obese women. Alcohol can interfere with metabolism of estrogen in the liver and increase its levels in the blood. The evidence suggests that estrogen is a promoter of cancer in sites that are estrogen-responsive, including breast tissue and the uterus.

The links between breast cancer and diet and exercise habits are still being investigated. Recent studies indicate that a high-fat diet alone may not increase the risk of breast cancer. However, research suggests that women may be more likely to get breast cancer if their diets are low in fiber, if they have a sedentary lifestyle, or if they are obese.

Although some of the risk factors for breast cancer—including heredity and some hormonal factors—cannot be changed, important lifestyle factors for breast cancer are under the control of the individual. Maintaining a normal weight by exercising regularly and eating a low-fat, high-fiber diet can minimize the chance of breast cancer. This is true even for women at risk due to family history or other factors.

Detecting and Treating Breast Cancer   The American Cancer Society advises a three-part personal program for early detection of breast cancer. Monthly breast self-examination is recommended for all women over 20, and a clinical breast exam performed by a physician should be part of a regular health checkup every three years. For women over 40, the odds of finding a tumor early can be improved by having the breasts examined with a sensitive low-dose x-ray technique called **mammography.** Mammograms are recommended every one to two years for women over 40 and once a year after 50, although a woman's individual health history and risk factors need to be considered along with these recommendations. These steps, consistently followed, will detect a majority of tumors at an early stage.

If a lump is detected, it may be scanned by **ultrasonography** and biopsied to see if it is cancerous. Nine times out of ten, the lump is found to be a cyst or other harmless growth and no further treatment is needed. If the lump does contain cancer cells, a variety of surgeries may be called for, ranging from a lumpectomy (removal of the lump and surrounding tissue) to a mastectomy (removal of the breast). To determine if the cancer has spread, lymph nodes from the armpit may be removed and examined. If cancer cells are found, tumor cells remaining in the body can often be slowed or killed by additional therapy, such as radiation, chemotherapy, or both.

The chance of survival in cases of breast cancer varies, depending both on the nature of the tumor and whether it has metastasized. If the tumor is discovered early, before it has spread to the adjacent lymph nodes, the patient has about a 92 percent chance of surviving more than 5 years.

Personal Insight   How do you feel about performing self-examinations for cancer? Do you do them regularly? If not, why not? Are you reluctant? If so, what do you think underlies your reluctance?

Carcinogen   Any substance that causes cancer.

Chemotherapy   Treatment of cancer with chemicals that selectively destroy cancerous cells.

Polyp   A small, usually harmless mass of tissue that projects from the inner surface of the colon or rectum.

Sigmoidoscope   A flexible fiber-optic probe used for examination of the lower bowel.

Mammography   Low-dose x-rays of the breasts used to check for early signs of breast cancer.

Ultrasonography   An imaging method in which sound waves are bounced off body structures to create an image on a TV monitor.

TERMS

All women over 20 should practice monthly breast self-examination (BSE) to assist in early detection of breast cancer. Examine your breasts when they are least tender, usually seven days after the start of your menstrual period. If you discover a lump or detect any changes, seek medical attention. Most breast changes are not cancerous.

For a complete BSE, remember these seven P's: positions, perimeter, **palpation**, pressure, pattern, practice with feedback, and plan of action.

1. *Positions.* The first part of BSE is a visual inspection while standing in front of a mirror. Examine your breasts with your arms raised. Look for changes in contour and shape of the breasts, color and texture of the skin and nipple, and evidence of discharge from the nipple. Repeat the visual examination with your arms at your side, with your hands on your hips, and while bending slightly forward.

   The remainder of the examination involves palpation of your breasts. Two positions are possible: *side-lying* or *flat.* The side-lying position is particularly recommended for women with large breasts: Lie on your side and rotate one shoulder back to the flat surface. You will be examining the breast on the side that is rotated back. If you use the flat position, place a pillow or folded towel under the shoulder of the breast to be examined.

2. *Perimeter.* The area you should examine is bounded by a line which extends down from the middle of the armpit to just beneath the breast, continues across along the underside of the breast to the middle of the breastbone, then moves up to and along the collarbone and back to the middle of the armpit. Most cancers occur in the upper outer area of the breast (shaded area).

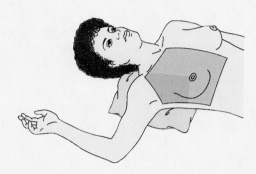

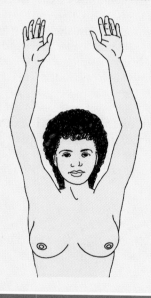

3. *Palpation.* Use your left hand to palpate the right breast, while holding your right arm at a right angle to the rib cage, with your elbow bent. Repeat the procedure on the other side. Use the pads of three or four fingers to examine every inch of your breast tissue. Move your fingers in circles about the size of a dime. Do not lift your fingers from your breast between palpations. You can use powder or lotion to help your fingers glide from one spot to the next.

4. *Pressure.* Use varying levels of pressure for each palpation, from light to deep, to examine the full thickness of your breast tissue. Using pressure will not injure the breast.

5. *Pattern of search.* Use one of the following search patterns to examine all of your breast tissue:

Prostate Cancer

The prostate gland is situated at the base of the bladder in men. It produces seminal fluid; if enlarged, it can block the flow of urine. Prostate cancer is the most common cancer in men and, after lung and colon cancer, the cause of the most deaths. There are over 240,000 new cases of prostate cancer in the United States each year. Prostate cancer is a disease that increases with age, and 80 percent of cases are diagnosed in men over the age of 65. One of 11 men will be diagnosed with prostate cancer during his lifetime. Diet and lifestyle probably influence the occurrence of this cancer, but compared to the other cancers we

TERMS

Palpation Examination by touch.

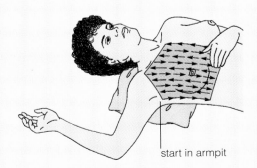

start in armpit

Vertical Strip: Start in the armpit and proceed downward to the lower boundary. Move a finger's width toward the middle and continue palpating upward until you reach the collarbone. Repeat this until you have covered all breast tissue. Make at least six strips before the nipple and four strips after the nipple.

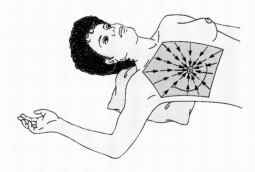

Wedge: Imagine your breast divided like the spokes of a wheel. Examine each separate segment, moving from the outside boundary toward the nipple. Slide fingers back to the boundary, move over a finger's width and repeat this procedure until you have covered all breast tissue. You may need between 10 and 16 segments.

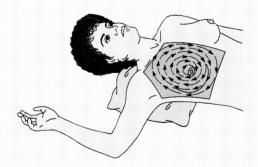

Circle: Imagine your breast as the face of a clock. Start at 12 o'clock and palpate along the boundary of each circle until you return to your starting point. Then move down a finger's width and continue palpating in ever-smaller circles until you reach the nipple. Depending on the size of your breast, you may need 8 to 10 circles.

Once you have completed the pattern, perform two additional exams: (1) squeeze your nipples to check for discharge (some women have a normal discharge), and (2) examine the breast tissue that extends into your armpit while your arm is relaxed at your side.

6. *Practice with feedback.* Have your BSE technique checked by your physician or another health care professional. Practice under supervision until you feel comfortable and confident.

7. *Plan of action:* Your personal breast health plan of action should include the following: (1) discuss the American Cancer Society breast cancer detection guidelines with your physician, (2) schedule clinical breast examination, and mammograms as appropriate, (3) do monthly BSEs, and (4) report any changes to your health care professional.

Source: American Cancer Society. 1992. *Breast Self-Examination: A New Approach,* May 1992.

---

have discussed, the risk factors are somewhat obscure. For reasons not completely understood, African Americans have the highest incidence of prostate cancer in the world.

The best method for controlling prostate cancer is through early detection, and the methods of screening are becoming increasingly sophisticated. Most cases are first detected by rectal examination during a routine physical exam. The physician can feel the prostate gland through the rectum and determine whether it is enlarged and whether lumps are present. Although a rectal exam is unpleasant, it is a quick, inexpensive, and practical way to detect the early stages of both prostate and rectal cancers.

A new blood test that measures the amount of prostate-specific antigen (PSA) in the blood can also be used to help diagnose prostate cancer. An elevated level or a rapid increase in PSA can signal trouble. A single measurement of PSA can help catch early prostate cancer,

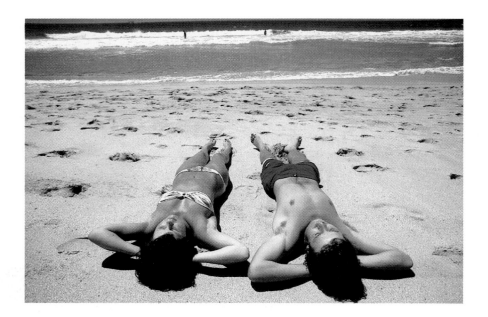

Cumulative exposure to sunlight, beginning in childhood, increases the risk of skin cancer later in life. Blistering sunburns are particularly dangerous, but tanning also poses a hazard. Sunscreens help protect the skin from the sun's radiation.

but it also registers benign conditions (about two-thirds of men over 50 have benign prostate disease). The PSA test is probably most useful if it is repeated over time to chart a rate of change; used in this way, it can more accurately distinguish between cancer and benign prostate disease.

Ultrasound is used increasingly as a follow-up, to detect lumps too small to be felt and to determine their size, shape, and properties. A needle biopsy of suspicious lumps can be performed relatively painlessly, and a **pathologist** can determine whether the biopsied cells are malignant or benign by examining them under a microscope. If they are malignant, the prostate is usually removed surgically; alternative or additional treatments include radiation, hormones, or anticancer drugs. Of course, early detection leads to a better outcome. Survival rates for all stages of this cancer have improved steadily since 1940—in the last 30 years, 5-year survival has increased from 50 percent to 80 percent.

Uterine, Cervical, and Ovarian Cancer

The uterus, uterine cervix, and ovaries are subject to similar hormonal influences, so the cancers of these organs can be discussed as a group. Uterine cancer is the most common cancer of the reproductive system, but ovarian cancer and cervical cancer are more deadly. Most early detection, however, is directed at cervical cancer.

Cancer of the body of the uterus, or **endometrium**, is usually a disease of mature women, and diagnosis is most often made between the ages of 55 and 69. The risk factors are a history of infertility, obesity, and prolonged estrogen therapy. Fortunately, endometrial cancer is often detectable during a standard pelvic exam, and it is curable

by surgery. About 83 percent of patients are living and apparently healthy 5 years after diagnosis.

Cervical cancer, in contrast, attacks younger women and eventually kills about one-third of those who are diagnosed with it. In a sense, cervical cancer is one of the great success stories of cancer control during the last few decades. As the use of the **Pap test** has become almost universal in the United States during the past 40 years, the death rate from cervical cancer has dropped by over 70 percent. Cells for the Pap test are collected during a routine gynecologic pelvic exam. Cells scraped from the cervix are placed on a slide and observed under the microscope. The early noninvasive form of cervical cancer can be identified by the presence of abnormal cells in these Pap tests. If abnormal cells are present, they can then be removed before they reach a dangerous invasive stage. The risk factors for cervical cancer include early age at first intercourse, multiple sex partners, cigarette smoking, and a history of sexually transmissible diseases. Infection of the cervical cells by human papillomavirus (the virus that causes genital warts) is strongly linked to the development of cervical cancer, and any infected woman should have regular Pap tests.

Even though ovarian cancer is rare compared to uterine and cervical cancer, it causes more deaths than the other two combined. It cannot be detected by a Pap test or any other simple screening method and is often noticed only late in its development, when surgery and other therapies are unlikely to be completely successful. Ovarian cancer incidence increases with age and reaches its peak at ages over 60 years. For women at high risk, particularly those with a family history of ovarian cancer, more frequent pelvic examinations and ultrasound imaging of the ovaries may be helpful.

Skin Cancer

Skin cancer is the most common cancer of all when cases of the highly curable forms are included in the count. (Usually these forms are not included, precisely because they are easily treated.) There were over 700,000 cases of all skin cancer in 1994, but only about 32,000 of these were the most serious type. Treatments are usually simple and successful when the cancers are caught early.

Almost all cases of skin cancer can be traced to excessive exposure to the ultraviolet rays of the sun, especially during the childhood years. Skin cancer may also be caused by exposure to coal tar, pitch, creosote, arsenic, and radioactive materials; but compared to sunlight, these agents account for only a small proportion of cases. Because of the link between severe sunburns in childhood and greatly increased risk of **melanoma** in later life, children in particular should be protected from traumatic sunburns. Men and women are equally at risk for skin cancer, but individuals with naturally heavy skin pigmentation have a considerable degree of protection. Conversely, people with fair skin have lower natural protection against skin damage from the sun and have a higher risk of developing certain skin cancers. Both severe, acute sun reactions (sunburns) and chronic low-level sun reactions (suntans) can lead to skin cancer.

Because of damage to the ozone layer, there is a chance that we may all be exposed to increasing amounts of ultraviolet radiation in the future. Take time now to understand the risks of excessive sun exposure, because the precautions suggested here will become increasingly critical if the ozone shield continues to thin.

Types of Skin Cancer   There are three main types of skin cancer, named for the types of skin cell from which they develop:

- **Basal cell** and **squamous cell carcinomas** together account for about 95 percent of the skin cancers diagnosed each year. They are usually found in chronically sun-exposed areas, such as face, neck, hands, and arms. They usually appear as pale, waxlike, pearly nodules, or red, scaly, sharply outlined patches. These cancers are often painless, although they may bleed, crust, and form an open sore on the skin.

- Melanoma is by far the most dangerous skin cancer because it spreads so rapidly. Since 1973, the incidence of melanoma has increased about 4 percent per year. It can occur anywhere on the body, but the most common sites are the back, chest, abdomen, and lower legs. A melanoma usually appears at the site of a preexisting mole. The mole may begin to enlarge, become mottled or varied in color (colors can include blue, pink, and white), or develop an irregular surface or irregular borders. Tissue invaded by melanoma may also itch, burn, or bleed easily.

Preventing and Detecting Skin Cancer   One of the major steps you can take to protect yourself against all forms of skin cancer is to avoid lifelong overexposure to sunlight. Blistering, peeling sunburns from unprotected sun exposure are particularly dangerous, but suntans also increase your risk of developing skin cancer later in life. Tanning salons cannot offer safe tanning because tanning in any form increases the risk of skin cancer. People of every age, including babies and children, need to be protected from the sun with **sunscreens** and protective clothing.

The only sure way to avoid a serious outcome from skin cancers is to make sure they are recognized and diagnosed early. In most successfully treated cases, patients themselves bring their melanoma or other skin cancer to their physician's attention. Make it a habit to examine your skin regularly. Most of the spots, freckles, moles, and blemishes on your body are normal; you were born with some of them, and others appear and disappear throughout your life. As you age, you may develop "liver" spots, patches of darkened skin that look like freckles—these are harmless. But if you notice an unusual growth, discoloration, or sore that does not heal, see your physician or a dermatologist immediately. The characteristics that may signal that a lesion is a melanoma—asymmetry, border irregularity, color change, and a diameter greater than 6 mm—are illustrated in Figure 12-6. Additionally, if someone in your family has had numerous skin cancers or melanomas, you may want to consult a dermatologist for a complete skin examination and discussion of your particular risk.

If you do have an unusual skin lesion, your physician will sometimes be able to determine whether it is benign, precancerous, or cancerous by a physical examination. In other cases, a biopsy is necessary for a definite diagnosis. If the lesion is cancerous, it is usually removed surgically. Even for melanoma, the outlook after removal in the early stages is good, with a 5-year survival rate of 95 percent and a 10-year rate of 90 percent. If the tumor is removed later, after it has begun to invade the surrounding tissues or other areas of the body, the survival rate drops sharply. Since prevention requires a minimum of time and attention, it pays to be alert.

TERMS

Pathologist   A specialist in the study of the origins, nature, and course of disease.

Endometrium   Tissue lining the uterus.

Pap test (Papanicolaou test)   A scraping of cells from the cervix for examination under a microscope to detect cancer.

Melanoma   A malignant tumor of the skin that arises from pigmented cells, usually a mole.

Basal cell carcinoma   Cancer of the deepest layers of the skin.

Squamous cell carcinoma   Cancer of the surface layers of the skin.

With proper clothing and use of sunscreens, you can lead an active outdoor life *and* protect your skin against most sun-induced damage.

Clothing

- Wear long-sleeved shirts made of tightly woven cotton fabric to protect the forearms, chest, and back. Thin, white shirts and wet clothing that clings to the body will not protect you sufficiently.

- Wear a wide-brimmed hat to protect the ears, forehead, and upper cheeks.

Sunscreen

- Use a sunscreen with an SPF (sun protection factor) of 15 or higher. (An SPF rating refers to the amount of time you can stay out in the sun before you burn, compared to using no sunscreen; for example, a product with an SPF of 15 would allow you to remain in the sun without burning 15 times longer, on average, than if you didn't apply sunscreen.) If you're fair-skinned or will be outdoors for long hours, use a sunscreen with a high SPF. Look for the seal of approval from the Skin Cancer Foundation, which tests sunscreens with SPF 15 or higher for safety and effectiveness.

- Choose a "broad spectrum" sunscreen for maximum protection against the full range of ultraviolet radiation from the sun. Many ingredient combinations work together to block a broader range of light waves and also wash off less easily.

- Apply sunscreen 30 to 45 minutes before exposure. This allows time for the sunscreen to penetrate the skin.

- Reapply sunscreen frequently and generously. Most people use less than half as much as they would need to attain the full SPF rating. Use a water-resistant sunscreen if you swim or sweat quite a bit.

- If you're taking medication, ask your physician or pharmacist about possible reactions to sunlight and interactions with sunscreens.

Time of Day/Location

- Try to avoid sun exposure between 10 A.M. and 3 P.M. when the sun's rays are most intense.

- Ultraviolet rays can penetrate at least three feet in water, so swimmers should wear water-resistant sunscreen.

- Locations near the equator have more intense sunlight, and so stronger sunscreens should be used and applied often. High elevations also have intense sunlight, because there is less atmosphere to filter the ultraviolet rays.

- Snow reflects the sun's rays, so don't forget to apply sunscreen before skiing and other snow activities. Sand and water also reflect the sun's rays, so you still need to apply a sunscreen if you are under a beach umbrella. Concrete and white-painted surfaces are also highly reflective.

Adapted from "Sunscreens: Everything New Under the Sun." *Consumer Reports on Health.* July 1994; "Protecting Yourself Against the Sun," *Healthline,* June 1992.

Oral Cancer

Oral cancer—cancers of the lip, tongue, mouth, and throat—can be traced principally to cigarette, cigar, or pipe smoking, use of smokeless or chewing tobacco, and excess use of alcohol. These risk factors work together to multiply the risk of oral cancer in an individual. The incidence of oral cancer is twice as great in men as in women and most frequent in men over 40. Some prominent sufferers of oral cancer have included Sigmund Freud and Fidel Castro, both notorious cigar smokers. Sports figures who have cultivated a taste for smokeless tobacco or "dipping snuff" are now also increasingly being diagnosed with oral cancer. Although cigarette smoking has declined over the past 25 years, there has been a resurgence in the use of all forms of smokeless tobacco. Among long-term snuff users, the excess risk of cancers of cheek, tongue, and gum is nearly fiftyfold.

Oral cancers do have the virtue of being fairly easy to detect, but they are often hard to cure. The principal methods of treatment are surgery and radiation. The 5-year survival rates vary from 91 percent for lip cancer to 26 percent for throat cancer. Overall 5-year survival is about 51 percent.

Testicular Cancer

Testicular cancer is relatively rare, accounting for only 1

TERMS

Sunscreen Substance used to protect the skin from ultraviolet rays; usually applied as an ointment or a cream.

A—Asymmetry: Is one half unlike the other?

B—Border irregularity: Does it have an uneven, scalloped edge rather than a clearly defined border?

C—Color variation: Is the color uniform, or does it vary from one area to another—from tan to brown to black, or from white to red to blue?

6mm D—Diameter larger than one-fourth inch: At its widest point, is the growth as large as or larger than a pencil eraser?

Figure 12-6 *ABCD test for melanoma.*

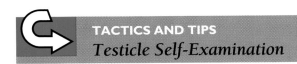
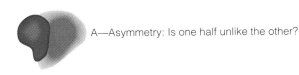
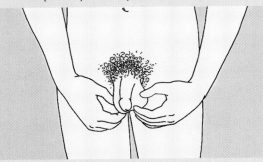
percent of cancer in men, but it is the most common cancer in men 29 to 35 years of age. Self-examination helps in early detection of testicular cancer. Men with undescended testicles are at increased risk for testicular cancer, and for this reason the condition should be corrected in early childhood. Treatment of this cancer has improved dramatically in the past 25 years; 5-year survival rates have risen from 63 percent to 93 percent.

Other Cancers

There were about 51,000 cases of bladder cancer in the United States in 1994. Bladder cancer is four times as common in men as in women, and smoking is responsible for about half of all cases in men. People living in urban areas and workers exposed to dye, rubber, or leather are at increased risk. The first symptoms are likely to be blood in the urine and/or increased frequency of urination. These symptoms should motivate a quick trip to your physician for a thorough exam, since the survival rate for early-stage bladder cancer is 88 percent.

Pancreatic cancer is the fifth leading cancer killer, with about 26,000 deaths in the United States in 1994. This cancer is both hard to detect and almost always deadly. The major environmental risk factor is, again, smoking. In addition, countries where the diet is high in fat have higher rates of pancreatic cancer. The disease often has a "silent" course, and by the time symptoms occur, the disease is usually far advanced. Very little is known about

this disease or how to prevent it. Better methods of imaging, as discussed in the final section of this chapter, may eventually allow earlier diagnosis.

A rare form of skin cancer, Kaposi's sarcoma, is seen almost exclusively in people with HIV infection, apparently as a result of the immune system's inability to function properly. It is discussed further in Chapter 13.

WHAT CAUSES CANCER?

Although scientists don't know everything about what causes cancer, they have identified genetic, environmental, and lifestyle factors. There are usually several steps in

The National Cancer Institute estimates that about one-third of all cancers are in some way linked to what we eat. This means that you can affect your risk of developing cancer by changing your diet in certain ways. The following changes in diet are recommended as a way to reduce your chances of getting cancer:

- Eat a varied diet.
- Eat more high-fiber foods such as fruits, vegetables, and whole-grain cereals, breads, and pasta.
- Eat dark-green and deep-yellow fruits and vegetables rich in vitamins A and C.
- Eat cruciferous vegetables such as cabbage, broccoli, brussels sprouts, and cauliflower.
- Be moderate in your consumption of salt-cured, smoked, and nitrite-cured foods.
- Cut down on your intake of fat and saturated fat.
- Maintain a healthy body weight.
- Be moderate in your consumption of alcoholic beverages.

Using the list of food components that offer protection from cancer, Susan Zarrow with the Rodale Food Center compiled a list of the 50 top anti-cancer foods. To make the list, a food had to be extremely high in one factor believed to prevent cancer, a good source of several factors, or a low-fat substitute for a common high-fat item. Her list includes the following foods:

Apricots	Broccoli
Bran cereal	Brown rice
Brazil nuts	Brussels sprouts

Butternut squash	Papaya
Cabbage	Peas (with edible pods)
Cantaloupe	Popcorn
Carrots	Potatoes
Cauliflower	Prunes
Chard	Pumpkin
Chicken breast	Raisins
Collard greens	Salmon (canned)
Corn and canola oil	Sardines (canned)
Evaporated skim milk	Skim milk
Figs (dried)	Spinach
Grapefruit	Strawberries
Great northern beans	Sunflower seeds
Kale	Sweet peppers
Kidney beans	Sweet potatoes
Kiwis	Swordfish
Mangoes	Tofu
Nonfat yogurt	Tuna (canned)
Nonfat yogurt cheese	Turnips and rutabagas
Oatmeal	Wheat germ
Oranges	Whole-wheat bread

Sources: American Cancer Society; S. Zarrow with the Rodale Food Center. 1989. "Eat to Beat Cancer: Our 50 Food Picks." *Prevention,* February.

the transformation of a normal cell into a cancer cell, and in many cases, different factors may work together in the development of cancer.

Take Good Care of Your DNA

Mutational damage to a cell's **DNA,** particularly to the DNA of the genes that control cell growth, can lead to rapid and uncontrolled division of cells. Environmental agents that produce mutational damage, known as **mutagens,** include radiation, viral infection, and chemical substances in the air we breathe and the food we eat. When these agents also cause cancer, we call them carcinogens. We know that several mutational changes are required before a normal cell takes on the properties of a cancer cell. Almost every month researchers identify new genes in which mutational changes are associated with the conversion of a normal cell into a cancer cell; these critical genes are known as **oncogenes.** Careful study of oncogenes will eventually lead to more precise and sensitive methods of determining who is at risk for certain cancers and to new methods of diagnosis and treatment.

Carcinogenic agents that cause mutational changes in the DNA of oncogenes are known as "initiators" of cancer. Ultraviolet rays from the sun or tanning lamps are an example of a cancer initiator. Other chemical agents are not capable of producing DNA mutations directly but can instead act as "promoters" of cancer. Promoters accelerate the growth of cells without damaging or permanently altering the cell's DNA. An example of a cancer promoter is estrogen, the female sex hormone, which acts as a growth stimulus to cells of female reproductive organs. By speeding up cell growth, promoters increase the odds that any damage done to DNA by initiators will be permanently preserved; they do so by stimulating the cell to replicate before damage can be repaired.

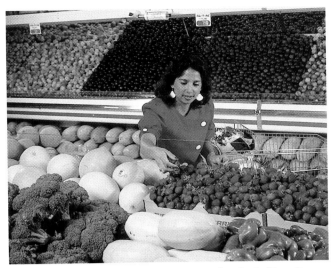

The American Cancer Society recommends a high-fiber diet containing cruciferous vegetables and rich in vitamins A and C. Broccoli, strawberries, and red and green peppers are all excellent choices.

Although much still needs to be learned about oncogenes, it's clear that minimizing mutational damage to our DNA will lower our risk of many cancers. Unfortunately, a great many substances produce cancer-causing mutations, and we can't escape them all. By identifying the important carcinogens and understanding how they produce their effects, we can help keep our DNA intact and avoid activating "sleeping" oncogenes.

Dietary Factors in Cancer

As noted above, agents that cause cancer are called carcinogens. **Anticarcinogens** are substances that protect us from cancer. The foods we eat contain both.

Fat and Fiber A "fatty" diet, high in saturated fats such as those found in red meats, appears to contribute to colon, prostate, and other cancers. Dietary fats stimulate the production of bile acids, which are necessary to break down and digest material in the colon. Once produced, these bile acids remove layers of cells from the intestinal epithelium, which in turn are replaced by growth of new cells. Newly formed and rapidly growing cells are particularly susceptible to cancer-causing agents. In addition, the animal fat we consume may contain fat-soluble synthetic pesticides, like dioxin and PCBs, that are themselves carcinogenic.

Some groups of people, particularly vegetarians, have little colorectal cancer. The vegetarian diet is typically low in fat and high in insoluble fiber. This link, backed up by laboratory evidence, suggests that colorectal cancer may also be related to lack of fiber in the diet. While fiber does not supply nutrition, it has many other useful properties. It provides bulk, which dilutes any carcinogens that may be present. It reduces the transit time of waste through the intestine, so that carcinogens have less time to act on the epithelial cells. Fiber also binds bile acids and other lipids that promote the development of colorectal cancer.

Alcohol Alcohol is associated with an increased incidence of several cancers. The link between alcohol intake and breast cancer is not well understood, but it is dramatic. An average alcohol intake of three drinks per day is associated with a doubling in the risk of breast cancer. As mentioned earlier, alcohol and tobacco (cigarettes or smokeless tobacco) interact as risk factors for oral cancer. The combination of the two multiplies the carcinogenic effect of each substance. Heavy users of both alcohol and tobacco have a risk for oral cancer up to 15 times greater than that of people who don't drink or smoke.

Anticancer Agents in the Diet Some dietary compounds have the ability to prevent carcinogenesis by environmental agents and so are known as anticarcinogens. An example is **beta-carotene,** a precursor of vitamin A that is present in carrots and other yellow and orange vegetables and in leafy green vegetables. Beta-carotene, carotenoids, and vitamin A itself seem to act as antipromoters, slowing the growth of epithelial cells throughout the body. Other anticarcinogens in your diet act at the level of cancer initiation. For example, **antioxidants** such as vitamin C and vitamin E can intercept and render harmless many of the chemical agents capable of causing mutagenic damage to DNA. Because it takes so long for most cancers to develop, it may be 10 to 20 years before researchers can tell us for sure whether we should add supplements of these vitamins to our diets. In addition, scientists have not yet identified all of the thousands of substances in fruits and vegetables that may be protective. So, be sure to include a variety of foods rich in these vitamins in your diet rather than relying on supplements.

People whose diet includes broccoli and other members of the **cruciferous** (cabbage) family of vegetables

DNA Deoxyribonucleic acid, a chemical substance that carries genetic information.

Mutagen Any factor (chemical, radiation, and so on) that can cause mutation.

Oncogene A gene involved in the transformation of a normal cell into a cancer cell.

Anticarcinogens Agents that destroy or otherwise block the action of carcinogens.

Beta-carotene A vitamin A precursor found in plants.

Antioxidants Substances that can react with potential carcinogens and render them harmless.

Cruciferous vegetables Vegetables of the cabbage family, including cabbage, broccoli, brussels sprouts, kale, and cauliflower; the flower petals of these plants form the shape of a cross, hence the name *cruciferous.*

TERMS

have a lower risk of a number of cancers. A potent anti-carcinogen, **sulforaphane,** has recently been purified from broccoli. Sulforaphane can induce, or turn on, the body's natural detoxifying enzymes, which are made by the colon, liver, and other tissues. These detoxifying enzymes are able to render many natural and synthetic dietary carcinogens harmless.

Additional protection against some cancers may be provided by vitamin D and calcium. Although the mechanism is still unclear, it appears that the combined presence of vitamin D and calcium slows the growth of cells in the bowel, thereby having an antipromoting effect on potentially cancerous cells. Low- and nonfat milk and milk products are excellent sources of both vitamin D and calcium.

Carcinogens in the Environment

Some carcinogens occur naturally in the environment, like the ultraviolet rays from the sun or the radioactive radon gas that seeps out of the earth and into houses in some regions. Others are manufactured or synthetic substances that show up occasionally in the general environment but more often show up in the work environments of specific industries.

Ingested Chemicals   Since World War II, new methods of distributing and marketing foods have greatly increased the length of time it takes food to travel from its source to the consumer. To prevent food from becoming spoiled or stale during this time, the food industry adds preservatives and numerous other additives. Some of these compounds are antioxidants and may actually decrease any cancer-producing properties the food might have. Other compounds, like the nitrates and nitrites found in processed meat, are potentially more sinister. While nitrates and nitrites are not themselves carcinogenic, they can combine with dietary amines in the stomach and be converted to **nitrosamines,** which are highly potent carcinogens. Foods cured with nitrites, as well as those cured by salt or smoke, have been linked to esophageal and stomach cancer, and they should be eaten only in modest amounts.

Environmental and Industrial Pollution   Pollutants in urban air have long been suspected of contributing to the incidence of lung cancer. The best available data indicate that less than 2 percent of cancer deaths are caused by general environmental pollution, such as substances in our air and water. Exposure to carcinogenic materials in the workplace is a more serious problem. Occupational exposure to specific carcinogens may account for up to 5 percent of cancer deaths.

Radiation   All sources of radiation are potentially carcinogenic—including medical x-rays, radioactive sub-stances (radioisotopes), and the ultraviolet rays of the sun. The most striking historical example of this has been the increased rates of cancer seen in the survivors of the atomic bombings of Hiroshima and Nagasaki in 1945. Most physicians and dentists are quite aware of the risk of radiation, and successful efforts have been made to reduce the amount of radiation needed for mammograms, dental x-rays, and other necessary medical x-rays.

Another source of environmental radiation is radon gas. Radon is a radioactive decomposition product of radium, which is found in small quantities in some rocks and soils. Since radon is inhaled with the air we breathe, it comes into intimate contact with the cells of the lung, where its radiation can produce mutations. Radon and smoking together create a more-than-additive risk of lung cancer. Fortunately, in most of our homes and classrooms, radon is rapidly dissipated into the atmosphere, where it presents no threat. But in enclosed spaces, such as mines, some basements, and airtight houses built of brick or stone, it can rise to dangerous levels.

Sunlight is a very important source of radiation, but since its rays penetrate only a millimeter or so into the skin, it could be considered a "surface" carcinogen. Most cases of skin cancers are the relatively benign and highly curable basal cell cancers, but a substantial minority are the potentially deadly malignant melanomas. As discussed earlier, all types of skin cancer are increased by early and excessive exposure to the sun, and severe sunburn early in childhood appears to carry with it excessive risk of melanoma later in life.

DETECTING, DIAGNOSING, AND TREATING CANCER

Early cancer detection often depends on our willingness to be aware of changes in our own body or to make sure we keep up with recommended diagnostic tests. Although treatment success varies with individual cancers, cure rates have increased—sometimes dramatically—in this century.

Detecting Cancer

Unlike those of some other diseases, early signs of cancer are usually not apparent to anyone but the victim. Even pain is not a reliable guide to early detection, since the initial stages of cancer may be painless. Self-monitoring is the first line of defense, and the American Cancer Society recommends that you pay close attention to the following signs, which you can remember with the acronym "CAUTION":

- **C**hange in bowel or bladder habits
- **A** sore that does not heal
- **U**nusual bleeding or discharge

TABLE 12-3 *Summary of Tests Recommended by the American Cancer Society for the Early Detection of Cancer in Asymptomatic People*

Site of Cancer	Test or Procedure	Sex	Population Age	Frequency
Colon or rectum	Sigmoidoscopy	M & F	Over 50	Every 3–5 years
	Stool occult blood test	M & F	Over 50	Every year
	Digital rectal examination	M & F	Over 40	Every year
Prostate	Digital rectal examination	M	50 and over	Every year
	PSA blood test	M	50 and over	Every year
Uterus or cervix	Pap smear	F	18–65; under 18 if sexually active	At least every three years after 3 negative exams 1 year apart
	Pelvic examination	F	18–39; under 18 if sexually active	Every 3 years
			40 and over	Every year
	Endometrial tissue sample	F	At menopause; women at high risk[a]	At menopause
Breast	Breast self-examination	F	20 and over	Every month
	Breast physical examination	F	20–40	Every 3 years
			Over 40	Every year
	Mammography	F	Under 40	Baseline
			40–49	Every 1–2 years
			50 and over	Every year
Lung	Chest x-ray		Not recommended	
	Sputum cytology		Recommended for people at risk	
Other[b]	Health counseling and cancer checkup	M & F	20–39	Every 3 years
		M & F	40 and over	Every year

[a]History of infertility, obesity, failure of ovulation, abnormal uterine bleeding, or estrogen therapy
[b]To include examination for cancers of the thyroid, testicles, prostate, ovaries, lymph nodes, oral region, and skin

- Thickening or lump in the breasts or elsewhere
- Indigestion or difficulty in swallowing
- Obvious change in a wart or mole
- Nagging cough or hoarseness

Although none of these signs is a sure indication of cancer, the appearance of any one should send you to see your physician. By being aware yourself of the risk factors in your own life, including the cancer history of your immediate family and your own past history, you can often bring a problem to the attention of a physician long before it would have been detected at a routine physical.

The American Cancer Society is probably the best authority on which tests for cancer detection should be

Sulforaphane A compound found in cruciferous vegetables that is able to turn on the body's detoxifying enzyme system.
Nitrosamines Chemical substances that can cause cancer.

TERMS

made routine. Their recommendations are summarized in Table 12-3. These routine tests are intended for people who have no signs of cancer. Self-examination of breast or testicles is probably the most useful self-screening procedure. Men and women over 40 should have a yearly rectal examination by a physician and a stool occult blood test every year after age 50.

Trends in Diagnosis and Treatment

Detection of a cancer by physical examination is only the beginning, and further diagnosis and treatment of cancer has become increasingly individualized. Methods for determining the exact location, type, and degree of malignancy of a cancer are sophisticated, and they continue to improve. Knowledge of the exact location and size of a tumor is necessary for precise and effective surgery or radiation therapy. This is especially true in cases where the tumor may be hard to reach, as in the brain. New high-technology diagnostic imaging techniques have replaced exploratory surgery for some patients. In magnetic resonance imaging (MRI), a huge electromagnet is used to detect hidden tumors by mapping, on a computer screen, the vibrations of different atoms in the body. Computerized tomography (CT) scanning uses x-rays to examine the brain and other parts of the body. Ultrasonography has also been used increasingly in the past few years to visualize tumors. It has several advantages: It can be used in the physician's office, it is less expensive than other imaging methods, and it is completely safe.

Treatment methods for cancers are based primarily on surgery (removing the tumor), chemotherapy, and radiation therapy. In the last two techniques, cancer cells that can't be surgically removed are killed either by interfering chemically with their growth or by killing them directly with concentrated ionizing radiation. Newer and still experimental methods of treatment are also showing promise. **Immunotherapy,** for instance, uses the body's own immune system to control cancer; interferon, interleukin-2, and several other biological-response modifiers that stimulate the immune system are under study.

All of these newer techniques offer the hope of reducing mortality from the common cancers and extending the lives of those who do have cancer. However, we should keep in mind that there are no technologies on the horizon that promise an all-encompassing cancer cure. As is the case with so many diseases, prevention remains your best protection against cancer.

Immunotherapy Experimental cancer treatment that uses various methods to stimulate the immune system to kill cancer cells.

TERMS

PREVENTING CANCER

Because your behaviors and behavior changes can radically lower your cancer risks, you can take a very practical approach to cancer prevention. Primary prevention involves measures you can take to avoid cancer-causing agents in the environment, such as those in the following list. Secondary prevention involves having cancers that do develop discovered as quickly as possible by following the cancer test recommendations of the American Cancer Society. Both levels of prevention are important to your long-term health. The primary prevention measures recommended by the American Cancer Society include the following:

- Stop smoking and avoid breathing the smoke from other people's cigarettes. Smoking is responsible for 80 to 90 percent of all lung cancers and for about 30 percent of all cancer deaths. People who smoke two or more packs of cigarettes a day have lung cancer mortality rates 15 to 25 times greater than those of nonsmokers. The carcinogenic chemicals in smoke are transported throughout the body in the bloodstream, making smoking a cocarcinogen for many forms of cancer other than lung cancer.

- Protect your skin from the sun. Almost all cases of nonmelanoma skin cancer are considered to be sun-related, and sun exposure is a major factor in the development of melanoma as well. Wear protective clothing when you're out in the sun and use a sunscreen with an SPF rating of 15 or higher. Don't go to tanning salons; they do not provide "safe tans."

- Drink alcohol only in moderation, if at all. Oral cancer and cancers of the larynx, throat, esophagus, and liver occur more frequently among heavy drinkers of alcohol. Risk is even higher among heavy drinkers who smoke.

- Avoid smokeless tobacco. Chewing tobacco and snuff, both highly habit-forming because of their nicotine content, are associated with cancer of the mouth, larynx, throat, and esophagus.

- Avoid excessive exposure to radiation. Most medical x-rays are adjusted to deliver the lowest dose possible without sacrificing image quality. Radiation from radon, on the other hand, may pose a threat. The American Cancer Society believes there is a problem with exposure to radon in some homes. Remedial steps should be taken in these cases.

- Avoid occupational exposure to carcinogens. A number of industrial agents are associated with cancer, including nickel, chromate, asbestos, vinyl chloride, and others. Risks increase greatly when combined with smoking.

- Watch your weight and exercise regularly. The risk for colon, breast, and uterine cancers increases for obese people. A high-fat diet may be a factor in the development of certain cancers, although the link between obesity and cancer hasn't been fully explained. Maintaining normal weight through a healthy diet and regular exercise lowers the risk.

- Control your diet. Choose a low-fat, high-fiber diet containing cruciferous vegetables and foods rich in vitamins A and C; avoid salt-cured, smoked, and nitrite-cured foods. See the specific suggestions in the box and table on dietary factors in cancer.

Although other factors are important, lifestyle is a strong predictor of cancer risk. Mormons and Seventh-day Adventists, for example, are much less likely to develop cancer than is the general population. Church doctrine of both groups forbids tobacco and alcohol use. Members also maintain a strong support network, which may influence both the incidence and the outcome of disease. A recent study determined that middle-aged Mormon men in the lay priesthood of that faith have reduced their risk of cancer to less than half that of the general population. Important factors in this risk reduction appear to be avoidance of tobacco and alcohol, regular exercise, and proper sleep. By making similar changes in lifestyle, other groups have every reason to expect to achieve the 50 percent cancer mortality reduction seen among Mormons and set as a goal for the nation by the National Cancer Institute for the year 2000.

Personal Insight Although many people are aware that certain behaviors help prevent cancer—such as using sunscreen and modifying their diets—a large percentage of them don't act on their knowledge. Do you follow through with behavior changes when you learn that certain things you do increase your risk of cancer? If so, how do you make the changes? If not, why do you think you don't?

SUMMARY

The Cardiovascular System

- The cardiovascular system pumps and circulates blood throughout the body.
- The heart beats when the ventricles contract (systole), pumping blood to the lungs via the pulmonary artery and to the body via the aorta and the entire arterial system. When the heart relaxes between beats (diastole), blood flows from the atria into the ventricles.

- The exchange of nutrients and waste products takes place between the capillaries and the tissues.

Risk Factors for Cardiovascular Disease

- Smoking greatly increases the risk for cardiovascular disease. ETS has also been linked to cardiovascular disease.
- High blood pressure weakens the heart and scars and hardens blood vessels; it often has no early warning signs.
- Cholesterol is crucial to the body's functioning, but high levels contribute to clogged arteries and increase the risk for CVD. High LDL and low HDL levels are associated with high risk.
- Dietary changes that can help improve cholesterol levels include limiting intake of fat, saturated fat, and cholesterol and increasing intake of fiber.
- Physical inactivity increases risk for CVD; as little as 90 minutes a week of mild exercise can reduce this risk.
- Other risk factors that contribute to CVD include overweight, diabetes, high levels of stress, a hostile personality, lack of social support, and low income and educational attainment.
- Risk factors for CVD that can't be changed include being over 65, being male, being African American, and having a family history of CVD.

Major Forms of Cardiovascular Disease

- Atherosclerosis is the process whereby arteries become narrowed by plaques and lose elasticity. Platelets may get stuck on a plaque and form a blood clot.
- Hypertension occurs when blood pressure exceeds normal limits most of the time. It can damage vital organs, including the heart, eyes, and kidneys. Possible causes of essential hypertension include diet, obesity, stress, and genetic factors.
- Heart attacks are the end result of a long-term disease process.
- Angina pectoris is the chest pain that occurs when—because of narrowed arteries—the heart doesn't get enough blood to supply the oxygen it needs.
- Arrhythmia is an abnormal heartbeat; if the heart's electrical system fails, sudden death can occur.
- Heart disease can be diagnosed through use of stress or exercise tests, electrocardiograms, magnetic resonance imaging, angiograms, and radioactive tracers.
- Nonsurgical treatments include a low-fat diet, regular exercise, smoking cessation, and small, regular doses

of aspirin. Surgical treatments include balloon angioplasty and coronary bypass surgery.

- A stroke occurs when the blood supply to the brain is cut off; injured brain cells cannot regenerate themselves.
- Strokes usually lead to some lasting disability. Effective treatment depends on prompt recognition of symptoms and correct diagnosis of the type of stroke.
- Congestive heart failure occurs when the heart's pumping efficiency is reduced and fluids build and collect in the lungs or other part of the body.
- Defects or malformations of the heart or major blood vessels at birth constitute congenital heart disease. These include holes in the wall that divides the chambers of the heart and a constricted aorta.

Protecting Yourself from Cardiovascular Disease

- To avoid CVD, it's important to have blood pressure checked regularly; have blood cholesterol measured; exercise regularly; quit smoking; alter diet to reduce intake of fat and saturated fat; increase intake of fiber; learn to handle stress and anger; monitor medical problems; and know personal and familial risk factors.

What Is Cancer?

- A malignant tumor can invade surrounding structures and spread to distant sites via the blood and lymphatic system, producing additional tumors.
- A malignant cell divides without regard for normal growth. As tumors grow, they produce signs or symptoms that are determined by their location in the body.
- The most common types of cancers are carcinomas, sarcomas, lymphomas, and leukemias.

Common Cancers

- Lung cancer is the most common cancer in the United States, and it kills more people than any other type of cancer. Smoking, the primary cause of lung cancer, also intensifies the effects of other causes like radon gas or asbestos.
- Long-term exposure to environmental tobacco smoke increases the risk of lung cancer for nonsmokers.
- Colorectal cancer is clearly linked to both diet and heredity. High-fiber diets can prevent and even reverse precancerous changes in colon cells. Most colon cancers arise from preexisting polyps.
- Breast cancer affects about one in nine women in the United States. Although there is a genetic component to breast cancer, diet and hormones are also risk factors.

- Early detection of breast cancer depends on monthly self-examination, clinical breast exams, and regular mammograms.
- Prostate cancer is chiefly a disease of aging; diet and lifestyle probably are factors in its occurrence. Early detection is possible through rectal examinations, blood tests, and sometimes ultrasound.
- Endometrial cancer is highly curable; risk factors include infertility, obesity, and prolonged estrogen therapy.
- Abnormal cervical cells can be detected with a Pap test and removed before they reach the invasive stage.
- Ovarian cancer is dangerous because it can't be detected by a Pap test or simple screening method.
- Abnormal cellular changes in the epidermis, often a result of exposure to the sun, cause skin cancers. Skin cancers occur as basal cell carcinoma, squamous cell carcinoma, and melanoma. Skin cancer prevention means avoiding overexposure to the sun.
- Oral cancer is caused primarily by cigarette and cigar smoking, excess alcohol consumption, and use of smokeless tobacco.
- Testicular cancer can be detected early through self-examination.

What Causes Cancer?

- Mutational damage to a cell's DNA can lead to rapid and uncontrolled growth of cells. Cancer initiators cause mutations in DNA; cancer promoters accelerate the growth of cells.
- A diet high in fat and low in fiber contributes to colon, prostate, and other cancers. Alcohol is associated with breast and oral cancers. Anticarcinogens in the diet include beta-carotene, vitamin C, vitamin E, and other antioxidants; cruciferous vegetables; dietary fiber; and vitamin D and calcium.
- A few food additives and preservatives react with other substances to become carcinogenic. Exposure to carcinogenic chemicals in the workplace puts workers in some industries at risk for cancer. All sources of radiation are potentially carcinogenic, including x-rays, radioisotopes, radon gas, and the ultraviolet rays of the sun.

Detection, Diagnosis, and Treatment

- Self-monitoring is essential to early cancer detection; the appearance of any early signs necessitates a visit to a physician. (The signs can be remembered by using the acronym CAUTION.)
- Magnetic resonance imaging and computerized tomography allow more precise visualization of

tumors than do standard x-rays. Ultrasound is also being used more frequently in cancer detection.

- Treatment methods consist of surgery, chemotherapy, and radiation therapy. Immunotherapy, vaccines, and genetic engineering also hold promise as effective treatments.

Preventing Cancer

- Primary prevention involves avoiding cancer-causing agents in the environment. Secondary prevention involves early detection of cancers that do occur.
- Primary prevention includes (1) not smoking and avoiding smoke, (2) protecting skin from the sun, (3) drinking alcohol in moderation, if at all, (4) avoiding smokeless tobacco, (5) avoiding excessive exposure to radiation, (6) avoiding occupational exposure to carcinogens, (7) watching one's weight and exercising, and (8) controlling one's diet.

TAKE ACTION

1. The CPR courses given by the Red Cross and other groups provide invaluable training that may help you save a life some day. Anyone can take these courses and become qualified to administer CPR. Investigate CPR courses in your community and sign up to take one.
2. Do some research into your family medical history. Is there cardiovascular disease or cancer in your family? Such a history is a risk factor for you. Keep that in mind as you consider whether you need to make lifestyle changes to avoid CVD and cancer.
3. Devise a plan for incorporating regular self-examinations for cancer (breast self-examination or testicle self-examination) into your life. What strategies can you use to help you remember to do your monthly exam? How can you keep yourself motivated?

JOURNAL ENTRY

1. If the hostility assessment in the chapter indicates that you may have a hostile personality, examine your thoughts and behavior more carefully. In your health journal, keep track of your cynical thoughts, angry feelings, and aggressive acts. For each entry, include the time, place, and cause of your cynical thoughts; what thoughts actually went through your head; the emotions you felt; and any actions you took. Review your journal at the end of a week to learn more about the frequency and kinds of situations that trigger these thoughts and behaviors.

2. In your health journal, list the positive behaviors that help you avoid cancer. How can you strengthen these behaviors? Also list the behaviors that tend to increase your risk of cancer. What can you do to change these behaviors?

3. *Critical Thinking:* How much responsibility does an individual have for his or her health? Do people have an obligation to take care of themselves as best they can to help avoid becoming a burden on their family and on society? Do people have a right to choose whatever lifestyle they want—no matter how unhealthy? In your health journal, write an essay describing your opinion about individual responsibility for health. Be sure to explain your reasoning.

4. Make a list of risk factors for cancer over which you have no control, including heredity and personal history. Do these risk factors increase your risk for any cancers? If so, make a list of behaviors you can adopt that will lower your risk for these cancers.

BEHAVIOR CHANGE STRATEGY

ADOPTING A DIET TO HELP PREVENT CVD AND CANCER

If you start now, you'll find that eating foods that reduce the risks of cardiovascular disease and cancer will soon be second nature.

Reducing the Saturated Fat in Your Diet

The American Heart Association recommends that no more than 10 percent of the calories in your diet come from saturated fat. The biggest sources of saturated fats are animal products, such as red meat, cheese, milk, cream, yogurt, and butter; the "tropical oils," such as palm and coconut oil; and heavily hydrogenated vegetable oils. To see how your diet measures up, monitor yourself for a week, keeping track of everything you eat. Keep your record in your health journal, writing the foods you eat (including meals and snacks) on the left side of the page and leaving room on the right for information about each food.

Information about the calorie and fat content of the foods you eat is available on many food labels and in books available in libraries and bookstores. For fast foods, use the appendix to Chapter 9 of this book.

Each day, after you have noted the foods you ate, enter the calories and the grams of saturated fat, and then compute the percentage of saturated fat for each food using the formula explained in Chapter 9. (Multiply grams of saturated fat by 9 and divide the product by the total calories. The result is the percentage of saturated fat.) Repeat the calculations for each day (based on total grams of saturated fat and total calorie intake) and for the week. How close do your daily and weekly percentages come to the goal of 10 percent or fewer calories from saturated fat?

You can also monitor and compute the percentages of monounsaturated and polyunsaturated fats in your diet. Foods high in polyunsaturated fat include corn oil, cottonseed oil, safflower oil, soybean oil, mayonnaise made with any of these oils, margarine, sunflower seeds, and walnuts. Foods high in monounsaturated fat include olive oil, peanut oil, sesame oil, almonds, cashews, hazelnuts, peanuts, pecans, pistachio nuts, and avocados. Try to keep each of these groups at or below about 10 percent of your total calories too.

If your diet includes more than your fair share of saturated fat, you can take steps to reduce it. Begin by looking at the tips in the box "Controlling Cholesterol Through Diet." Start to become more aware of what type of food you order in restaurants, buy at the supermarket, and prepare for meals. Do you usually go for hamburgers, hot dogs, steaks, and chops? Choose lean meat, chicken, or fish instead, and broil or bake it instead of frying it. Do you have salami and cheese on rye for lunch? Try turkey for a change. Is ice cream your downfall? Sliced fruit in season with low-fat yogurt and honey is a delicious alternative. Put your best effort into finding attractive, satisfying, and enjoyable activities as substitutes, such as trying out restaurants that serve low-fat dishes.

Phasing in a Healthier Diet

Is it hard to break bad eating habits? Of course, and it doesn't happen in a day. But two nutritional scientists at the Oregon Health Sciences University in Portland have devised a plan for improving eating habits in three phases. Although Dr. William Connor and Sonja Conner designed their diet (described in their book *The New American Diet*) to reduce the risk of heart disease, their plan and many of their specific suggestions work as an anticancer diet as well. The guiding principle is to avoid doing anything radical, but instead to increase gradually your consumption of fruits, vegetables, and grains while you reduce your intake of fat, cholesterol, and known and suspected carcinogens.

Begin by monitoring your diet for one or two weeks, noting in your health journal both the health-protecting and the cancer-promoting foods you eat (see the box "A Dietary Defense Against Cancer").

After you have recorded your diet, analyze it to see how often you consume the foods listed. Do you have cruciferous vegetables two or three times a week? Are carrots, peaches, or apricots part of your diet? Do you eat bacon only occasionally? Do you limit your intake of alcohol? Once you have some idea of how much your diet protects you against cancer and how much it puts you at

risk, try implementing the following three-phase diet-change plan:

Phase I: Substitutions Avoid egg yolks, butter, lard, organ meats, bacon and other cured meats, and any burnt meat. Start using vegetable oils for all purposes rather than animal fats. Switch to low-fat or nonfat milk products and other low-fat foods. Discard chicken skin and meat fat. Reduce consumption of beer and wine. Keep using favorite recipes, but decrease salt and fat content.

Phase II: New Recipes Reduce the amount of red meat and cheese you eat; replace with chicken and fish. Cut down on fats, including vegetable fats. Begin to replace meats and fats with grains, beans, fruits, and vegetables, especially those high in vitamins A and C and members of the cabbage family. Choose low-fat dishes when eating out. Replace recipes that cannot be altered.

Phase III: A New Way of Eating Eat meats and cheeses as side dishes, in small amounts, rather than as main courses. Increase consumption of beans and grains as protein and fiber sources. Save rich foods such as chocolate and bakery goods for special treats only, no more than once a month. Make a habit of trying new grains and beans, fruits, and vegetables (select some from the lists given in the chapter, or see what the supermarkets and ethnic stores in your community offer). Keep developing a new repertory of recipes.

A diet like this can provide benefits to your cardiovascular system, help you lose weight gradually and permanently, and give you some insurance against cancer later in life. Try making these changes over the course of a few months to improve your overall health and your chances for a cancer-free future.

Adapted from "Phasing in a Healthier Diet." *University of California at Berkeley Wellness Letter*, October 1987.

SELECTED BIBLIOGRAPHY

American College of Cardiology. 1992. 41st Annual Scientific Session, Dallas, Texas. *Supplement A:* 1A–395A.

American Heart Association. 1994. *Heart and Stroke Facts.*

———. 1992. *Physicians' Cholesterol Education Handbook.*

———. 1995. *Heart and Stroke Facts: 1995 Statistical Supplement.*

American Medical Association. 1992. *Position Paper on Exercise.*

Andriole, G. L., and W. J. Catalona. 1991. The diagnosis and treatment of prostate cancer. *Annual Reviews of Medicine* 42: 9–15.

Banks, B. A., and others. 1992. Attitudes of teenagers toward sun exposure and sunscreen use. *Pediatrics* 89(1): 40–42.

Bates, M. N. 1991. Extremely low frequency electromagnetic fields and cancer: The epidemiologic evidence. *Environmental Health Perspectives* 95:147–56.

CeBallos, P. I., and others. 1995. Current concepts: Melanoma in children. *New England Journal of Medicine* 332(10): 656–62.

Centers for Disease Control and Prevention. 1994. Advance report of final mortality statistics, 1992. *Monthly Vital Statistics Report* 43(6): 51.

Coronary Artery Disease: Diagnosis and Treatment. 1994. *Harvard Heart Letter, A Special Report*, November.

"Fat and Cancer: A Clear Picture at Last." *Consumer Reports on Health*. December 1992.

Douglas, P. S., and others. 1992. Exercise and atherosclerotic heart disease in women. *Medicine and Science in Sports and Exercise* 6 Suppl.: S266–76.

Glantz, S. A., and W. W. Parmley. 1992. Passive smoking causes heart disease and lung cancer. *Journal of Clinical Epidemiology* 45(8): 815–919.

Harris, J. R., and others. 1992. Breast cancer: Medical progress. *New England Journal of Medicine* 327(5): 319–27.

Haskell, W. L., and others. 1992. Cardiovascular benefits and assessment of physical activity and physical fitness in adults. *Medicine and Science in Sports and Exercise* 6 Suppl.: S201–20.

———. 1992. Role of water-soluble dietary fiber in the management of elevated plasma cholesterol in healthy subjects. *American Journal of Cardiology* 69(5): 433–39.

Hirayama, T. 1992. Life-style and cancer: From epidemiological evidence to public behavior change to mortality reduction of target cancers. *Monographs/National Cancer Institute* 12:65–74.

Howard, J., and others. 1992. A collaborative study of differences in the survival rates of black patients and white patients with cancer. *Cancer* 69(9): 2349–60.

Keil, J. E., and others. 1992. Does equal socioeconomic status in black and white men mean equal risk of mortality? *American Journal of Public Health* 82(8): 1133–36.

Kolonel, L. N., and M. T. Goodman. 1992. Racial variation in cancer incidence: Fact or artifact? *Journal of the National Cancer Institute* 84(12): 915–16.

La Vecchia, C. 1992. Cancers associated with high-fat diets. *Monographs/National Cancer Institute* 12:79–85.

Leaf, A. 1992. Health claims: Omega-3 fatty acids and cardiovascular disease. *Nutrition Reviews* 50(5): 150–54.

Mayo Clinic Heart Book. 1993. New York: William Morrow.

More on Aspirin. 1995. *Harvard Heart Letter* 5(5): 2, January.

Musante, L., and others. 1992. Hostility: Relationship to lifestyle behaviors and physical risk factors. *Behavioral Medicine* 18(1): 21–26.

Vail-Smith, K., and D. M. White. 1992. Risk level, knowledge, and preventive behavior for human papillomaviruses among sexually active college women. *Journal of American College Health* 40(5): 227–30.

Wynder, E. L. 1992. Cancer prevention: Optimizing life-styles with special reference to nutritional carcinogenesis. *Monographs/National Cancer Institute* 12:87–91.

Zhang, Y., and others. 1992. A major inducer of anticarcinogenic protective enzymes from broccoli: Isolation and elucidation of sulforaphane structure. *Proceedings of the National Academy of Sciences of the United States of America* 89(6): 2399–2403.

RECOMMENDED READINGS

American Cancer Society. 1995. *Cancer Facts and Figures—1995*. New York: American Cancer Society. *Available in every library, this is a condensed and authoritative summary of the current cancer statistics, renewed each year.*

Dollinger, M., E. H. Rosenbaum, and G. Cable. 1991. *Everyone's Guide to Cancer Therapy: How Cancer Is Diagnosed, Treated, and Managed Day to Day*. Toronto: Somerville House. *An authoritative lay guide to cancer diagnosis and treatment written by top cancer specialists.*

Grundy, S. 1989. *American Heart Association Low-Fat, Low-Cholesterol Cookbook: An Essential Guide for Those Concerned About Their Cholesterol Levels*. New York: Random House. *Recipes and easy-to-follow advice for heart-healthy eating.*

Moser, M. 1989. *Lower Your Blood Pressure and Live Longer: A Simple and Effective Program Developed by a Leading Specialist in Hypertension*. New York: Villard Books. *Comprehensive advice on lifestyle changes to reduce blood pressure without drugs. Helpful charts list sodium content of common foods. Also covers hypertension medications, their uses, and side effects.*

Ornish, D. 1990. *Reversing Heart Disease*. New York: Ballantine Books. *A revolutionary approach to treating and preventing heart disease using diet, stress reduction, group support, and exercise.*

Selzer, A. 1993. *Understanding Heart Disease*. Berkeley: University of California Press. *A comprehensive guide to help patients with heart disease communicate with health professionals.*

Smith, J. S., and S. D. Smith. 1993. *The Low-Fat Supermarket*. Lancaster, Pa.: Starburst Publications. *A registered dietitian and a physician compiled this pratical guide to cutting down on fat.*

Whelan, E. 1994. *The Complete Guide to Preventing Cancer*. New York: Prometheus Books. *Provides up-to-date information in non-technical language.*

Williams, R., and V. Williams. 1993. *Anger Kills: Seventeen Strategies for Controlling the Hostility That Can Harm Your Health*. New York: Times Books. *Dr. Williams, an expert in behavioral medicine, discusses the biological correlates of anger and hostility that can lead to heart disease, and suggests strategies for recognizing and controlling hostility.*

American Cancer Society (1-800-ACS-2345) publishes a wide range of materials on the prevention and treatment of cancer, all available free of charge. Titles include: *Nutrition and Cancer, How to Examine Your Breasts, Cancer Facts for Women, Facts on Ovarian Cancer,* and *Sexuality and Cancer.*

The National Cancer Institute (NCI) maintains a database of the latest published information about cancer. Operators will perform a search for callers on specific subjects and send along relevant materials (1-800-4-CANCER). NCI also publishes a wide range of cancer materials, available free of charge. Sample titles: *Cancer Prevention, Cancer Rates and Risks, Breast Biopsy: What You Should Know, What You Need to Know About Colon and Rectal Cancer, When Someone In Your Family Has Cancer, The Future of Cancer Therapy.* Publications may be ordered by writing: Public Inquiries Section, Office of Cancer Communications, NCI, Bldg. 31, Room 10A16, 9000 Rockville Pike, Bethesda, MD 20892.

13

Immunity and Infection

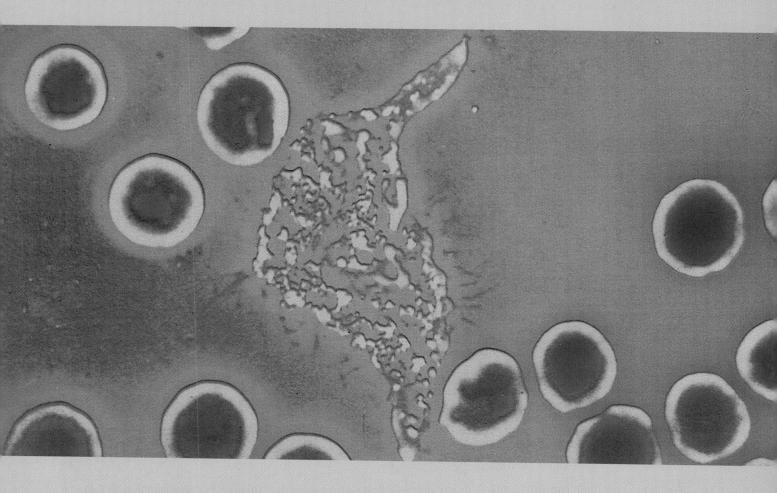

CONTENTS

One consequence of the AIDS epidemic has been to make many people more aware of the incredible job constantly being performed by the human immune system—and of the equally incredible devastation that occurs when the system falters. There are countless, unseen microscopic organisms that live around, on, and in us. Many of them would like nothing better than to consume the very tissues and organs they call home. Only constant vigilance on the part of our immune system keeps these microorganisms at bay and our bodies intact and healthy. The immune system works to keep the body from being overwhelmed not just by invaders from the outside (infection) but also by changes on the inside, such as cancer.

Most people don't pay much attention to any of these internal skirmishes unless they become sick and find themselves deprived of their usual feelings of well-being. Clearly, it's best to keep your immune systems working well and to do whatever you can to keep yourself from being infected. This chapter provides information that will help you understand immunity, infection, and how to keep yourself well in a world of hungry microorganisms.

THE BODY'S DEFENSE SYSTEM

Our bodies have very effective ways of protecting themselves against invasion by foreign organisms, especially **pathogens,** microorganisms that cause disease. Pathogens can enter the body in one of three ways: (1) by penetration of the skin (for example, through an insect bite or cut) or by direct contact (for example, when mucous membranes come into contact with a herpes or syphilis lesion), (2) by inhalation of particles, or (3) by ingestion of contaminated food or water. The body's first line of defense is a formidable array of physical and chemical barriers. When these barriers are breached, the body's immune system comes into play. Together, these defenses provide an effective response to nearly all the challenges and invasions our bodies will ever experience.

Physical and Chemical Barriers

The skin, the body's largest organ, prevents many microorganisms and particles from entering the body. Although many bacterial and fungal organisms live on the surface of the skin, very few can penetrate it except through a cut or break. Wherever there is an opening in the body, or an area without skin, other barriers exist. The mouth, the main entry to the gastrointestinal system, is lined with mucous membranes, which contain cells designed to prevent the passage of unwanted organisms and particles. These surfaces and the fluids that cover them (for example, tears, saliva, and vaginal secretions) are rich in antibodies (discussed in detail later in the chapter) and in **enzymes** that destroy many microorganisms.

The respiratory tract is lined not only with mucous membranes but also with cells having hairlike protrusions called **cilia.** The cilia sweep foreign matter up and out of the respiratory tract. Particles that are not caught by this mechanism may be expelled from the system by a cough. If the ciliated cells are damaged or destroyed, as they are by smoking tobacco, a cough is the body's only way of ridding the airways of foreign particles. This is one reason why smokers generally have a chronic daily cough— they're compensating for damaged airways.

> *Personal Insight* How do you feel when you get sick? Do you feel "weak"? Guilty? Angry? Are you impatient to get back on your feet, or do you want to prolong the time you can legitimately be excused from your normal obligations? When you were sick as a child, was it unpleasant or did it have certain pleasant aspects, such as getting extra attention or staying home from school? How have your childhood experiences affected your current feelings about being sick?

The Immune System

Once the body has been invaded by a foreign organism, an elaborate system of responses is activated. The immune system operates through a remarkable information network involving billions of cellular defenders who rush to protect the body when a threat arises. We discuss here two of the body's responses: the inflammatory response and the immune response. But before we cover these specific defenses, let's turn to a brief description of the defenders themselves and the mechanisms by which they work.

The Immunological Defenders and How They Work

The immune response is carried out by different types of white blood cells, all of which are continuously being produced in the bone marrow. **Neutrophils,** one type of white blood cell, travel in the bloodstream to areas of invasion, attacking and ingesting pathogens. **Macrophages,** or "big eaters," take up stations in tissues and act as scav-

Infection Disease caused by a pathogen.

Pathogens Organisms that cause disease.

Enzymes Chemicals necessary for energy production and protein synthesis in normal animal cells.

Cilia Microscopic hairlike structures that sweep mucus and foreign substances up out of the bronchial tubes.

Neutrophil A type of white blood cell that engulfs foreign organisms and infected, damaged, or aged cells; they are particularly prevalent during the inflammatory response.

Macrophages Large phagocytic ("cell-eating") cells that devour foreign particles.

TERMS

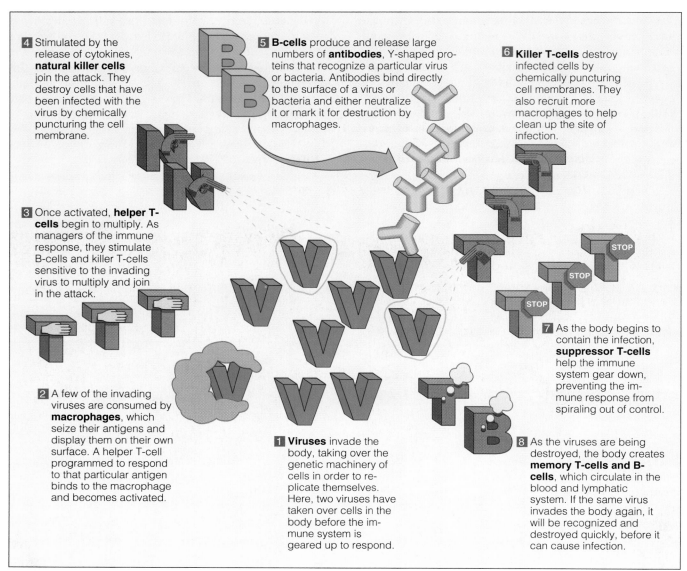

4 Stimulated by the release of cytokines, **natural killer cells** join the attack. They destroy cells that have been infected with the virus by chemically puncturing the cell membrane.

5 **B-cells** produce and release large numbers of **antibodies**, Y-shaped proteins that recognize a particular virus or bacteria. Antibodies bind directly to the surface of a virus or bacteria and either neutralize it or mark it for destruction by macrophages.

6 **Killer T-cells** destroy infected cells by chemically puncturing cell membranes. They also recruit more macrophages to help clean up the site of infection.

3 Once activated, **helper T-cells** begin to multiply. As managers of the immune response, they stimulate B-cells and killer T-cells sensitive to the invading virus to multiply and join in the attack.

2 A few of the invading viruses are consumed by **macrophages**, which seize their antigens and display them on their own surface. A helper T-cell programmed to respond to that particular antigen binds to the macrophage and becomes activated.

1 **Viruses** invade the body, taking over the genetic machinery of cells in order to replicate themselves. Here, two viruses have taken over cells in the body before the immune system is geared up to respond.

7 As the body begins to contain the infection, **suppressor T-cells** help the immune system gear down, preventing the immune response from spiraling out of control.

8 As the viruses are being destroyed, the body creates **memory T-cells and B-cells**, which circulate in the blood and lymphatic system. If the same virus invades the body again, it will be recognized and destroyed quickly, before it can cause infection.

Figure 13-1 *The immune response.*
Once invaded by a pathogen, a complex series of reactions takes place to eliminate the invader. Pictured here are the principal elements of the immune response to a virus; not shown are the many types of cytokines that help coordinate the actions of the different types of defenders.

engers, devouring pathogens and worn-out cells. **Natural killer cells** directly destroy virus-infected cells and cells that have turned cancerous. **Lymphocytes,** of which there are several types, are white blood cells that travel in both the bloodstream and the **lymphatic system.** At various places in the lymphatic system there are lymph nodes (or glands), where macrophages congregate and filter bacteria and other substances from the lymph. When these nodes are actively involved in fighting an invasion of microorganisms, they fill with cells; physicians use the location of swollen lymph nodes as a clue to the location and cause of an infection.

The two kinds of lymphocytes are known as **T-cells** and **B-cells.** T-cells are further differentiated into **helper T-cells, killer T-cells,** and **suppressor T-cells.** B-cells are lymphocytes that produce **antibodies.** The first time T-cells and B-cells encounter a specific invader, some of them are reserved as **memory T- and B-cells,** enabling the body to mount a rapid response should the same invader appear again in the future. These cells and cell products—macrophages, natural killer cells, T-cells (helper T-cells, killer T-cells, and suppressor T-cells), B-cells and antibodies, and memory cells—are the principal players in the body's immune response.

The immune system is built on a remarkable feature possessed by these defenders—the ability to distinguish foreign cells from the body's own cells. Since the lymphocytes are capable of great destruction, it's essential that they not attack the body itself. When they do, they cause **autoimmune diseases,** such as lupus and rheumatoid arthritis.

How do the lymphocytes know when they've encountered an enemy? All the cells of an individual's body display markers on their surfaces—tiny molecular shapes—that identify them as "self" to lymphocytes who encounter them. Lymphocytes also recognize the markers displayed on the surfaces of invading microorganisms and know they've encountered "not self." Markers that are recognized by lymphocytes as foreign and that trigger the immune response are known as **antigens.**

The Inflammatory Response   When the body has been injured or infected, one of the body's responses is the inflammatory response. Special cells in the area of invasion or injury release **histamine** and other substances that cause blood vessels to dilate and fluid to flow out of capillaries into the injured tissue. This produces increased heat, swelling, and redness in the affected area. White blood cells, including neutrophils and macrophages, are drawn to the area and attack the invaders, in many cases destroying them. At the site of infection there may be pus, a collection of dead white blood cells and debris resulting from the encounter.

The Immune Response   Another bodily response to invasion is the immune response (Figure 13-1). For convenience, we can think of this response as having four critical phases: (1) recognition of the invading pathogen, (2) amplification of defenses, (3) attack, (4) slowdown. In each of these phases, crucial actions occur that are designed to destroy the invader and restore the body to health.

1. In the first phase, macrophages are drawn to the site of the injury and consume the foreign cells; they then provide information about the enemy by displaying its antigen on their surfaces. Helper T-cells, the "commanders-in-chief" of the immune response, read this information and rush to respond.

2. Now the second phase of the immune response gets underway. Multiplying rapidly, helper T-cells trigger the production of killer T-cells and B-cells in the spleen and lymph nodes. **Cytokines,** chemical messengers secreted by lymphocytes, help regulate and coordinate the immune response. **Interleukins** and **interferons** are two examples of cytokines. They stimulate increased production of T- and B-cells and antibodies, promote the activities of natural killer cells, produce fever, and have special antipathogenic properties themselves.

3. With its forces constantly amplifying, the immune system launches its attack, the third phase of its response. Killer T-cells strike at foreign cells and cells of the body that have been invaded and infected,

identifying them by the antigens displayed on the surface of the cells. (They destroy body cells that have mutated and become cancerous in the same way.) Puncturing the cell membrane, they sacrifice body cells in order to destroy the foreign organism within. This type of action is known as a *cell-mediated immune response,* because the attack is carried out by cells. Killer T-cells also trigger an amplified inflammatory response and recruit more macrophages to help clean up the site.

B-cells work in a different way. Stimulated to multiply by helper T-cells, they produce large quantities of antibody molecules, which are released in the bloodstream and tissues. Antibodies are Y-shaped protein molecules that bind to antigen-bearing targets and mark them for destruction by macrophages. This type of response is

Natural killer cell   A type of white blood cell that directly destroys virus-infected cells and cancer cells.

Lymphocytes   White blood cells continuously made in lymphoid tissue as well as in bone marrow.

Lymphatic system   A system of vessels and organs that picks up excess fluid, proteins, lipids, and other substances from the tissues; filters out disease-causing organisms and other waste products; and returns the cleansed fluid to the general circulation.

T-cell   One kind of lymphocyte; arises in bone marrow, and some progeny move into thymus (giving its name).

B-cells   Lymphocytes that produce antibodies.

Helper T-cells   Lymphocytes that stimulate other lymphocytes to increase.

Killer T-cells   Lymphocytes that kill cells of the body that have been invaded by foreign organisms; also can kill cells that have turned cancerous.

Suppressor T-cells   Lymphocytes that discourage the growth of other lymphocytes.

Antibodies   Specialized proteins, produced by white blood cells, that can recognize and neutralize specific microbes.

Memory T- and B-cells   Lymphocytes that are generated during an initial infection and circulate in the body for years, "remembering" the specific antigens that caused the infection and quickly destroying them if they appear again.

Autoimmune disease   Disease in which an individual's immune system attacks the individual's own body or body parts.

Antigen   A molecule that marks an invading particle; can be recognized and neutralized by an antibody.

Histamine   A chemical responsible for the dilation and increased permeability of blood vessels in allergic reactions.

Cytokines   Chemical messages released by immune system cells that help amplify and coordinate the immune response.

Interleukins   A class of cytokines that alert immune system cells to the presence of foreign organisms and stimulate them into action.

Interferons   A class of cytokines that bind to cell membranes, increasing their resistance to many viruses; they also stimulate the activities of macrophages and natural killer cells.

known as an *antibody-mediated immune response.* Antibodies work against bacteria and against viruses and other substances when they are in the body but outside cells. They don't work against infected body cells or viruses that are replicating inside cells.

4. Now that the invading microorganism has been destroyed or incapacitated, the body has to call off the attack. The last phase of the immune response is the slowdown of activity. A third type of T-cell, the suppressor T-cell, regulates the levels of lymphocytes in the body and controls their activities. When the danger is over, suppressor T-cells halt the immune response and restore homeostasis. Dead cells, killed pathogens, and other debris that result from the immune response are scavenged by certain types of white blood cells; filtered out of circulation by the liver, spleen, and kidneys; and excreted from the body.

Immunity   In many infections, survival confers **immunity;** that is, an infected person will never get the same illness again. This is because some of the lymphocytes created during the amplification phase of the response are reserved as memory T- and B-cells. They continue to cir-

culate in the blood and lymphatic system for years or even for the rest of the person's life. If the same antigen enters the body a subsequent time, the memory T- and B-cells recognize and destroy it before it can cause illness. This subsequent response takes only a day or two, whereas the original response lasted several days, during which time the individual suffered the symptoms of illness. The ability of memory lymphocytes to remember previous infections is known as **adaptive** or **acquired immunity.**

Symptoms and Contagion   The immune system is operating at the cellular level within your body all the time, maintaining its vigilance when you're well and fighting invaders when you're sick. How does it all feel to you, the host and playing field for these activities? How do your symptoms relate to the course of the infection and the immune response?

During **incubation**—when a virus is multiplying in the body or when bacteria are actively multiplying before the immune system has gathered momentum—you may not have any symptoms of the illness, but you may be contagious. During the second and third phases of the immune response, you may still be unaware of the infection, or you may "feel a cold coming on."

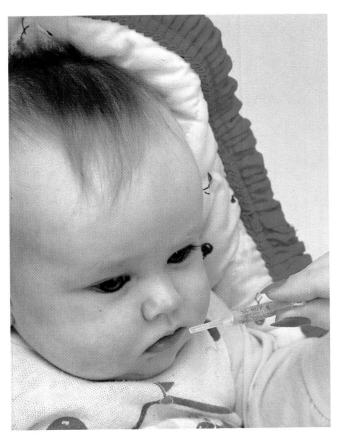

Before polio vaccines were developed by Jonas Salk and Albert Sabin in the 1950s, many people, especially children, were paralyzed or killed by this viral infection. This 1-year-old is being given oral polio vaccine as part of the standard series of childhood immunizations.

Many of the symptoms of an illness are actually due to the immune response of the body rather than to the actions or products of the invading organism. For example, fever is thought to be caused by the release and activation of certain cytokines in macrophages and other cells during the immune response. Cytokines travel in the bloodstream to the brain, where they cause the body's thermostat to be "reset" to a higher level. An elevated temperature is thought to assist in fighting pathogens by enhancing many immune responses. (During an illness, it is only necessary to lower a fever if it is uncomfortably high [over 101.5° F] or if it occurs in an infant who is at risk for seizures from fever.)

Similarly, you get a runny nose when your lymphocytes destroy infected mucosal cells, leading to increased mucus production. You get a sore throat when your lymphocytes destroy infected throat cells. The malaise and fatigue of the "flu" may be caused by interferons.

You are contagious when there are active organisms replicating in your body and they can gain access to another person. This may be before a vigorous immune response has occurred, so at times you may be contagious before experiencing any symptoms. This means that you can transmit an illness without knowing you're infected or catch an illness from someone who doesn't appear to be sick. On the other hand, your symptoms may continue after the invading organisms have been mostly destroyed, when you are no longer infectious.

Immunization

The ability of the immune system to remember previously encountered organisms and retain its strength against them is the basis for immunization. When a person is immunized against a disease, the immune system is "primed" with an antigen that's similar to the disease-causing organism but not as dangerous. The body responds by producing antibodies to the organism, which prevent serious infection if the person is exposed to the disease itself. The preparations used to manipulate the immune system this way are known as **vaccines.**

Vaccines are made in several ways. In some cases, organisms are cultured in the laboratory in a way that weakens (attenuates) them. These "live, attenuated" organisms are used in vaccines against such diseases as measles, mumps, and rubella (German measles). In other cases, when it's not possible to breed attenuated organisms, vaccines are made from pathogens that have been killed in the laboratory but that still retain their ability to stimulate the production of antibodies. Vaccines composed of "killed" viruses are used against influenza viruses, among others. A third type of vaccine has been developed to protect against tetanus. This disease is caused by a bacterium that thrives in deep puncture wounds and produces a deadly toxin. The vaccine is made from a "toxoid" that resembles the toxin—that is, lymphocytes recognize it as being the same—but that doesn't produce the same effects. Tetanus shots are normally needed every ten years, but in the case of a deep wound, a tetanus shot may be needed if five years have elapsed since the last shot. Immunizations available in the United States are listed in Table 13-1.

Vaccines confer what is known as *active immunity*—that is, the vaccinated person produces his or her own an-

TABLE 13-1 Immunizations Available in the United States

Type of Immunization	Who Should Be Immunized	Effectiveness of Immunization and Frequency of Booster Doses
Chicken pox	Children over the age of 12 months and adults who have not had the disease	About 70 to 90 percent effective; renewal every 6–10 years may be needed
Diphtheria	All children	Highly effective; renew every 10 years
Gamma globulin	Travelers to nonindustrialized countries	Effective for 6 months
German measles (rubella)	All children	Highly effective; need for boosters not established
Hemophilus influenza	All children	Very effective against meningitis
Hepatitis B	All children; health care workers; sexual partners and newborns of hepatitis B carriers	Very effective; may need booster if exposed
Influenza	Adults over age 65; anyone with chronic disease of the heart, respiratory tract, or endocrine system	Renew every year (because viral strains change easily)
Japanese encephalitis	Long-term visitors to endemic areas	About 85 percent effective; renew every 2 years if needed
Measles	All children. Adults born after 1956 should get a booster.	Highly effective; some states now require booster for school entry
Mumps	All children	Believed to confer lifetime immunity
Pneumococcus	Adults over age 65; anyone with chronic heart or lung disease or who doesn't have a spleen	About 70 percent effective
Polio	All children; all adults, particularly travelers, those exposed to children, and those in health and sanitation industries	Long-lasting immunity; no booster necessary unless exposure anticipated
Rabies	Only those bitten by rabid animal	Five doses are given over a 4-week period
Tetanus (lockjaw)	Everyone	Very effective; renew every 10 years or when treated for a contaminated wound if more than 5 years have elapsed since last booster
Typhoid fever	Travelers to endemic areas	About 80 percent effective
Whooping cough (pertussis)	Essential for children by age 3 to 4 months	Highly effective
Yellow fever	Travelers to endemic areas	Highly effective; renew every 10 years

tibodies to the microorganism. Another type of injection confers *passive immunity*. In this case, a person exposed to a disease is injected with the antibodies themselves, produced by other human beings or animals who have recovered from the disease. Injections of **gamma globulin**—a product made from the blood plasma of many individuals, containing all the antibodies they have ever made—are sometimes given to people exposed to a disease against which they haven't been immunized. Such injections create a rapid but temporary immunity and are useful against certain viruses, such as **hepatitis** A. Gamma globulin is also sometimes used to treat antibody deficiency syndromes.

Allergy—The Body's Defense System Gone Haywire

You probably know someone with **allergies,** or perhaps you have an allergy yourself. Allergic reactions are a response of the immune system, but in this case the response is inappropriate, annoying, and sometimes even life-threatening. Allergic reactions occur when the body recognizes a relatively harmless substance, such as dust, pollen, or animal hair, as a dangerous antigen and mounts an immune response to it. B-cells multiply, antibodies are produced, and quantities of histamine and other substances are released from cells near the location of the invasion. The resulting inflammatory response produces such symptoms as runny nose, red, itchy eyes, sneezing, congestion, hives, and asthma.

THE TROUBLEMAKERS—PATHOGENS AND DISEASE

Now that we've discussed the beautiful and intricate system that protects us from disease, let's consider some pathogens, those disease-producing organisms that live within us and around us. When they succeed in gaining entry to body tissue, they can cause illness and sometimes death to the unfortunate host. They include bacteria, viruses, fungi, protozoa, and parasitic worms.

Personal Insight How do you feel when you hear that someone has HIV infection? Herpes? Chicken pox? Bronchitis? If you feel differently about these cases, what is the basis for the difference?

Bacteria

Among the microorganisms that exist everywhere in our environment are one-celled organisms called **bacteria.** Essential for life as we know it, bacteria break down dead organic matter, allowing it to be restructured for use by other organisms so that life can go on. They also perform a similar task in our intestines, helping digest food for better absorption by the body. If we view the entire digestive tract as a long hollow tube beginning in the mouth and moving down the esophagus, stomach, small and large intestine to the anus, we see that even though bacteria reside inside the intestine, they are not really a part of the body. Underneath the skin, within the bloodstream, tissues and organs, the body is devoid of bacteria, or "sterile." Bacteria found in these areas are almost always pathogenic, or disease-producing. It is here that the immune system keeps up its constant surveillance, seeking out and destroying any invaders.

Because of their tiny size, bacteria can be seen only using a microscope. Bacteria are grouped according to their shape: cocci (spheres), bacilli (rods), and spirochetes (spirals). Common sphere-shaped bacteria that can cause disease include streptococcus (which can inflame the tonsils and throat and cause pneumonia) and staphylococcus (which is responsible for toxic shock syndrome and some

types of skin infections). The rod-shaped bacteria include the organisms responsible for many urinary tract infections and for Legionnaire's disease. Different spirochetes cause **syphilis** and Lyme disease. Different species of bacteria are also responsible for tuberculosis (TB), Rocky Mountain spotted fever, and typhus.

To fight bacteria, we use antibiotics, which are both naturally occurring and synthetic substances having the ability to kill bacteria. Most of the natural antibiotics are produced by molds. **Penicillin,** for example, was discovered by Alexander Fleming in 1929 when he noticed that bacteria growing on a culture were inhibited by a mold left in the laboratory overnight. Since that time thousands of naturally occurring substances have been screened for antibiotic activity, and many have been marketed for use in treating infected patients. Other antibiotics have been created completely in the test tube. However they originated, most antibiotics work in a similar fashion: They interrupt the production of new bacteria by damaging some part of their reproductive cycle or by causing faulty parts of new bacteria to be made. Antibiotics are useful mainly against bacteria; against most viruses, they are ineffective.

When antibiotics inhibit a specific bacteria's growth, these bacteria are said to be "sensitive." Unfortunately, when bacteria are repeatedly exposed to small doses of antibiotics, a few develop a resistance to the drug and can survive and multiply even when the drug is present. Antibiotic-resistant bacteria can develop if antibiotics are overused or if people don't finish their entire course of medication. In recent years, antibiotic-resistant strains of gonorrhea, salmonella, tuberculosis, streptococcus, and many other bacteria have been identified.

Viruses

Visible only with an electron microscope, **viruses,** the smallest of the pathogens, are on the borderline between living and nonliving matter. Viruses lack all the enzymes essential to energy production and protein synthesis in

Gamma globulin Serum containing specific antibodies, injected to provide temporary immunity to specific antigens.

Hepatitis Inflammation of the liver caused by one of a group of viruses that can be transmitted through certain types of sexual and nonsexual contact.

Allergies Diseases caused by the body's own exaggerated response to foreign chemicals and proteins.

Bacteria Organisms about 100–1,000 times larger than viruses, about 100 species of which can cause disease in humans.

Syphilis A sexually transmissible disease caused by a spiral-shaped, corkscrew bacteria called a spirochete.

Penicillin An antibiotic substance produced by the fungus *penicillium.*

Viruses The smallest pathogenic organisms; cannot grow or reproduce by themselves.

TERMS

Lyme disease is caused by a spirochete bacteria transmitted by the deer tick, which makes its home on deer and mice (except in California, where the culprit is the closely-related black-legged tick, which also lives on wood rats). Ticks acquire the spirochete by feasting on the blood of an infected animal and then may transmit it to their next meal.

Symptoms of Lyme disease vary from person to person, but usually appear in three stages. In the first stage an expanding red rash develops from the area of the tick bite, usually about two weeks after the bite occurs; some people develop flu-like symptoms as well. The second stage occurs weeks to months later in about 10 to 20 percent of untreated patients. Symptoms include impaired motor coordination, partial facial paralysis, and heart rhythm abnormalities. These symptoms usually disappear within a few weeks. The third stage, which occurs in about half of untreated people, can occur years after the tick bite and usually consists of chronic or recurring arthritis (inflammation of the joints), usually affecting the knees. Lyme disease can also cause fetal damage or death at any stage of pregnancy.

If you live in an area where Lyme disease is prevalent and spend time in the woods or even in your yard—especially between May and September—take these steps:

- Wear light-colored, long-sleeved, long-legged clothing outdoors, preferably with elastic wrist and ankle bands or with pants tucked into your shoes or socks. Wear closed shoes and a hat to protect your feet and scalp.

- Check yourself occasionally for ticks, especially if you're in the underbrush or forest. When you get home, do a thorough check of your entire body, clothes, and gear. Deer ticks and black-legged ticks are smaller than dog ticks (see below); when engorged with blood these eight-legged ticks look like blood blisters. The immature ticks, called nymphs, are even smaller (about the size of a pinhead), and are responsible for up to 90 percent of all cases of Lyme disease. A nymph

Deer tick (actual size)

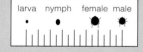

will feed on you for two to three days, an adult tick for up to a week. *The sooner you remove it, the better your chance of avoiding infection. Recent studies reveal that if the tick is on you for less than 24 hours, it is improbable that you'll develop the disease.*

- Inspect children daily, especially during the summer, when they spend lots of time outdoors.

- Check pets after they've been outdoors. They can carry ticks to your home or property or develop the disease themselves.

- Use an insect repellent containing DEET (short for N, N-diethyltoluamide) on your skin and a spray containing the insecticide permethrin on your clothing. (DEET has caused allergic reactions in some children and should be used with caution.)

- Remove a tick with fine-tipped tweezers—always carry a pair with you when outdoors. (It is almost impossible to remove a small tick with your fingers.) Exert a slow, steady pull. Don't twist the tick.

- Put the tick in a small jar containing alcohol (carry one with you if you're out hiking) so you can take it to your doctor or health department for identification.

- If you have been in an area where Lyme disease is a problem and you notice any symptoms—a rash or a flulike illness within the next two to three weeks—call your physician (see the text for a full description of symptoms). Lyme disease is treatable and almost always curable with antibiotics, especially in its early stages.

If you take these precautions and know what to watch for, you can still enjoy the outdoors without taking a chance of getting Lyme disease.

Source: M. Castleman. 1994. "Seasons of the Tick." *Sierra,* July/August; "Lyme Disease Update," *University of California at Berkeley Wellness Letter,* August 1992.

---

normal animal cells, and they cannot grow or reproduce by themselves. They must lead a **parasitic** existence inside a cell, borrowing what they need for growth and reproduction from the cells they invade. Once a virus is inside the host cell, it sheds its protein covering and its genetic material takes control of the cell and tricks it into

manufacturing more viruses like itself. The normal functioning of the host cell is thereby disrupted.

Different viruses affect different kinds of cells, and the seriousness of the disease they cause depends greatly on which kind of cell is affected. The viruses that cause colds, for example, attack upper respiratory tract cells, which are constantly cast off and replaced. The disease is therefore mild. Poliovirus, in contrast, attacks nerve cells that cannot be replaced and the consequences, such as paralysis, are severe.

Illnesses caused by viruses are the most common forms of **contagious disease.** They include most of the

TERMS

Parasitic Invading and surviving in the living tissue of other organisms.

Contagious disease Disease that can be transmitted from one carrier to another.

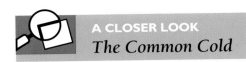
A cold is an inflammation of the upper respiratory tract caused by a viral infection. More than 200 different viruses cause colds, but many cold-causing viruses fall into one of three families—rhinoviruses, coronaviruses, and adenoviruses. Like all viruses, those that cause colds trick cells in the body into ingesting them and then take over the cells' reproductive machinery to make new viruses. When an infected cell dies, new virus particles are released and go on to infect other cells.

Some of the symptoms of a cold are caused by the actions of the virus. For example, destruction of cells lining the respiratory tract or throat can cause sore throat, cough, and runny nose. Other symptoms are caused by the body's immune reaction to the virus. When the body recognizes the viruses as foreign, immune cells release interferons and leukotrienes, which help mobilize the body's defenses but also cause fever, aches, and fatigue.

Colds are usually spread by simple hand-to-hand contact with another person or with inanimate objects such as doorknobs and telephones. People with colds often touch their mouth or nose, contaminate their hands, and then unknowingly infect others. The best way to interrupt this mode of transmission is to wash your hands frequently with soap and warm water. Viruses can also be transmitted in the small airborne particles produced by a cough or sneeze, but this requires very close contact and is relatively rare. Whether you come down with a cold once you've been exposed to the virus depends on a variety of factors, including age, genetics, type and amount of exposure, whether you smoke, and whether you've developed antibodies to that particular virus.

There is no cure for the common cold. Consumers spend more than $1 billion every year on nonprescription treatments for coughs and colds, but these products provide only temporary relief:

- *Antihistamines* decrease nasal secretions by blocking the effects of histamine, which causes swelling of small blood vessels and results in sneezing and runny nose. Antihistamines are most useful in treating allergies, which are associated with high levels of histamine. Caution—antihistamines can make you drowsy.

- *Decongestants* shrink nasal blood vessels, relieving swelling and congestion, but may dry out mucous membranes in the throat and make a sore throat worse.

- *Cough medicines* may be helpful when your cough is nonproductive (not bringing up mucus) or if it disrupts your sleep or work. Expectorants make coughs more productive by increasing the volume of mucus and decreasing its thickness; this helps remove irritants from the respiratory airways. Suppressants (antitussives) reduce the frequency of coughing.

- *Analgesics*—aspirin, acetaminophen (the ingredient in Tylenol), ibuprofen (the ingredient in Advil and Motrin), and naproxen sodium (the ingredient in Aleve)—help lower fever and relieve muscle aches. Some evidence suggests that aspirin may prolong the time a person sheds the virus in his or her secretions, thereby lengthening both the contagious phase and the duration of the illness. Aspirin is also associated with an increased risk for Reye's syndrome in children; for this reason, aspirin should not be given to children. Some studies suggest that ibuprofen in combination with a decongestant actually decreases the time of viral shedding and reduces the duration of symptoms.

- *Antibiotics* aren't necessary for a cold unless a bacterial infection such as strep throat is present.

What about chicken soup? This favorite home remedy is an effective treatment for some of your cold symptoms—the steam soothes a sore throat and loosens secretions, and the liquid and salt help prevent dehydration.

So, although there's no cure for a cold, you can make yourself more comfortable while your body fights off the infection. When you have a cold, the best plan may be to rest, drink plenty of hot liquids, and get what relief you can from appropriate nonprescription cold remedies.

Adapted from "Pain Relievers." *Mayo Clinic Health Letter*, April 1994; "The Common Cold." *Mayo Clinic Health Letter*, September 1992; and R. Baxter. 1988. "Uncommon Facts About the Common Cold." *Healthline*, October.

---

minor ailments that cause short-lived illness and are rarely precisely diagnosed. Among these are the common cold, a variety of brief and undiagnosed respiratory infections, **influenza**, gastrointestinal upsets that cause diarrhea, and assorted aches and pains. More serious are the diseases that occur mainly in childhood and frequently cause a severe rash, such as measles, chicken pox, and mumps.

Infectious mononucleosis (mono) is caused by a herpesvirus called **Epstein-Barr virus (EBV)**. This disease is spread by close contact and usually affects children and young adults. The virus attacks white blood cells, and its symptoms may even look like leukemia. About three weeks after contact, the infected person has a severe sore throat with painful swelling of lymph nodes in the neck,

Influenza   The flu—a usually mild viral disease, highly infective and adaptable; the form changes so easily that every year new strains arise, making treatment difficult.

Epstein-Barr virus   A member of the herpesvirus family associated with infectious mononucleosis.

TERMS

- Eat a balanced diet and maintain moderate weight. Consume a variety of low-fat foods to obtain the recommended amount of nutrients every day (see Chapter 9). No particular vitamin or mineral, including vitamin C, has been shown conclusively to prevent or cure the common cold or any other infectious disease.

- Get enough sleep—six to eight hours per night. Sleep is extremely important in helping the body replenish itself. Adequate sleep allows the proper production of all immune-related cells and products. Insufficient sleep predisposes you to a great number of illnesses and more severe infections.

- Exercise (but not while you're sick). Moderate aerobic exercise is an excellent way to reduce stress and strengthen the body, thereby preventing infection. However, exercise while you are sick—such as with a virus causing an upper respiratory infection—actually decreases your immunity and can prolong the infection, probably by facilitating the replication of the viruses.

- Don't smoke—smoking decreases the levels of some immune cells.

- Drink alcohol only in moderation. Heavy and long-term drinking interferes with the normal functioning of the immune system.

- Wash your hands frequently. Since most viral illnesses are transmitted by hand-to-hand contact, proper hand washing with soap and warm water can often prevent transmission of disease.

- Avoid contact with people who are infectious with diseases transmitted via the respiratory route, such as influenza, chicken pox, and tuberculosis.

- Don't eat raw meats, poultry, seafood, eggs, or milk; don't drink water from streams or lakes near campsites or hiking trails.

- Avoid contact with ticks, rodents, and other disease carriers.

- Practice "safer sex" and don't inject drugs to protect yourself against diseases such as hepatitis and HIV infection.

lethargy, and fever. Antibiotics have no effect on the disease process, which is usually self-limited. Some infected people may experience fatigue for weeks or even months.

More severe infections caused by viruses include HIV infection and hepatitis. There is no cure for either HIV infection or hepatitis, but there is an effective vaccine for the most common type of hepatitis (hepatitis B). Another serious viral infection is **poliomyelitis,** or polio, which attacks muscle-controlling nerves; in some cases, it leads to permanent paralysis. Fortunately, there is an effective vaccine and polio is now rare in the United States.

Most viral diseases cannot be treated and must simply run their course. Over-the-counter cold remedies and pain relievers treat symptoms, not their viral cause. If you want to take an OTC medication for your cold or flu, it's probably better to avoid the "shotgun" approach—taking all medications at once. Take medication only for those symptoms you actually have.

Fungi, Protozoa, and Parasitic Worms

The organisms referred to as **fungi** are primitive plants that may be multicellular (like molds) or unicellular (like yeasts). Mushrooms and the molds that form on bread and cheese are all examples of fungi. Only about 50 fungi out of many thousands of species cause disease in humans, and these diseases usually are restricted to the skin, mucous membranes, and lungs. Common fungal maladies include **candidiasis,** a yeast infection of the vagina that can also occur in other areas of the body; athlete's foot; jock itch; and ringworm, a disease of the scalp. These three conditions are usually easy to cure and rarely give rise to major problems. However, some fungal diseases are extremely difficult to treat.

Another group of pathogens are the **protozoa,** microscopic single-celled animals, which are associated with such tropical diseases as **malaria, African sleeping sickness,** and **amoebic dysentery.** Many protozoa-based diseases are recurrent. The pathogen remains in the body, alternating between activity and inactivity. Hundreds of millions of Asians, Africans, and South Americans suffer from protozoal infections. The most common protozoal disease in the United States is trichomoniasis, a relatively mild vaginal infection. Another protozoal disease, which

TERMS

Poliomyelitis A disease of the nervous system, sometimes crippling; vaccines now prevent most polio.

Fungi Molds, mushrooms, and yeasts—primitive plants.

Candidiasis A sexually transmissible disease caused by the fungus *Candida albicans,* producing vaginitis and infant thrush (mouth sores); an opportunistic infection often accompanying AIDS.

Protozoa Microscopic single-celled animals, often producing recurrent, cyclical attacks of disease.

Malaria Severe, recurrent, mosquito-borne protozoal disease.

African sleeping sickness Severe, recurrent, insect-borne protozoal disease marked by lassitude.

Amoebic dysentery Protozoal infection of the intestines.

can be contracted by drinking untreated water even in pristine wild areas, is giardiasis, characterized by diarrhea, nausea, and abdominal cramps.

Finally, the parasitic worms are the largest organisms that can enter the body to cause infection. The tapeworm, for example, can grow to a length of several feet. Worms, including such intestinal parasites as the tapeworm, hookworm, and pinworm, cause a great variety of relatively mild infections. Smaller worms known as **flukes** infect such organs as the liver and lungs and, in large numbers, can be deadly. Generally speaking, worm infections originate from contaminated food or drink and can be controlled by careful attention to hygiene.

Other Immune Disorders: Cancer and Autoimmune Diseases

The immune system has evolved to protect the body from invasion by foreign microorganisms. Sometimes, as in the case of cancer, the body comes under attack by its own cells. Cancer cells cease to cooperate normally with the rest of the body and multiply uncontrollably. The immune system can often detect cells that have recently become malignant and then destroy them just as they would a foreign microorganism. But if the immune system breaks down, as it may when people get older or when they have certain immune disorders (including HIV infection), the cancer cells may multiply out of control before the immune system recognizes the danger.

Another immune disorder occurs when the body confuses its own cells with foreign organisms. As described earlier, the immune system must be able to recognize many thousands of antigens as foreign and then be able to recognize the same antigens again and again. Our own tissue cells also are antigenic; that is, they would be recognized by another person's immune system as foreign. A delicate balance must be maintained to ensure that one's immune system recognizes only truly foreign antigens as enemies; erroneous recognition of one's own cells as foreign produces havoc.

This is exactly what happens in what are known as "autoimmune" disorders. In this type of malady, the immune system seems to be a bit too sensitive and begins to misapprehend itself as "not-self." Rheumatoid arthritis is one such disease; the immune system attacks the joints, sometimes causing crippling arthritis. Systemic lupus erythematosus is another autoimmune disease, in which blood vessels, or the lining of the heart, lungs, or brain become inflamed when the body attacks itself.

SEXUALLY TRANSMISSIBLE DISEASES

No single health issue has commanded as much public attention in recent years as **acquired immunodeficiency syndrome,** or **AIDS.** This fatal, incurable disease cur-

rently ranks eighth as a cause of death among Americans, and the epidemic of **HIV infection** is considered the number one health priority in the United States. Although recent public education campaigns have focused primarily on HIV infection, they deserve to be repeated for all the **sexually transmissible diseases (STDs)** because their incidence also continues to climb among Americans.

What are the most severe and dangerous STDs? In general, seven different diseases pose major health threats: HIV infection/AIDS, hepatitis, syphilis, chlamydia, gonorrhea, herpes, and human papillomavirus (HPV), which causes genital warts. These diseases are considered "major" because they are serious in themselves, cause serious complications if left untreated, and/or pose risks to a fetus or newborn. Additionally, pelvic inflammatory disease (PID) is a common complication of gonorrhea and chlamydia and merits discussion as a separate disease.

> ***Personal Insight*** How would you feel if your sexual partner told you he or she exposed you to an STD? How would you feel if you contracted an STD?

HIV Infection/AIDS

HIV infection is one of the most serious and challenging problems facing the United States and the world today. Despite the intense efforts of health professionals all around the world, HIV infection continues to spread and a cure is yet to be found. By the end of 1994, nearly 500,000 Americans had been diagnosed with AIDS, and over a million were believed to be infected with HIV. Worldwide, over 17 million people are believed to have been infected with HIV; and by the year 2000, it's estimated that 40 to 120 million people will be infected. According to the World Health Organization, someone is infected with HIV every 15 to 20 seconds.

What Is HIV Infection? HIV infection is a chronic disease that progressively damages the body's immune system, making an otherwise healthy person susceptible to a variety of infections and disorders. Under normal conditions, when a virus or other disease-causing agent enters

Flukes Parasitic worms that can infest lungs and liver; can cause death.

AIDS, acquired immunodeficiency syndrome A fatal, incurable, sexually transmissible viral disease.

HIV infection A chronic, progressive disease that damages the immune system; caused by the human immunodeficiency virus (HIV).

Sexually transmissible diseases (STDs) Diseases that can be transmitted by sexual contact; some can also be transmitted by other means.

TERMS

Although first detected among heterosexuals in Africa, AIDS captured world attention in the early 1980s as a disease occurring primarily among homosexual men in the United States and Europe. Since then, AIDS has spread around the world. HIV infections have been reported in virtually all countries of the world, and actual AIDS cases have been documented in 164 countries. Over 17 million people worldwide have been infected with HIV since the epidemic began. The World Health Organization predicts that 40 million people will be infected with HIV by the year 2000. The Harvard-based Global AIDS Policy Coalition predicts that the number will be much higher, perhaps as high as 110 million.

As AIDS education and prevention programs take hold in developed countries, the vast majority—70 to 90 percent—of new infections are expected to occur in developing countries, where heterosexual contact is the main means of transmission. In the developed world, too, the pattern of infection is shifting away from homosexual males and toward the larger heterosexual population. Women are the fastest-growing group of newly infected people in the industrialized world.

Currently, more than 7 million of those infected with HIV are in Africa, where, in some cities, one-third of all adults carry the virus. Sub-Saharan Africa remains the hardest hit of all areas of the world. However, experts believe that Asia is now at the same stage of the disease that Africa was 10 years ago. As in Africa, the principal means of transmission is heterosexual contact. In Asia, however, many more people are at risk, since Asia accounts for more than 50 percent of the world's population. The World Health Organization hopes that education campaigns can prevent India, China, and Southeast Asia from following the same path followed in Africa.

Efforts to combat AIDS are complicated by political, economic, and cultural barriers in many parts of the world. Education and prevention programs are often hampered by resistance from social and religious institutions and by taboos on open discussion of sex. Condoms are unfamiliar in many countries, for example, and when their use has been proposed as a way to prevent disease, responses have ranged from hostility on the part of political leaders to confusion and indignation on the part of members of the general population. Additionally, women in many societies do not have sufficient power over their lives to demand that men use condoms during sex.

Despite these obstacles, education and prevention remain the best hope for slowing the spread of AIDS. Although many countries still deny the extent of infection among their populations, many others are overcoming their reluctance to discuss sensitive subjects and embracing campaigns that include graphic descriptions of safer sex practices. Some leaders are aggressively leading discussions about AIDS and encouraging their governments to set up national educational programs. In some Asian countries, strategies to block the disease are already in place. Until there is a cure for AIDS, efforts must continue to focus on widespread educational campaigns and prevention through behavior change.

Sources: D. C. Weeks. 1992. "The AIDS Pandemic in Africa." *Current History*, May; J. Frank. 1992. "Focus of World AIDS Prevention Is Shifting from Africa to Asia." *San Francisco Chronicle*, 16 December; "AIDS Crisis Hits Asia, Grows Rapidly," *The Wall Street Journal*, 30 December 1991; L. Garrett. 1992. "The Call for an Aggressive New AIDS Strategy." *Washington Post*, 21 July.

Estimated Adult HIV Infections for 1995
(Cumulative Numbers)

Geographic Area	Number of Infections
North America	1,495,000
Western Europe	1,186,000
Oceania	40,000
Latin America	1,407,000
Sub-Saharan Africa	11,449,000
Caribbean	474,000
Eastern Europe	44,000
Southeast Mediterranean	59,000
Northeast Asia	80,000
Southeast Asia	1,220,000
Total	17,454,000

Source: Global AIDS Policy Commission

the body, it is targeted and destroyed by the body's immune system. But the human immunodeficiency virus (HIV) attacks the immune system itself, invading and taking over the cells that initiate and control the body's system of defense. Once these cells have been sidetracked from their duties, the immune system can no longer respond adequately to infection.

The incubation period of HIV—the time between the initial infection with the virus and the onset of disease symptoms—may range from 2 to 20 years. Among adults, the average is 10 years. About 30 percent of infected people experience flulike symptoms shortly after the initial infection, but the rest have no symptoms at all. Most people infected with the virus remain generally healthy for

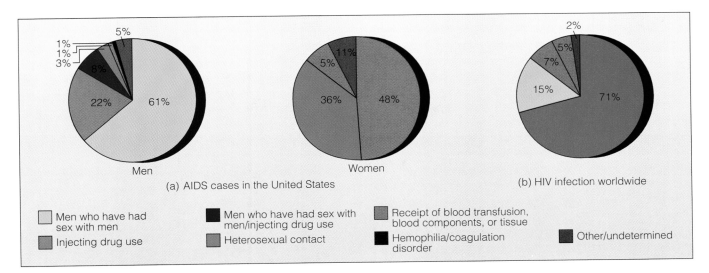

(a) AIDS cases in the United States

(b) HIV infection worldwide

- Men who have had sex with men
- Injecting drug use
- Men who have had sex with men/injecting drug use
- Heterosexual contact
- Receipt of blood transfusion, blood components, or tissue
- Hemophilia/coagulation disorder
- Other/undetermined

VITAL STATISTICS

Figure 13-2 *Routes of HIV transmission among adults.*

Sources: Centers for Disease Control and Prevention. 1995. *MMWR* 44(13):257; Centers for Disease Control and Prevention. 1995. *HIV/AIDS Surveillance Report,* March, pp. 10–12; Mann, J., D. J. M. Tarantola and T. W. Netter, eds. 1992. *AIDS in the World.* Cambridge, Mass.: Harvard University Press, p. 33.

years; but during this time, the virus is progressively infecting and destroying the cells of the immune system. People infected with HIV can pass the virus to others—even if they have no symptoms and do not know they have been infected.

The destruction of the immune system by HIV is signaled by the loss of a certain type of white blood cell, called the **CD4 lymphocyte,** or T4 cell, which is vital to the functioning of the immune system. As the number of CD4 cells declines, an infected person may begin to experience mild to moderately severe symptoms. A person is diagnosed with "full blown" AIDS when he or she develops one of the conditions defined as a marker for AIDS or when the number of CD4 cells in the blood drops below a certain level (200/mm³). People with AIDS are vulnerable to a number of serious, often fatal secondary, or "opportunistic," infections.

How Is the Virus Transmitted? HIV lives only within cells and body fluids, not outside of the body. It is transmitted by blood and blood products, semen, and vaginal and cervical secretions. It cannot live in air, in water, or on objects or surfaces such as toilet seats, eating utensils, or telephones. The three main routes of HIV transmission are (1) from particular kinds of sexual contact, (2) from direct exposure to infected blood, and (3) from an HIV-infected woman to her fetus during pregnancy or childbirth or, possibly, to her infant during breastfeeding.

Among different types of sexual contact, HIV is more likely to be transmitted by unprotected anal or vaginal intercourse than by other sexual activities. HIV can be transmitted through minute tears in the fragile lining of the vagina, cervix, penis, anus, and mouth and through direct infection of cells in some of these areas. The pres-

ence of lesions or blisters from other sexually transmissible diseases in the genital, anal, or oral areas makes it easier for the virus to be transmitted. During vaginal intercourse, male-to-female transmission is more likely to occur than female-to-male transmission. HIV has been found in preejaculatory fluid, so transmission can occur before ejaculation.

Direct, bloodstream contact with the blood of an infected person is the second major route of HIV transmission. Needles used to inject drugs (including heroin, cocaine, and anabolic steroids) are routinely contaminated by the blood of the user. If needles are shared, small amounts of one person's blood are directly injected into another person's bloodstream. HIV may also be transmitted through subcutaneous and intramuscular injection as well, from needles or blades used in acupuncture, tattooing, ritual scarring, and piercing.

HIV has been transmitted in blood and blood products used in the medical treatment of **hemophilia,** injuries, and serious illnesses, resulting in about 20,000 cases of AIDS. The blood supply in all licensed blood banks and plasma centers in the United States is now screened for HIV. The Centers for Disease Control and Prevention estimate that the current risk of transfusion-related HIV transmission is about 1 in 340,000 to 420,000 transfusions, or about 43 blood recipients per year.

CD4 lymphocyte A type of white blood cell that helps coordinate the activity of the immune system; it is the primary target for HIV infection. A decrease in the number of these cells correlates with the risk and severity of HIV-related illness.

Hemophilia A hereditary blood disease in which blood fails to clot and abnormal bleeding occurs, which requires transfusions of blood with a specific factor to aid coagulation.

TERMS

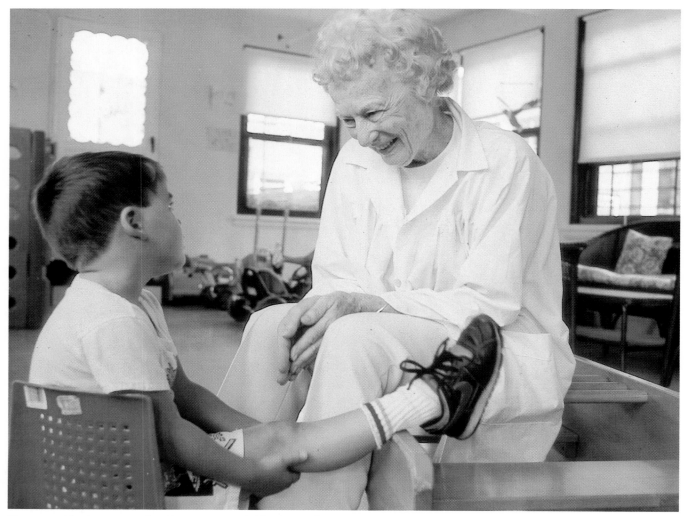

The ever-widening net cast by STDs ensnares children as well as adults. This boy with
AIDS, being cared for in a group home for children infected with HIV, is part of a growing
population of children infected with HIV in the womb.

The final major route of HIV transmission is mother-to-child, also called *vertical transmission*. About 25 to 30 percent of infants born to untreated HIV-infected mothers are also infected with the virus. Most of these infections occur during pregnancy, but a few may happen during childbirth or through breastfeeding. By 1995, over 6,000 cases of AIDS among children infected by their mothers had been reported in the United States.

What about contact with other body fluids? Trace amounts of HIV have been found in the saliva and tears of some infected people. However, researchers believe that these fluids don't carry enough of the virus to infect another person, and no cases of HIV infection have been traced to exposure to tears or saliva. HIV has been found in urine and feces, and contact with the urine or feces of an infected person may carry some risk. Contact with an infected person's sweat is not believed to carry any risk.

Among Americans with AIDS, the most common means of exposure to HIV has been sexual activity between men; injecting drug use and heterosexual contact are the next most common (Figure 13-2). Changes in the sexual behavior of homosexual men and the screening of all donated blood have slowed the rate of infection from these sources. Women—infected through injecting drug use or sexual activity—and children born to infected mothers make up an increasingly large proportion of new cases of HIV infection.

HIV is not spread through casual contact. A person is not at risk of getting HIV infection by being in the same classroom, dining room, or even household with someone who is infected. Before this was generally known, many people with HIV infection, including children, were the targets of ostracism, hysteria, and outright violence. Today, it is an acknowledged responsibility of all to treat people with HIV infection with respect and compassion, regardless of their age or how they became infected.

Symptoms of HIV Infection/AIDS

Signs and symptoms suggesting HIV infection include persistent swollen glands; lumps, rashes, sores, or other growths on or under the skin or on the mucous membranes of the eyes, mouth, anus, or nasal passages; persistent yeast infections; unexplained weight loss of more than 10 pounds or 10 percent of body weight in less than two months (unrelated to illness, dieting, or increased physical activity); fever and drenching night sweats; dry cough and shortness of breath; persistent diarrhea; easy bruising and unexplained bleeding; profound fatigue, sometimes accompanied by lightheadedness or dizziness; loss of memory; loss of sense of balance, tremors, or seizures; changes in vision, hearing, taste, or smell; difficulty in swallowing; changes in mood and other psychiatric symptoms; and persistent or recurrent pain. Obviously some of these symptoms can also occur with minor colds or flu.

Because the immune system is weakened, people with HIV infection are highly susceptible to infections, both common and uncommon. The infection most often seen among people with HIV is *Pneumocystis carinii,* a protozoal infection that produces pneumonia. **Kaposi's sarcoma,** a rare form of cancer, is common among HIV-infected men. More and more cases of tuberculosis (TB) are also being reported among people with HIV; in Africa, drug-resistant strains of TB are now the most deadly infection among people with AIDS. Most of the infections associated with HIV are rare among people with healthy immune systems and are not contagious; however, tuberculosis is spread through the air and may pose a risk for non-HIV-infected people, especially medical personnel who come into contact with infected patients.

Diagnosis

Early diagnosis of HIV infection is important to minimize the impact of the disease, medically, psychologically, and socially. Up until a few years ago, there were no known ways to combat the disease. Now, drugs exist that can be used to slow the progress of the virus and to fight specific infections, especially if they are discovered early.

The surest diagnosis of HIV infection is the detection of the virus itself in human tissues through laboratory tissue culture procedures, but the techniques for this method are expensive and not available everywhere. The most commonly used screening test is the **HIV antibody test.** This test, developed by the National Cancer Institute, consists of an initial screening called an **ELISA test,** and a more specific confirmation test called the **Western blot.** These tests determine whether a person has antibodies to HIV circulating in the bloodstream, a sign that the virus is present in the body. If an individual repeatedly tests positive on the HIV antibody test and the diagnosis is confirmed in follow-up tests, the person is considered both infected (**HIV-positive**) and infectious.

The FDA has recently approved the HIV-1 antigen test for use. This test measures the HIV particles in the bloodstream and is known as the P-24 antigen test. It can be used as a diagnostic tool for the presence of HIV and as a way for physicians to monitor the effectiveness of treatments.

As mentioned earlier, AIDS is the most severe form of HIV infection. The criteria for a diagnosis of AIDS reflect the stage of HIV infection at which a person's immune system becomes dangerously compromised. Since January 1993, a diagnosis of AIDS is made if a person is HIV-positive and either has developed an infection defined as an AIDS indicator or has a severely damaged immune system (as measured by CD4 cell counts).

Reporting

All cases of AIDS, as defined by the CDC, must be reported to public health authorities. This measure is meant to help public health officials track the disease and keep their records of its progress up-to-date. Reporting requirements vary from state to state; although all states require that cases of AIDS be reported, most do not require that incidences of positive HIV tests alone be reported.

Treatment

There is no known cure for HIV infection, but new drugs have been developed to slow the advance of the virus and to treat some of the opportunistic infections. People infected with HIV usually live ten years or more before becoming sick with AIDS. Researchers hope that before too long, AIDS may be a manageable chronic disease that people will be able to control with medication.

Current research is focused on two categories of anti-HIV drugs—antivirals and drugs that stimulate or regulate the immune system. Antivirals are agents that kill the virus directly or limit its growth. To date, none of these

---

TERMS

Pneumocystis carinii   An organism that causes a particular type of pneumonia common in people infected with HIV.

Kaposi's sarcoma   A form of cancer characterized by purple or brownish lesions that are generally painless and occur anywhere on the skin; usually appears in men infected with HIV.

HIV antibody blood test   A test currently being used to determine if an individual has been infected by the human immunodeficiency (HIV) virus.

ELISA (or Enzyme Linked Immune Sorbant Assay)   A test that detects the presence of antibodies produced against HIV by an infected person's immune system.

Western blot   A test that detects the presence of HIV antibodies. It is a more accurate and more expensive test, so it is used to confirm positive results from an ELISA test.

HIV-positive   A person who has tested positive for the presence of HIV in his or her bloodstream; also referred to as seropositive.

agents has been able to eradicate HIV from an infected person, but they can help delay the onset of severe symptoms. The most widely known and used is **zidovudine (AZT),** and many people with HIV take AZT regularly. Other antivirals include didanosine (ddI), dideoxycytidine (ddC), and Compound Q. Another group of drugs under study is those designed to stimulate, regulate, or modulate the immune system. These include naltrexone, anti-interferon, globulin, disulfiram, and interleukin-2. Although the ideal approach to reducing transmission of HIV to infants is to prevent HIV infection among women, giving AZT to infected women can reduce the risk of perinatal transmission of HIV by nearly two-thirds.

Depending on the type of infection, treatment for HIV-related conditions may include antibiotics, chemotherapy, and radiotherapy. Researchers are also working to develop drugs to help prevent the occurrence of some common HIV-related infections. For example, Septra (Bactrim), Dapsone, or aerosolized pentamidine can help prevent *Pneumocystis carinii* pneumonia. To treat pneumonia and tuberculosis, antibiotics are typically used; chemotherapy may be used for Kaposi's sarcoma and cervical cancer.

The cost of treatment for HIV continues to be an area of major concern. Medications alone for a person with AIDS average about $3,000 to $4,000 per month. The average cost of treatment for a person infected with HIV is about $10,000 per year; for someone diagnosed with AIDS, treatment may cost more than $40,000 per year.

What about a vaccine? No vaccine has ever been developed for a virus like HIV, and the difficulties—scientific, political, industrial, and financial—are considerable. The virus's ability to mutate poses a major challenge to researchers attempting to develop a vaccine. Successful vaccines have been developed against the simian version of HIV, but a vaccine for the human version is not expected to be ready in the foreseeable future.

Prevention   Although AIDS is currently fatal and incurable, it is a preventable disease. You can protect yourself by avoiding behaviors that may bring you into contact with HIV. This means making careful choices about sexual activity and not sharing needles to inject drugs.

Make Careful Choices About Sexual Activity   For anyone not involved in a long-term, mutually monogamous relationship, abstinence from any sexual activity that involves the exchange of body fluids is the only sure

way to prevent HIV infection. Safer sex includes many activities that carry virtually no risk of HIV infection, like hugging, massaging, closed-lip kissing, rubbing bodies together, kissing your partner's skin, and mutual masturbation.

Anal and vaginal intercourse are the sexual activities associated with the highest risk of HIV infection. If you have intercourse, always use a latex condom. Condoms are not perfect, and they do not provide risk-free sex; however, used properly, a latex condom provides a high level of protection against HIV. Condoms should also be worn during oral sex. Some experts also suggest the use of latex squares and dental dams, rubber devices that can be used as barriers during oral-genital or oral-anal sexual contact. In 1993, the FDA approved the use of the female condom, which is made of polyurethane. While it has been proven effective in reducing the risk of STD transmission, it is not yet widely used.

Limiting the number of sexual partners you have—particularly partners who have engaged in risky behaviors in the past—can also lower your risk of exposure to HIV. Take the time to talk with a potential new sexual partner about HIV and safer sex, and take precautions with every partner. Don't agree to have intercourse or give up precautions as a way to show your love or commitment to a relationship. Your specific sexual practices can be just as important as the number of partners you have.

Removing alcohol and other drugs from sexual activity is another crucial component of safer sex. The use of alcohol and mood-altering drugs may lower inhibitions and affect judgment, making you more likely to engage in unsafe sex.

Don't Share Drug Needles   People who inject drugs should avoid sharing needles, syringes, or anything that might have blood on it. Any injectable drug, legal or illegal, can be associated with HIV transmission. Needles can be decontaminated with a solution of bleach and water, but it is not a foolproof procedure. (Boiling needles and syringes does not necessarily destroy HIV either.) If you are an injecting drug user, your best protection against HIV is to obtain treatment and refrain from using drugs.

Participate in an HIV Education Program   What can you do to reinforce what you know about HIV? Many schools and colleges have peer counseling and education programs about preventing HIV. These programs give you a chance to practice skills in communicating with potential sexual partners and negotiating safer sex, to engage in role-playing to build self-confidence, and, although controversial, even to learn about how to use condoms.

Hepatitis

An inflammation of the liver, hepatitis is usually caused by one of three common hepatitis viruses. Infection with

TERMS

Zidovudine (AZT)   A drug used in the treatment of HIV infection that inhibits the reproduction of HIV.

Jaundice   Increased bile pigment levels in the blood, characterized by yellowing of the skin and the whites of the eyes.

For those who don't have a long-term monogamous relationship with an uninfected partner, abstinence is the only truly safe option. Individuals should remember that it is OK to say no to sex and drugs.

"Safer sex" activities that allow intimate skin-to-skin contact without exposure to body fluids carry virtually no risk of HIV infection. These include fantasy, hugging, massage, rubbing bodies together, mutual masturbation, and kissing with lips closed. (Although no cases of HIV infection have been traced to kissing, transmission of HIV through deep-mouth kissing is thought to be possible.)

If you choose to be sexually active, talk with potential sexual partners about HIV, safer sex, and the use of condoms before you begin a sexual relationship. The following behaviors will help lower your risk of exposure to HIV during sexual activities:

- Limit the number of your sexual partners. Avoid sexual contact with people who have HIV or who have engaged in risky behaviors in the past, including unprotected sex and injecting drug use.

- Use latex condoms during every act of intercourse and oral sex.

- Use condoms properly to obtain maximum protection (refer back to the detailed instructions for condom use given in Chapter 6). Use a water-based lubricant; don't use oil-based lubricants such as petroleum jelly or baby oil. Unroll condoms gently to avoid tearing them, and smooth out any air bubbles.

- Avoid sexual contact that could cause cuts or tears in the skin or tissue.

- Get prompt treatment for any STDs you contract.

- Don't drink or use drugs in sexual situations. Mood-altering drugs can affect your judgment and make you more likely to engage in risky behaviors.

If you inject drugs of any kind, don't share needles, syringes, or anything that might have blood on it. Decontaminate needles and syringes with household bleach and water.

If you are at risk for HIV infection, don't donate blood, sperm, or body organs. Don't have unprotected sex or share needles or syringes. Consider being tested for HIV.

---

hepatitis viruses can be transmitted sexually as well as through nonsexual contact. The Centers for Disease Control and Prevention estimate that between 200,000 and 300,000 Americans become infected with hepatitis each year and that between 750,000 and 1 million people are carriers (capable of infecting others) of the most common form—hepatitis B. There is no known cure for hepatitis, and hepatitis can cause death in severe cases. The disease is preventable, however, and a vaccine for hepatitis B is available.

Transmission   Three different agents have been identified as primary causes of viral hepatitis. Hepatitis A virus causes the mildest form of the disease and is usually transmitted by food or water contaminated by sewage or an infected person. Anal-oral contact is the primary means of sexual transmission of hepatitis A.

The hepatitis B virus is found in all body fluids and is easily transmitted through any sexual activity that involves the exchange of body fluids, the use of contaminated needles, and any blood-to-blood contact, including the use of contaminated razor blades, toothbrushes, and eating utensils. The primary risk factors for acquiring hepatitis B are heterosexual exposure and injecting drug use; having multiple sexual partners greatly increases risk. In addition, a pregnant woman can transmit hepatitis B to her unborn child.

The hepatitis C virus used to be the leading cause of hepatitis following blood transfusions, but the blood supply is now screened for both hepatitis B and C. Hepatitis C virus is transmitted in the same way as hepatitis B, but sexual transmission has not been confirmed.

Symptoms   Many people infected with hepatitis never develop symptoms. Mild cases of hepatitis cause flulike symptoms such as fever, body aches, chills, and loss of appetite. As the illness progresses, there may be nausea, vomiting, dark-colored urine, abdominal pain, and **jaundice**. Some people with hepatitis also develop a skin rash and joint pain or arthritis. Most cases of hepatitis A tend to be of short duration, but people with hepatitis B or C, even when they recover completely, can become chronic carriers of the virus, capable of infecting others for the rest of their lives. Chronic hepatitis can cause cirrhosis of the liver, liver failure, and a deadly form of liver cancer. Hepatitis kills about 6,000 Americans each year.

Diagnosis and Treatment   Blood tests can be used to diagnose hepatitis through analysis of liver function and detection of the specific organism causing the infection. There is no cure for hepatitis, and treatment is designed to minimize damage to the liver. Researchers are investigating the use of corticosteroids and interferon.

Prevention   To reduce your risk of contracting hepatitis A, avoid contaminated water and infected food, wash your hands frequently, and avoid oral-anal sexual contact. Preventive measures for the B and C forms of hepatitis are similar to those for HIV infection: Avoid sexual contact that involves sharing of body fluids, including saliva; use condoms during intercourse; and don't share hypodermic needles.

The vaccine for hepatitis B is safe and highly effective. All pregnant women should be tested for hepatitis B and infants of infected mothers vaccinated immediately after birth. Many physicians recommend routine immunization of all infants and adolescents as part of the normal set of childhood vaccinations. Immunizations are also recommended for adults in high-risk groups. A vaccine for hepatitis A is currently being tested and may be available within the next five years.

Syphilis

Although death and disability from syphilis declined dramatically after the introduction of penicillin treatment, there are about 100,000 new cases every year in the United States. Syphilis is caused by a spirochete called *Treponema pallidum.* It requires warmth and moisture to survive and dies very quickly outside the human body. The disease is usually acquired through sexual contact, although unborn children can contract it through the placenta from an infected mother. The organism passes through any break or opening in the skin or mucous membranes and can be transmitted by kissing, vaginal or anal intercourse, or oral-genital contact.

Symptoms   Syphilis is characterized by sores or lesions known as **chancres** (pronounced "shang-kers") containing large numbers of bacteria; they make the disease highly contagious when they are present. Left untreated, an individual can remain contagious for as long as 18 months. In later stages, when the lesions have disappeared and the person is no longer contagious, the disease can cause devastating damage to almost any system of the body. Syphilis progresses through three stages as the organism becomes established in the body.

First Stage: Primary Syphilis   Within ten to ninety days (usually about three weeks) of contact with an infected partner, a single chancre less than the size of a dime appears at the site where the organism entered the body, most commonly the genital area. These sores are painless

unless they become infected and may not even be noticed. They generally heal within a few weeks.

Second Stage: Secondary Syphilis   Approximately six weeks after a chancre first appears, an untreated person begins to show signs and symptoms of secondary disease. These include fever, malaise, sore throat, headache, hoarseness, a depressed appetite, swollen lymph glands, and loss of hair. The second stage may also be characterized by a rash that appears anywhere on the body but most typically on the palms of the hands and the soles of the feet. The rash may also affect the mucous membranes of the lips, cheeks, tongue, tonsils, throat, and vocal cords, where grayish-white patches of mucus surrounded by dull red borders appear. These sores break down and ooze a clear fluid that contains large numbers of bacteria, making this stage highly contagious. With or without antibiotic treatment, skin lesions of secondary syphilis usually heal in two to ten weeks. However, if the disease remains untreated, relapses can occur.

Third Stage: Latent Syphilis   By definition, people without symptoms but with evidence of having had syphilis in the past have latent syphilis. In this stage of the disease, the organism invades the internal organs and the central nervous system. The principal manifestation of central nervous system damage is a condition called **paresis,** which involves partial or complete paralysis and chronic, progressive mental degeneration leading to death. Symptoms may include facial tremors, slurred speech, impaired vision, headaches, epileptic convulsions, exaggerated reflexes, defective memory, delusions, depression, and dementia (insanity).

In infected pregnant women, the syphilis organism can cross the placenta after the tenth week of gestation. If the mother is not treated before the eighteenth week, the probable result is stillbirth or congenital deformity.

Diagnosis and Treatment   To diagnose primary syphilis, clinicians take a specimen from the surface of the chancre. Diagnosis of secondary syphilis is made from blood tests and clinical observation of the symptoms. Penicillin remains the drug of choice for the treatment of syphilis in all stages. For those allergic to penicillin, tetracycline and erythromycin can be effective substitutes. Sexual partners must be treated as well, and follow-up tests are necessary.

Chlamydia

Gonorrhea and chlamydia have similar symptoms and are often mistaken for each other, but chlamydia is now the more common disease. In fact, *Chlamydia trachomatis* currently causes the most prevalent bacterial infection in the United States, with 3 to 4 million new cases occurring every year.

TERMS

Treponema pallidum   The spiral-shaped organism that causes syphilis.

Chancre   The sore produced by syphilis in its earliest stage.

Paresis   Central nervous system damage, sometimes a result of syphilis, involving paralysis and mental degeneration.

Chlamydia trachomatis   A sexually transmissible organism that produces a wide variety of sometimes acute infections; now reaching epidemic scale in the United States.

Although everyone is susceptible to chlamydia, women bear the greatest burden because of the possible complications and consequences of the disease. In men, chlamydia is the leading cause of urinary tract infection and is also responsible for approximately 50 percent of the 500,000 cases of **epididymitis** (inflammation of the testicles) seen annually in the United States. *In most women, chlamydial infection produces no early symptoms,* a factor that contributes to the devastation it can cause. If left undetected for two months or more, it can lead to a severe condition known as pelvic inflammatory disease (PID).

Infants of infected mothers can acquire the infection through contact with the organism in the birth canal during delivery. In newborns, chlamydia can cause eye infections, pneumonia, and (less often) ear infections. Screening pregnant women and treating those with chlamydia is a highly effective way to prevent infection of babies during birth.

Symptoms   In men, chlamydia symptoms include painful urination and a slight watery discharge from the penis. In women, symptoms include a discharge from the cervix, painful urination, and painful inflammation of the oviducts, which is symptomatic of PID at this point. However, most people experience few or no symptoms, increasing the likelihood that they will inadvertently spread the infection to their partners.

Diagnosis and Treatment   Physicians often diagnose chlamydia only after they have excluded the presence of gonorrhea during an examination. A definitive diagnosis is made after the organism is grown in tissue culture or through a microscopic antibody test. Because of the seriousness of an undetected infection, some physicians may add a laboratory test for chlamydia to a routine Pap test.

Once chlamydia has been diagnosed, the infected person and his or her sexual partner or partners are given antibiotics, either tetracycline, doxycycline, or erythromycin. *Penicillin is not effective against chlamydia.* As with all antibiotics, it is essential that the entire course of medication be completed. It is also important to refrain from sexual intercourse until the treatment is completed.

Gonorrhea

In the United States, between 400,000 and 600,000 new cases of **gonorrhea** are reported every year. The highest incidence is among 20- to 24-year-olds. Like chlamydia, untreated gonorrhea can cause PID in women and epididymitis in men, leading to sterility. It can also cause **dermatitis** (inflammation of the skin) and a type of arthritis. An infant passing through the birth canal of an infected mother may contract **gonococcal conjunctivitis,** an infection in the eyes that can cause blindness if left

untreated. In some states, all newborn babies are routinely treated with antimicrobial eye drops to prevent infection.

Gonorrhea is caused by the bacterium *Neisseria gonorrhoeae,* which grows well in mucous membranes. It cannot live long outside the warm, moist environment of the human body and dies within moments of exposure to light and air. Consequently, gonorrhea cannot be contracted from toilet seats, towels, or other objects.

Symptoms   In men, the incubation period for gonorrhea is brief, generally about five days. The first symptoms are a form of urethritis (inflammation of the urethra) that causes discomfort on urination and a thick, yellowish-white or yellowish-green discharge from the penis. The lips of the urethral opening may become inflamed and swollen. In some men, the lymph glands in the groin become enlarged and swollen. A small percentage of men—10 to 30 percent—will have very minor symptoms or none at all.

Approximately 80 percent of women with gonorrhea have no symptoms whatsoever and therefore don't know when they are infected. Additionally, some women with symptoms mistake the discharge from a gonorrhea infection for a normal preovulation mucus discharge. When symptoms do appear in women, they are similar to those in men, including an irritating discharge and discomfort on urination. When the infection has been established for a longer period of time, generally two months or more, symptoms may include lower abdominal cramping or pain, fever, and vaginal bleeding, indicating that the woman may have PID. Any woman with discomfort and an unusual discharge should see a physician immediately to be tested for gonorrhea.

Gonorrhea bacteria can also infect the throat or rectum in individuals with the disease who engage in oral or anal sex. The symptoms of gonorrhea in the throat may be a sore throat or pus on the tonsils, and those of gonorrhea in the rectum may be pus in the feces or rectal irritation, pain, and itching. As with other infections, gonorrhea is often accompanied by a fever and swollen glands.

Diagnosis and Treatment   The test for gonorrhea consists of a smear test or a culture of the discharge. Accurate diagnosis of gonorrhea is especially important because

---

TERMS

Epididymitis   An inflammation of the small body of ducts that rests on the testes.

Gonorrhea   A sexually transmissible disease caused by a type of bacteria that usually affects mucous membranes.

Dermatitis   An inflammation of the skin evidenced by itching, redness, and various skin lesions.

Gonococcal conjunctivitis   An inflammation of the mucous membrane lining of the eyelids, caused by the gonococcus bacterium.

new strains of the gonococcal organism are antibiotic-resistant.

When gonorrhea is diagnosed early, treatment with broad-spectrum antibiotics is relatively easy and effective. *Using drugs prescribed for friends or sexual partners or left over from other illnesses is not a safe and effective way to treat gonorrhea or any other STD.* As mentioned earlier, the entire course of medication must be taken, and if two people share a prescription, neither will be cured. Following treatment, sexual activity should not be resumed until follow-up testing shows no evidence of the disease.

Pelvic Inflammatory Disease

A major complication in 10 to 15 percent of women who have been infected with either gonorrhea or chlamydia, or both, is **pelvic inflammatory disease (PID).** An infection of the oviducts that may extend to the ovaries, PID is often serious enough to require hospitalization and sometimes surgery. Even if the disease is treated successfully, the woman has a continuing susceptibility to recurrent infection, ectopic (tubal) pregnancy, sterility, and chronic menstrual problems. PID is the leading cause of infertility in young women, often undetected until later when the desire to have a child leads to further testing.

Both infectious agents may be transmitted sexually by an infected partner. During or just after menstruation, these organisms appear to rise into the uterine cavity, where they may cause inflammation, or they may pass directly into the oviducts. This inflammatory process spreads easily into the pelvic cavity, causing further infection and in some cases pelvic abscess.

Symptoms   Most women remain asymptomatic for some time, usually until the next menstrual cycle. Once the organisms reach the oviducts, symptoms can develop within seven days. Women with rapid onset of symptoms most often have chills, fever, loss of appetite, nausea, and/or vomiting. Most complain of abdominal pain on one or both sides. Some women may also have abnormal vaginal bleeding, prolonged menstruation, or abnormal vaginal discharge.

Diagnosis and Treatment   Diagnosis of PID is usually made on the basis of symptoms. Laparoscopy may be used to isolate the suspected organism and grow it in a culture medium. Treatment is more effective when the causative organism is identified, but since gonorrhea and chlamydia are often both present, a broader-spectrum approach to treatment is usually initiated. Commonly used drugs include penicillin and tetracycline. Repeat cultures are done to ensure that the bacteria have been eradicated. All sexual partners need to be treated for infection.

Complications of PID are serious and irreversible. Scarring of the oviducts, often as a result of abscesses, can result in adhesions, chronic pelvic pain, and ectopic pregnancies.

Genital Warts

The incidence of **genital warts,** or condyloma, has increased rapidly in recent years and is now exceeded only by that of gonorrhea and chlamydia. Condyloma is the most common STD for which diagnosis and treatment is sought in student health services; the disease appears to be most prevalent in young people aged 16 to 25. This increase has serious implications, since the precancerous condition known as cervical dysplasia often occurs among women with untreated genital warts. Identification of the causative agent of condyloma has revealed a family of viruses known as **human papillomavirus (HPV).**

Symptoms   Genital warts are dry, painless growths, rough in texture and gray or pink in color. They can be flat or raised, and they vary in size. Untreated warts can grow together to form a cauliflowerlike mass. In males, they appear on the penis, more commonly in circumcised men. They often involve the urethra, appearing first at the opening and then spreading as a complication. The growth may cause irritation and bleeding, leading to painful urination and a urethral discharge. Warts may also appear around the anus or within the rectum.

In women, warts may appear on the labia, vulva, and may spread to the perineum, the area between the vagina and the rectum. They may also appear on the cervix. If the warts are small and flat, they can be difficult for the physician to see.

Diagnosis and Treatment   A genital wart infection is very contagious through contact with the lesions, but infected people can transmit the disease to their sex partners without having any symptoms themselves. Early diagnosis and effective treatment are often impeded by a long incubation period (which averages two to three months), a lack of awareness of symptoms in women, and a complex, not-always-effective treatment approach. Although the risks are not clear, newborns can be infected during delivery. To treat genital warts effectively, the

TERMS

Pelvic inflammatory disease (PID)   An infection that progresses from the vagina and cervix to infect the pelvic cavity and oviducts.

Genital warts   A sexually transmissible disease caused by a virus and characterized by the appearance of growths on the genital area of men and women.

Human papillomavirus   The organism that causes genital warts.

Podophyllin   An acid used in the treatment of warts.

Acyclovir   A drug used in the treatment of recurrent herpes infection.

physician has to differentiate the lesions from those of other diseases, particularly those of secondary syphilis. The virus lives within the lesion itself and does not travel throughout the body. Therefore, HPV is diagnosed by the physical appearance of the lesion and the presence of the virus in it.

All treatments currently available are physically destructive, and none can assure removal of HPV. The traditional treatment for genital warts is application of **podophyllin,** a toxic agent, directly to the lesion. Other treatment options include removal of the lesion by electrocautery, cryosurgery (freezing), surgery, and, recently, CO_2 laser therapy. In 1989 the FDA approved a new drug, alpha interferon, to treat genital warts. The drug is administered in a series of injections; the long-term effects of the treatment are still being studied.

Even when treated, however, genital warts can recur. Because of the relationship of HPV to increased risk of cervical cancer, women who have had genital warts should have Pap tests every six months.

Herpes

Infection with the herpesvirus type II is considered a serious STD in part because of its extremely high incidence—more than 500,000 new cases each year and over 20 million total cases in the United States—and in part because of its serious impact on newborns. Additionally, there is no cure, nor is there a vaccine available. Despite research and efforts to develop treatments, vaccines, and specific preventive approaches, the "arsenal" to combat this relatively common STD remains quite small.

After an initial herpes infection is over, new outbreaks can be triggered by a variety of factors. Each time the infection recurs, the person is contagious again, making it a difficult disease to deal with and to prevent from spreading to others. Two of the different viruses in the herpes family that infect human beings are the following:

- *Herpes simplex, type I,* which usually causes cold sores and fever blisters around the lips, mouth, and facial area.

- *Herpes simplex, type II,* also known as genital herpes, which is usually seen in the genital area.

Symptoms   Typically, herpes infections (both types I and II) appear two to twenty days after initial exposure. Both types are highly contagious. Symptoms can include one or more blisterlike sores on or around the mouth, the face, or the genitals. The sores are painful, fluid-filled lesions and may be accompanied by swollen glands, general muscle aches and pains, fever, a mild burning sensation during urination in men, and a vaginal discharge in women. Some women may have internal lesions on the vagina or the cervix. Because the cervix has no nerve endings, an infected woman may be completely unaware that lesions are present.

Although a direct relationship between the herpesvirus and cancer is yet to be established, women with genital herpes are five times more likely to develop cancer of the cervix. It is recommended that women who have had genital herpes inform their physicians and be sure to have a Pap test every six months.

Herpes infections are particularly dangerous to newborns because of their immature immune systems and their somewhat restricted ability to fight off a virulent virus like herpes simplex I or II. Newborns should not have direct contact with adults with cold sores, and pregnant women with herpes have to be monitored near the time of delivery to ensure that the newborn isn't exposed to the virus. If the woman's infection becomes active, the baby will usually be delivered by cesarean section to protect it from contact with lesions in the birth canal or genital area. There is no effective treatment for babies who contract the herpesvirus, which can cause severe brain damage and sometimes death in newborns.

One of the most frustrating aspects of a herpes infection is its ability to recur. After the first infection, which can last as long as three to four weeks, the virus lies dormant along nerve pathways in the area of initial infection. A recurrence may be triggered by exposure to sun, temperature extremes, high levels of stress, certain foods (chocolate, seeds, and nuts, for example), acute illness, lowered resistance from poor general health, or some other factor. Because herpes is chronic, it has a long-lasting effect on sexuality. A person with an active infection is contagious and has an obligation to prevent the spread of the disease to others. Maintaining good general health and avoiding factors that may trigger new outbreaks can help prevent repeated bouts of infection.

Diagnosis and Treatment   Most cases of herpes are diagnosed on the basis of the presence of lesions, medical history, and other symptoms. If doubt exists that the infection is caused by the herpesvirus, a sample smear can be obtained from the lesion and grown in live tissue culture to determine the type of virus.

There is no cure for herpes, and at present treatment is directed at relieving pain, itching, and burning, avoiding secondary infection of lesions, and preventing the infection from spreading to other parts of the body. The drug **acyclovir** is sometimes used to treat genital herpes, with varying degrees of effectiveness for different individuals.

Other STDs

Although they are far less serious than the diseases already described, a few other diseases are transmitted sexually and are therefore included in this discussion. More annoying than threatening, these STDs still require responsible sexual behavior to prevent their spreading to others. They include trichomoniasis, a protozoal infec-

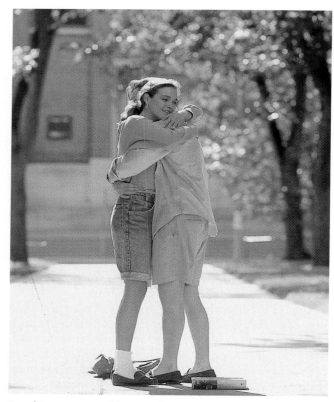

By taking a responsible attitude toward STDs, people show respect and concern for themselves and their partners. This couple's plans for the future could be seriously disrupted if one of them contracted an STD like gonorrhea or chlamydia. Either of these diseases, if untreated, could result in pelvic inflammatory disease, the leading cause of sterility in young women.

tion; *Candida albicans,* a fungal (yeast) infection; and pubic lice and scabies, parasitic infections.

WHAT CAN YOU DO?

You can take responsibility for your health and contribute to a general reduction in the incidence of STDs in three major areas: education, prevention, and diagnosis and treatment.

Education

Education efforts targeted at increasing public awareness about AIDS through the media have included public service announcements, dramatic presentations, and support from well-known public figures. However, the continuing controversy over the proper timing and nature of sex education still hinders active discussion of sexuality in schools, in churches, and on television. From a public health perspective, it has become a public health risk not to talk about sexuality, including the risks of STDs and the use of condoms.

In addition to public awareness campaigns, there are other opportunities for education about STDs in our society. Colleges offer courses in human sexuality. Free pamphlets and other literature are available from public health departments, health clinics, physicians' offices, student health centers, and Planned Parenthood; and easy-to-understand books are available in libraries and bookstores. Several national hot lines have been set up to provide free, confidential information and referral services to callers anywhere in the country.

- *National STD hot line,* sponsored by the Centers for Disease Control and the American School Health Association, provides confidential information and referrals about sexually transmissible diseases. Call 1-800-227-8922, between 8 A.M. and 11 P.M. (Eastern time), Monday through Friday.

- *National AIDS hot line,* sponsored by the Centers for Disease Control, provides confidential information about HIV infection and referrals for testing and treatment. Call 1-800-342-AIDS, 1-800-344-SIDA (Spanish), or 1-800-243-7889 (TTY, deaf access).

Prevention

STDs *are* preventable. As discussed earlier, the only sure way to avoid exposure to STDs is to abstain from sexual activity. Should you decide not to abstain, the key is to think about prevention *before* you have a sexual encounter or find yourself in the "heat of the moment." Find out what your partner thinks before you become sexually involved. Remember, you can become infected with an STD from just one unprotected encounter.

Most people don't want to think, talk, or ask questions about STDs for a variety of reasons. They may think it detracts from the appeal and excitement of the moment, that it takes away from the spontaneity of the experience, or that it will be perceived as a personal insult. For others, simply not knowing how to talk about STDs and safer sex may prevent them from bringing up the issue with a partner.

Plan ahead for safer sex. Know what sexual behaviors are risky. Find out about your partner's sexual history and practices. Be honest and ask your partner to do the same. By thinking and talking about STDs, you are expressing a sense of caring for yourself, your potential partner, and your future children. Taking STDs seriously is practical, courageous, and loving; it means giving yourself the respect you deserve.

Everyone can reduce the risk of infection by practicing responsible sexual behaviors. After abstinence, the next most effective approach to preventing STDs is having sex with one mutually faithful uninfected partner. If you are sexually active, use a condom during every act of intercourse to reduce your risk of contracting a disease. Although not foolproof, a properly used condom provides an effective barrier against disease-causing organisms, including HIV. A disease can be transmitted if there is contact with an infected area that isn't protected by the condom, however, such as the scrotum, the perineum, or the anal area. The use of a barrier over the cervix (diaphragm or cervical cap) in addition to a condom can help further lower the risk of STDs for women; as discussed in Chapter 6, these methods may provide some protection against the organisms that cause gonorrhea, genital warts, and chlamydia.

Approaches to STD prevention that are not safe include urinating or douching after intercourse, engaging in oral sex, or practicing genital play without full penetration. Birth control pills and sterilization protect you against conception and unwanted pregnancy but not against STDs.

Personal Insight Do you feel comfortable about having a frank discussion with a new sexual partner about your sexual histories? Under what circumstances do you feel such a discussion would be appropriate or inappropriate?

Diagnosis and Treatment

If you are sexually active, be alert for any sign or symptom of disease, such as a rash, a discharge, sores, or unusual pain, and don't hesitate to have a professional examination if you notice such a symptom. (You can obtain a copy of the genital self-examination guide developed by the Burroughs Wellcome Company by calling 1-800-234-1124.) Be alert for these signs or symptoms in your sexual partner too, and don't hesitate to question him or her if you notice something unusual.

If you are diagnosed as having an STD, you should begin treatment as quickly as possible. Inform your partner(s) to prevent further spread of the infection and to protect him or her from the complications that can occur when treatment is delayed. Avoid any sexual activity until your treatment is complete and testing indicates that you are cured. If your sexual partner tells you that he or she has contracted an STD, you need to be tested immediately, even if you don't have any symptoms.

Despite the awkwardness and difficulty, it's crucial that your partners be informed about a disease they may have been exposed to and urged to seek testing and/or treatment as quickly as possible. Because it is awkward and difficult, you can get help telling your partner if you should need it. Public health departments will notify sexual partners of their possible exposure while maintaining your confidentiality and anonymity. Peer counseling and student health programs often assist students with practice in role-playing in these circumstances, and concerned health care personnel can also provide assistance.

The decision to have a sexual relationship carries with it certain uncertainties and risks, both physical and emotional. It also carries the responsibility of safeguarding one's own health and that of others. You and your partner need mutual respect and honesty to make good decisions together. Caring about yourself and your partner means asking questions and being aware of signs and symptoms. It may be a bit awkward, but the temporary embarrassment of asking intimate questions is a small price to pay to avoid contracting or spreading disease. If your partner thinks less of you for being concerned, you may want to reconsider the relationship in terms of your personal values. Concern about STDs is part of a sexual relationship, not an intrusion into it, just as sexuality is part of life, not separate from it.

Personal Insight How do you feel about seeking examination or treatment for an STD? Do you feel differently than you would about other symptoms?

SUMMARY

The Body's Defense System

- Foreign organisms may enter the body by penetration of the skin, inhalation, or ingestion. The body's defense system against outside organisms consists of physical and chemical barriers, backed up by the immune system.

- Physical and chemical barriers to microorganisms include skin, mucous membranes, and the cilia lining the respiratory tract.

- The immune response is carried out by white blood cells that are continuously produced in the bone marrow. These include neutrophils, macrophages, natural killer cells, and lymphocytes.

- Lymphocytes recognize the antigens of invading organisms as foreign. When a foreign organism appears in the body, the appropriate lymphocyte locks onto it and sets off the immune response.

- The inflammatory response occurs when cells in the area of invasion or injury release histamines and other substances that cause blood vessels to dilate and fluid to flow out of capillaries.

- The immune response has four critical stages: recognition of the invading pathogen; rapid replication of killer T-cells and B-cells; attack by killer T-cells and macrophages; suppression of the immune response.

- Memory T- and B-cells recognize and destroy an antigen that enters the body a subsequent time.

- Immunization is based on the body's ability to remember previously encountered organisms and retain its strength against them. Vaccines are preparations made of antigens similar to a disease-causing organism but not so dangerous.
- Allergic reactions occur when the immune system responds to harmless substances as if they were dangerous antigens.

The Troublemakers—Pathogens and Disease

- Bacteria are one-celled organisms that break down dead organic matter; in the human digestive tract, they help digest food. Anywhere else in the body they are pathogenic. They occur as bacilli, cocci, and spirochetes.
- Although the immune system can fight off many bacterial infections, damage can be caused by both the bacteria and the body's immune defenses.
- Most antibiotics work by interrupting production of new bacteria. Bacteria can become resistant to antibiotics.
- Viruses, the smallest pathogens, cannot grow or reproduce by themselves; they live a parasitic existence in the cells they invade. The seriousness of diseases caused by viruses depends on which kind of cell is infected.
- About 50 species of fungi can cause diseases in humans, usually restricted to the skin, mucous membranes, and lungs.
- Protozoa cause several tropical diseases as well as giardiasis and trichomoniasis.
- Parasitic worm infections generally originate in contaminated food or drink.
- The immune system often detects malignant cells and destroys them as if they were pathogens. If the immune system breaks down, cancer cells can multiply before the immune system recognizes danger.
- Autoimmune diseases occur when the body identifies its own cells as foreign.

Sexually Transmissible Diseases

- HIV affects the immune system, making an otherwise healthy person susceptible to a variety of infections.
- HIV is carried in blood and blood products, semen, and vaginal and cervical secretions. HIV is transmitted through the exchange of these fluids, through sexual activity, the sharing of hypodermic needles used to inject drugs, blood transfusions (prior to 1985) and from mother to child during pregnancy, birth, or breastfeeding.
- Because HIV weakens the immune system, infected people are susceptible to serious opportunistic infections.
- Diagnosis of HIV infection depends upon detecting antibodies to HIV circulating in the bloodstream.
- There is currently no cure or vaccine for HIV infection. Drugs have been developed to slow the course of the disease and to prevent or treat particular infections.
- HIV infection can be prevented by making careful choices about sexual activity, not sharing drug needles, and learning as much as possible about protecting yourself from the disease.
- Hepatitis is usually caused by a viral infection of the liver that can be transmitted through sexual and nonsexual contact.
- There is no cure for hepatitis, but there is a vaccine for hepatitis B.
- Syphilis is contracted through sexual contact or through the placenta of an infected mother. If untreated, syphilis can lead to mental degeneration, paralysis, and death.
- Chlamydia is the most prevalent bacterial infection in the United States. It causes urinary tract infection and epididymitis in men; in women, it can lead to PID if untreated.
- Untreated, gonorrhea can cause PID in women and epididymitis in men, leading to sterility; infants exposed to the bacteria during birth may develop an infection that can cause blindness if untreated.
- Pelvic inflammatory disease is an infection of the oviducts that may extend to the ovaries. It can lead to chronic infections, sterility, and menstrual problems.
- Genital warts, caused by the human papillomavirus, are associated with cervical cancer. An infection is contagious through contact with the dry, painless growths.
- Herpes has a high incidence in the United States, can be fatal to newborns, and is incurable. After an initial infection, the herpesvirus lies dormant in the area of the infection. Recurrences can be triggered by environmental, health, and personal factors.

What Can You Do?

- All STDs are preventable; the key is practicing responsible sexual behaviors—which requires planning. Those who are sexually active are safest with one mutually faithful uninfected partner. Using a condom properly with every act of sexual intercourse helps protect against STDs.
- Successful treatment of STDs on an individual basis means being alert to symptoms in oneself and one's partners, seeing a physician if symptoms occur,

getting treatment, informing partners, and avoiding sexual activity until treatment is complete.

TAKE ACTION

1. Find out from your parents or your health records which immunizations you have had, including when you last had a tetanus shot. Are your immunizations up-to-date? If they aren't, or if you're not sure, check with the health center about what they recommend.

2. Go to your local pharmacy and examine the cold and cough remedies. Exactly which symptoms does each one claim to alleviate, and with what active ingredient? If possible, ask the pharmacist which ones he or she recommends for various symptoms.

3. Go to a drugstore and examine the over-the-counter contraceptives. Which ones provide protection against STDs? If you are sexually active, make sure you use the best protection available.

4. More and more communities have treatment and support programs for people with HIV infection. Look in the yellow pages or contact local health agencies to find out what services are available where you live. If any of these agencies use volunteers, consider donating some of your time to help.

JOURNAL ENTRY

1. In your health journal, list the positive behaviors that help you avoid or resist infection, including sexually transmissible diseases. Consider how you can strengthen those behaviors. Then list the behaviors that tend to block your positive behaviors and put you at risk for contracting infection. Consider which of these you can change.

2. *Critical Thinking:* Does the government have the right to quarantine people who have serious infectious diseases such as tuberculosis, HIV infection, or measles? Which should take precedence—concerns about public safety or the rights of individuals? Are there aspects of an illness—such as the seriousness of the illness or the mode of transmission—that should be considered in making this decision? Write an essay outlining your position on this issue; describe what circumstances, if any, you feel would warrant quarantining an infectious person.

3. Monitor yourself the next time you feel a cold coming on, keeping a record like the one shown in Chapter 1 for eating behavior. Note the symptoms, how they felt, the time and date of their occurrence, what you were doing, how you were feeling emotionally, and what you did in response to the symptoms. Keep the record until the cold is gone, noting how long it takes to run its course. Is there an association between your emotional state and how you experienced the symptoms? Between your emotional state and the length of the cold? Does taking medication (decongestant, cough syrup, etc.) make a difference in the symptoms or the duration of the cold?

SELECTED BIBLIOGRAPHY

Adimara, A. A., and others. 1994. *Sexually Transmitted Diseases: Companion Handbook,* 2nd ed. New York: McGraw-Hill.

Altman, L. 1995. *AIDS is now the leading killer of Americans from 24 to 44. The New York Times Science.* 31 January.

American College Health Association. 1990. *HIV Infection and AIDS: What Everyone Should Know.* Baltimore, Md.: American College Health Association.

Aral, S. O., and K. K. Holmes. 1990. Epidemiology of STDs. In *Sexually Transmitted Diseases,* 2nd ed., ed. K. K. Holmes and others, 19–36. New York: McGraw-Hill.

Balows, A., W. J. Hausler, and E. H. Lennette, eds. 1988. *Laboratory Diagnosis of Infectious Disease, Principles and Practice.* New York: Springer-Verlag.

Basen-Enquist, K. 1992. Psychosocial predictors of safer sex behaviors in young adults. *AIDS Education and Prevention* 4(2): 120–34.

Centers for Disease Control. 1991. *Health Information for International Travel.* Atlanta: Centers for Disease Control, Bureau of Epidemiology.

———.1992. National action plan to combat multidrug-resistant tuberculosis: Report from the U.S. Department of Health and Human Services. *Morbidity and Mortality Weekly Report* 41 (RR-11).

———. 1993. Update: Barrier protection against HIV infection and other sexually transmitted diseases. *Morbidity and Mortality Weekly Report* 42:589–91, 597.

———. 1994. Lyme disease—United States, 1993. *Morbidity and Mortality Weekly Report* 43(31).

———. 1995. Update: AIDS among women—United States, 1994. *Morbidity and Mortality Weekly Report* 44:5.

Cohen, S., D. A. J. Tyrrell, and A. P. Smith. 1991. Psychological stress and susceptibility to the common cold. *New England Journal of Medicine* 325:606–12.

Corey, L. 1990. Genital herpes. In *Sexually Transmitted Diseases,* 2nd ed., ed. K. K. Holmes and others, 391–414. New York: McGraw-Hill.

Evans, A. S., ed. 1991. *Bacterial Infections of Humans: Epidemiology and Control,* 2nd ed. New York: Plenum.

———. ed. 1991. *Viral Infections of Humans: Epidemiology and Control,* 3rd ed. New York: Plenum.

Felts, W. M., and S. M. Knight. 1992. The nature and prevention of viral hepatitis: What health educators should know. *Journal of Health Education* 23(5): 267–74.

Goldsmith, M. F. 1992. Critical moment at hand in HIV/AIDS pandemic, new global strategy to arrest its spread proposed. *Journal of the American Medical Association* 268(4): 445.

Hatcher, R. A., and others, eds. 1990. *Contraceptive Technology, 1990–1992. With Two Special Sections: AIDS and Condoms,* 15th rev. ed. New York: Irvington Press.

Holmes, K. K., P. Mardh, P. F. Sparling, and P. J. Weisner, eds. 1990. *Sexually Transmitted Diseases,* 2nd ed. New York: McGraw-Hill.

Hook, E. W. III, and H. Handsfield. 1990. Gonorrhea infection in the adult. In *Sexually Transmitted Diseases,* 2nd ed., ed. K. K. Holmes and others, 149–60. New York: McGraw-Hill.

Mandell, G. B., and others. 1990. *Principles and Practice of Infectious Diseases,* 3rd ed. New York: Churchill Livingstone.

Markell, E. K., M. Voge, and D. T. John. 1992. *Medical Parasitology,* 7th ed. New York: W. B. Saunders.

Murphy, J. W., H. Friedman, and M. Bendinelli, eds. 1992. *Fungal Infections and Immune Responses.* New York: Plenum.

O'Leary, A., F. Goodhart, L. S. Jermmott, and D. Boccher-Lattimore. 1992. Predictors of safer sex on the college campus: A social-cognitive theory analysis. *Journal of American College Health,* vol. 40, May.

Oriel, D. 1990. Genital human papillomavirus infection. In *Sexually Transmitted Diseases,* 2nd ed., ed. K. K. Holmes and others, Chap. 38. New York: McGraw-Hill.

Rahn, D. W., and S. E. Malawista. 1991. Lyme disease: Recommendations for diagnosis and treatment. *Annals of Internal Medicine* 114:472–81.

Russell, S. 1992. Definition of AIDS broadens tomorrow. *San Francisco Chronicle,* 31 December.

Ryan, K. ed. 1994. *Sherris Medical Microbiology: An Introduction to Infectious Diseases.* 3rd ed. Norwalk, Conn.: Appleton and Lange.

Sarracco, A., and others. 1993. Man-to-woman sexual transmission of HIV: Longitudinal study of 343 steady partners of infected men. *Journal of Acquired Immune Deficiency Syndrome* 6:497–502.

Schochetman, G., and J. R. George. 1994. *AIDS Testing: A Comprehensive Guide to Technical, Medical, Social, Legal, and Management Issues.* 2nd ed. New York: Springer-Verlag.

Stoeckle, M. Y., and R. G. Douglas, Jr. 1992. Infectious diseases. *Journal of the American Medical Association* 268(3).

San Francisco AIDS Foundation. 1992. *AIDS Medical Guide,* 3rd ed. San Francisco: Impact AIDS.

Squires, S. 1992. Hepatitis B vaccinations. *Washington Post Health,* 5 May.

Voeller, B., J. M. Reinisch, and M. Gottlieb, eds. 1990. *AIDS and Sex: An Integrated Biomedical and Behavioral Approach.* New York: Oxford University Press, Kinsey Institute Series.

Warren, K. S., and A. F. Mahmoud. 1990. *Tropical and Geographical Medicine,* 2nd ed. New York: McGraw-Hill.

World Bank. *World Development Report 1993.* New York: Oxford University Press.

White, D. O., and F. J. Fenner. 1994. *Medical Virology.* 4th ed. San Diego, Calif.: Academic Press.

RECOMMENDED READINGS

Bollet, A. J. 1987. *Plagues and Poxes: The Rise and Fall of Epidemic Diseases.* New York: Demos Publications. *Includes descriptions of the history and epidemiology of famous epidemics.*

Brock, T., ed. 1990. *Microorganisms—From Smallpox to Lyme Disease: Readings from* Scientific American *Magazine.* New York: W. H. Freeman. *A collection of articles from* Scientific American *on medical microbiology and communicable diseases.*

Burroughs Wellcome Co. 1990. *What You Need to Know About Sexually Transmitted Diseases, HIV Disease and AIDS.* Distributed at the American Medical Association Conference on STDs: Risk Assessment, Diagnosis and Treatment. Research Triangle Park, N.C.: Burroughs Wellcome, November. *An easy-to-read survey of the STDs.*

Channing L. Bete Co., Inc. 1995. *What Do You Know About HIV?* South Deerfield, Mass.: Channing L. Bete Co., Inc. *Contains basic information, written for the general public.*

Department of Health and Human Services. 1993. *Surgeon General's Report to the American Public on HIV Infection and AIDS.* Washington, D.C.: U.S. Public Health Service.

Garrett, L. 1994. *The Coming Plague: Newly Emerging Diseases in a World Out of Balance.* New York: Farrar, Straus, and Giroux. *The author traces the emergence of new and drug-resistant microbes over the past 50 years, pinpoints conditions that promote their spread, and proposes solutions.*

Levy, S. B. 1992. *The Antibiotic Paradox: How Miracle Drugs Are Destroying the Miracle.* New York: Plenum. *An easy-to-understand description of the effects of misuse and overuse of antibiotics, with suggestions for changing current practices to protect the effectiveness of antibiotics.*

Sacks, S. L. 1989. *The Truth About Herpes.* West Vancouver: Gordon Soules. *A complete overview of the disease that makes a good reference for self-care information.*

Shilts, R. 1987. *And the Band Played On: Politics, People and the AIDS Epidemic.* New York: St. Martin's Press. *A highly readable account of the AIDS epidemic and the political response it has evoked, written by a concerned and committed reporter. This book is as powerful now as it was in 1987.*

The Challenge of Aging

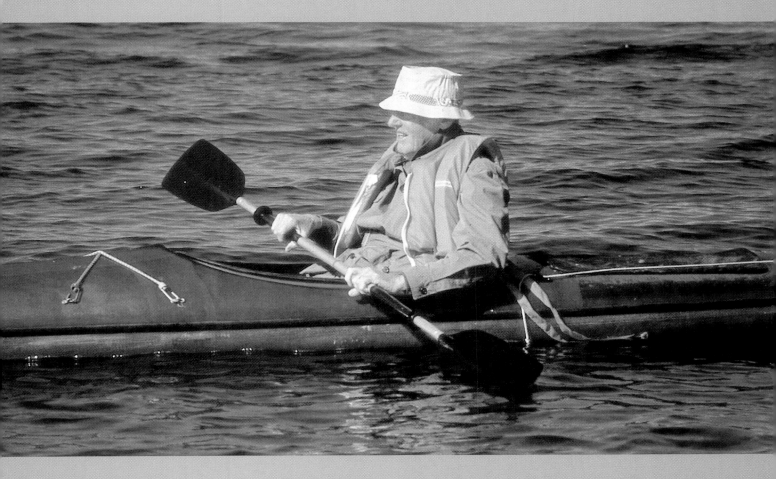

CONTENTS

Many people would like to live for a long time and never grow old and die. When we see that old age has taken us in its grip, we're stunned. We regard old age as something alien, a foreign species. But aging is a normal process of development that occurs over the entire lifetime. It happens to everyone, but at different rates for different people. Some people are "old" at 25; others are still young at 75.

Learning to accept and deal with aging and death is a difficult but important part of life, a process that requires information, insight, and commitment, just as simpler life tasks do. Although youth is not entirely a state of mind, your attitude toward life and your attention to your health significantly influence the satisfaction you will derive from life, especially when new physical, mental, and situational challenges occur in later years. If you take charge of your health during young adulthood, you can exert great control over the physical and mental aspects of aging, and you can better handle your response to events that might be out of your control. With foresight and energy you can shape a creative, graceful, and even triumphant old age.

GENERATING VITALITY AS YOU AGE

Circumstances, bodies, and mental faculties change. Some changes occur gradually, over a lifetime. **Biological aging,** for example, includes all the normal, progressive, irreversible changes to one's body that begin at birth and continue until death. Psychological and social aging usually involve more abrupt changes in circumstance and emotion: relocating, changing homes, losing a spouse and friends, retiring, having a lower income, and changing roles and social status. These changes represent opportunities for growth throughout life.

> *Personal Insight* How do you envision your old age? How will it resemble the old age of elderly people you know now, and how will it differ? What external events could affect your control of your lifestyle when you're older?

What Happens as You Age?

Many of the characteristics associated with aging aren't due to aging at all. They are due rather to neglect and abuse of our bodies and minds. These assaults lay the foundation for later mental problems and chronic conditions like arthritis, heart disease, diabetes, hearing loss, and high blood pressure. We sacrifice our optimal health by smoking, eating a poor diet and overeating, abusing alcohol and drugs, bombarding our ears with excessive noise, and exposing our bodies to too much ultraviolet ra-

diation from sun rays. We also jeopardize our bodies through inactivity, encouraging our muscles and even our bones to wither and deteriorate. And we endure abuse from the toxic chemicals in our environment.

But even with the best behavior in the best environment, aging does occur. It results from biochemical processes that we don't yet fully understand. The physiological changes in organ systems are caused by a combination of gradual aging and injury from disease.

Life-enhancing Measures: Age Proofing

You can prevent, delay, lessen, or even reverse some of the changes associated with aging through good health habits. A few simple things you can do every day will make a vast difference to your appearance, your health, your energy and vitality. The following suggestions have been mentioned throughout this text, but are profoundly related to health in later life and so are highlighted here.

Challenge Your Mind Creativity and intelligence remain stable in healthy individuals. Develop interests and hobbies that you can enjoy throughout your life. Staying involved in learning as a lifelong process can help you remain sharp and keep your mental abilities.

Develop Physical Fitness Exercise enhances both mental and physical health. Enough cannot be said for the positive effects of appropriate exercise throughout your life, particularly when weighed against the physical and mental deterioration of the elderly who have not kept their minds and bodies fit. The benefits of an active and vigorous lifestyle include the following:

- Increased resiliency and suppleness of arteries
- Better protection against heart attack and much increased chance of survival should one occur
- Sustained capacity of lungs and respiratory reserves
- Weight control through less accumulation of fat
- Maintenance of physical flexibility, balance, agility, reaction time
- Greatly preserved muscle strength
- Protection against ligament injuries, dislocation strains in the knees, spine, shoulders
- Protection against osteoporosis
- Increased effectiveness of the immune system
- Maintenance of mental agility and flexibility, response time, memory, hand-eye coordination

Eat Wisely Health at every age is helped by a varied diet with special attention to lower fat and calorie intake.

- Eat meals low in fat and high in complex carbohydrates. Concentrate on fresh fruits and vegetables, whole grains, and pasta.

- Eat fish and poultry (no skin) instead of eggs and fatty meats.
- Use no-fat or low-fat dairy products. Substitute olive oil for other oils and fats.
- If you frequently salt your food, reduce your intake.
- Maintain calcium intake of 850–1,000 mg per day.

Maintain Healthy Weight   People can control their weight, although it takes time and can be stressful; it's especially difficult for people who have been overweight most of their lives. A sensible program of using more calories through exercise and perhaps cutting calorie intake or a combination of both will work for most people who want to lose weight. Obesity is not physically healthy, and it leads to premature aging. Recommended caloric intake declines with age to 1,600 per day for women and 2,050 for men over age 75. Protein, vitamin, and mineral requirements remain the same.

Control Drinking and Overdependence on Medications   Alcohol abuse ranks with depression as a common hidden mental health problem, affecting 20 percent of the elderly. The problem is often not identified because the effects of alcohol or drug addiction can mimic disease, such as Alzheimer's. Signs of potential alcohol or drug dependence include unusual or frequent accidents, forgetfulness, depression, and malnutrition. Problems can be avoided by not using alcohol to relieve anxiety or emotional pain and not taking medication when safer forms of treatment are available.

Don't Smoke   The average pack-a-day smoker can expect to live about 12 years less than a nonsmoker. Worse, smokers suffer more illnesses that last longer, and they are subject to respiratory disabilities that limit their total vigor for many years before their death. Even young cigarette smokers suffer respiratory impairment, some within a year of starting to smoke. Premature balding and skin wrinkling have been linked to cigarette smoking. Smokers at age 50 have the wrinkles of a person of 60.

Schedule Physical Examinations to Detect Treatable Diseases   When detected early, many diseases, including hypertension, diabetes, and many types of cancer, can be successfully controlled by medication and lifestyle changes. Regular testing for **glaucoma** after age 40 can prevent blindness from this eye disease. And keeping your immunizations up-to-date can protect you from preventable infectious diseases (see Chapter 13).

Recognize and Reduce Stress   Stress-induced physiological changes increase wear and tear on your body. Cut down on the stresses in your life. Don't wear yourself out too fast through lack of sleep, abuse or misuse of drugs, or workaholism. Practice relaxation, using the techniques described in Chapter 2. If you contract a disease, consider it your body's attempt to interrupt your life pattern and permit you to reevaluate your lifestyle, perhaps to slow down.

Ironically, the health behaviors you practice now weigh more heavily in determining how long you will live than will your behaviors at a later age. Retiring from your life's occupation with a physically healthy body will allow far more options for enjoying yourself than will retiring with frail health or disabilities. Poor health that could have been prevented drains finances, emotions, and energy and contributes to poor mental health. By attending to yourself now, you're buying some insurance for the future.

CONFRONTING THE CHANGES OF AGING

The changes that occur with aging have repercussions that must be grappled with and resolved. Just as you can act now to prevent or limit the physical changes of aging, you can also begin preparing yourself mentally, socially, and financially for changes that may occur later in life. These developmental tasks of aging are determined by biological, social, and perhaps economic changes and may require significant lifestyle adjustments. Although aging puts unique demands on each person, the changes cut across ethnic and socioeconomic variables. If you have aging parents, grandparents, and friends, the following information may give you insight into their lives and encourage you to begin cultivating appropriate and useful behaviors now.

Planning for Social Changes

Retirement marks a major change in the second half of life. As the longevity of Americans has increased, individuals spend a larger proportion of their lives in retirement—15 years or more. This has implications for reestablishing important relationships, developing satisfying interests outside work, and saving for an adequate retirement income.

Changes in social roles are a major feature of middle age. Children become young adults and leave home, putting an end to day-to-day parenting. Parents experiencing this "empty nest syndrome" must adapt to changes in their customary responsibilities and personal identities. And though retirement is a wished-for landmark for most people, it may also be viewed as a threat to prestige,

Biological aging   Changes in body structure and function that result from the passage of time.

Glaucoma   Disease in which fluid inside the eye is under abnormally high pressure; can lead to blindness.

TERMS

Aging and Changing: Your Body Through Time

Skin   Skin becomes looser as you get older—it stretches more easily and doesn't snap back as well after stretching. Long-term exposure to ultraviolet light from the sun produces wrinkles and areas of spotty pigmentation ("age spots"). Hats, gloves, sunglasses, and sunscreen provide protection from the sun. Skin also becomes drier as you age, as sweat and oil glands quit working. Overuse of soaps and antiperspirants can worsen dry skin.

Body Fat   You can expect an increase in body fat and reduction in body size from a decrease in muscle mass and body water content. However, changes in muscle tone and body composition (the ratio of fat to muscle) can be kept to a minimum through regular exercise. Deposits of fat in the waist are associated with a higher incidence of disease. Weight management is important throughout life.

Hearing   The ability to hear high-pitched and sibilant (hissing) consonant sounds such as s, z, sh, and ch declines for most people as they age, enough so that hearing loss is now the fourth most common chronic physical disability in the United States. Even by age 35, you may not hear as well as you did at 25. Most people don't notice the progressive muffling until their sixties, when they may begin to have difficulty following speech. These losses may be due to abuse rather than to aging, however. Extremely loud noise, such as from stereo earphones or loud machines may contribute to hearing loss. In less industrialized and quieter societies, hearing is almost as keen in old age as it is in youth. A high-fat diet has been linked to clogging of the blood vessels that nourish the hearing organs.

Eyesight   By your mid-forties you will develop **presbyopia**—a gradual decline in the ability to focus on objects close to you. This occurs because the ocular lens no longer expands and contracts as readily. You will need brighter lights for reading and close work. Slowed light-to-dark adaptation and distorted depth perception make night driving more difficult and require compensating driving techniques. **Cataracts,** a clouding of the lens caused by lifelong oxidation damage (a by-product of normal body chemistry), may dim vision by the sixties. Visual defects in the elderly often go undetected. Annual eye exams can help to prevent injury from falls and automobile crashes.

Taste and Smell   Sensations of taste and smell diminish with age. About two-thirds of the taste buds in the mouth die by age 70, as do many of the sensory receptors in the nose. Some medications can further interfere with taste, and long-term exposure to smoke lessens the ability to smell.

Hair   As you age, cells at the base of hair follicles produce progressively less pigment and eventually die. By age 50 half of Americans are partially gray, and hair loss in men becomes apparent. Twelve percent of men are balding by age 25; 65 percent by age 65. Thickest at age 20, individual hair shafts shrink after that; by age 70, your hair will probably be as fine as when you were a baby.

Bones, Muscles, and Teeth   Bones maintain themselves through a cyclic process called remodeling in which old bone is absorbed and new bone develops. By the mid-thirties, more bone is being absorbed than developed. Loss of bone mass is generally not a problem for men because they have denser bones than women to begin with. For women, bone loss accelerates after menopause. One out of every four women over age 60 develops **osteoporosis**, in which bones become weaker, more porous, and more prone to fractures. Adequate calcium in your diet and regular weight-bearing exercise will help build strong bones while you're young and slow the loss of bone as you age (see Chapter 9).

Muscles become weaker, too, although you can retard your loss of muscle strength and mass through regular physical work and play. As you age, more protein is being broken down and less is being synthesized, so muscle fibers atrophy and lose their ability to contract; some are lost; fat and collagen accumulate. Aging muscles are less flexible and more susceptible to strains, pulls, and cramps. After the mid-forties, strength usually declines: A man may lose 10 to 20 percent of his maximum strength by age 60, and a woman even more.

Height also decreases with age—about 1 to 4 inches are lost after young adulthood. Factors contributing to this decrease in height include loss of bone mass, weakening back muscles, and deterioration of the discs between the bones in the spine.

Your teeth, with proper care, can last a lifetime. Not aging, but disuse, abuse, and chronic degenerative disease

---

Presbyopia   The inability of the eyes to focus sharply on nearby objects, caused by a loss of elasticity of the lens that occurs with advancing age.

Cataracts   Opacity of the lens of the eye that impairs vision and can cause blindness.

Osteoporosis   Loss of bone density that causes bones to become weak, porous, and more prone to fractures.

Periodontitis   Disease of the bone, tissue, and gum that support the teeth, caused by the accumulation of plaque.

purpose, and self-respect—the loss of a valued or customary role—and will probably require a period of adjustment.

If you have developed diverse interests, retirement can be a joyful and fulfilling period of your life. Retirement can provide opportunities for expanding your horizons by giving you the chance to try new activities, make trips you never had time for before, take classes, and meet new people. Volunteering in your community can enhance cause teeth problems. Teeth and all their support systems respond well to the stress and stimulation of chewing crunchy foods. **Periodontitis** is a common agent in tooth loss after age 35; it is caused by the buildup of plaque. You can prevent it with proper dental care, including brushing and flossing each day.

Heart Your resting heartbeat stays about the same throughout your life, but the heart pumps less blood with each beat as you get older. This effect is most pronounced during exercise because your pulse can no longer rise as high, nor return as rapidly to its resting rate, as it once did. The dramatic problems of the cardiovascular system associated with aging—heart attack and stroke—are usually caused by atherosclerosis and high blood pressure, which can be largely controlled with diet and exercise. People who have high blood cholesterol, who smoke, or who have diabetes or a family history of coronary artery disease may wish to discuss aspirin therapy with their physician.

Lungs Good news: Your respiratory system resists change, and your respiratory tract actually grows stronger with age. After a lifetime of exposure to viruses, people build up immunity and catch fewer and less severe colds by middle age. Your vital capacity—the amount of air you can expel from your lungs—should not decline if you keep fit and don't smoke. Regular vigorous exercise can increase vital capacity.

Digestive System and Kidneys With age, your stomach will secrete less acid and smaller amounts of the enzymes that aid digestion. Digesting a meal takes longer and may be more difficult. Kidneys filter wastes more slowly, causing decreased drug clearance. Fewer calories are required to maintain body weight.

Immune System With age your defense system may become less efficient, but the decline varies greatly among people. Only the progressive atrophy of the thymus gland seems invariably linked to advancing age. The consequences of immune system decline are increased rates of cancer and autoimmune and infectious diseases but better tolerance of tissue and organ transplants. Both good diet and exercise benefit the immune system. People who are in good physical shape rid themselves of respiratory infections much faster than do those who are not.

Brain and Nervous System Only half as much blood travels to the brain of a 50-year-old as to that of a 10-year-old, with most of the reduction occurring before age 30. By age 85, the brain has lost 10 to 20 percent of its weight, mainly through nerve cell atrophy. These **neuron** losses are selective: Some sites show no loss, while in the **cerebral cortex**, the site of higher mental activities, loss is significant. Your mental ability will not necessarily decline with the loss of neurons, partly because the brain continues to sprout new **dendrites**, communication lines to other neurons. They may be one way the brain compensates for neuron loss.

Sleep patterns change with age, although troubled sleep may be a sign of an emotional or physical disorder rather than of age. The deepest stage of non-REM sleep decreases as you age, which may explain why older people are considered light sleepers. Reliance on sleeping medications should be avoided because they interfere with REM sleep (see Chapter 2 for more information on sleep).

Sexual Organs and Sexual Response An active and satisfying sex life can continue as you age. Women do not ordinarily lose their capacity for orgasm nor men their capacity for erection and ejaculation. A slowing of response, especially in men, is considered a part of the normal aging process.

For women, menopause (cessation of menstruation) usually occurs between the ages of 47 and 50. The common symptoms of menopause, including hot flashes and sweating, can be treated with hormone therapy. Women may experience a drying and thinning of the vaginal walls due to lower levels of ovarian-produced estrogen after menopause; use of an estrogen cream and/or a water-soluble lubricant can usually treat the problem. A hysterectomy or mastectomy does not have to affect sexual activity. Monthly breast self-exams and mammograms every two years are important.

As they age, men may take longer to attain an erection and the erection may not be as firm or as large as when they were younger. The prostate gland may become enlarged after middle age, causing problems with urination. This condition can now usually be treated without affecting sexual response.

---

self-esteem and allow you to be a contributing member of society.

Retirement often also brings a new economic situation. It may mean a severely restricted budget or possibly even financial disaster if you don't take stock of finances and plan ahead. People in their twenties and thirties should estimate how much money they need to meet their standard of living, calculate their projected income, and begin a savings program. The earlier such a program is begun, the more money will be saved for retirement and the more interest that money will accrue.

TERMS

Neuron A nerve cell.
Cerebral cortex The outer layer of the brain, which controls the behavior and mental activity of humans.
Dendrites A branched part of a nerve cell that transmits impulses toward the cell body.

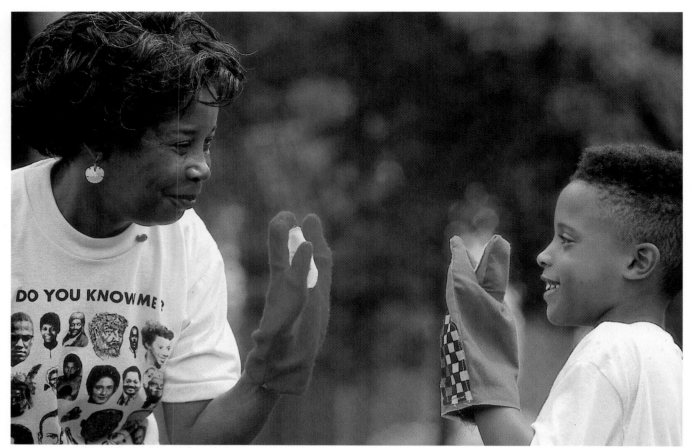

One of the challenges of aging is finding satisfying activities that provide meaningful connections with others. This retired woman is using hand puppets to help teach refusal skills as part of a substance abuse prevention project.

Adapting to Physical Changes

Decreased energy and changes in health mean that older people have to develop priorities for how to use their energy. Rather than curtailing activities to conserve energy, they need to learn how to generate energy. This usually involves saying "yes" to enjoyable activities and paying close attention to needs for rest and sleep.

Adapting, rather than giving up, favorite activities may be the best strategy for dealing with physical limitations. For example, if **arthritis** interferes with piano playing, a person can continue to enjoy music by attending concerts or checking out music from the local library. Obtaining treatment for medical problems such as arthritis and glau-

coma can also help limit the effects of aging on day-to-day activities.

One common physical disability—hearing loss—can have a particularly strong effect on the lives of elderly people. Hearing loss affects a person's ability to interact with others and can lead to a sense of isolation and depression. If someone you know complains that words are difficult to understand, that another person's speech sounds slurred or mumbled, or that people are not speaking loudly enough, that person may have suffered some hearing loss. You may also notice that the person sets the volume of a radio or TV very high. Hearing loss should be assessed and treated by a health care professional; in some cases, hearing can be completely restored by dealing with the underlying cause of hearing loss. In other cases, hearing aids may be prescribed to help with hearing.

There are many strategies for dealing with the gradual decline in vision that occurs with aging. The first is to treat any underlying medical problems, such as cataracts or glaucoma. Older people may need about a 30 percent increase in light in order to work more effectively; in-

TERMS

Arthritis   Inflammation of a joint or joints causing pain and swelling.

Dementia   Deterioration of intellectual faculties (including memory, concentration, and judgment) resulting from a disease or disorder of the brain; often accompanied by emotional disturbances and changes in personality.

In the early 1900s, a German neurologist named Alois Alzheimer performed an autopsy on a patient in her mid-fifties whom he had diagnosed several years earlier with presenile dementia, a condition marked by mental deterioration, loss of memory, and unpredictable behavior and occurring before aging has advanced very far. Alzheimer had assumed that the cause was hardening of the arteries. On autopsy, however, he discovered no signs of arteriosclerosis. What he did discover was massive damage to nerve cells in the brain. The condition known as presenile dementia is now referred to as Alzheimer's disease.

Alzheimer's is a fatal brain disorder that causes physical and chemical changes in the brain. As nerve cells are destroyed in the brain, the system that produces the neurotransmitter acetylcholine breaks down, and communication among parts of the brain deteriorates. Autopsies reveal two other important characteristics: Nerve cells are packed with shriveled filaments known as tangles, and the tips of their branches are mired in plaques, clusters of degenerating nerve fibers.

To the layperson, Alzheimer's disease is synonymous with dementia, which literally means "deprived of mind." Among the elderly, Alzheimer's probably accounts for most cases of dementia, but there are at least 50 known disorders that can cause this condition. Some cases can be attributed to strokes or to Parkinson's disease. Limited healing or reversal of damages is sometimes possible in these cases. Less common causes of dementia include brain injuries or tumors, chronic alcoholism, depression, vitamin B-12 deficiency, thyroid disease, reaction to drugs taken for kidney or heart disease, and improper use of medication. Dementia from many of these causes can be reversed with treatment.

The first symptom of Alzheimer's disease is loss of memory. This doesn't mean that simple forgetfulness—forgetting a friend's birthday or where you left the car keys—is a sign. Rather, an afflicted person is likely to forget the identity of a familiar person or how to operate a familiar appliance such as a washing machine.

Other symptoms of the disease include confusion or disorientation, depression, anxiety, sleep disorders, and aggressive behavior. As the disease progresses, afflicted people lose the ability to function mentally. They experience a change in personality, a loss of identity. Eventually, they lose control of physical functioning, becoming incontinent and completely dependent on caregivers to feed and clothe them. On average, a person will live eight to ten years from the development of the first symptoms. Autopsy is the only certain way currently of diagnosing the disease.

Scientists do not yet know what causes Alzheimer's disease. Some researchers believe that a slow-acting virus is the cause. Others are investigating a link to environmental toxins; abnormal accumulations of aluminum found in the brain cells offer evidence for this theory. Still others believe that Alzheimer's is caused by a prion—a "proteinaceous infectious particle" that affects the genetic structure of cells.

Indeed, the disease does seem to have a genetic link, especially the form known as early-onset Alzheimer's disease (also called "familial Alzheimer's disease"). People who have early-onset Alzheimer's usually show symptoms before the age of 57; people with late-onset Alzheimer's on the other hand, may not show symptoms until well into their sixties. The early-onset form of the disease accounts for 10 to 30 percent of all cases. The chance of inheriting early-onset Alzheimer's disease is much greater than that of inheriting late-onset Alzheimer's.

According to the National Institute on Aging, about 10 percent of the adult population over the age of 65 has Alzheimer's disease, and about 47 percent of people over 85 have the disease. At any given time, an estimated 1.5 million to 4 million Americans suffer from the disease. Currently, it is the fourth leading cause of death for adults. As the population of aging Americans continues to grow, the disease will become more significant. By the year 2050 there may be 14 million Americans with Alzheimer's. Although there is no cure or treatment right now, research holds promise. Scientists are working on drugs to slow the progress of the disease and thus halt the decline of mental ability. When such drugs are developed, the burden of this tragic disease will be eased for both families and society.

Sources: K. Flieger. 1992. "Despite New Clues, Alzheimer's Mystery Remains Unsolved." *Healthline,* September; S. B. Prusiner. 1991. "Molecular Biology of Prion Diseases." *Science,* June; D. Chase and D. Lumpe. 1991. "Not All Memory Loss is Alzheimer's." *New Choices,* September.

creasing the number of light sources and painting rooms in a lighter, paler color helps. Increasing light sources in darkened areas such as stairwells can reduce falls from the slower light-to-dark accommodation that occurs with age. Hats and sunglasses worn outside help reduce glare. If visual losses are more severe, large-print books, magnifying glasses, and a variety of electronic devices are available to help an individual adapt to limitations in eyesight.

Handling Psychological and Mental Changes

Many people associate old age with forgetfulness, and slowly losing one's memory was once considered an inevitable part of growing old. However, we now know that most elderly people in good health remain mentally alert. Severe and significant brain deterioration in elderly individuals, called senility or **dementia,** affects only about 7

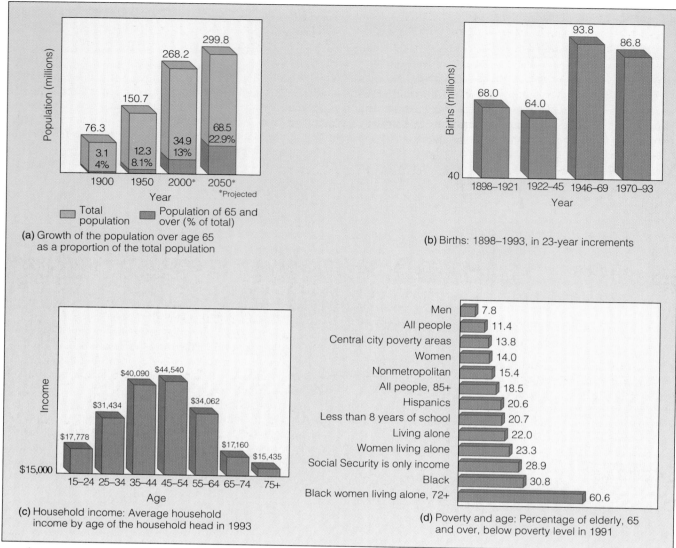

VITAL STATISTICS

Figure 14-1 *A statistical look at the elderly in America.*

Sources: U.S. Bureau of the Census. 1994. *Statistical Abstract of the United States,* 114th ed. (Washington, D.C.: U.S. Government Printing Office). U.S. Senate Special Committee on Aging. 1991. *Aging America: Trends and Projections.* (Washington, D.C.: U.S. Department of Health and Human Services). U.S. Bureau of the Census. 1989. *Historical Statistics of the United States, Colonial Times to 1970,* 3rd ed. (Washington, D.C.: U.S. Government Printing Office).

percent of people under age 80 (the incidence rises sharply for people in their eighties and nineties).

Dementia can be caused by many different factors, some of which are treatable, so it's important to have any symptoms evaluated by a health professional. Even for **Alzheimer's disease** and other incurable forms of dementia, appropriate treatment may greatly improve an afflicted person's quality of life.

Repeatedly telling stories about the past—something older people often do—doesn't indicate dementia. Reminiscence, the recollection of past personal experiences

and significant events, is a normal part of development. Repeatedly telling the same stories allows an older person to integrate life by making past events meaningful in the present. Reminiscence can be of great significance to members of the younger generations because it is a rich source of social, cultural, and family history.

Another psychological and emotional challenge of aging is dealing with grief and mourning. Aging is associated with losses—friends, peers, physical appearance, possessions, and health. Grief is the work of getting through the pain of loss, and it can be one of the most lonely and intense times in a person's life. It can take a year or two to completely come to terms with the loss of a loved one and to establish a new model of the self without the loved one.

One of the most important ways of dealing with the changes associated with aging is to adopt a flexible attitude toward whatever life brings you. Self-enjoyment and acceptance can help make the later years more meaningful and enjoyable. The right attitude can also help stave off the negative effects of some circumstances. Acceptance of limitations, an optimistic outlook, and a sense of humor are tools that can help you cope with all of life's changes.

Personal Insight What kinds of contact with older people did you have when you were growing up? Were these experiences positive or negative? How have they affected your current attitudes toward aging and elderly people?

AGING AND LIFE EXPECTANCY

Human **life expectancy** is the average length of time we can expect to live. It is calculated by averaging mortality statistics—the ages of death of a group of people over a certain period of time. A female born in the United States in 1993 has a longer life expectancy (78.7 years) than does her male counterpart (72.0 years). Individuals who reach their sixty-fifth birthday can expect to live even longer—17 more years or longer—because they have already survived hazards to life in the younger years. The reason for the gender gap in life expectancy is not known, but estrogen production and other factors during a woman's fertile years appear to protect her from heart disease. Her risks increase after menopause. Increased male mortality can also be traced to smoking (lung cancer, heart, and respiratory disease), more accidents, and more alcoholism. Where these factors are not operative, as among the Amish, men live as long as women. Life expectancy also varies among racial and ethnic groups; reasons for these differences include socioeconomic, genetic, and lifestyle factors.

How long can humans expect to live in the best of circumstances? It now seems possible that our maximum potential **life span** is about 100 or 110 years. (Although there are reports of very long-lived individuals, there is little evidence that anyone lives past age 110.) Failure to achieve that span in good health results to some degree from destructive environmental and behavioral factors—factors over which we can exert considerable control. Long life doesn't necessarily mean a longer period of disability, either. People often live longer because they have been well longer. A healthy, productive old age is very often an extension of a healthy, productive middle age. However, behavior changes cannot extend the maximum human life span, which seems to be built into our genes.

LIFE IN AN AGING AMERICA

As life expectancies increase, a larger proportion of the population will be in the later years; this change will necessitate new government policies and changes in our general attitudes toward elderly people.

America's Aging Minority

People over 65 are a large minority in the American population—over 30 million people, 12 percent of the total population in the 1990s. (For a statistical look at the elderly in America, see Figure 14-1.) As birth rates drop, the percentage is increasing dramatically. Many older people are happy, healthy, and self-sufficient. Changes that come with age, even negative ones, normally occur so gradually that most people adapt, some even gracefully.

Today the status of the aging is improving more than ever before. People now in their forties and fifties will probably benefit from new knowledge about the aging process. And the enormous increase in the over-55 population is markedly affecting our stereotypes of what it means to grow old. The misfortunes associated with aging—frailty, forgetfulness, poor health, isolation—occur to fewer people in their sixties and seventies and are shifting instead to burden the very old, those over 85.

Changing the Public's Idea of Aging

Aging people may be one of our least used and least appreciated resources. How can we employ the knowledge and productivity of our growing numbers of older citizens, particularly those now leaving the workforce through mandatory early retirement?

First, we must change our thinking about what aging means. We must learn to judge productivity rather than age. Capacity to function should replace age as a criterion for usefulness. Most people today are vigorous, in good health, mentally alert, and capable of making a productive contribution until they are at least 75 years old. The costs of losing what these people can contribute to our national productivity and quality of life are too high. Through their early retirement we forfeit substantial income-tax and Social Security tax revenues on earnings.

Alzheimer's disease A disease characterized by progressive loss of mental faculties caused by degeneration of brain cells.

Life expectancy The average length of life of members of a species.

Life span Theoretically projected length of life based on maximum potential of the human body in the best environment.

TERMS

Most people associate a visit to their physician with an illness or injury. But physicians can also play a crucial role in helping healthy people stay healthy. There are three primary components of preventive medical care: counseling about lifestyle and disease risks, appropriate immunizations, and screening tests for various diseases. Working together, you and your physician can help prevent many health problems and lessen the impact of any diseases you do develop. Preventive medicine is an important part of a healthy lifestyle.

Counseling

During periodic health checkups, your physician should counsel you about your disease risks, especially in areas where they are increased because of heredity, environment, or lifestyle. Your physician can reinforce the importance of many healthy behaviors, including eating a low-fat, high-fiber diet that contains adequate amounts of essential nutrients; controlling body fat; not smoking; using alcohol only in moderation and not in potentially dangerous situations; exercising regularly; practicing safer sex; avoiding unintended pregnancy (through abstinence or contraception); and not abusing drugs, illegal or prescription. Your physician might also advise you to wear a helmet while riding a motorcycle or bicycle, protect your back from injury on the job, or use sunscreen while outdoors. Although many of these behaviors are widely known as important parts of a healthy lifestyle, information and encouragement from a physician have been shown to be effective in motivating people to adopt healthy behaviors.

Immunizations

As discussed in earlier chapters, appropriate immunizations are an easy and effective way to protect yourself from certain infectious diseases. The need for immunization doesn't end with childhood. Everyone should receive a tetanus-diphtheria booster every 10 years. Anyone over age 65 should be immunized against influenza every year and receive a one-time pneumococcal vaccine. Physicians can help identify people in high-risk groups who may also need immunization against rubella, hepatitis B, or other diseases.

Screening Tests

Many tests are currently available to screen for early signs of disease. For a screening test to be truly useful, it must reliably detect a significant disease before symptoms develop, and the treatment for the disease must be more effective when begun before symptoms arise. A good example of a useful screening test is the Pap smear, which can identify cervical cancer before symptoms appear, when it is most easily cured. A test for an incurable form of lung cancer would not be a particularly useful test—if a person doesn't survive longer as a result of early diagnosis and treatment, it serves little purpose. The risk and cost of tests and treatment are also important issues to consider when evaluating screening tests.

Despite disagreements and limitations, some rough guidelines can be offered to help you select which medical tests to have and approximately how often they should be performed. These guidelines represent the minimum tests recommended for people *without symptoms*. If you have symptoms or are at risk for certain conditions, additional tests may be advised. Use the guidelines in the table below as a starting point, and discuss your particular needs with your physician. And remember, don't rely on medical testing to protect your health—a healthy lifestyle will do more to protect and promote your health than all the tests in the world.

Screening Test	Frequency
Medical and family history	Periodically
Total blood cholesterol	Every 5 years
Blood pressure	Every 2 years
Weight	Periodically
Sigmoidoscopy (a visual examination of the lower colon to detect colorectal cancer)	Every 5–10 years for anyone over age 50. Anyone at higher risk due to personal or family history should discuss appropriate screening with a physician.

Preventive Medicine for Healthy Adults (continued)

Screening Test	Frequency
Fecal occult blood test (a test for hidden blood in the stool to detect colon cancer)	Every 1–2 years. Anyone at increased risk for colon cancer due to personal or family history should discuss appropriate screening with a physician. (This test is of uncertain benefit for average-risk people age 50 and older.)
Skin examination	Periodically for anyone with history of excessive sun exposure or severe sunburns, skin cancer or precancerous skin conditions, family history of malignant melanoma.
Blood glucose (sugar) (a blood test for diabetes)	Periodically for anyone more than 50 pounds overweight, with a family history of diabetes or a history of diabetes during pregnancy, or of American Indian heritage.
Clinical breast exam (physical examination of breasts by health professional for breast cancer detection)	Every 1–2 years for all women over the age of 40; women at higher risk due to history of previous breast cancer or family history of breast cancer should have an exam every year beginning at age 35.
Breast self-exam (a self-examination for breast cancer detection)	Every month for all women over the age of 20
Mammogram (x-ray examination used to detect breast cancer)	Every 1–2 years for women age 50 to 75 who are of average risk (the test has less certain benefit between the ages of 40–50 and over age 75). Every year beginning at age 35 for women at higher risk due to personal or family history.
Pap test (an examination of the cells of the cervix for detection of cervical cancer)	Every 1–3 years for women ages 18–65 (less certain benefit after age 65 if previous tests normal)
Rubella antibodies (blood test for immunity to German measles)	Once for women of childbearing years who are fertile and do not know from previous blood tests if they are immune.
Sexually transmitted disease tests (gonorrhea, chlamydia, and syphilis)	Periodically for anyone with multiple sexual partners or history of other recent sexually transmitted diseases.
HIV testing (blood test for AIDS virus antibodies)	Periodically for anyone at risk (see Chapter 13).
Tuberculin skin test (PPD) (to detect infection with tuberculosis)	Periodically for anyone with close contact in the last two years with someone known to have tuberculosis or anyone who recently moved to the United States from Asia, Africa, Central America, South America, or Pacific Islands where TB is more common.
Testicular self-exam (a self-examination for testicular cancer)	Every month for men ages 18–45.

Recommendations adapted from U.S. Task Force Staff. 1989. *Guide to Clinical and Preventive Services: Report of the U.S. Preventive Services Task Force.* Baltimore: Williams and Wilkins; and H. C. Scott. 1994. Preventive health services in adults. *New England Journal of Medicine* 330(22): 1589–95.

Words of Wisdom: Attitudes Toward Aging Among Native Americans and Hispanic Americans

The following is excerpted from an article written by Dr. Robert Coles, a professor of psychiatry and medical humanities at Harvard Medical School.

Why are so many Americans afraid of growing old? This question occurred to me often during the three years my wife and I lived in New Mexico and Arizona. Not a day went by when we weren't reminded of how much Native American and Hispanic families value old age. These are cultures that grant dignity and authority to their elders.

One young Hispanic woman described to us her relationship with her parents, both in their seventies, in this way: "When I am wondering what to do about a problem, I turn to my mother or my father. Even if they are not here, I still turn to them. I picture them in my mind and I hear them saying words that make good sense." One day, this woman's father made a show of his humorous and practical good sense before his young grandson. "You know what my son said to me that night when he was going to bed?" the woman asked. "He told me he wished he could be old like his grandpapa!"

In another town, a Pueblo woman told us, "When my children ask me what it means to be a Pueblo Indian, I point to my parents, and I don't even talk." The woman went on to describe how her mother enhanced her own life. "She wants me to remember that the land, our land, was here before I came, and it will be here after I have left. 'We are visitors,' she always says, 'so we should be grateful for every day and not waste time with stupid things.' That is why old people

are here, to remind us of what is important and what is not."

To be old is to "last" oneself—to go through ups and downs, to survive bad luck and avoid successfully all sorts of hazards. To be old, then, is to be blessed by fate, by chance and circumstance. Pueblo Indians know that. One Hopi child drew me a picture of an old woman shaking hands with the moon. Then she explained, "When you're old, you're a full moon; you make the night a little less dark." For Hopi children, an older person is a source of encouragement, instruction, inspiration, a part of nature's awesome presence.

For many young people living in other parts of America, old age is regarded not as a major achievement but rather as a last, sad, brief way station. One boy in Boston commented, "It's no fun to be old; it's the worst thing in the world, except to die." To many of us, old age means abandonment, rejection, loneliness, a loss of respect from others, and subsequently a loss of self-respect. This is not the case, though, in Hispanic and Native American cultures. The elders we met in New Mexico and Arizona showed a great deal of self-confidence, and in general they seemed contented with their lives. In their contentment and harmony with nature lies a lesson for all of us.

Adapted from R. Coles. 1989. "Full-Moon Wisdom," in *New Choices for the Best Years*, September.

Those who retire at 62 start using their **Social Security** benefits earlier than otherwise.

A far better arrangement would be to make available full- and part-time volunteer and paid employment. We would benefit by providing retraining programs for both occupational and leisure time activities. We need more community-sponsored classes in remunerative activities such as real estate selling and management, horticulture, and library work, and in recreational and self-improvement activities such as music, writing, and health maintenance. Volunteer opportunities, such as preparing recordings for the blind, helping with activities for the retarded, and performing necessary tasks in hospitals, could be expanded. At the same time we could possibly change both public and private pension programs to make partial retirement possible. In such cases we could allow people to borrow against their Social Security benefits to finance their retraining or enrollment in wholly new educational programs.

There can be benefits to aging, but they don't come automatically. They require planning and wise choices ear-

lier in life. One octogenarian, Russell Lee, founder of a medical clinic in California, perceived the advantages of aging as growth: "The limitations imposed by time are compensated by the improved taste, sharper discretion, sounder mental and esthetic judgment, increased sensitivity and compassion, clearer focus—which all contribute to a more certain direction in living. The later years can be the best of life for which the earlier ones were preparation."

WHAT IS DEATH?

Death, like life, is change. When the body is no longer able to resist unhealthy changes in itself or is mechanically broken beyond repair, it ceases to function and dies.

Defining Death

Traditionally, death has been defined in clinical terms as occurring when the heart stops beating and breathing

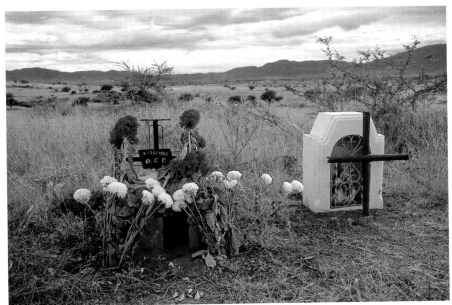

Death can challenge our sense of emotional and intellectual security, particularly the sudden death of a young person. These roadside markers were placed in memory of people killed in an automobile crash at this site.

ceases. Defining death in this way—as cessation of the flow of vital bodily fluids—is adequate for determining death in most cases. However, the use of respirators and other **life-support systems** in modern medicine allows some bodily functions to be artificially sustained. To determine death in such cases requires investigating the presence or absence of a physical response other than heartbeat or breathing.

Medical scientists now agree that the brain is the physical locus for determining whether a person is alive or dead. Thus, when a body is being kept alive on a respirator, for example, death is determined by measuring brain-wave activity. According to the standards published in 1968 by a Harvard Medical School committee, four characteristics describe **brain death:** (1) lack of receptivity and response to external stimuli, (2) absence of spontaneous muscular movement and spontaneous breathing, (3) absence of observable reflexes, and (4) absence of brain activity, signified by a flat **electroencephalogram** (EEG). The Harvard criteria call for a second set of tests to be performed after 24 hours have elapsed. They also exclude cases of hypothermia (body temperature below 90° F) as well as situations involving the presence of central nervous system depressants, such as barbiturates. Most states have adopted legislation that redefines death according to these criteria when conventional methods of determining death prove inconclusive.

In contrast to **clinical death,** which is determined according to the criteria just discussed, **cellular death** refers to a gradual process that takes place when heartbeat, respiration, and brain activity have stopped. It en-compasses the breakdown of metabolic processes in the cells, resulting in the complete cessation of function at the cellular level. Death can be defined biologically as the cessation of life resulting from irreversible changes in cell metabolism.

Why Is There Death?

Ultimately, no answer to the question of why death exists can be completely satisfying. Although we acknowledge that every living thing eventually dies, that recognition is of little comfort. Nor are we comforted by being told that

Social Security A government program that provides financial assistance to people who are unemployed, disabled, or retired (and over a certain age); financed through taxes on business and workers.

Life-support systems Medical technologies, such as the artificial respirator, used to keep alive patients who would otherwise die.

Brain death A medical definition of death that indicates final cessation of activity in the central nervous system as determined by the use of various diagnostic criteria, particularly a flat electroencephalogram reading.

Electroencephalogram (EEG) A tracing of electrical activity in the brain (brain waves) recorded by an electroencephalograph.

Clinical death A determination of death made according to accepted medical criteria.

Cellular death The total breakdown of metabolic processes at the level of the cell.

TERMS

matter and energy are never destroyed but simply changed. Most of us want our conscious self to continue. The notion of being reborn, with another consciousness, is not especially attractive.

Looking at the big picture, we see that death promotes variety. It permits the renewal and evolution of species. From a personal point of view, however, death challenges our sense of emotional and intellectual security—especially when it involves seemingly needless, accidental, or sudden death or the deaths of children or adults in the prime of life.

Attitudes Toward Death

Death is absolute loss. The death of a best friend, parent, mate, or child typically evokes feelings of confusion and pain. The prospect of our own death can be emotionally devastating. We prefer not to think about it—not so much because we don't know what will happen after death, but because death is the relinquishment, the letting go, of everything and everyone dear to us. Death forces us to puzzle out an understanding of its meaning in our lives. We may choose not to ponder some issues, such as the possibility of an afterlife, but we cannot refrain from facing the reality of death itself. Regardless of our explanations and efforts to minimize its effect, death is painful—both to the person who is dying and to those left behind.

Our attitudes toward death change as we grow and mature, as does our understanding of it. Very young children recognize death as an interruption and an absence, but their lack of a mature time perspective means they don't understand death is final. This view of death evolves considerably from about ages 5 to 9. Children come to understand that death is final, although initially this recognition applies only to others, not to themselves. They think they will somehow escape the universality of death (an illusion that even adults sometimes display by their risk-taking activities). By age 10 or so, most children do recognize that death is universal, inescapable, and irreversible. During the years of adolescence and young adulthood, the mature understanding of death is further refined by contemplating the impact of death on close relationships and the value of religious or philosophical answers to the enigma of death.

Personal Insight Think back to your first encounter with dying and death in your childhood. Who or what died—a pet, a relative, a neighbor? What were your feelings at the time, and what are your feelings as you recall the incident now? What were you told about death when you were a child? What would you tell your own children?

Once we acknowledge the inevitability of death, we can plan for it and thereby ease what otherwise could be difficult decisions for both our survivors and ourselves. Preparing for death requires completing unfinished business, dealing with medical care needs, allocating our time and other resources, and helping our survivors plan tasks that will be carried out after we die. People who unexpectedly find themselves in the midst of a painful and debilitating terminal illness may be so drained physically and emotionally that they are unable to make prudent decisions that could have easily been made before the onset of crisis.

Indeed, some decisions can be made while you are young. Decisions about a will, for example, can and should be made as early as the college years. Adequate planning can help to ensure that a sudden, unexpected death is not made even more difficult for survivors. Although some decisions cannot be made until one is actually in a particular situation, other decisions can be anticipated and discussed with close relatives and friends.

Making a Will

A will is a legal document expressing a person's intentions and wishes for the disposition of his or her property after death. It is a declaration of how a person's estate—that is, everything he or she owns—will be distributed upon that person's death. During the life of the **testator** (the person making the will), a will can be changed, replaced, or revoked.

When a person dies **intestate**—that is, without having left a valid will—his or her property is distributed according to rules set up by the state. A court-appointed administrator supervises the distribution and is awarded a commission taken directly from the estate. Although the distribution may be just the way you would have done it, chances are it will not be.

To avoid having property undergo **probate**—the process of settling an estate—in addition to making a will, you might want to consider transferring title to property or adding names for joint ownership. Sensible, legal steps can be taken to avoid probate or at least minimize its cost. It is usually helpful to involve family members in the process of will making and financial planning to prevent problems that might arise when such actions are taken without the knowledge of those who will be affected.

Choosing Where to Die

Would you prefer to spend your last days at home tended by relatives and friends? Or would you rather have access to the sophisticated medical techniques available in the hospital setting? Would hospice care, with its emphasis on alleviation of pain and family involvement, be your choice for care at the end of life? Although the place where we die is not always something we can choose, we can and should consider the alternatives.

Home   Until well into the early decades of this century, virtually everyone died at home. Now, however, most deaths occur in an institutional setting, usually a hospital or nursing home. Although few Americans now spend their last days at home, advocates of home care believe that a person's home is the preferred setting for terminal care at the end stage of an illness. Among the advantages of home care, the most obvious is that the dying person is in a familiar setting, one intimately connected with family and friends. However, home care requires support not only from the patient's family and friends, but also from skilled, professional caregivers who supervise the care being provided at home and provide relief when necessary.

Hospital   Hospitals are organized to provide short-term intensive treatment for acute injury and illness. Highly specialized care is provided to patients who usually stay in the hospital only briefly before returning to normal life. Because of this emphasis on acute care, hospitals are generally not well suited to meet the needs of patients expected to die from terminal disease. However, some medical institutions have instituted **palliative care** programs to care for patients who are not expected to recover. Unlike acute care, which involves active measures to sustain life, palliative care is focused on providing relief from pain while acknowledging that further treatment is futile.

Hospice   The concept of **hospice** care grew out of the perception that the care of the dying within conventional hospital settings was inadequate. Hospice care is an alternative to both home care—especially when families need relief—and hospital care. Its goals are to help provide a dignified, comfortable death and to care for the patient and family together. Most hospice programs are based on home care and offer support to the family members and friends who are providing the primary care; hospice programs can also be administered in a hospital or other institutional setting.

How does hospice care differ from other types of health care? The goal of hospice care is to relieve pain and symptoms rather than to cure the disease. Sophisticated pain management techniques are used to maximize comfort and alertness. The emphasis is on enhancing the quality of life rather than extending its length. The focus is on the person rather than the disease, and the interdisciplinary hospice team addresses the medical, emotional, psychological, and spiritual needs of both the patient and his or her family.

Deciding Whether to Prolong Life

If you were diagnosed with a terminal illness, would you want to be kept alive on life-support systems? Framing an answer to this question could determine the quality of the final phase of your life. Many people are alive today because of advanced medical technology, such as the heart pacemaker and the kidney dialysis machine. In spite of successes, however, modern medical innovations do not always clearly confer benefits.

The medical approach that strives to keep people alive by all means and at any expense is being questioned. The human organism often can be kept alive despite the cessation of normal heart, brain, respiratory, or kidney function. Should a patient without any hope of recovery be kept alive by means of artificial life support? What if the patient has fallen into a **persistent vegetative state**—that is, profound unconsciousness, lacking any sign of normal reflexes and unresponsive to external stimuli, with no reasonable hope of improvement?

Ethical questions about the "right to die" have become widespread in American society since the landmark case of Karen Ann Quinlan; in 1975 at age 22 she was admitted in a comatose state to an intensive care unit where her breathing was soon being sustained by a respirator. When she remained unresponsive in a persistent vegetative state, her parents requested that the respirator be disconnected, but this request was denied by the medical staff responsible for Karen's care. Eventually, the request reached the New Jersey Supreme Court, which ruled that artificial respiration could be discontinued.

More recently, courts in various parts of the country have ruled on requests to remove other forms of life support, including artificial feeding mechanisms that provide nutrition and hydration to comatose patients who are able to breathe on their own. The case of Nancy Beth Cruzan was heard before the U.S. Supreme Court in 1990. As a result of injuries she received in 1983, Cruzan was in a persistent vegetative state. Physicians had implanted a feeding tube to provide nourishment, the only form of life support she was receiving. As in the case of Karen Quinlan, when Nancy Cruzan's parents requested that artificial life support be withdrawn, hospital person-

TERMS

Testator   A person who dies with a will in force.

Intestate   Situation in which a person dies having made no legal will.

Probate   The legal process of establishing a will as valid and settling an estate.

Palliative care   Measures taken to reduce the intensity of a disease, especially those involving control of pain and other symptoms.

Hospice   A facility or program designed to provide care and support for terminally ill patients.

Persistent vegetative state   A condition of profound unconsciousness caused by disease or injury in which an individual lacks normal reflexes and is unresponsive to external stimuli, lasting for an extended period with no reasonable hope of improvement.

nel refused, arguing that the state had an inherent interest in preserving life.

The Supreme Court ruled that states are justified in making a requirement that only the patient can decide to withdraw treatment. Since Nancy apparently had not provided a clear expression of her wishes on the matter before her accident, the state was not bound to honor the wishes of her parents. However, a few months later, in light of new testimony from several of Nancy's friends that she had expressed her wishes "not to live like a vegetable," a state court ruled that the "clear and convincing" evidence standard now had been met and permission was obtained for removal of the feeding tube. This case points up the value of expressing one's wishes regarding life-sustaining measures, preferably in writing, before the need for such a statement arises.

Allowing Someone to Die   When suffering outweighs the benefits of continued existence, many people argue that individuals have a "right to die," whether or not they choose to exercise that right. Withdrawing or not initiating treatments that could potentially sustain life is sometimes termed **passive euthanasia**, although many medical practitioners and ethicists reject this term because it tends to confuse the generally unacceptable and unlawful practice of actively causing death with the fairly well-established practice of withholding or withdrawing useless treatments. It is increasingly considered good medical practice not to artificially prolong the life and suffering of a person whose condition is inevitably fatal. Courts also seem to be coming to a consensus that mentally competent, informed patients have the right to refuse medical treatment, including life support provided by mechanical or artificial means.

TERMS

Passive euthanasia   The practice of withholding (not initiating) or withdrawing (removing) life-prolonging but ultimately futile treatment, thereby allowing a terminally ill person to die naturally.

Active euthanasia   The practice of intentionally hastening the death of a person who requests it to avoid a painful or prolonged dying.

Lethal injection   The administering, by injection, of a drug intended to result in death.

Living will   A document enabling individuals to provide instructions about the kind of medical care they wish to receive or refuse, including the use of life-sustaining procedures, should they become unable to participate in treatment decisions. A living will often states that the individual's life should not be sustained by artificial means or medical heroics if recovery is impossible.

Power of attorney   A legal instrument allowing one person to act as the agent of another person.

Active Euthanasia   In contrast to withdrawing or withholding treatment, **active euthanasia** refers to the practice of intentionally hastening the death of a terminal patient who requests it in order to avoid a painful and prolonged dying. Death in such cases is usually hastened by a **lethal injection.** The distinction between passive and active euthanasia is sometimes characterized as the difference between "letting die" and "killing" (although advocates of active euthanasia prefer the phrase "helping to die").

In most countries, including the United States, taking active steps to end someone's life is a crime, even if the motive is based on good intentions. Thus, active euthanasia, which has been called "the most compassionate of crimes," must also be the most secret. As a result, few cases of active euthanasia are reported. Also, because dying patients are often heavily dosed with painkilling drugs that have potentially lethal side effects, the immediate cause of death may not be entirely certain.

Many people who endorse the philosophy of hospice and palliative care argue that adequate treatment for pain and depression usually eliminates the need to consider active measures to end a patient's life. According to this view, the distinction between active euthanasia and allowing to die ought to be maintained. However, a patient who is surrounded by an array of machinery and tubes may seem less a human being than an extension of medical technology. In such situations the claims in favor of a human being's "right to die" are most clearly and emotionally rendered. If we wish to avoid the burden on ourselves and on medical practitioners of actively hastening patients' deaths, it follows that we must actively seek better ways of lifting the burden of suffering experienced by the dying.

Living Wills   Since the mid-1970s, most American states have enacted legislation that allows people to complete a **living will** or other form of advance directive to express their wishes regarding medical care in the event of a terminal condition. Most such documents state that if the person is suffering from a terminal illness or injury that is certified by one (sometimes two) physicians, his or her life should not be sustained by artificial means or heroic measures.

In light of the increasingly widespread judicial standard of "clear and convincing evidence" of a patient's wishes regarding life-sustaining treatment, it may be prudent to complete both a living will and a **power of attorney** for health care. While the living will, as an advance directive, allows you to specify your wishes in case you become unable to speak for yourself, the power of attorney for health care allows you to designate a proxy—that is, a trusted friend or relative—who can act on your behalf to make a broad range of medical decisions and to see that your wishes are carried out should the need arise.

Helping Terminally Ill Patients Die: Is It Legal? Is It Ethical?

In 1990, a 54-year-old teacher named Janet Adkins was diagnosed with Alzheimer's disease. Although the disease was still in its early stages, Adkins decided she could not face a future of increasing dementia and personality loss. With the help of Jack Kevorkian, a Detroit physician, Adkins ended her own life swiftly and calmly with a lethal injection of potassium chloride. The device she used was invented by Kevorkian and is endorsed by some advocates of the "right to die" movement. Kevorkian's role in Adkins's death, and in others since then, has been hotly debated in the medical and legal communities, fueling the arguments for and against legalized euthanasia.

Many patients facing a terminal illness may wish to end their pain and suffering by refusing medical treatment that prolongs life. As of 1990, this choice is sanctioned by law. In the case of *Cruzan vs. Missouri,* the Supreme Court decided that a person has the right, according to the Constitution, to refuse life-sustaining medical treatment. Subsequently, Congress passed the Patient Self-Determination Act, which requires that all government-funded health care providers inform patients of their right to refuse medical treatment. Hospitals and physicians, then, are permitted to withhold or withdraw treatment when a patient is in a persistent vegetative state, with no chance of recovery, and when there is evidence that the person wants no life-prolonging treatment—for example, if the person communicated these wishes through a living will or other advance directive. In fact, perhaps as a result of the *Cruzan vs. Missouri* case, living wills have become more popular.

Although the 1990 Supreme Court ruling permits withdrawal or non-initiation of treatments, it does not enable health care workers to assist actively in a patient's choice to die, as in the case of Janet Adkins. Many "right to die" advocates want physician-assisted suicide to be legalized, and the issue of euthanasia has found a political forum. In 1991 and 1992, voters in Washington and California rejected initiatives that would legalize physician-assisted suicide. In 1994, an Oregon initiative that allows physicians to prescribe lethal drugs so that terminally ill patients can end their own lives passed by a narrow margin. About half of the states consider assisted suicide to be a crime; in others there are no legal statutes that define the act of assisted suicide.

The issue of suicide—whether assisted or not—is a complex one. On the whole, Americans value quality of life, humane treatment for pain and suffering, and the right of free choice for individuals. At the same time, society places a high value on the very nature of life, and Americans tend to fear the consequences of condoning suicide. To many people, it simply seems unethical to accept death as a solution, because it devalues human life. Attitudes toward suicide are also shaped by religion. Christian doctrine holds that humans have no inherent right to control their own death. So suicide, whether assisted or not, runs contrary to most religious belief in America.

Attitudes are also shaped by our views toward physicians and the health care system in America. Some people fear that if assisted suicide becomes legal, health care workers may abuse patients' trust or that errors in judgment will result in unnecessary deaths. Many people believe that sanctioning assisted suicide will negate the advances in medical science that offer hope to terminally ill patients. Cures may arrive before a patient dies, or advances in pain management may sufficiently relieve a patient's discomfort and enhance his or her quality of life. Finally, there is concern that the growing "right to die" movement may be a response to rising health care costs: Patients may look to death as a solution only because the expense of medical treatment may be burdensome.

In spite of these attitudes, many Americans seem to believe that people have the right to terminate their lives and to seek help in doing so. In a recent Gallup Poll, 58 percent of the respondents said that a person with an incurable disease has the moral right to end his or her life; 66 percent said that a person in great pain and with no hope of improvement has such a right; and 65 percent said that physicians should be allowed to end a patient's life if requested to do so by the patient and the patient's family. With strong feelings on both sides of this issue, physician-assisted suicide is certain to remain a subject of heated debate in the years ahead.

Adapted from "The Final Chapter." *Harvard Health Letter,* February 1995; R. L. Worsnop. 1992. "Assisted Suicide." *CQ Researcher,* 21 February, pp. 147–51; "Euthanasia: What Is the 'Good Death'?" *The Economist,* 20 July 1991, pp. 21–24.

Personal Insight   How do you think you would feel if someone you loved were terminally ill and in pain and asked to be allowed to die? What would you do? How do you think you would feel if a close friend told you he or she wanted to die because of depression and an inability to cope with life's problems? What would you do?

Donating Organs

A human body is a valuable resource. Of all the recent advances in medical techniques for helping patients who were formerly considered beyond recovery, probably the best known and most widely accepted is the transplantation of human organs. Eye corneas can be transplanted to give sight to the blind. Kidneys can give years of vigorous life to people whose own have stopped working. Human

UNIFORM DONOR CARD

of _____
(print or type name of donor)

In the hope that I may help others, I hereby make this anatomical gift, if medically acceptable, to take effect upon my death. The words and marks below indicate my wishes.

I give: (a)_____any needed organs or parts
(b)_____only the following organs or parts

_____
(specify the organ(s), tissue(s) or part(s))

for the purposes of transplantation, therapy, medical research or education;

(c)_____my body for anatomical study if needed

Limitations or special wishes, if any: _____

Signed by the donor and the following two witnesses in the presence of each other:

_____   _____
Signature of Donor   Date of Birth of Donor

_____   _____
Date Signed   City and State

_____   _____
Witness   Witness

This is a legal document under the Anatomical Gift Act or similar laws.
☐ Yes, I have discussed my wishes with my family.
For further information consult your physician or

THE NATIONAL KIDNEY FOUNDATION
30 East 33rd Street   New York, NY 10016

Figure 14-2 *A sample organ donor card.*

skin is the best dressing for burn wounds. Bones can be used for grafting. In some parts of the world, undiseased blood from dead bodies is used for transfusions. Perhaps the most dramatic organ transplants are those involving the heart. Although some people may find the thought of donating organs unsettling, the procedures aren't very different from those used in routine autopsies and normal preparation for burial.

The Uniform Anatomical Gift Act, approved in 1968 and enacted in some form in all 50 states, provides for the donation of the body or specific body parts upon the donor's death. The most widely used method for donating body parts is through the **Uniform Donor Card,** which is available from the National Kidney Foundation (Figure 14-2). In some states, the desire to donate organs can be communicated by use of a card attached to a person's driver's license. Besides specifying how one's body may be used after death, the donor may also specify the final disposition of his or her remains once the donation has been

completed. Many donations are authorized by relatives at the time of a loved one's death. Plans for organ or body donation should be discussed with members of your family so that they are aware of your wishes and can help see that they are fulfilled.

Deciding What to Do with the Body

Most people have a preference about how their body will be disposed of when they die. For Americans, this decision usually involves either burial or cremation. Burial can be in a single grave dug into the soil or entombment in a multitiered mausoleum. Cremation involves burning a body to its bones by intense heat. Cremated remains can be buried, entombed, kept by the family, or scattered at sea or on land, in accordance with state and local laws. If a body or organ donation has been made, burial or cremation will take place once the donation procedures have been completed. Depending on the type of funeral ceremony desired, a body destined for burial or cremation may or may not be embalmed.

Plans for body disposition may be made explicit by executing a preplanned (or "pre-need") arrangement with a funeral home or memorial society. Decisions about how one's body will be disposed of after death are best considered early in life while a person is healthy and able to gather the necessary information about available choices.

Planning a Funeral or Memorial Service

It is generally agreed that bereaved persons benefit from participating in a ceremony to mark the death of a loved one. The choice of funeral rites may involve a traditional funeral ceremony or a simple memorial service. The tone of the rites might reflect a somber remembrance of the deceased or a more upbeat wake or party. Some people express the preference for no services, although bereaved friends and relatives generally benefit from the opportunity to mark their grief through ritual and ceremony. Ideally, last rites and body disposition will be planned in agreement with the wishes and needs of one's survivors.

A typical American Christian funeral ceremony involves **embalming** the corpse, viewing the body in the funeral home before the funeral service, a religious ceremony with the body present, and a processional to the graveside where a brief final ceremony is held. Other religious traditions follow different practices, as do other ethnic groups. In a pluralistic society like the United States, there are many ways of constructing a meaningful funeral or memorial service.

Some people choose a minimal role in caring for their dead loved ones; others seek more active participation. A ceremony can develop in whatever way is appropriate and meaningful for those involved. It may be held indoors or outside in natural surroundings. The participants may choose to voice their feelings about the deceased or simply share their loss in silence. A member of

TERMS

Uniform Donor Card A consent form authorizing the use of the signer's body parts for transplantation or medical research upon his or her death.

Embalming Removing blood and other fluids from a body and replacing them with chemicals to disinfect and temporarily retard deterioration of the corpse.

the clergy or other leader may be called upon to officiate, or the participants may create their own form of ritual to mark the deceased's passing from the community. The sharing of grief may be expressed in a common meal, dancing, singing, or prayer.

THE EXPERIENCE OF LIFE-THREATENING ILLNESS

People with life-threatening illness face costly medical care, loss of earnings, repeated and often lengthy hospitalization, and the emotional havoc that accompanies the news of a potentially terminal condition. The emotional response to life-threatening illness can include anguish, a sense of hopelessness, depression, and feelings of isolation and loneliness. Gathering information about the disease and its treatment, sharing one's experience in settings where mutual support can be provided, and finding ways of communicating more clearly with caregivers as well as with family and friends are all examples of positive approaches to dealing with life-threatening illness.

Coping with Dying

How do individuals come to terms with the prospect of dying? In his book *Dying,* John Hinton noted that about half of the dying people he observed openly acknowledged their death and accepted it. Of the remaining half, about a quarter spoke with undisguised anguish about their impending death, and the other quarter denied it entirely and did not speak about it at all. When death confronts us squarely, even if we have come to some degree of acceptance, we may yet hope for a last-minute reprieve. The way each of us copes with dying will likely resemble the ways we've coped with living and with other losses in our lives.

After talking with hundreds of dying people, Elisabeth Kübler-Ross identified several common, although not inevitable, psychological stages that people experience while coping with the prospect of imminent death. She described this coping process in her landmark study *On Death and Dying.* In an idealized model, an early period of shock, disbelief, and denial eventually gives way to some degree of acceptance. It should be emphasized that not everyone experiences each of the psychological stages, or states, listed below, nor are they necessarily experienced in the same order or for the same duration. Indeed, some reactions may be experienced simultaneously, and there is a cycling between the various states during different phases of the illness. Dealing with these intense emotions can enable the dying person to arrive at a personal sense of acceptance with respect to his or her impending death.

- *Denial and isolation.* The initial stage of coping with terminal illness is characterized as a temporary state of shock in which people deny the fact of death and isolate themselves from further confrontation with it. They insist "It can't be." Denial is a useful coping mechanism because it acts as a buffer against shock and allows time for the mobilization of other defenses.

- *Anger.* When the truth can no longer be denied, anger often follows. People ask "Why me?" and may lash out at family members, their physicians, and the hospital staff—blaming them for the situation. Anger is a normal response to disability and the loss of control over one's life and situation.

- *Bargaining.* As a means of marshaling what hope remains, people often try to find a way out. A common scenario involves making promises to God in exchange for a prolonged life. The intense desire to find an "out" can also cause people to grasp at straws, becoming vulnerable to so-called miracle cures promoted by quacks and charlatans.

- *Depression.* When people begin to accept their fate and face the reality of their impending death, they may become depressed about things that will be left unfinished in their lives and all they are leaving behind. Depression is a natural part of grief as a person strives to prepare for separation from this world. Although depression is emotionally painful, it is an appropriate step in the process of coming to terms with loss; it is eased when people are allowed to express their sorrow in an atmosphere of nonjudgmental support and compassion.

- *Acceptance.* People facing their own death may eventually come to some resolution about their situation. They are no longer angry or depressed, nor are they searching for some kind of miracle to change their fate. They accept the reality that nothing is certain until it happens, and they are willing to live to the fullest extent possible in the time that remains to them. It often seems that they are able to suspend judgment or expectations about the future and simply appreciate the present. Acknowledging that they are ultimately not in control of their future, they seem content to make the best of what comes their way. At the end, when death is near, they may choose not to talk much with visitors, even family members and close friends. This, too, is part of letting go.

Again, this list is a general description of the coping process, not a schedule to be strictly followed or imposed on a particular situation. Each person's patterns of coping should be respected.

Personal Insight If you were told you had a short time to live, what would you do—withdraw, try to tie up loose ends, try to satisfy unfulfilled desires or have new experiences, try to take care of others, make no changes? Why do you think you would react this way?

Supporting a Dying Person

Most people feel somewhat uncomfortable in the presence of a person who has been diagnosed with a terminal illness. What can we say? How should we act? It may seem that any attempt to provide comfort results in words that are little more than stale platitudes. Nevertheless, we want to express our concern and make meaningful contact. Perhaps the most important gift we can bring to the person who is confronting his or her own death is the gift of listening. Giving the person an opportunity to speak honestly and openly about his or her experience is crucial, even though talking about death may be painful at first.

Although we sometimes tend to place dying people in a special category, the reality is that their needs are not fundamentally different from anyone else's, although their situation is perhaps more urgent. As is true of anyone, dying people want to know that they are valued, that they are not alone, that they are not being unfairly judged, and that those close to them are also trying to come to terms with a difficult situation. As with any relationship, there are opportunities for growth on both sides.

COPING WITH LOSS

Even if we have not experienced the death of someone close, all of us are survivors of the various losses that have occurred in our lives. Death is not the only kind of loss that calls upon our resources for coping; everyone experiences the losses that accompany changes and endings. The loss of a job, the ending of a relationship, transitions from one neighborhood or school to another—all these are examples of the kinds of losses that fill our lives. Some people call these losses "little deaths," and our response to them, although less painful perhaps, includes many of the mental and emotional reactions that occur in connection with the deaths of loved ones.

Grieving

Grief encompasses a person's emotional response to the event of loss. It can include feelings of sadness, longing, loneliness, and sorrow, as well as feelings of guilt, anger, and rage. When we recognize that many kinds of feelings occur in grief—not just feelings of sadness—then we are likely to be better able to accept our grief and move toward its resolution. Grieving is the means to healing.

When a loved one dies after a long period of illness, survivors may experience feelings of relief that the ordeal is over as well as anguish at the ending of a beloved relationship. When death takes someone close to you, anger may be felt over unresolved issues in the relationship. The emotions that occur in grief are much like those experienced by a dying person: shock, disbelief, denial, anger, guilt, vulnerability, depression. The bereaved person is

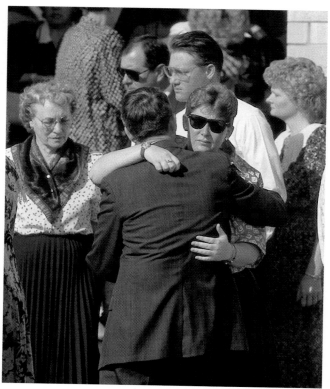

Funeral or memorial services give friends and relatives of the deceased the opportunity to mark their grief through ritual and ceremony.

likely to experience many different feelings, often conflicting ones.

Talking and crying, even yelling in rage, are ways of resolving the intense feelings of grief. Don't try to hold back feelings or to be "strong" and "brave." Those who offer such advice do not understand the dynamics of grief, nor the necessity for grief to be expressed as a way of healing. On the other hand, you needn't pretend to grieve or exaggerate your emotions if the strong feelings that often accompany grief simply aren't present in your experience.

Although various models have been proposed to summarize the processes associated with grief, each person's actual experience is highly individual. We can use such models as an aid to understanding grief, but it is important that we do not try to superimpose a rigid structure on our own or another's experience.

In the aftermath of a death, the early period of grief is characterized by shock and numbness, often with strong feelings of disbelief and denial. We can't believe that the devastating loss has happened; it can't be real. The sense of disorganization that pervades our mental and emotional life during this period is challenged by the need to attend to the various actions and decisions surrounding the disposition of the deceased's body. Being forced to engage in such activities is therapeutic; it helps us accept the reality of the death, thereby taking us beyond the initial

- Realize and recognize the loss.
- Take time for nature's slow, sure, stuttering process of healing.
- Give yourself massive doses of restful relaxation and routine busy-ness.
- Know that powerful, overwhelming feelings will lessen with time.
- Be vulnerable, share your pain, and be humble enough to accept support.
- Surround yourself with life: plants, animals, and friends.
- Use mementos to help your mourning, not to live in the dead past.
- Avoid rebound relationships, big decisions, and anything addictive.

- Keep a diary and record successes, memories, and struggles.
- Prepare for change, new interests, new friends, solitude, creativity, growth.
- Recognize that forgiveness (of ourselves and others) is a vital part of the healing process.
- Know that holidays and anniversaries can bring up the painful feelings you thought you had successfully worked through.
- Realize that any new death-related crisis will bring up feelings about past losses.

Source: The Centre for Living with Dying

period of shock and into the intense grief work that is at the heart of coping with loss.

The middle phase of grief, then, is a period of intense grief work as we experience the pain of separation. The bustle of activities that takes place immediately after a death begins to lessen, and friends are usually not as accessible as they had been during the initial crisis. This is often a time of intense yearning for the lost loved one, an intense reexamination of the whole relationship as the bonds of attachment are slowly relinquished. Survivors experience fantasies of somehow "undoing" the loss, making everything as it was before. Varying considerably among survivors and depending, too, on the circumstances of the loss, this phase of grief generally lasts from several weeks to several months. It is during this period that many physiological symptoms associated with intense grief are experienced: lethargy, restlessness, disturbed sleep, lack of appetite, and weight loss.

As survivors and as caring helpers, we need to keep in mind that social support is every bit as critical during this phase of grief as during the early days following the loss. To go through the psychological process of mourning, the bereaved person needs to express his or her feelings. As the reality of the loss is absorbed, the predominant feeling will likely be sadness. By gradually undoing the bonds of the lost relationship through intense grieving, emotions are slowly freed for reinvestment in life.

The last phase of "active" grief is characterized as a period of resolution, a time of reestablishing our physical and emotional balance, of reintegration. The acute feelings and emotional turmoil of grief are no longer experienced constantly. Our sadness doesn't go away completely, but it recedes into the background. Reminders will stimulate the pain of loss from time to time, but we begin to move ahead with life and focus more on present concerns, not past memories. This new-found sense of freedom can be difficult to admit at first; it may feel like a betrayal of the deceased loved one. In fact, it indicates a healthy willingness to engage once again in the outside world. Coming to terms with grief does not mean forgetting the loved one or denying the significance of the lost relationship. At various times throughout our lives, reminders of the loss can stimulate a recurrence of grief; as time passes, however, this happens with diminishing frequency and intensity.

Supporting a Grieving Person

A variety of activities, rituals, and social institutions can help survivors cope with loss. Social support provided by relatives and friends can be a major source of strength for the bereaved. The simple gift of listening can be extremely helpful, since talking about a loss is an important way that survivors cope with their changed reality. The key to being a good listener is to refrain from making judgments about whether the feelings expressed by the survivor are "right" or "wrong," "good" or "bad." The feelings generated by a loss are not necessarily the ones we might expect. However, they are valid in terms of a particular survivor's total response to bereavement. We are endowed with two ears and one mouth, and that ratio between listening and speaking can guide our conversations with recently bereaved friends and relatives.

COMING TO TERMS WITH DEATH

Encountering death can help make us more aware of the preciousness of life. In facing death, we find that relationships are more important than things; priorities are reordered as we cope with the painful reality of loss. Realizing that life offers no guarantees, we find ourselves able to overcome our own anxieties and petty concerns as well as the social structures that prevent us from living our lives more fully.

Examining our assumptions about death leads us to a discovery of its meaning in our own lives. Denying death eventually results in denying life. This denial is inherent in our news reports, where only the deaths of the famous or violent deaths get attention, and then only for a fleeting moment. In societies where each individual is considered to be important and irreplaceable, death is not ignored but is marked by community-wide grief for a genuine social loss. When we stop avoiding death, we find that it is an event whose significance touches not only the individual and his or her family and friends, but also the wider community of which we are all part.

SUMMARY

- People who take charge of their health in youth have greater control over the physical and mental aspects of aging.

Generating Vitality as You Age

- Many characteristics traditionally considered to be consequences of aging are due rather to neglect and abuse of body and mind. Nevertheless, aging is inevitable, a result of biochemical processes.
- A lifetime of interests and hobbies helps maintain creativity and intelligence.
- Exercise throughout life enhances physical and mental health.
- A low-fat, high-carbohydrate diet that includes a variety of foods promotes health at every age. Obesity leads to premature aging.
- Alcohol abuse is a common but often hidden problem, as is overdependence on medications. Tobacco use not only shortens life but also may cause severe health impairment for many years.
- Regular physical examinations help detect conditions that can shorten life and make old age less healthy. Immunizations protect against preventable infectious diseases.
- Stress increases wear and tear on the body; getting enough sleep, avoiding drugs, and practicing relaxation help reduce stress.

Confronting the Changes of Aging

- Retirement can be a fulfilling and enjoyable time of life for those who adjust to their new roles, enjoy participating in a variety of activities, and have planned ahead for financial stability.
- Decreased energy levels require older people to set priorities for their activities. Successful aging involves anticipating and accommodating physical limitations.
- Slight confusion and forgetfulness are not signs of a serious illness; severe symptoms may indicate Alzheimer's disease or another form of dementia.
- Resolving grief and mourning and dealing with depression are important tasks for older adults; adopting a flexible attitude can help.

Aging and Life Expectancy

- Life expectancy, which has risen dramatically in the 1900s, is generally greater among women. Life expectancy increases with age.
- The maximum potential human life span seems to be 100 to 110 years; environmental and behavioral factors prevent most people from achieving it.

Life in an Aging America

- People over 65 form a large minority in the United States, and their status is improving.
- The aged represent an underused resource; society needs to learn to consider productivity and capacity to function rather than age.

What Is Death?

- Brain death is characterized by lack of receptivity and response to external stimuli; absence of spontaneous muscular movement and spontaneous breathing; absence of observable reflexes; and absence of brain activity, signified by a flat electroencephalogram.
- Clinical death refers to a determination of death made according to either the traditional signs of death or the criteria used in defining brain death. Cellular death refers to the breakdown of metabolic processes in the cells when heartbeat, respiration, and brain activity cease.
- Although death is logical in terms of species survival and evolution, no answer to the question of why death exists can ever be completely satisfying.
- From about age 10, most children understand that death is universal, inescapable, and irreversible.

Planning for Death

- A will is a legal instrument governing the distribution of a person's property after his or her death.

- Dying at home requires considerable time and energy from relatives or friends.
- Palliative care devoted to making dying patients comfortable and pain-free is available in many hospitals.
- The hospice philosophy of care stresses a team approach in providing palliative care to dying patients and relies to a large extent on volunteer help.
- Passive euthanasia refers to the practice of withdrawing or withholding life-sustaining treatment. Active euthanasia refers to the practice of intentionally hastening the death of a patient.
- Living wills, powers of attorney for health care, and other advance directives are vehicles for expressing one's wishes about the use of life-sustaining measures.
- All states have legal provisions that allow people to donate their bodies or individual organs for use after death.
- For Americans, the decision about what to do with the body after death usually involves either burial or cremation.

The Experience of Life-threatening Illness

- Facing death is a difficult and painful experience. Responses to one's own imminent death vary greatly, although periods of denial and isolation, anger, bargaining, depression, and acceptance are commonly experienced.
- Those who wish to offer support to a dying person should consider that person's unique needs. Giving the dying person opportunities to speak openly is crucial.

Coping with Loss

- Grieving is the emotional process of healing the pain of loss, and it can include a variety of feelings.
- Social support provided by relatives and friends is a major source of strength for the bereaved.

Coming to Terms with Death

- Encountering death can help make a person more aware of the preciousness and precariousness of life.
- Death touches not only the individual and his or her family and friends, but also the wider community.

TAKE ACTION

1. Interview your parents or grandparents to find out how they want to spend their old age. Do they want to live at home, in a retirement community, with a relative? Do they plan to live on a pension, retirement account, Social Security? Have they made any concrete plans, or have they not yet confronted those decisions?

2. Interview several people from different cultural backgrounds about their attitudes toward aging and elderly people. How do they view the aging process? How are elderly people treated or viewed in their culture? Do you notice any significant differences between their attitudes and yours?

3. In some states, the motor vehicle department now sends organ donor forms to residents along with auto registration materials. Individuals can fill them out and keep them with their driver's license. If your state doesn't provide them, you can also request a Uniform Donor Card from the National Kidney Foundation (30 East 33rd St., New York, NY 10016). When you receive the donor form, consider the advantages and disadvantages of being a donor. If you decide to be a donor, fill out the card and keep it with your driver's license.

4. Obtain sample copies of a living will and a durable power of attorney for health care that are appropriate for the state you live in. Check with your local hospital or health services organization for these forms or request them from Choice in Dying (200 Varick Street, New York, NY 10014). After you have reviewed the forms, consider the advantages and disadvantages of their use. If you decide to execute a living will or durable power of attorney for health care, discuss your decision with members of your family to make them aware of your wishes.

JOURNAL ENTRY

1. Imagine that you are very old and are looking back on your life. What will have given you satisfaction—a successful career, parenthood, happiness, travel, self-knowledge? Make a list in your health journal of your life goals and priorities. What actions can you take now to work toward your goals? Choose one goal and take an action this week that moves you toward it.

2. What do you believe happens after death—heaven or hell, eternal sleep, nothingness, return to life in another form, union with a higher consciousness, something mysterious and unknowable? Write a brief essay explaining your concept or belief. Where did it come from? Is it what you wish would happen after death?

3. *Critical Thinking:* Research the issue of physician-assisted suicide (active euthanasia). Write a brief essay that presents the main arguments on both sides of the issue; conclude your essay with a statement of your

own opinion. Be sure to explain your reasoning. What are the most important factors in your decision? Why do you think you hold the opinion you do?

SELECTED BIBLIOGRAPHY

Adler, L. 1991. *Centenarians: People over 100 a Triumph of Will and Spirit.* New York: Heal Press.

Annas, G. J. 1991. *The Rights of Patients: The Basic ACLU Guide to Patients' Rights,* 2nd ed. Clifton, N.J.: Humana Press.

Aging successfully: How to succeed at the business of growing older. 1992. *Mayo Clinic Health Letter.* November.

Callahan, D. 1990. *What Kind of Life: The Limits of Medical Progress.* New York: Simon and Schuster.

Cox, H. 1991. *Annual Editions: Aging.* New York: Dushkin.

DeSpelder, L. A., and A. L. Strickland. 1996. *The Last Dance: Encountering Death and Dying,* 4th ed. Mountain View, Calif.: Mayfield.

Douglass, R. L., and L. Pearson. 1992. *Domestic Mistreatment of the Elderly: Toward Prevention.* Washington, D.C.: AARP.

Duda, D. 1982. *A Guide to Dying at Home.* Santa Fe, N. Mex.: John Muir.

Enders, R. 1991. *A Country Lawyer's Essays on Estate Planning and Aging.* New York: SOS.

Feinstein, D., and P. E. Mayo. 1990. *Rituals for Living and Dying: From Life's Wounds to Spiritual Awakening.* San Francisco: HarperCollins.

Hinton, J. 1972. *Dying,* 2nd ed. Baltimore, Md.: Pelican.

Kübler-Ross, E. 1968. *On Death and Dying.* New York: Macmillan.

Macklin, R. 1987. *Mortal Choices: Bioethics in Today's World.* New York: Pantheon Books.

Morgan, E. 1988. *Dealing Creatively with Death: A Manual of Death Education and Simple Burial,* 11th ed. Burnsville, N.C.: Celo Press.

Porter, S. 1991. *Planning Your Retirement.* New York: Prentice Hall.

Porterfield, J. D., and R. St. Pierre. 1992. *Healthful Aging.* New York: Dushkin.

Sanders, C. M. 1989. *Grief, the Mourning After: Dealing with Adult Bereavement.* New York: John Wiley.

Sherman, C. 1992. The aging process: How to cope with growing older. *San Francisco Chronicle,* 20 October, G1, G6.

U.S. Department of Health and Human Services. 1994. *The Medicare Handbook.* Washington, D.C.: Health Care Financing Administration.

———. 1994. *Guide to Choosing a Nursing Home.* Publication No. HCFA-02174. Baltimore: HCFA.

Williams, M. E. 1994. *The American Geriatrics Society Book on Aging.* New York: Harmony.

Winslade, W. J., and J. W. Ross. 1986. *Choosing Life or Death: A Guide for Patients, Families, and Professionals.* New York: Free Press.

RECOMMENDED READINGS

Beresford, L. 1993. *The Hospice Handbook: A Complete Guide.* Boston: Little, Brown. *Addresses practical questions, such as knowing when hospice care is needed, insurance coverage, and Medicare benefits, and describes different kinds of hospice care.*

Biracree, T., and N. Biracree. 1991. *Over 50: The Resource Book for the Better Half of Your Life.* New York: HarperCollins. *Offers comprehensive advice and information on finances, health care, recreation, housing, and social life; includes directories of government agencies and private organizations.*

Birkedahl, N. 1991. *Older and Wiser: A Workbook for Coping with Aging.* Oakland, Calif.: New Harbinger Publications. *Exercises and activities for self-reflection about money, diet, exercise, family, stress, and health.*

DeSpelder, L. A., and A. L. Strickland. 1995. *The Path Ahead: Readings in Death and Dying.* Mountain View, Calif.: Mayfield. *An anthology of articles that reflects the evolving understanding of dying and death in today's multicultural environment and encourages readers to examine their own feelings and beliefs.*

Humphreys, H. 1989. *Take Charge! A Step-by-Step Guide to Managing Your Money.* Ashland, Oreg.: Gatehouse Books. *A workbook with worksheets and information to help people plan for retirement.*

Kastenbaum, R., and B. Kastenbaum, eds. 1989. *Encyclopedia of Death.* Phoenix: Oryx Press. *Provides broad coverage of topics relating to dying and death; most entries include references for further study.*

McGivney, S. A., and J. H. McGivney. 1989. *Eternally Young: A Guide to Aging Well.* New York: Ageless Publishing. *A practical guide to optimizing quality of life for people over age 50 and their families.*

McGuire, S. 1993. Promoting positive attitudes toward aging: Literature for young children. *Childhood Education* 69(4): 204–211. *Good resource for teachers K–12. Lists books containing positive depictions of the elderly.*

McKenzie, R. 1993. The pleasures of age. *New Choices for Retirement Living* 33(2): 96. *Focuses on things that get better with time.*

Rando, T. A. 1988. *Grieving: How to Go on Living When Someone You Love Dies.* Lexington, Mass.: Lexington Books. *An outstanding and sensitive guide to coping with loss.*

Veatch, R. M. 1989. *Death, Dying, and the Biological Revolution: Our Last Quest for Responsibility,* rev. ed. New Haven, Conn.: Yale University Press. *Provides a comprehensive and useful discussion of the issues important to an understanding of medical ethics.*

Veninga, R. L. 1991. *Your Renaissance Years: Making Retirement the Best Years of Your Life.* Boston: Little, Brown. *Shows how to prepare for retirement financially, physically, and emotionally.*

For more information about retirement planning and other issues that affect the lives of older people, contact the American Association of Retired Persons, 601 E Street, N.W., Washington, D.C. 20049.

15

Environmental Health

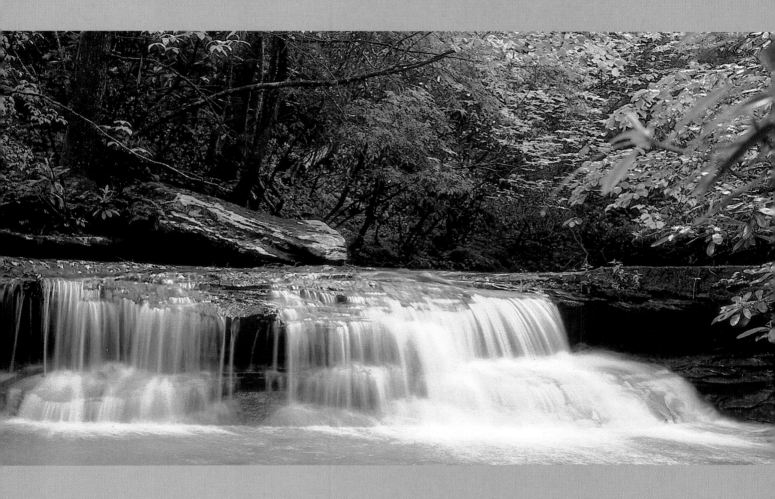

CONTENTS

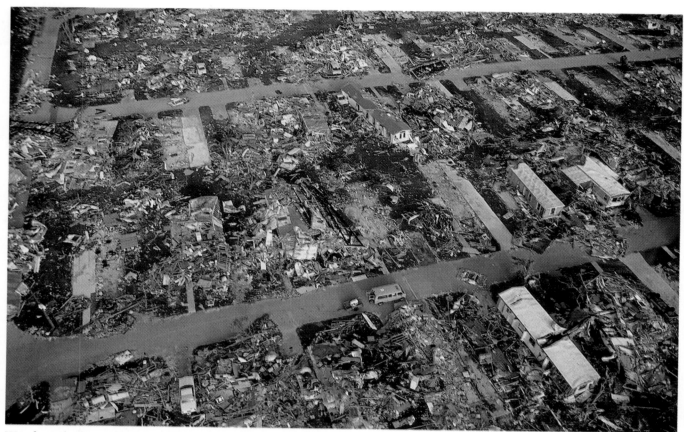

We often take for granted the well-organized system responsible for environmental health in our society, but natural disasters remind us of its fragility. In 1992, Hurricane Andrew disrupted essential services, including the delivery of clean drinking water.

Environmental health has historically focused on preventing infectious diseases spread by water, waste, food, rodents, and insects. Although these problems still exist, the focus of environmental health has expanded and become more complex, for several reasons. First, we now recognize that environmental pollutants contribute not only to infectious diseases but to many chronic diseases as well. Additionally, technological advances have increased our ability to affect and damage the environment. And finally, rapid population growth—which has resulted partly from past environmental improvements—means that far more people are consuming and competing for resources than ever before, magnifying the effect of humans on the environment.

CLASSIC ENVIRONMENTAL HEALTH CONCERNS

Every time we venture beyond the boundaries of our everyday world, whether traveling to a less developed country or camping in a wilderness area, we are reminded of the importance of the basic elements of a healthy environment—clean water, sanitary waste disposal, safe food, and insect and rodent control.

Clean Water

Few things are as important to human health as adequate quantities of safe, clean drinking water. In the latter half of the nineteenth century, the United States and Great Britain both began building complex water systems that brought clean water to cities, right into buildings. Governments took on the role of inspecting water, and in most instances governments provided it too. As a result, the incidence of water-borne diseases fell sharply by 1900 and remains virtually nil today in areas that have adequately treated water from municipal supplies.

Many cities still rely at least in part on wells that tap local groundwater, but often they have to find lakes and rivers to supplement wells. Because such surface water is more likely to be contaminated with both organic matter and disease-causing microorganisms, it is purified in water treatment plants before being piped into the community.

As we move toward the year 2000, water has once again become a worldwide environmental concern. Many supplies of water, both on the surface and in the ground, are becoming polluted with hazardous chemicals. Manufacturing and agriculture are responsible for part of this

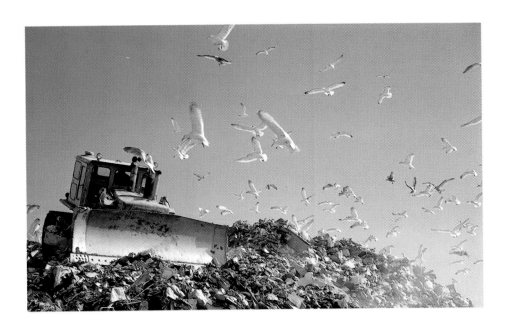

Many existing landfills are reaching their limits at the same time that people are becoming more resistant to the opening of new ones in their communities. The solution to the waste problem lies in less consumption of disposable items and more recycling.

toxic waste, but the accumulated hazardous waste from individual households also contributes to the problem. Increased incidence of cancer is just one of the health problems associated with chemical pollution of the water supply.

Water shortages are also a growing concern. Some parts of the United States are experiencing rapid population growth that outstrips the ability of local systems to provide adequate water to all. According to the World Health Organization, only about 35 percent of the world's people have an adequate water supply. Groundwater pumping and the diversion of water from lakes and rivers for irrigation are further reducing the amount of water available to local communities. Problems of this scope obviously demand long-range solutions on both the national and the international level.

Waste Disposal

Humans generate large amounts of waste, which must be handled in an appropriate manner if the environment is to be safe and sanitary. Some of this waste is sewage composed of human excrement, some is garbage from food materials, and some is solid waste, a by-product of our "throw-away" society.

Sewage   Most cities have sewage treatment systems that separate fecal matter from water in huge tanks and ponds and stabilize it so that it cannot transmit infectious diseases. Once treated and biologically safe, the water is released back into the environment. The sludge that remains behind may be spread on fields as fertilizer if it is free from **heavy metal** contamination, or it may be burned or buried. If incorporated into the food chain, heavy metals, such as lead, cadmium, copper, and tin, can cause illness and death.

In addition to regulating industrial discharge, many cities have now begun to treat sewage further to remove heavy metals and other hazardous chemicals. This action has resulted from many studies linking exposure to such chemicals as mercury, lead, and **polychlorinated biphenyls (PCBs)** with long-term health consequences, including cancer and central nervous system damage. Sewage treatment systems that collect and concentrate these chemicals from an entire city should not dump them back into the environment where they might contaminate a present or future water source.

Solid Waste   The bulk of the organic food garbage produced in American kitchens is now dumped in the sewage system by way of the mechanical garbage disposal. The garbage that remains is not very hazardous from the standpoint of infectious disease, since there is very little food waste in it, but it does represent an enormous disposal and contamination problem.

Since the 1960s much of this solid waste has been buried in **sanitary landfill** disposal sites. Layers of solid waste are covered with thin layers of dirt on a regular basis until the site is filled. Some communities then plant grass and trees and convert the site into a park. Landfill is relatively stable; almost no decomposition occurs in the solidly packed waste.

Burying solid waste in sanitary landfills has several disadvantages. Much of this waste contains chemicals that

Heavy metal   A metal with a high specific gravity, such as lead, copper, or tin.

Polychlorinated biphenyl (PCB)   An industrial chemical used as an insulator and linked to cancers in humans.

Sanitary landfill   A disposal site where solid wastes are buried.

TERMS

should not be released indiscriminately into the environment. Despite precautions, buried contaminants do leak into the surrounding soil and groundwater. Burial is also expensive and requires huge amounts of space. Over two-thirds of the country's landfills have closed since the late 1970s; the range of years remaining is between 3 (Georgia) and 50 (Oregon). At the same time that disposal is becoming more restricted, the amount of garbage is growing all the time. The average American produces more than 4.3 pounds of solid waste per day, up 80 percent since 1960 and 20 percent greater than the objectives set in *Healthy People 2000*. The biggest single component of this trash is paper products. Solid waste is not limited to household products. Manufacturing, mining, and other industries all produce large amounts of potentially dangerous materials that cannot simply be dumped.

Because of the expense and potential chemical hazards posed by any form of solid waste disposal, many communities today encourage individuals and businesses to recycle their trash. By following recommended disposal procedures and participating in recycling, people can help the nation gain time to develop more environmentally efficient methods of disposal and packaging.

> **Personal Insight** Are you ever tempted to throw toxic substances down the drain or in the trash? If so, what do or can you tell yourself in order to resist?

Food Inspection

Most people would be surprised at the number of agencies that inspect food at the various points of production. On the federal level, the Department of Agriculture inspects grains and meats, and the Food and Drug Administration is responsible for ensuring the wholesomeness of foods and regulating the chemicals that can be used in food, drugs, and cosmetics. On the state level, public health departments inspect dairy herds, milking barns, storage tanks, tankers that transport milk, and processing plants. Local health departments inspect and license restaurants.

Considering the number of meals eaten outside the home and the number of meals prepared at home with purchased food, it is remarkable how few instances there are of food-borne illness or death. The food distribution system in the United States is very safe and efficient. Recalls of ice cream, cheese, and tuna in recent years have usually been based on a potential for illness because of processing error, not on actual illness or death. In fact, most food-associated illnesses are caused by contamination in the home, such as from salmonella bacteria or from **staphylococcus** poisoning (see Chapter 13). It is estimated that each person in the United States suffers an average of two to three episodes of food poisoning every year, although these episodes are usually assumed to be caused by a 24-hour virus.

Insect and Rodent Control

A great number of illnesses can be transmitted to humans by animal and insect vectors. In recent years we have seen outbreaks of **encephalitis** transmitted by mosquitoes, **Lyme disease** from ticks in the Northeast, Midwest, and Pacific states, **Rocky Mountain spotted fever** from another type of tick in the Southeast, and **bubonic plague** from fleas on wild mammals in the West. Rodents carry forms of typhus, hantavirus, and even **salmonella**. Disability and death from these diseases is prevented by spraying insecticides when necessary, wearing protective clothing, and exercising caution in infested areas.

POPULATION GROWTH

Throughout most of history, humans have been a minor pressure on the planet. About 200 million people were alive in A.D. 1; by the time Europeans were settling in the United States 1,600 years later, the world population had increased gradually to 500 million. But then it began rising exponentially—zooming to 1 billion by about 1830, more than doubling by 1950, and then doubling again (Figure 15-1). This rapid expansion of population, particularly in the last 50 years, is generally believed to be responsible for most of the stress humans put on the environment. A large and rapidly growing population makes it more difficult to provide the basic components of environmental health discussed earlier, including clean and disease-free food and water; it is also a driving force behind many of the newer environmental health concerns.

The world's population, currently about 5.6 billion people, is increasing at a rate of over a quarter of a million people a day. The United Nations now projects that even if fertility stabilizes at a replacement rate, world population will reach 10 billion by the year 2050 and level off at around 11.6 billion in about 2200. Most of this growth will take place in the developing world, where the population growth rates, although falling, are still double and even triple those of more affluent, developed countries.

Although it's apparent that population growth must be controlled, population trends are difficult to influence and manage. A variety of interconnecting factors fuel the current population explosion, including high fertility rates, lack of family planning resources, and lower death rates due to improved health care.

To be successful, population management must change the condition of people's lives to remove the pressures for large families, especially poverty. Research indicates that the combination of improved health, better education, and increased literacy and employment opportunities for women works together with family planning to cut fertility rates.

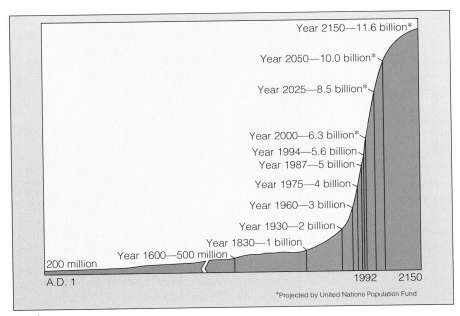

VITAL STATISTICS

Figure 15-1 *World population growth.*

POLLUTION

The term *pollution* refers to any unwanted contaminant in the environment that may pose a health risk. When we are talking about health risks, the level of concentration of a particular pollutant is very important. In typical concentrations, many environmental pollutants don't seem to harm our general health in the short term. The long-term effects are harder to evaluate.

Air Pollution

Air pollution is not a human invention or even a new problem. The air is "polluted" naturally with every forest fire, pollen bloom, and dust storm, as well as with countless other natural pollutants. To these natural sources, human beings have always contributed the by-products of their activities. However, two recent developments have changed our attitudes toward air pollution. First, we are living long enough to experience both the short-term and the long-term consequences. Second, increased population growth, combined with more industrialization using old technologies, concentrates the problems and makes them more visible to the public and possibly more dangerous.

Air pollution can be more than just unsightly; it can cause illness and death if pollutants become concentrated for a period of several days or weeks. Increased amounts of carbon monoxide and air-borne acids and decreased amounts of oxygen all put excess strain on people suffering from heart or respiratory disease, as well as on the very young and the elderly.

Conditions for an Air Pollution Emergency   Before an air pollution emergency can occur, three conditions must be present. First, there must be a source of pollution. Today, this is most frequently the burning of fossil fuels, such as coal in industry or gasoline in cars. Second, there must be a topographical feature, such as a mountain range or a valley, that prevents the prevailing winds from pushing stagnant air out of the region. Third, there must be a weather event called a **temperature inversion**, which occurs when a layer of warm air traps a layer of cold air next to the ground. The effect is like covering an area with a dome that traps all the pollutants and prevents vertical dispersion. If this condition persists for several

TERMS

Staphylococcus   A bacterium found on the skin that can cause food-borne infections if allowed to multiply in foods.

Encephalitis   An inflammation of the brain sometimes caused by insect-borne diseases.

Lyme disease   A disease spread by a deer tick that can lead to fever and arthritis-like conditions if untreated.

Rocky Mountain spotted fever   A wood-tick-borne disease causing high fevers and found primarily in the Southeast.

Bubonic plague   A virulent infectious disease carried by fleas on wild mammals, marked by characteristic discolored swellings.

Salmonella infection   A bacterial infection often caused by eating food contaminated with fecal matter, such as improperly cleaned and cooked chicken.

Temperature inversion   A weather condition in which a cold layer of air is trapped by a warm layer so that pollutants cannot be dispersed.

days, the buildup of pollutants may reach dangerous levels and threaten people's health.

Concern about air pollution in the 1960s was one of several factors that led to the establishment of the U.S. Environmental Protection Agency (EPA), which has the task of setting standards and monitoring pollution levels. The EPA reports improved air quality as measured by decreased levels of smog and several airborne chemicals in many areas. How this improvement translates specifically into improved health status has yet to be determined.

The Greenhouse Effect and Global Warming

The temperature of the earth's atmosphere depends on the balance between the amount of energy the earth absorbs from the sun (mainly as high-energy ultraviolet radiation) and the amount of energy radiated back into space as lower-energy infrared radiation. Key components of temperature regulation are carbon dioxide, water vapor, methane, and other "greenhouse gases"—so-called because, like a pane of glass in a greenhouse, they let through visible light from the sun but trap some of the resulting infrared radiation and reradiate it back to the earth's surface. This reradiation causes a buildup of heat that raises the temperature of the earth's lower atmosphere, a natural process known as the **greenhouse effect**. Without it, the atmosphere would be far cooler and considerably more hostile to life.

Human activity may be tipping this balance toward global warming. The concentration of greenhouse gases is increasing due to human activity, especially the combustion of oil, gasoline, coal, and natural gas. Carbon dioxide levels in the atmosphere have increased rapidly since the onset of the Industrial Revolution, and current levels are higher than at any time in the past 100,000 years. Deforestation, often by burning, also sends carbon dioxide into the atmosphere and reduces the number of trees available to convert carbon dioxide into oxygen. But energy use in the developed world is the primary cause of increases in the concentrations of greenhouse gases. The United States alone is responsible for over 20 percent of the world's total emission of greenhouse gases.

Many experts predict that this increase in greenhouse gases will cause temperatures on earth to rise and climates all over the planet to become warmer. Such a temperature rise, they say, may melt the polar ice caps, raise the level of the sea, and change ocean currents and weather patterns, affecting seacoasts and food-producing areas of the world. Some experts predict a rise of 4 to 7° F worldwide in the next 70 years; others predict a milder warming of 1 to 2° F. Whatever the outcome, the full implications of this type of climate change are unknown.

Depletion of the Ozone Layer

A second air pollution problem is the thinning of the **ozone layer** of the atmosphere—a fragile, invisible layer about 10 to 30 miles above the earth that shields the surface of the planet from the sun's hazardous ultraviolet (UV) rays. Since the mid-1980s, scientists have observed the seasonal appearance and growth of a "hole" in the ozone layer over Antarctica. More recently, thinning over the Arctic and other areas of the north, including Canada, Scandinavia, the northern United States, and parts of the former Soviet Union, has been noted. The ozone layer is being destroyed primarily by **chlorofluorocarbons (CFCs)**, industrial chemicals used as coolants, foaming agents, propellants, and solvents. When CFCs rise into the atmosphere, they can destroy ozone under certain conditions.

The ozone hole in the Antarctic in late 1992 was the largest to date—roughly equal to the size of North America. Since 1979 about 15 percent of Antarctic ozone has been destroyed, although locally and seasonally up to 95 percent of the ozone disappears (forming the "hole"). In the Northern Hemisphere, ozone levels have declined 2 to 10 percent in the past decade, and certain regions may be temporarily depleted in late winter and early spring by as much as 40 percent.

The loss of ozone is of concern because without the ozone layer to absorb ultraviolet radiation from the sun, life on earth would be impossible. The potential effects of increased long-term exposure to UV light for humans include skin cancer, wrinkling and aging of the skin, cataracts and blindness, and reduced immune response.

Worldwide production and use of CFCs and other ozone-destroying substances have declined rapidly since the danger to the ozone layer was recognized. But even if all use of CFCs stopped today, future ozone losses are inevitable because CFCs can persist in the atmosphere for more than a century.

Acid Rain

A by-product of many industrial processes, **acid rain** occurs when atmospheric pollutants combine with moisture in the air and fall to earth as highly acidic rain or snow. It occurs especially when coal containing large amounts of sulfur is burned and sulfur dioxide, sulfur trioxide, nitrogen dioxide, nitric acid, and other chemicals are released into the atmosphere. These concentrations can be carried great distances by the prevailing winds and form a highly acidic mixture containing sulfuric acid and nitric acid. Most of the pollutants in acid rain are produced by coal-burning electric power plants. Other sources include motor vehicles and certain industrial activities, such as smelting.

Many trees and some aquatic life can tolerate only a very narrow range of acidity and are either weakened or killed by acid rain. Currently, acid rain seems to be affecting forests, lakes, and streams in Canada, the northeastern United States, southern Sweden, Norway, and parts of central Europe. Thousands of lakes in Sweden are now so acidified that fish stocks have been severely reduced, and in Bavaria and other areas of central Europe, whole forests are dying. As for damage in the United States, the National Acid Precipitation Assessment Program found that acid rain has adversely affected aquatic life in about 10 percent of eastern lakes and streams, contributed to the decline of red spruce at high elevations, and contributed to erosion and corrosion of buildings and materials. There is also concern that long-term exposure to acid rain could cause nutrient deficiencies in soil, endanger food chains, and activate heavy metals such as mercury, contaminating water supplies.

> ***Personal Insight*** If you found out you could get a smog certificate without having to get your car fixed, what would you do? Would the convenience be worth the pollution?

Chemical Pollution

New chemicals are constantly being created and introduced into the environment, whether as pesticides, herbicides, solvents, cleaning fluids, flame retardants, or any of hundreds of other products. Although chemical pollution is not a new problem, many more chemicals are in use, in more concentrated forms, and larger numbers of people are exposed to them than ever before.

Chemical pollutants have been responsible for several environmental disasters. The Hudson River in New York and the Housatonic River in Massachusetts have both been contaminated with polychlorinated biphenyls (PCBs), carcinogenic compounds used in the manufacture of electrical appliances. In 1984, thousands of people in Bhopal, India, were killed and injured when a powerful chemical used in manufacturing the insecticide Sevin was released from a plant. Catastrophes illustrate the short-term potential for disaster, but the long-term health consequences may be just as deadly. The following are brief descriptions of just a few current problems.

Asbestos A mineral-based compound, asbestos was widely used for fire protection and insulation in buildings until the late 1960s. When first introduced, asbestos was hailed as a great advance in fire safety. As long as it stayed where it was applied and its protective coating was not disturbed, there was no problem. However, microscopic asbestos fibers can be released into the air when this material is applied or when it later deteriorates or is damaged. These fibers can lodge in the lungs, causing **asbestosis**, lung cancer, and other serious lung diseases. Similar conditions are risks in the coal mining industry, from exposure to coal dust (black lung disease), and in the textile industry, from exposure to cotton fibers (brown lung disease).

Lead Lead poisoning continues to be a serious problem, particularly among children living in older buildings and adults who are exposed to lead in the workplace.

When lead is ingested or inhaled, it can damage the central nervous system, cause mental retardation, hinder oxygen transport in the blood, and create digestive problems. Severe lead poisoning may cause coma or even death. Some symptoms of lead poisoning, including anemia, headaches, and abdominal pain, may cease if exposure stops, but neurological impairment can be permanent. Lead damage to the brain can start even before birth if a pregnant woman has elevated levels of lead in her body.

Lead-based paints are believed to be the chief culprit in lead poisoning of children. They were banned from residential use in 1978, but as many as 57 million American homes still contain lead paint. The use of lead in plumbing is now also banned, but some old pipes and faucets contain lead that can leach into drinking water. Lead gets into the air from industrial and vehicle emissions, from tobacco smoke and paint dust, and from the burning of solid wastes that contain lead. Other sources include foods stored or served in lead-glazed pottery or lead crystal as well as processed foods sold in lead-soldered cans.

Pesticides and Other Chemical Pollutants Pesticides are used primarily for two purposes—to prevent the spread of insect-borne disease and to maximize food production by killing insects that eat crops. Most pesticide hazards have been a result of overuse and abuse, but there are concerns about the health effects of long-term exposure to small amounts of pesticide residues in foods.

The list of real and potential chemical pollution problems may well be as long as the list of known chemicals. To the preceding list we can add recent concern about mercury in fish, **formaldehyde** in synthetic building materials, and other by-products of our industrial age. As mentioned earlier, hazardous wastes are also found in the home and should be handled and disposed of properly. They include automotive supplies (motor oil, antifreeze, transmission fluid), paint supplies (turpentine, paint thinner, mineral spirits), art and hobby supplies (oil-

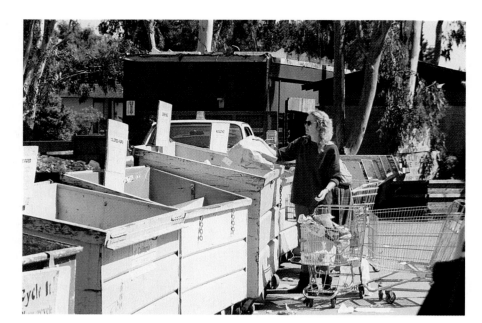

Recycling paper, cans, bottles, and plastics conserves resources, saves energy, and keeps large amounts of solid wastes out of landfills. Some communities have curbside pickup recycling, while others have a system of drop-off sites.

based paint, solvents, acids and alkalis, aerosol sprays), insecticides, batteries, and household cleaners containing sodium hydroxide (lye) or ammonia. These chemicals are dangerous when inhaled or ingested, when they contact the skin or the eyes, or when they are burned or dumped. Many communities provide guidelines about approved disposal methods for household chemicals and have special hazardous waste collection days.

Radiation

Many people are afraid of **radiation**, in part because they don't understand what it is. Basically, radiation is energy. It can come in different forms, such as ultraviolet rays, microwaves, or x-rays, and from different sources, such as the sun, uranium, and nuclear weapons. Although radiation can't be seen, heard, smelled, tasted, or felt, its health effects can include **radiation sickness** and death at high doses and chromosome damage, sterility, tissue damage, cataracts, and cancers at lower doses.

Recently, there has been concern about the electromagnetic radiation associated with such common modern devices as microwave ovens, computer video display terminals (VDTs), microwave telephones, and even high-voltage power lines. We know that these forms of radiation do have effects on health. For example, new bone growth at the point of a fracture can be stimulated by a slight electric current. But current research is contradictory and inconclusive about the health effects of this type of radiation.

Another recent area of concern is **radon**, a form of radiation that is found in certain soils, rocks, and building materials. An unknown number of homes have been built on or with these substances. Well-insulated homes retain radon and allow higher concentrations to develop. Radon gas increases the incidence of lung cancer. Most state health departments can now test for radon gas concentrations, but the short- and long-term health consequences of radon are still poorly quantified.

Noise Pollution

We are increasingly aware of the health effects of loud or persistent noise in the environment. Concerns focus on two areas, hearing loss and stress. Prolonged exposure to sounds above 80–85 **decibels** (a measure of the volume of sound) can cause permanent hearing loss. The scream of an infant, the noise in a machine shop, and freeway traffic sounds can all exceed the safe range. Two common potential sources of excessive noise are the workplace and large gatherings of people at sporting events, rock concerts, and so on.

Most hearing loss occurs in the first two hours of exposure, and hearing usually bounces back within two hours after the noise stops. But if exposure continues or is

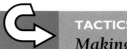

It takes only a few minutes to write to an elected official, but it can make a difference on an environmental issue you care about. When elected officials receive enough letters on a particular issue, it will influence their votes—they want to be reelected and your vote counts!

To help give your letter the greatest possible impact:

- Use your own words and your own stationery.

- Be concise, but try to write more than just one or two sentences. A one-page letter is a good length.

- Identify your subject clearly—refer to legislation by its name or number.

- Discuss only one issue in each letter—different issues are handled by different staff members, so stick to one subject to ensure your letter goes to the right person.

- Ask the legislator to do something specific—to vote a particular way on a particular bill, request hearings, cosponsor a bill, etc.

- Ask for a reply.

- Try not to use form letters.

- Don't be unnecessarily critical. Never threaten or insult.

To find out the current status of legislation pending in the House or Senate, call the legislative status line: 202-225-1772.

Your phone book has addresses of all state and local representatives. United States senators and representatives can be reached at the following addresses:

The Honorable _____
United States Senate
Washington, DC 20510

Dear Senator_____:

The Honorable_____
U.S. House of Representatives
Washington, DC 20515

Dear Representative _____:

Adapted from R. Wild, ed. 1990. *The Earth Care Annual 1990.* Emmaus, Penn.: National Wildlife Federation and Rodale Press.

---

repeated frequently, hearing loss may be permanent. The employees of a club where rock music is played loudly are at much greater risk than the patrons of the club, who might be exposed for only two hours at a time. Another possible effect of exposure to excessive noise is **tinnitus**, a condition of more or less continuous ringing or buzzing in the ears.

To prevent hearing loss and protect your general well-being, follow these key safety tips for dealing with noise:

- Wear ear protectors when working around noisy machinery.

- When listening on a headset with the volume numbered 1 through 10, keep the volume no louder than 4; your headset is too loud if you are unable to hear people around you speaking in a normal tone of voice.

- Avoid loud music. Don't sit or stand near speakers or amplifiers at a rock concert and don't play a car radio or stereo so high that you can't hear the traffic.

- Avoid any exposure to painfully loud sounds and avoid repeated exposure to sounds above 80 decibels.

WHAT CAN YOU DO?

Faced with a vast array of confusing and complex ecological issues, you as an individual may feel overwhelmed.

You may conclude that there isn't anything you can do about global problems. But this isn't true. If everyone made individual changes in his or her life, the impact would be tremendous.

At the same time, it's important to recognize that large corporations and manufacturers are the ones primarily responsible for environmental degradation. Many of them have jumped on the "environmental bandwagon" with public relations and advertising campaigns designed to make them look good, but they haven't changed their practices. To influence them, people have to become educated, demand changes in production methods, and elect people to office who consider both environmental concerns and business profits.

Large-scale changes and individual actions complement each other. What you do every day *does* count; the following is just a sampling of some of the ways that you can make a difference.

- Cut back on driving. Ride your bike, walk, use public transportation, or carpool in a fuel-efficient vehicle.

- Keep your car tuned up and well-maintained. Use only unleaded gas and keep your tires inflated at recommended pressures. Stay within the speed limit and don't use your air conditioner when opening the window would suffice.

- Use less electricity and less heat. Make sure your home is well-insulated; use shades and curtains to keep heat in during winter and out during summer.

- Buy energy-efficient appliances and use them only when necessary. Run the washing machine, the dryer, and dishwasher only when you have full loads, and do laundry in warm or cold water instead of hot water; don't overdry your clothes.

- Plant and care for trees in your own yard and neighborhood. Trees recycle carbon dioxide, provide shade, and cool the air so less air conditioning is needed.

- Keep your car's air conditioner in good working order and have it serviced by a service station that recycles, rather than releases, CFCs. (Auto air conditioners are a major source of CFC emissions.)

- Check labels on aerosol cans and avoid those that contain CFCs (some products, including VCR-head cleaners and drain plungers, are still allowed to contain CFCs).

- Don't use foam plastic insulation in your home, unless it is made with ozone-safe agents. Buy an energy-efficient refrigerator and keep it in good working order. Don't buy a halon fire extinguisher for home use (halons are as much as 10 times more destructive to ozone than are CFCs).

- Buy products with the least amount of packaging you can, or buy products in bulk. Buy products packaged in glass, paper, or metal containers; avoid plastic and aluminum (unless it's recycled).

- Buy recycled or recyclable products. Use long-lasting or reusable products such as refillable pens and rechargeable batteries.

- When shopping, take along your own bag. Reuse paper and plastic bags.

- To store food, use glass jars and reusable plastic containers rather than plastic wrap.

- Recycle your newspapers, glass, cans, paper, and other recyclables. If you receive something packaged with foam pellets, take them to a commercial mailing center that accepts them for recycling.

- Take showers, not baths, to cut water consumption. Don't let water run when you're not actively using it while brushing your teeth, shaving, or hand-washing clothes. Don't run a dishwasher or washing machine until you have a full load.

- Install sink faucet aerators and water-efficient showerheads, which use two to five times less water with no noticeable decrease in performance.

- Put a displacement device in your toilet tank to reduce the amount of water used with each flush. A plastic bottle or bag filled with water works well.

- Make sure your friends and family are informed about environmental issues. Share what you learn.

- Join, support, or volunteer your time to organizations working on environmental causes that are important to you.

- Contact your elected representatives and communicate your concerns.

These are just a few of the steps you can take to improve the quality of the environment. As with personal health behaviors, the crucial step is to get started, today. Let the size and scope of the problems be a call to action, not an excuse for apathy.

> ***Personal Insight*** Do you recycle? If you don't, why don't you? How convenient would it have to be to get you to recycle?

SUMMARY

- The combination of increased population and modern technology has increased the impact of humans on the environment.

Classic Environmental Health Concerns

- Basic elements of a healthy environment include clean water, sanitary waste disposal, safe food, and insect and rodent control.

- Water used in municipal systems must be purified because it's likely to be contaminated with organic matter and disease-causing microorganisms.

- Concerns with water today center on hazardous chemicals from industry and households as well as on water shortages.

- Most cities have sewage treatment systems. Such systems must also deal with heavy metals and hazardous chemicals.

- The amount of garbage is growing all the time; paper is the biggest component. Recycling of trash can help solid waste disposal problems.

- Illness and death associated with food-borne disease and toxic food additives have decreased substantially.

- Disability and death from diseases transmitted by insects and rodents can be prevented by spraying insecticides, wearing protective clothing, and avoiding infested areas.

Population Growth

- The world's population is increasing rapidly and is expected to reach 10 billion by 2050.

- Many factors influence population growth, including high fertility rates, lack of family planning resources, and decreasing death rates. Successful population management requires elimination of the pressures for large families.

Pollution

- People today live long enough to experience the long-term consequences of air pollution, and increased population and industrialization make the problems more visible and dangerous.

- Increased amounts of air pollutants are especially stressful to those with heart and lung problems. Air pollution emergencies occur when (1) fossil fuels are burned, (2) a topographic feature prevents prevailing winds from pushing stagnant air away, and (3) a temperature inversion exists.

- Carbon dioxide and other natural gases act as a "greenhouse" around the earth. Levels of these gases are rising through human activity; as a result, the world's climate could change.

- The ozone layer shields the earth's surface from the sun's ultraviolet rays, but a "hole" over Antarctica has been found seasonally since the 1980s. One cause is the release of chlorofluorocarbons.

- Acid rain or snow occurs when certain atmospheric pollutants combine with moisture in the air. Trees and aquatic life can be damaged or killed by acid rain.

- Chemical pollutants include asbestos, lead, pesticides, and hundreds of other chemical products.

- Radiation can cause radiation sickness, chromosome damage, and cancers, among other health risks. Radon, found in certain soils, rocks, and building materials, can concentrate in homes; it increases the incidence of lung cancer.

- Loud or persistent noise can lead to hearing loss and/or stress; two common sources of excessive noise are the workplace and rock concerts.

What Can You Do?

- Most health advances today must come from lifestyle changes and improvements in the global environment. The impact of personal changes made by every concerned individual could be tremendous.

TAKE ACTION

1. Do an inventory to find out what hazardous chemicals you have in your household. Read the labels for disposal instructions. If there aren't any instructions, call your local health department and ask how to dispose of specific chemicals. Also ask if there are hazardous waste disposal sites in your community or special pickup days. If possible, get rid of some or all of the hazardous wastes in your home.

2. Investigate the recycling facilities in your community. Find out how materials are recycled and what they are used for in their recycled state. If recycling isn't available in your community, contact your local city hall to find out how a recycling program can be started.

3. Junk mail is an environmental hazard coming and going—millions of trees are cut down to produce the paper it's printed on, and millions of pieces of junk mail clog the nation's landfills. Keep your name from being sold to any more mailing list companies by writing to Mail Preference Service, Direct Marketing Association, 6 East 43rd Street, New York, NY 10017. Recycle the junk mail you still get; newspaper can be recycled with newspapers, paper and envelopes (without windows) with paper.

JOURNAL ENTRY

1. In your health journal, list the positive behaviors that help you protect the environment. What can you do to reinforce and support these behaviors? Then list the behaviors that may harm the environment. How can you change one or more of them?

2. *Critical Thinking:* Some developing nations want to "catch up" with the West in terms of economic development and standard of living by using the same kinds of industrial practices that developed nations have used to get where they are. They are cutting down forests to raise cattle for beef, using pesticides that have been banned in the developed nations on export crops, and polluting their water and air with industrial and agricultural wastes. Do you think it's fair to expect them to be environmentally conscious when the developed nations weren't? Do they have a right to the same standard of living that Americans have, no matter what the environmental costs? Write a short essay that makes a case for or against their continuing use of these practices.

SELECTED BIBLIOGRAPHY

Allison, M. 1992. Lead poisoning: Not just for kids. *Harvard Health Letter,* May.

Clark, S. L. 1991. *Fight Global Warming: 29 Things You Can Do.* New York: Consumer Reports Books.

Cohen, J. 1992. How many people can earth hold? *Discover,* November, pp. 114–19.

Easterbrook, G. 1990. Everything you know about the environment is wrong. *The New Republic,* 20 April.

Ehrlich, P. R., and A. H. Ehrlich. 1991. *Healing the Planet: Strategies for Solving the Environmental Crisis*. Reading, Mass.: Addison-Wesley.

Elmer-Dewitt, P. 1992. Summit to save the earth: Rich vs. poor. *Time,* 1 June, pp. 42–58.

Freed, V. H. 1986. Hazards in the physical environment. *The Oxford Textbook of Public Health*, vol. 1, eds. V. W. Holland, R. Detels, and G. Knox. Oxford: Oxford University Press.

Hunter, L. M. 1989. *The Healthy Home: An Attic-to-Basement Guide to Toxin-Free Living*. Emmaus, Penn.: Rodale Press, pp. 69–103.

Johnson, O., ed. 1994. *1995 Information Please® Almanac*. Boston: Houghton Mifflin.

Monastersky, R. 1991. Antarctic ozone hole sinks to a record low. *Science News* 140:244–45.

Myers, N., ed. 1993. *Gaia: An Atlas of Planet Management*, Rev. ed. New York: Anchor Books.

Naar, J. 1990. *Design for a Livable Planet: How You Can Help Clean Up the Environment*. New York: Harper and Row, pp. 85–89.

News about noise. 1992. *Healthline,* March.

Okun, D. A. 1986. Water and waste disposal. In *Public Health and Preventive Medicine,* 12th ed., ed. Maxcy-Rosenau. Norwalk, Conn.: Appleton-Century-Crofts.

Polar "ozone hole" grows to record size. 1992. *Facts on File,* 1 October.

Sadik, N. 1991. Healthy people—in numbers the world can support. *World Health Forum* 12:347–55.

The science and politics of ozone depletion. 1992. *Star Tribune,* 28 June.

Stevens, W. K. 1992. Humanity confronts its handiwork: An altered planet. *The New York Times,* 5 May, pp. B5–B7.

U.S. Bureau of the Census. 1994. *Statistical Abstract of the United States: 1994*. 114th ed. Washington, D.C.: U.S. Government Printing Office.

Warde, J. 1992. Home improvement: Cleaning up the air inside your home. *The New York Times,* 26 November.

Wright, J. W., ed. 1993. *The Universal Almanac 1994*. Kansas City: Andrews and McMeel.

RECOMMENDED READINGS

The Bennet Information Group. 1990. *The Green Pages: Your Everyday Shopping Guide to Environmentally Safe Products*. New York: Random House. *A practical guide covering over 900 items by brand name, including detergents, cleansers, shampoo, paper towels, flea collars, and many more.*

Carson, R. 1962. *Silent Spring*. Boston: Houghton Mifflin. *The classic that awakened people to the dangers of wide-scale insecticide spraying.*

Chivian, E., ed. 1993. *Critical Condition: Human Health and the Environment*. Cambridge, Mass.: MIT Press.

The Earth Works Group. 1989. *50 Simple Things You Can Do to Save the Earth*. Berkeley, Calif.: Earthworks Press. *Full of useful information, practical advice, sources, and resources, this slim volume is an indispensable guide to improving the environment. Includes names and addresses of organizations that can provide further information on specific issues.*

Ehrlich, P. R. 1990. *The Population Explosion*. New York: Ballantine Books. *An update of Ehrlich's landmark 1971 book calling attention to the problems associated with population growth.*

McMichael, A. J. 1993. *An Endangered Species: Global Environmental Change and Human Health*. Cambridge: Cambridge University Press.

Moeller, D. W. 1992. *Environmental Health*. Cambridge: Harvard University Press. *New survey text by a Harvard professor who has taught environmental health for 25 years.*

Myers, N., ed. 1993. *Gaia: An Atlas of Planet Management,* Rev. ed. New York: Anchor Books. *A beautifully illustrated and informative guide to environmental problems and possible solutions.*

World Health Organization. 1994. *Ultraviolet Radiation: An Authoritative Scientific Review of the Health Effects of UV, With Reference to Global Ozone Layer Depletion*. Geneva: World Health Organization.

There are many national and international organizations working on environmental health problems. A few of the largest and best-known are listed below.

Greenpeace, USA, Inc.
1436 U Street NW
Washington, DC 20009
202-462-1177

National Audubon Society
700 Broadway
New York, NY 10003
212-979-3000

National Wildlife Federation
1400 16th Street NW
Washington, DC 20036
202-797-6800

The Nature Conservancy
1815 North Lynn Street
Arlington, VA 22209
703-841-5300

Sierra Club
730 Polk Street
San Francisco, CA 94109
415-776-2211

Index

Boldface numbers indicate pages on which glossary definitions appear.

"*t*" indicates that the information is in a table.

Carcinogens, **131**, 267
Carcinomas, **265**, 271
Cardiac myopathy, 146, **147**
Cardiopulmonary resuscitation (CPR), **259**
Cardiorespiratory endurance, **234–235**
Cardiorespiratory endurance exercise, 231–233, 234
Cardiovascular disease (CVD), **250–263**
   protecting against, 263
   risk factors for, 251–257
   stress and, 23, 25, 254–256
   types of, 257–263
   See also Heart disease; Stroke
Cardiovascular system, 145–146, **250–251**
Cataracts, **314**
Caucasians, osteoporosis among, 190
CD4 lymphocytes, **297**
Celibacy, 80, **81**
Cell-mediated immune response, 287
Cellular death, **323**
Central nervous system, **161**
Central nervous system depressants, 142, **143**, **162–164**
Central nervous system stimulants, 142, **143**, 164, **165–167**
Cerebral cortex, **131**, **315**
Cerebral embolism, **261**
Cerebral hemorrhage, **261**
Cerebral thrombosis, 260–**261**
Cerebrovascular accident (stroke), 7, 16, 256, 260–262, **261**
Cervical cancer, 270
Cervical cap, 110, **111**
Cesarean section, 97, **98**
Chancres, **302**
Chemotherapy, **267**
Chicken pox, 290*t*, 293
Childbirth, 89, 94, 95
Chlamydia trachomatis, **302–303**
Chlorofluorocarbons (CFCs), 340, **341**
Cholesterol, **183**, 191
   cardiovascular disease and, 252–254, 252*t*, 263
   dietary, 252–254, 252*t*
   serum, 182, 232
Chorionic villi, 90, **91**
Chorionic villus sampling, 92, **93**
Chronic bronchitis, 133
Chronic obstructive lung disease, 8*t*, 133, 140*t*
Cigarettes, 131, 135. *See also* Smoking
Cigarette tar, 130–**131**
Cigar smoking, 134–135
Cilia, **285**
Circumcision, 74
Clinical death, **323**
Clitoris, **71**
Clove cigarettes, 135
Coarctation of the aorta, **262**
Cocaine, 92, 164–166
Cocarcinogens, **131**
Codependency, 171
Cognitive stress-management techniques, 29–30
Cohabitation, **56**
Colds, 293
Collateral circulation, **259**
Colon cancer, 184, 266
Colostrum, **89**, 98
Communication, 42, 59, **60–61**
Compulsions, 42, **43**
Computerized tomography (CT scan), **262**
Conception, **85**, 87, **103**
Condoms, 107–109
   female, 109, 113
   male, **107–108**, 113, 300, 301

Condyloma, 304–305
Conflict resolution, 61
Congenital heart disease, **262**
Congenital malformations, **93**
Congestive heart failure, **262**
Conjunctivitis, gonococcal, 303
Consciousness, altered states of, **169**
Contagious disease, 292–293
Contraceptive methods, **103–124**
   abstinence, **112**, 114, 300, 301
   barrier methods, **107–111**
   cervical cap, 110, **111**
   choosing, 117
   combining, 112
   condoms, 107–109, 300, 301
   continuation rate for, **103**
   culture and, 116
   Depo-Provera, 106
   diaphragm, **109–110**, 111
   effectiveness of, 103, 113
   failure rate of, **103**, 113
   fertility awareness method (FAM), **111**–112
   intrauterine devices (IUDs), **106–107**
   new, 115, 117
   Norplant implants, 105–106
   oral, 103–105, **104**
   reversibility of, 103
   spermicides, **109–110**, 111
   sponge, 110
   sterilization, 112–115
   withdrawal, **112**
Contract(s), personal, 12–13, 32, 247
Contractions
   Braxton Hicks, **89**
   during labor, 95
Coronary arteries, 250, **251**
Coronary bypass surgery, 260, **261**
Coronary heart disease (CHD), **131**–132. *See also* Heart disease
Coronary occlusion, **259**
Coronary thrombosis, **259**
Corpus luteum, **75**, 76, **103**
Cortisol, **21**
Cough medicines, 293
Counselors, 47
Cowper's glands, 72
CPR (cardiopulmonary resuscitation), **259**
Crack, 165
Cremation, 328
Cross-training, **244**
Cruciferous vegetables, **275–276**
CT scan, 262
Culture
   attitudes toward aging and, 322
   circumcision and, 74
   contraception and, 116
   HIV infection and, 296
Cunnilingus, 80
Cytokines, **287**, 289

Daily Values, **188–189**
Date rape, 82, **83**
Dating, 56
Death/dying, 322–332
   attitudes toward, 324
   coping with, 329–332
   definitions of, 322–323
   disposal of body, 328
   leading causes of, 5, 8*t*
   planning for, 324–329
   right to die, 325–326, 327
Death rates, 3, 16, 94–95, 230
Decibel, **342**
Decongestants, 293

Defense mechanisms
   of body, 285–291
   mental, 41–42, **43**
Deliriants, 169–170
Delirium, **169**
Delirium tremens (DTs), **148**, 149
Delusions, 46
Dementia, **316**, 317–318
Demoralization, 40–41
Dendrites, **315**
Dependency. *See* Addiction/dependency
Depersonalization, 168, **169**
Depo-Provera, 106
Depressants, 142, **143**, **162–164**
Depression, 44–46
   postpartum, 98, 99
Dermatitis, **303**
DES (diethylstilbestrol), **87**
Designer drugs, 170, **171**
Diabetes mellitus, 5, 8*t*, 254, **257**
Diaphragm, **109–110**, 111
Diastole, 250, **251**
Diet(s)
   aging and, 312–313
   cancer and, 274, 275–276, 279, 281–282
   composition of, 180
   eating disorders and, 217, 221–225
   guidelines for, 187–194
   heart disease and, 252–254, 252*t*, 263, 281–282
   improving, 198–199, 207*t*, 252, 253–254, 281–282
   stress and, 26–27
   vegetarian, 193–194
   See also Weight management
Diet aids, 219–220
Dietary Guidelines for Americans, **187**, 190–193
Diethylstilbestrol (DES), **87**
Dietitians, 196
Digestion, 182, **183**
Digitalis, 262
Distillation, **139–140**
Distress, **20**
Diuretics, 262
Diverticulitis, 183
Divorce, 63
DNA (deoxyribonucleic acid), **274–275**
Domestic violence, 61–63
Dose-response function, 160, **161**
Dose-response relationship, **143**
Douche, 111
Drug(s), 156, **157**
   antihypertensive, **259**
   dependence on, 158–159, 162–164, 165, 167, 169, 172–174
   designer, 170, **171**
   dose-response function and, 160, **161**
   generic vs. brand name, 163
   pharmacological properties of, **159–160**
   pregnancy and, 93, 165–166
   psychoactive. *See* Psychoactive drugs
   safe use of, 163
   testing for, 171–172
   time-action function and, 160, **161**
Drug abuse, 158, **159**. *See also* Psychoactive drugs
DTs (delirium tremens), **148**, 149
Dying. *See* Death/dying
Dysentery, amoebic, **294**
Dysmenorrhea, 76

Eating disorders, **217**, 221–225
Eclampsia, 94, **95**
Ectopic pregnancy, 94, **95**
Ejaculation, 79, **107**

CHAPTER 1
Taking Charge of Your Health

Multiple Choice

1. Which of the following is NOT associated with lifestyle choices common to Americans?
   a. osteoporosis
   b. high blood pressure
   c. heart disease
   d. sickle cell anemia

2. Which of the following is NOT part of a personal contract for behavior change?
   a. the date you will start changing your behavior
   b. the steps you will use to measure success in changing your behavior
   c. the date you expect to reach your final goal
   d. the consequences of not reaching your final goal

3. The MOST important contributor to personal health for most people is:
   a. environment.
   b. health care.
   c. health behavior.
   d. heredity.

4. The MOST likely cause of death in the last part of the twentieth century is:
   a. heart disease.
   b. infection.
   c. childhood disease.
   d. physician neglect.

5. The health determinant LEAST under your personal control is:
   a. heredity.
   b. environment.
   c. access to health care.
   d. behavioral choices.

6. Probably the LEAST effective health behavior change strategy is:
   a. changing several behaviors at once.
   b. charting health behaviors.
   c. setting up short-term reward systems.
   d. selecting the easiest-to-change behavior as the first target for change.

7. While monitoring the target behavior you want to change you also want to gather data about all of the following EXCEPT:
   a. what other things you do when you engage in the behavior
   b. when and where you engage in the behavior
   c. what your feelings are at the time you engage in the behavior
   d. who is displeased when you engage in the behavior

8. A habit you want to change with behavior self-management is called a:
   a. program behavior.
   b. behavior event.
   c. informed behavior.
   d. target behavior.

9. When you encounter obstacles and disappointments while working on a behavior change project, do all of the following EXCEPT:
   a. be persistent.
   b. revise your program if necessary.
   c. blame yourself.
   d. evaluate progress to date.

10. The term most closely associated with wellness is:
    a. vitality.
    b. hostility.
    c. passivity.
    d. longevity.

True or False

T F 1. If you live longer you will automatically be healthier.

T F 2. The only rewards that effectively motivate a person to make behavior change are external.

T F 3. The value of using the "buddy system" in pursuing behavior change is the support and encouragement that the buddy can provide.

T F 4. A good role model is a person who has reached the goal you are striving for.

T F 5. Wellness requires learning about and protecting yourself from environmental hazards.

T F 6. Today, the most serious threats to health are chronic illnesses such as heart disease and cancer.

T F 7. One of the values of a health journal is that it allows you to record the feelings that accompany your success or lack of progress.

T F 8. Scientific research is continually revealing new connections between our habits and emotions and the level of health we enjoy.

T F 9. Most people are likely to be motivated by long-term goals such as avoiding disease some 20 or 30 years from now.

T F 10. The incidence of heart disease, this country's leading cause of death, has continued to rise in the last quarter of this century.

ANSWERS: Multiple Choice: 1. d; 2. d; 3. c; 4. a; 5. a; 6. a; 7. d; 8. d; 9. c; 10. a
True/False 1. F; 2. F; 3. T; 4. T; 5. T; 6. T; 7. T; 8. T; 9. F; 10. F

WELLNESS WORKSHEET 1.1

Evaluate your lifestyle

All of us want optimal health. But many of us do not know how to achieve it. That's what this brief test, adapted from one created by the U.S. Public Health Service, is all about. The behaviors covered in the test are recommended for most Americans. (Some of them may not apply to people with certain diseases or disabilities, or to pregnant women, who may require special advice from their physicians.) After you take the quiz, add up your score for each section.

	Almost Always	Sometimes	Never
Tobacco Use			
If you never use tobacco, enter a score of 10 for this section and go to the next section.			
1. I avoid using tobacco.	2	1	0
2. I smoke only low-tar-and-nicotine cigarettes, or I smoke a pipe or cigars, or I use smokeless tobacco.	2	1	0
Tobacco Score: _____			
Alcohol and Other Drugs			
1. I avoid alcohol, or I drink no more than 1 or 2 drinks a day.	4	1	0
2. I avoid using alcohol or other drugs as a way of handling stressful situations or problems in my life.	2	1	0
3. I am careful not to drink alcohol when taking medications, such as for colds or allergies, or when pregnant.	2	1	0
4. I read and follow the label directions when using prescribed and over-the-counter drugs.	4	1	0
Alcohol and Other Drugs Score: _____			
Nutrition			
1. I eat a variety of foods each day, including 5 or more servings of fresh fruits and vegetables.	3	1	0
2. I limit the amount of fat and saturated fat in my diet.	3	1	0
3. I avoid skipping meals.	2	1	0
4. I limit the amount of salt and sugar I eat.	2	1	0
Nutrition Score: _____			
Exercise/Fitness			
1. I engage in moderate exercise for 15 to 60 minutes, three to five times a week.	4	1	0
2. I maintain a healthy weight, avoiding overweight and underweight.	2	1	0
3. I do exercises to develop muscular strength and endurance at least twice a week.	2	1	0
4. I spend some of my leisure time participating in physical activities such as gardening, bowling, golf, or baseball.	2	1	0
Exercise/Fitness Score: _____			

(over)

Emotional Health

1. I enjoy being a student and I have a job or do other work that I like.	2	1	0
2. I find it easy to relax and express my feelings freely.	2	1	0
3. I manage stress well.	2	1	0
4. I have close friends, relatives, or others I can talk to about personal matters and call on for help.	2	1	0
5. I participate in group activities (such as church and community organizations) or hobbies that I enjoy.	2	1	0

Emotional Health Score: _____

Safety

1. I wear a seat belt while riding in a car.	2	1	0
2. I avoid driving while under the influence of alcohol or other drugs.	2	1	0
3. I obey traffic rules and the speed limit when driving.	2	1	0
4. I read and follow instructions on the labels of potentially harmful products or substances, such as household cleaners, poisons, and electrical appliances.	2	1	0
5. I avoid smoking in bed.	2	1	0

Safety Score: _____

Disease Prevention

1. I know the warning signs of cancer, diabetes, heart attack, and stroke.	2	1	0
2. I avoid overexposure to the sun and use sunscreens.	2	1	0
3. I get recommended medical screening tests (such as blood pressure checks and Pap smears), immunizations, and booster shots.	2	1	0
4. I practice monthly breast/testicle self-exams.	2	1	0
5. I am not sexually active *or* I have sex with only one mutually faithful, uninfected partner *or* I always engage in "safer sex" (using latex condoms) *and* I do not share needles.	2	1	0

Disease Prevention Score: _____

What Your Scores Mean

Scores of 9 and 10   Excellent! Your answers show that you are aware of the importance of this area to wellness. More important, you are putting your knowledge to work for you by practicing good health habits. As long as you continue to do so, this area should not pose a serious health risk. It's likely that you are setting an example for your family and friends to follow. Since you earned a very high test score on this part of the test, you may want to focus on other areas where your scores indicate room for improvement.

Scores of 6 to 8   Your health practices in this area are good, but there is room for improvement. Look again at the items you answered with a "Sometimes" or "Never." What changes can you make to improve your score? Even a small change can often help you achieve better health.

Scores of 3 to 5   Your health risks are showing! You may need more information about the risks you are facing and about why it is important for you to change these behaviors. Perhaps you need help in deciding how to successfully make the changes you desire.

Scores of 0 to 2   Your answers show that you may be taking serious and unnecessary risks with your health. Perhaps you are not aware of the risks and what to do about them. You can easily get the information and help you need to improve, if you wish. The next step is up to you.

CHAPTER 2
Stress: The Constant Challenge

Multiple Choice

1. Which of the following is LEAST influential in determining the effect of stress on a person?
   a. intensity of the stress
   b. coping skills
   c. available support system
   d. age

2. Hans Selye is
   a. an oncologist.
   b. an otolaryngologist.
   c. an endocrinologist.
   d. a philosopher.

3. Which of the following is one of the stages of the general adaptation syndrome?
   a. anxiety
   b. ambivalence
   c. stabilization
   d. alarm

4. Eustress is triggered by:
   a. getting a bad grade.
   b. winning the lottery.
   c. having your parents get a divorce.
   d. homeostasis.

5. When a person's adaptive energy resources have been depleted, the person goes into:
   a. exhaustion.
   b. resistance.
   c. recovery.
   d. alarm.

6. A disease that Selye believed to be a disease of adaptation in some cases is:
   a. chicken pox.
   b. ulcers.
   c. diphtheria.
   d. glaucoma.

7. Which of the following is an emotional sign of stress?
   a. depression
   b. sleep disturbances
   c. dry mouth
   d. sexual problems

8. Repetitive-stress injury (RSI) is MOST likely to impact the sense of:
   a. hearing.
   b. sight.
   c. touch.
   d. smell.

9. The alarm reaction produces:
   a. bronchial constriction.
   b. skeletal muscle relaxation.
   c. increased digestion.
   d. increased respiration.

10. The biggest single time management problem for most people is:
    a. procrastination.
    b. overcommitment.
    c. not being able to say "no."
    d. poor planning.

True or False

T F   1. All stress in one's life is not healthy.

T F   2. The sympathetic nervous system mobilizes the body for action.

T F   3. High-potency formulations of vitamins C, E, and B-complex have been proven useful in combatting psychological or emotional stress.

T F   4. The body has an unlimited reserve of adaptive energy.

T F   5. An adaptive reaction is the body's attempt to restore homeostasis.

T F   6. Cortisol is a natural opiate produced in the brain.

T F   7. The scientist who conceptualized the general adaptation syndrome is Linus Pauling.

T F   8. The most dangerous stage of the general adaptation syndrome is exhaustion.

T F   9. Progressive relaxation is primarily a mental process.

T F   10. Diseases of adaptation include cardiovascular disease.

ANSWERS: Multiple Choice: 1. d; 2. c; 3. d; 4. b; 5. a; 6. b; 7. a; 8. c; 9. d; 10. a
True/False 1. F; 2. T; 3. F; 4. F; 5. T; 6. F; 7. F; 8. T; 9. F; 10. T

WELLNESS WORKSHEET 2.1

Identify your stressors

Signals of Stress

To identify sources of stress in your life you must first be able to identify the signals of stress. Put a check next to any of the listed signs that you have experienced in the last month.

Physical Signs

_____ Pounding heart
_____ Trembling or nervous tics
_____ Grinding of teeth
_____ Dry mouth
_____ Excessive perspiration
_____ Gastrointestinal problems (diarrhea, constipation, indigestion, queasy stomach)
_____ Stiff neck or aching lower back
_____ Migraine or tension headaches
_____ Frequent colds or low-grade infections
_____ Cold hands and feet
_____ Allergy or asthma attacks
_____ Skin problems (hives, eczema, psoriasis)

Emotional Signs

_____ Tendency to be irritable or aggressive
_____ Tendency to feel anxious, fearful, or edgy
_____ Hyperexcitability, impulsiveness, or emotional instability
_____ Depression
_____ Frequent feelings of boredom
_____ Inability to concentrate
_____ Fatigue

Behavioral Signs

_____ Increased use of alcohol, tobacco, or other drugs
_____ Excessive TV watching
_____ Sleep disturbances (e.g., insomnia) or excessive sleep
_____ Overeating or undereating
_____ Sexual problems

Possible Stressful Events

Listed below, in order of probable severity of effect, are thirty-five life events you may experience that cause stress. Put a check next to any item that you have experienced recently or expect to experience soon. If you find you have checked several items, take time out to develop and cultivate your coping skills.

_____ Death of a close family member
_____ Divorce or separation from mate
_____ Detention in jail or other institution
_____ Major personal injury or illness
_____ Death of a close friend
_____ Divorce between parents
_____ Marriage
_____ Being fired from job or expelled from school
_____ Retirement
_____ Change in health of a family member
_____ Pregnancy
_____ Being a victim of a crime
_____ Sexual difficulties
_____ Gaining new family members (through birth, adoption, older person moving in, and so on)
_____ New boy- or girlfriend

_____ Major business or academic readjustment (merger, change of job or major, failing important course)
_____ Major change in financial state (a lot worse or a lot better off than before)
_____ Taking out a loan or mortgage for school or a major purchase
_____ Trouble with parents, spouse, or girl- or boyfriend
_____ Outstanding personal achievement
_____ Graduation
_____ First quarter/semester in college
_____ Denied admission to program or school
_____ Change in living conditions
_____ Serious argument with instructor, friend, or roommate

(over)

_____ Lower grades than expected

_____ Major change in working hours or conditions or increased workload at school

_____ Major change in recreational, social, or church activities

_____ Major change in sleeping or eating habits

_____ Denied admission to required course

_____ Taking out a loan for a lesser purchase (for a car, TV, or freezer, for example)

_____ Chronic car trouble

_____ Change in number of family get-togethers

_____ Vacation

_____ Minor violation of the law (traffic tickets and so on)

Weekly Stress Log

Now that you are familiar with the signals of stress, complete the weekly stress log to map patterns in your stress levels and identify external and internal sources of stress.

	AM							PM											Total
	6	7	8	9	10	11	12	1	2	3	4	5	6	7	8	9	10	11	12	
Monday																				
Tuesday																				
Wednesday																				
Thursday																				
Friday																				
Saturday																				
Sunday																				
Total																				

CODE
1. No anxiety; general feeling of well-being
2. Mild anxiety; no interference with activity
3. Moderate anxiety; specific signal(s) of stress present
4. High anxiety; interference with activity
5. Very high anxiety and panic reactions; general inability to engage in activity

Identifying Sources of Stress

External stressors: List several persons, places, or things that caused you a significant amount of discomfort this week.

Internal stressors: Make a list of any recurring thoughts or worries that produced feelings of discomfort this week.

CHAPTER 3
Mental Health

Multiple Choice

1. Mental health workers who have completed a Ph.D. degree are:
   a. clinical psychologists.
   b. social workers.
   c. psychiatrists.
   d. analysts.

2. The scientist/author associated with self-actualization is:
   a. Maslow.
   b. Skinner.
   c. McCluan.
   d. Toffler.

3. A phobia is:
   a. an unfounded fear of a specific thing.
   b. a heart attack symptom.
   c. a common response to stress.
   d. uncommon among panic patients.

4. An example of negative self talk is:
   a. I overdid it last night. Next time I'll make different choices.
   b. It may not be the best speech I'll ever give, but it was good enough to earn a grade of "B."
   c. I wonder why my boss wants to see me? I'll just have to wait and see.
   d. I wouldn't feel so lousy today if someone had stopped me from drinking so much last night.

5. A common defense mechanism in which a person removes an unpleasant feeling or memory from awareness or refuses to acknowledge it is:
   a. projection
   b. repression
   c. rationalization
   d. sublimation

6. Recognizing your own favorite defense mechanisms can be difficult, because:
   a. they probably have not become automatic habits.
   b. they occur outside of your conscious awareness.
   c. people cannot look at themselves objectively.
   d. an outside observer is required to analyze your thoughts.

7. The first concern of humans, according to Maslow's hierarchy of needs is/are:
   a. food and shelter
   b. safety
   c. being loved
   d. maintaining self-esteem

8. Giving a false, acceptable reason for behavior when the real reason is unacceptable is called:
   a. repression.
   b. rationalization.
   c. projection.
   d. denial.

9. Shyness is:
   a. a social anxiety.
   b. relatively uncommon.
   c. not inherited.
   d. seldom outgrown.

10. Mental health workers who are medical doctors are:
   a. clinical psychologists.
   b. social workers.
   c. psychiatrists.
   d. analysts.

True or False

T F 1. To be mentally healthy is to be normal.

T F 2. Anyone who seeks help from a mental health professional is of unsound mental health.

T F 3. It is easy to tell the status of a person's mental health by appearances.

T F 4. Mental health can be defined as the absence of mental illness.

T F 5. Being an inner-directed person is a sign of mental health.

T F 6. Capacity for emotional intimacy is an indicator of mental health.

T F 7. Simple phobias and social phobias are the same.

T F 8. There is a strong relationship between severe depression and suicide.

T F 9. Children need to develop a sense of being loved, but a sense of being able to give love comes only with adulthood.

T F 10. A primary task beginning in adolescence is the development of an adult identity.

ANSWERS: Multiple Choice: 1. a; 2. a; 3. a; 4. d; 5. b; 6. b; 7. a; 8. b; 9. a; 10. c
True/False 1. F; 2. F; 3. F; 4. T; 5. T; 6. T; 7. F; 8. T; 9. F; 10. T

Name _____   Section _____   Date _____

WELLNESS WORKSHEET 3.1

Maslow's characteristics of a self-actualized person

In the spaces given below, describe yourself in relation to each of Maslow's characteristics of a self-actualized person. How closely does the description fit you? Where would you like to make changes?

1. **Clear perception of reality and comfortable relations with it.** The self-actualized person judges others accurately and is capable of tolerating uncertainty and ambiguity.

2. **Acceptance of self and others.** Self-actualizers accept themselves as they are and are not defensive. They have little guilt, shame, or anxiety.

3. **Natural and spontaneous.** Self-actualizers are spontaneous in both thought and behavior.

4. **Focus on problems rather than self.** Self-actualizers focus on problems outside themselves; they are concerned with basic issues and eternal questions.

5. **Need privacy; tend to be detached.** Although self-actualizers enjoy others, they do not mind solitude and sometimes seek it.

6. **Autonomous.** Self-actualizers are relatively independent of their culture and environment, but they do not go against convention just for the sake of being different.

7. **Continued freshness of appreciation.** Self-actualizers are capable of fresh, spontaneous, and nonstereotyped appreciation of objects, events, and people. They appreciate the basic pleasures of life.

(over)

8. **Mystic experience.** Self-actualizers have had peak experiences or experiences in which they have attained transcendence.

9. **Social interest.** Self-actualizers have feelings of identification, sympathy, and affection for others.

10. **Interpersonal relations.** Self-actualizers do on occasion get angry, but they do not bear long-lasting grudges. Their relationships with others are few but are deep and meaningful.

11. **Democratic character structure.** Self-actualizers show respect for all people irrespective of race, creed, income level, etc.

12. **Discrimination between means and ends.** Self-actualizers are strongly ethical with definite moral standards. They do not confuse means with ends; they relate to ends rather than means.

13. **Sense of humor.** Self-actualizers have a sense of humor that is both philosophical and nonhostile.

14. **Creativeness.** Self-actualizers are original and inventive, expressive, perceptive, and spontaneous in everyday life. They are able to see things in new ways.

15. **Nonconformity.** Self-actualizers fit into their culture, but they are independent of it and do not blindly comply with all its demands. They are open to new experiences.

CHAPTER 4
Intimate Relationships

Multiple Choice

1. Our gender role is defined for us by our:
   a. genetics.
   b. culture.
   c. decisions.
   d. sexual experiences.

2. One of the first elements to begin to cause attraction between two people is:
   a. social status.
   b. personality traits.
   c. general behavior.
   d. political persuasion.

3. Cohabitation is:
   a. more popular among senior citizens than young singles.
   b. increasing in popularity.
   c. remaining the same in popularity.
   d. undetermined as to popularity.

4. What percent of married women are in the workforce?
   a. more than 10 percent
   b. more than 20 percent
   c. more than 40 percent
   d. more than 50 percent

5. The most destructive way of dealing with anger is probably to:
   a. suppress it.
   b. talk about your feelings.
   c. give yourself some space until your anger subsides.
   d. negotiate and explore alternatives.

6. After divorce, the recovery period usually does not start for about:
   a. one year.
   b. two years.
   c. three years.
   d. four years.

7. Which of the following is NOT one of the three characteristics that assist couples in avoiding marital dissatisfaction after the birth of a baby?
   a. The couple had developed a strong relationship before the baby is born.
   b. Each parent has a satisfying career.
   c. The child was planned and wanted.
   d. The couple communicates about their feelings and expectations.

8. Which of the following tends to be TRUE about strong families:
   a. They are without problems.
   b. Some may be seen at counseling centers.
   c. They avoid talking about disagreements.
   d. They know they care for one another without having to show it.

9. Recent studies have shown that cancer patients are more likely to be less depressed and to feel less pain if they:
   a. receive "alternative" treatment.
   b. participate in a support group.
   c. are single.
   d. become vegetarian.

10. Which one of the following statements about marriage is TRUE?
   a. Less than a quarter of marriages in the U.S. end in divorce.
   b. The primary functions and benefits of marriage are very different from other personal relationships.
   c. People are marrying at younger ages than in the past.
   d. Today, people marry more for personal, emotional reasons.

True or False

T F   1. Successful intimate relationships are more likely for people who have high self-esteem.

T F   2. It is more likely that life partners will be different than similar.

T F   3. The less religious a person is, the less likely it is that the person will participate in cohabitation.

T F   4. A large number of people in all age groups are single.

T F   5. About half of all American marriages end in divorce.

T F   6. Nonverbal communication is only a small part of the overall communication that occurs between two people.

T F   7. "Blended family" is another term for cohabitation.

T F   8. About half of all marriages are first marriages.

T F   9. For most people, love sustains the relationship and sex intensifies the relationship.

T F   10. The high rate of divorce in the United States indicates that most Americans don't believe in marriage anymore.

ANSWERS: Multiple Choice: 1. b; 2. a; 3. b; 4. d; 5. a; 6. a; 7. b; 8. b; 9. b; 10. d
True/False 1. T; 2. F; 3. F; 4. T; 5. T; 6. F; 7. F; 8. T; 9. T; 10. F

Name _____   Section _____   Date _____

WELLNESS WORKSHEET 4.1

Rate your family's strengths

This Family Strengths Inventory was developed by researchers who studied the strengths of over 3,000 families. To assess your family (either the family you grew up in or the family you have formed as an adult), circle the number that best reflects how your family rates on each strength. A 1 represents the lowest rating and a 5 represents the highest.

1. Spending time together and doing things with each other	1	2	3	4	5
2. Commitment to each other	1	2	3	4	5
3. Good communication (talking with each other often, listening well, sharing feelings with each other)	1	2	3	4	5
4. Dealing with crises in a positive manner	1	2	3	4	5
5. Expressing appreciation to each other	1	2	3	4	5
6. Spiritual wellness	1	2	3	4	5
7. Closeness of relationship between spouses	1	2	3	4	5
8. Closeness of relationship between parents and children	1	2	3	4	5
9. Happiness of relationship between spouses	1	2	3	4	5
10. Happiness of relationship between parents and children	1	2	3	4	5
11. Extent to which spouses make each other feel good about themselves (self-confident, worthy, competent, and happy)	1	2	3	4	5
12. Extent to which parents help children feel good about themselves	1	2	3	4	5

Scoring   Add the numbers you have circled. A score below 39 indicates below-average family strengths. Scores between 39 and 52 are in the average range. Scores above 53 indicate a strong family. Low scores on individual items identify areas that families can profitably spend time on. High scores are worthy of celebration but shouldn't lead to complacency. Like gardens, families need loving care to remain strong.

What do you think is your family's major strength? What do you like best about your family?

What about your family would you most like to change?

Inventory used with permission. N. Stinnet and J. DeFrain. 1986. *Secrets of Strong Families*. Boston: Little, Brown, pp. 167–169.

CHAPTER 5
Sexuality, Pregnancy, and Childbirth

Multiple Choice

1. Puberty is first marked by:
   a. the development of differentiated genitalia.
   b. an equalization of the capabilities of the sexes.
   c. an ability to reproduce.
   d. the development of secondary sex characteristics.

2. The reproductive maturation of girls precedes that of boys by about _____ years.
   a. two
   b. three
   c. four
   d. five

3. A contemporary definition of impotence is:
   a. erectile dysfunction.
   b. premature ejaculation.
   c. retarded ejaculation.
   d. orgasmic dysfunction.

4. All of the following are characteristic of fetal alcohol syndrome EXCEPT:
   a. low birth weight.
   b. mental retardation.
   c. congenital heart defects.
   d. spina bifida.

5. Home pregnancy tests are usually _____ percent reliable.
   a. 40–50
   b. 50–75
   c. 85–95
   d. 100

6. Each trimester of pregnancy is approximately ____ weeks long.
   a. 10
   b. 11
   c. 12
   d. 13

7. Just after fertilization, the fertilized egg is called a (an):
   a. embryo.
   b. zygote.
   c. fetus.
   d. blastocyst.

8. Which of the following is a symptom of eclampsia, but not preeclampsia?
   a. high blood pressure
   b. fluid retention
   c. swollen legs
   d. blurred vision

9. If the egg is not fertilized, it lasts about _____ hours and then disintegrates.
   a. two
   b. twelve
   c. twenty-four
   d. thirty

10. Which of the following circumstances is a contraindication for exercise during pregnancy?
    a. Mother is under 25 years of age.
    b. Exercise will occur in hot, humid weather.
    c. Preferred exercise is swimming.
    d. Exercise bout will be shorter than 15 minutes.

True or False

T F   1. Preejaculatory fluid may contain some sperm.

T F   2. The sexual organs of males and females develop from the same structures and perform similar functions.

T F   3. Hegar's sign is an indication that birth is imminent.

T F   4. Women of normal weight gain approximately 18–25 percent of their normal weight during pregnancy.

T F   5. Alpha-fetoprotein screening is performed earlier in the pregnancy than any other test.

T F   6. Symptoms of toxemia of pregnancy can include increased appetite and higher levels of energy.

T F   7. The number of babies born to mothers who are regular cocaine users has increased dramatically in recent years.

T F   8. Ultrasound is the only prenatal test that provides reliable information about the unborn infant.

T F   9. One of the risks associated with sexually transmissible diseases is infertility.

T F 10. Colostrum is thin, milklike fluid secreted by mammary glands around the time of pregnancy.

ANSWERS: Multiple Choice: 1. d; 2. a; 3. a; 4. d; 5. c; 6. d; 7. b; 8. d; 9. c; 10. b
True/False 1. T; 2. T; 3. F; 4. T; 5. F; 6. F; 7. T; 8. F; 9. T; 10. T

Name _____   Section _____   Date _____

Creating a family health tree

Knowing that a specific disease runs in your family allows you to watch closely for the early warning signs and get appropriate screening tests. It can also help you target important health habits to adopt. You can put together a simple family health tree by compiling key facts on your primary relatives; siblings, parents, aunts and uncles, and grandparents. If possible, have your primary relatives fill out a family health history record like the one below.

Family Health History

Name: _____   Date of birth: _____

Blood and Rh type: _____   Occupation: _____

Please note any serious or chronic diseases you have experienced, with special attention to the following:

_____ Alcoholism

_____ Allergies

_____ Arthritis

_____ Asthma

_____ Blood diseases (hemophilia, sickle cell anemia, thalassemia)

_____ Cancer (i.e., breast, bowel, colon, ovarian, skin, and stomach)

_____ Cystic fibrosis

_____ Diabetes

_____ Epilepsy

_____ Familial high blood cholesterol levels

_____ Hearing defects

_____ Heart defects

_____ Huntington's disease

_____ Hypertension (high blood pressure)

_____ Learning disabilities (dyslexia, attention deficit disorder, autism)

_____ Liver disease (particularly hepatitis)

_____ Lupus

_____ Mental illness (manic depressive disorders; schizophrenia)

_____ Mental retardation (Down's syndrome, fragile X, etc.)

_____ Migraine headaches

_____ Miscarriages or neonatal deaths

_____ Multiple sclerosis

_____ Muscular dystrophy

_____ Myasthenia gravis

_____ Obesity

_____ Phenylketonuria (PKU)

_____ Respiratory disease (emphysema, bacterial pneumonia)

_____ Rh disease

_____ Skin disorders (particularly psoriasis)

_____ Thyroid disorders

_____ Tay-Sachs disease

_____ Tuberculosis

_____ Visual disorders (dyslexia, glaucoma, retinitis pigmentosa)

_____ Other (please list):

(over)

List any important health-related behaviors (including tobacco use, dietary and exercise habits, and alcohol use):

Please note names of your relatives below, along with indications of any illnesses, such as those listed above, which affected them. If deceased, list age and cause. Also make note of lifestyle habits such as smoking.

Father: _____

Mother: _____

Brothers and sisters: _____

Children of brothers and sisters: _____

If you don't have enough information on past generations, you can get clues by requesting death certificates from state health departments or medical records from relatives' physicians or hospitals where they died. Once you've collected the information you want, plug it into the tree format as shown in your text.

Adapted from "What's Lurking in Your Family Tree?" *Consumer Reports on Health,* September 1992; and March of Dimes Birth Defects Foundation. 1992. "Genetic Counseling."

CHAPTER 6
Contraception and Abortion: Current Issues

Multiple Choice

1. The typical failure rate of IUDs during the first year of use is:
    a. 1–2 percent.
    b. 8 percent.
    c. 15 percent.
    d. 22 percent.

2. The oral contraceptive user who is most likely to suffer a stroke is a:
    a. smoker.
    b. woman who has not had any children.
    c. woman who started using the pill after the age of twenty-five.
    d. small-framed woman.

3. Depo-Provera is administered:
    a. by skin patch.
    b. by injection.
    c. by implantation.
    d. orally.

4. Oral contraceptives prevent pregnancy by:
    a. creating a sperm barrier.
    b. causing spontaneous abortion.
    c. stopping ovulation.
    d. an unknown mechanism.

5. A method of contraception that is more popular in the United States than male condoms is:
    a. IUDs.
    b. oral contraceptives.
    c. Norplant implants.
    d. diaphragms.

6. The pro-life position argues that:
    a. women ought to have the right to have an abortion under any circumstances.
    b. abortion ought to be permitted up to the sixth week of pregnancy.
    c. abortion is morally wrong.
    d. their position is essentially consistent with the pro-choice position.

7. Amniocentesis is a procedure for:
    a. diagnosing birth defects.
    b. abortion.
    c. late abortion.
    d. dilating the cervix in preparation for abortion.

8. According to the Supreme Court's Casey decision, which of the following is NOT judged to be an "undue burden" for women seeking abortion?
   a. requiring women to tell husbands of the intention to seek an abortion
   b. requiring women to register with an adoption agency until after the abortion has been performed
   c. requiring women to wait until after the twelfth week of pregnancy before undergoing an abortion
   d. requiring women to hear educational information about fetal development and alternatives to abortion

9. The earliest date when abortion was universally legal in the United States is:
   a. 1973.
   b. 1850.
   c. 1960.
   d. 1981.

10. One of the most severe restrictions that the Supreme Court's Webster decision let stand was a requirement that:
   a. viability tests be done if the fetus is judged to be more than 20 weeks old.
   b. women seeking abortions wait for 24 hours.
   c. minors obtain parental permission.
   d. women seeking abortions look at photos of developing fetuses.

True or False

T F   1. There is no proven relationship between taking birth control pills and contracting breast cancer.

T F   2. The contraceptive method that is most like the cervical cap is the IUD.

T F   3. The Billings method of contraception requires that sexual partners abstain from intercourse on fertile days.

T F   4. A woman can reduce her risks of complications due to taking oral contraceptives if she has regular checkups of her blood pressure.

T F   5. Norplant implants were invented and used for the first time in the United States.

T F   6. The literal and popular definitions of abortion are the same.

T F   7. In the United States, the vast majority of abortions are performed during the first twelve weeks of pregnancy.

T F   8. The risks associated with childbirth are higher than those associated with abortion.

T F   9. The risk of death of the mother associated with abortion increases with the length of pregnancy.

T F 10. Psychological side effects of abortion are clearly defined and patient responses are quite predictable.

ANSWERS: Multiple Choice: 1. a; 2. a; 3. b; 4. c; 5. b; 6. c; 7. a; 8. d; 9. a; 10. a
True/False 1. T; 2. F; 3. T; 4. T; 5. F; 6. F; 7. T; 8. T; 9. T; 10. F

W E L L N E S S   W O R K S H E E T 6.1

Your position on the legality and morality of abortion

To help define your own position on abortion, answer the following series of questions.

		Agree	Disagree
1.	The fertilized egg is a human being from the moment of conception.	___	___
2.	The rights of the fetus at any stage take precedence over any decision a woman might want to make regarding her pregnancy.	___	___
3.	The rights of the fetus depend upon its gestational age: further along in the pregnancy, the fetus has more rights.	___	___
4.	Each individual woman should have final say over decisions regarding her health and body; politicians should not be allowed to decide.	___	___
5.	In cases of teenagers seeking an abortion, parental consent should be required.	___	___
6.	In cases of married women seeking an abortion, spousal consent should be required.	___	___
7.	In cases of late abortion, tests should be done to determine the viability of the fetus.	___	___
8.	The federal government should provide public funding for abortion to ensure equal access to abortion for all women.	___	___
9.	The federal government should not allow states to pass their own abortion laws; there should be uniform laws for the entire country.	___	___
10.	Does a woman's right to choose whether or not to have an abortion depend upon the circumstances surrounding conception or the situation of the mother? In which of the following situations, if any, would you support a woman's right to choose to have an abortion (check where appropriate):		

_____ An abortion is necessary to maintain the woman's life or health.

_____ The pregnancy is a result of rape or incest.

_____ A serious birth defect has been detected in the fetus through amnio-centesis or chorionic villus sampling.

_____ The pregnancy is a result of the failure of a contraceptive method or device.

_____ The pregnancy occurred when no contraceptive method was in use.

_____ A single mother, pregnant for the fifth time, wants an abortion because she feels she cannot support another child.

_____ A pregnant 15-year-old high school student feels having a child would prove to be too great a disruption in her life and keep her from reaching her goals for the future.

(over)

_____ A pregnant 19-year-old college student does not want to interrupt her education.

_____ The father of the child has stated he will provide no support and is not interested in helping raise the child.

_____ Parents of two boys wish to terminate the mother's pregnancy because the fetus is male rather than female.

On the basis of your answers to the questions on the previous page, write out your position on abortion. Should it be legal or illegal? Are there certain circumstances in which it should or should not be allowed? What sorts of rules should govern when it can be performed?

CHAPTER 7
Tobacco and Alcohol

Multiple Choice

1. Smokers who change to low-tar cigarettes are likely to:
   a. puff less frequently.
   b. inhale less deeply.
   c. smoke less of each cigarette.
   d. smoke more cigarettes.

2. Children of mothers who smoked during pregnancy are more likely to:
   a. score lower on school reading tests.
   b. become lower-income adults.
   c. drop out of high school.
   d. suffer from eating disorders.

3. The most widespread cause of death among cigarette smokers is:
   a. coronary heart disease.
   b. lung cancer.
   c. pancreatic cancer.
   d. cancer of the thoracic cavity.

4. The material that blocks the arteries of a patient with atherosclerosis is:
   a. plaque.
   b. catecholamines.
   c. macrophages.
   d. tar.

5. Male smokers are more likely than nonsmokers to suffer all of the following cancers EXCEPT:
   a. prostate cancer.
   b. pancreatic cancer.
   c. bladder cancer.
   d. stomach cancer.

6. High concentrations of alcohol (high blood alcohol content) are MOST likely to produce:
   a. diminished motor skill.
   b. increased intellectual function.
   c. increased verbal performance.
   d. increased coordination.

7. The disease most closely associated with alcohol abuse is:
   a. cirrhosis.
   b. glaucoma.
   c. gout.
   d. hypotension.

8. All other things being equal, which of the following people is going to get intoxicated most quickly?
   a. 200-lb. male
   b. 150-lb. female
   c. 150-lb. male
   d. 125-lb. female

9. The best way to reduce the intoxicating effects of alcohol is to:
   a. drink at a steady rate.
   b. space one's drinks.
   c. drink on an empty stomach.
   d. drink a 50-proof beverage instead of a 40-proof beverage.

10. Below-normal birth weights occur in babies born to women who drank as few as _____ beers per day during pregnancy.
   a. two
   b. three
   c. one
   d. four

True or False

T F 1. Almost all deaths from coronary heart disease can be attributed to cigarette smoking.

T F 2. Due to smoking, lung cancer has surpassed breast cancer as the leading cause of cancer death among women.

T F 3. Cigarettes with low tar and nicotine have reduced the incidence of lung cancer among smokers.

T F 4. Mainstream smoke contains lower concentrations of toxic and carcinogenic compounds than does sidestream smoke.

T F 5. Smoking is the primary cause of emphysema.

T F 6. The common psychoactive ingredient in beer is hops.

T F 7. Alcohol is a depressant.

T F 8. According to the text, fraternity members drink less frequently and less heavily than other college students.

T F 9. There is a positive relationship between academic performance and the amount of alcohol consumed.

T F 10. One enabling behavior is to make excuses for an alcoholic's intoxication.

ANSWERS: Multiple Choice: 1. d; 2. a; 3. a; 4. a; 5. a; 6. a; 7. a; 8. d; 9. b; 10. a
True/False 1. F; 2. T; 3. F; 4. T; 5. T; 6. F; 7. T; 8. F; 9. F; 10. T

WELLNESS WORKSHEET 7.1

Personal drinking guide

Evaluate Your Reasons for Drinking

Be honest with yourself. It is necessary for you to know why you drink in order to control your alcohol-related behavior. Put a check next to the statements that are true for you.

I drink to tune myself in to

_____ enhance enjoyment of people, activities, special occasions

_____ promote social ease by relaxing inhibitions, aiding ability to talk and relate to others

_____ complement and add to enjoyment of food

_____ relax after a period of hard work and/or tension

I drink to tune myself out to

_____ escape problems

_____ mask fears when courage and self-confidence are lacking

_____ block out painful loneliness, self-doubt, feelings of inadequacy

_____ substitute for close relationships, challenging activity

_____ mask a sense of guilt about drinking

Alcohol Content

Drinks differ in the amount of pure alcohol they contain; therefore, a "drink" means different amounts of liquid depending on the type of drink. A proof value indicates concentration of alcohol in a particular drink; the proof value is equal to twice the percentage of alcohol in a drink. To calculate the number of ounces of pure alcohol in a drink, multiply the size of the drink by the percentage of alcohol it contains (one-half proof value). For example, a 12 oz. beer (10 proof) has 0.6 oz. of pure alcohol (10 proof = 5% alcohol concentration; 0.05×12 oz. = 0.6 oz.).

Calculate the number of ounces of pure alcohol in each of the following drinks.

Drink	Size (oz.)	Proof value	Oz. of pure alcohol
beer	12	10	_____
wine	6	24	_____
sherry	4	40	_____
liquor	1.5	80	_____

Try the calculations on different size drinks and drinks of different alcohol content.

_____	_____	_____	_____
_____	_____	_____	_____
_____	_____	_____	_____
_____	_____	_____	_____

(over)

Maintenance Rate (or how long to sip a drink)

Remember that the effects of alcohol will be greater when your BAC is rising than when you keep it stable or allow it to fall. BAC is directly proportional to the rate of ethyl alcohol intake. Assuming a general maintenance rate (rate at which the body rids itself of alcohol) of 0.1 oz. of pure alcohol per hour per 50 pounds of body weight, you can calculate the approximate length of time it takes you to metabolize a given drink by applying the following formula:

$$\frac{2.5 \times \text{proof of drink} \times \text{volume (size in oz.) of drink}}{\text{body weight}} = \text{time in hours per drink}$$

For example, to calculate how long it should take to drink one can (12 oz.) of 10 proof beer for a person weighing 150 pounds:

$$\frac{2.5 \times 10 \times 12}{150} = 2 \text{ hours}$$

So, it takes this 150-pound individual 2 hours to completely metabolize one 12 oz. can of 10 proof beer.

Choose your favorite three drinks (or choose three of the examples from the previous page) and use this formula to calculate your maintenance rate for each drink.

1. $$\frac{(\quad) \times (\quad) \times (\quad)}{(\quad)} = \boxed{\qquad \text{hours/drink}}$$

2. $$\frac{(\quad) \times (\quad) \times (\quad)}{(\quad)} = \boxed{\qquad \text{hours/drink}}$$

3. $$\frac{(\quad) \times (\quad) \times (\quad)}{(\quad)} = \boxed{\qquad \text{hours/drink}}$$

In Case of Excess

To sober up, the only remedy that works is to stop drinking and allow time. For any given type of drink, the amount of time would be the number of drinks you have consumed multiplied by your maintenance rate for that drink. For the example given above, if the 150-pound individual had consumed three 12 oz. cans of 10 proof beer, he or she would have to wait 6 hours before the alcohol would be metabolized. Calculate the amount of time that would have to elapse for you to metabolize all the alcohol if you had consumed three of one of the types of drinks you calculated a maintenance rate for above:

$$3 \times (\quad) = \underline{\qquad} \text{ hours}$$

Given this consumption level, your answer here indicates the number of hours you should wait before driving.

CHAPTER 8
The Use and Abuse of Psychoactive Drugs

Multiple Choice

1. The most likely physical reaction to amphetamine ingestion is:
   a. lethargy.
   b. fatigue.
   c. boredom.
   d. alertness.

2. The effects of cocaine most closely resemble the effects of:
   a. alcohol.
   b. deliriants.
   c. hallucinogens.
   d. amphetamines.

3. All of the following are common consequences of using marijuana EXCEPT:
   a. an increase in the heart rate.
   b. a decreased inclination to participate in physical activities.
   c. constriction of the blood vessels of the eye.
   d. euphoria.

4. Information learned in a drug-induced state that is difficult to recall when not intoxicated is a description of:
   a. setting.
   b. learning discrimination.
   c. state dependency.
   d. neurosis.

5. The most widely used ILLICIT drug in the United States is:
   a. alcohol.
   b. crack.
   c. heroin.
   d. marijuana.

6. Which of the following is a drug user factor?
   a. body mass
   b. pharmacological characteristics
   c. setting
   d. time-action function

7. Which of the following is a drug factor?
   a. dose-response function
   b. set
   c. other drugs consumed by user
   d. drug use during pregnancy

8. Opiates:
    a. relieve pain.
    b. stimulate activity.
    c. induce alertness.
    d. do all of the above.

9. The children of women who use amphetamines during pregnancy have a higher incidence of:
    a. impaired vision.
    b. impaired hearing.
    c. misshapen head.
    d. cleft palate.

10. The effects of caffeine include stimulation of:
    a. appetite.
    b. respiration.
    c. mental activity.
    d. aggressiveness.

True or False

T F   1. Drugs that stimulate the central nervous system are called BAC stimulants.

T F   2. Dependence is not related to tolerance.

T F   3. The effects of a single dose of heroin last longer than a single dose of cocaine.

T F   4. The first half of the twentieth century was a period during which rates of drug use and addiction dropped in America.

T F   5. Drug dependence is exclusively a physical experience.

T F   6. Cocaine is a central nervous system stimulant.

T F   7. Most central nervous system depressants can lead to classic physical dependence.

T F   8. Marijuana is a drug for which a regular user is likely to develop a high degree of tolerance.

T F   9. The effects of amphetamine abuse, while serious, are almost all completely reversible when amphetamine consumption is stopped.

T F 10. Methadone is a synthetic drug used in medical drug rehabilitation as a less debilitating substitute for heroin.

ANSWERS: Multiple Choice: 1. d; 2. d; 3. c; 4. c; 5. d; 6. a; 7. a; 8. a; 9. d; 10. b
True/False 1. F; 2. F; 3. T; 4. T; 5. F; 6. T; 7. T; 8. T; 9. F; 10. T

CHAPTER 9
Nutrition Facts and Fallacies

Multiple Choice

1. A good source of omega-3 fatty acids is:
   a. bread.
   b. rice.
   c. vegetables.
   d. salmon.

2. Carbohydrates are divided into which of the following groups?
   a. simple and complex
   b. complex and complete
   c. complete and incomplete
   d. incomplete and simple

3. If you consume more carbohydrates than you need, the excess will be:
   a. excreted in urine.
   b. expired during respiration.
   c. stored as fat.
   d. stored as muscle.

4. Nutritionists classify dietary fiber as:
   a. soluble and complete.
   b. complete and incomplete.
   c. simple and insoluble.
   d. soluble and insoluble.

5. Vitamin A deficiency can cause:
   a. allergies.
   b. loss of lean body mass.
   c. mental retardation in fetuses.
   d. blindness.

6. Which one of the following foods has the lowest water content?
   a. apples
   b. celery
   c. beef
   d. cherries

7. Muscles and bones are formed by:
   a. carbohydrates.
   b. fiber.
   c. fat.
   d. protein.

8. The building blocks of protein are called:
   a. soluble fiber.
   b. complex carbohydrates.
   c. amino acids.
   d. fatty acids.

9. Health experts recommend that we reduce our fat intake to _____ of total calories.
   a. 10 percent or less
   b. 30 percent or less
   c. 50 percent or less
   d. 70 percent or less

10. An increase in carbohydrate consumption should take place at the expense of:
    a. vitamin intake.
    b. fat intake.
    c. vegetable consumption.
    d. water consumption.

True or False

T F   1. The potential fuel in food is expressed in kilometers.

T F   2. The body's main structural components are made up of calcium.

T F   3. Another name for fats is lipids.

T F   4. Some amino acids are essential nutrients.

T F   5. Consuming large amounts of swordfish may put you at risk for mercury poisoning.

T F   6. The primary source of energy for the body during heavy exercise is fat.

T F   7. Americans should increase their intake of carbohydrates.

T F   8. Vitamin deficiencies can cause blindness.

T F   9. The nutrient content of foods is given on food labels as a percentage of Daily Values.

T F   10. Most Americans need to take nutrient supplements to obtain needed vitamins and minerals.

ANSWERS: Multiple Choice: 1. d; 2. a; 3. c; 4. d; 5. d; 6. c; 7. d; 8. c; 9. b; 10. b
True/False 1. F; 2. F; 3. T; 4. T; 5. T; 6. F; 7. T; 8. T; 9. T; 10. F

Name _____ Section _____ Date _____

WELLNESS WORKSHEET 9.1

Nutrition checklist

The Food Guide Pyramid provides a general basis for good nutrition. Your choice of foods within each group and methods of food preparation are also important. Evaluate some of your dietary habits by answering the following questions with yes (Y) or no (N). A "no" answer indicates a behavior you might want to change.

_____   1. I rarely add salt to my food when cooking or eating.

_____   2. I take time to read food labels when shopping.

_____   3. I choose foods that are fresh and unprocessed whenever possible.

_____   4. I eat a wide variety of foods.

_____   5. I remove fat and skin before cooking meat, poultry, or fish.

_____   6. I sometimes have meatless days, substituting healthy alternatives to meat.

_____   7. I broil, boil, or bake rather than fry meat, fish, and poultry.

_____   8. I choose nonfat or low-fat milk and milk products.

_____   9. I eat sherbet or frozen yogurt rather than ice cream.

_____ 10. I use vegetable oil instead of butter or margarine.

_____ 11. I choose whole-grain breads rather than white.

_____ 12. I choose cereals that are high in fiber.

_____ 13. I choose cereals, crackers, bread, and other foods that are low in added sugar and low in fat.

_____ 14. I have at least one serving of a citrus fruit each day.

_____ 15. I have at least one serving of a dark green or orange vegetable every day.

_____ 16. I eat fresh or frozen fruits and vegetables rather than canned whenever possible.

_____ 17. When I cook vegetables, I generally steam them.

_____ 18. I avoid frequent consumption of salt-cured, smoked, or nitrate-cured foods.

_____ 19. I consume alcohol in moderation.

_____ 20. I use nonstick pans or sprays when cooking to avoid adding extra fat to my food.

Choose one of your "no" answers and devise a behavior change program around it. List five strategies that might help you change the behavior you've chosen.

1. _____

2. _____

3. _____

4. _____

5. _____

WELLNESS WORKSHEET 9.2

Fast food

Use the information in the fast-food appendix in your text to complete the chart below for the last fast-food meal you ate. (If you haven't recently been to one of the restaurants listed, fill in the chart for any sample meal you might eat.) Compare the values for fat, protein, carbohydrate, cholesterol, and sodium content with the levels suggested by the Dietary Guidelines for Americans.

Food items

	Dietary Guidelines									** Total
Calories										
Fat (9 cal./gram)* saturated	10%									
monounsaturated	10%									
polyunsaturated	10%									
Total	30%									
Protein* (4 cal./gram)	15%									
Carbohydrate* (4 cal./gram)	55%									
Cholesterol (300 mg/day/3) ***	100 mg									
Sodium (6 g/day/3) ***	2000 mg									

* To calculate the % calories from each food element, use the following formula:

$$\frac{(\text{# grams of food element}) \times (\text{# calories per gram of food element})}{(\text{Total # of calories})}$$

For example, the % calories from protein in a 150-calorie dish containing 10 grams of protein would be:

$$\frac{(10 \text{ grams of protein}) \times (4 \text{ calories per gram})}{(150 \text{ calories})} = \frac{40}{150} = 27\% \text{ calories from protein}$$

** For the totals column, add up the total grams of fat, carbohydrate, and protein contained in your sample meal and calculate the percentages based on the total calories in the meal. For cholesterol and sodium values, add up the total number of milligrams.

*** Recommended daily levels of cholesterol and sodium are divided by 3 here to give an approximate recommended level for a single meal.

STUDY GUIDE

CHAPTER 10
Weight Management

Multiple Choice

1. Which of the following types of activity is best for burning fat?
   a. stretching
   b. resistance training
   c. endurance exercise
   d. weight lifting

2. The lowest rate at which the body burns calories is:
   a. resting metabolic rate.
   b. post–exercise metabolic rate.
   c. fasting metabolic rate.
   d. post-prandial metabolic rate.

3. Satiety is a feeling of:
   a. hunger.
   b. fullness.
   c. nausea.
   d. guilt felt by bulimics/anorexics.

4. Which type of exercise best helps maintain lean body mass during diet-induced weight loss?
   a. endurance exercise
   b. resistance training
   c. flexibility exercise
   d. walking

5. A good source of complex carbohydrates is:
   a. chicken.
   b. beef.
   c. potatoes.
   d. Gatorade.

6. Which of the following is the most accurate method of measuring percentage of body fat?
   a. height–weight tables
   b. underwater weighing
   c. body mass index
   d. waist-to-hip ratio

7. If you want to lose weight your exercise bouts should be:
   a. short and high intensity.
   b. long and moderate intensity.
   c. short and moderate intensity.
   d. high intensity and high duration.

8. For an obese person, losing as little as _____ can reduce blood pressure.
   a. 5 pounds
   b. 10 pounds
   c. 15 pounds
   d. 20 pounds

9. The most frequently occurring consequence of excess sugar in the diet is:
   a. tooth decay.
   b. diabetes.
   c. obesity.
   d. hyperactivity.

10. The text suggests that it might be time for a radical idea to answer the question of what one "should" weigh:
   a. Use the body composition approach.
   b. Let a healthy lifestyle determine your weight.
   c. Use percent of body fat as your guide.
   d. Don't worry about weight at all.

True or False

T F 1. Most Americans get less exercise than did their grandparents.

T F 2. More men than women are overweight.

T F 3. A history of dieting may cause resting metabolic rate to decline.

T F 4. Height and weight tables take body fat into consideration.

T F 5. A woman is increasing her health risks if her percent body fat is reduced to less than 8 percent.

T F 6. When a woman's percent body fat is too low she may stop menstruating.

T F 7. The risk of cancer is increased by being obese.

T F 8. "Normal" healthy values for body fat content are lower for women than for men.

T F 9. Successful dieting strategies include limiting food choices.

T F 10. There is only one way to assess body weight scientifically.

ANSWERS: Multiple Choice: 1. c; 2. a; 3. b; 4. b; 5. c; 6. b; 7. b; 8. b; 9. a; 10. b
True/False 1. T; 2. F; 3. T; 4. F; 5. T; 6. T; 7. T; 8. F; 9. F; 10. F

WELLNESS WORKSHEET 10.1

What triggers your eating?

This test is designed to provide you with a score for five factors that describe many people's eating. This information will put you in a better position to manage your eating behavior and control your weight. Circle the number that indicates to what degree each situation is likely to make you start eating.

	Very Unlikely					Very Likely			

Social

1. Arguing or having conflict with someone — 1 2 3 4 5 6 7 8 9 10
2. Being with others when they are eating — 1 2 3 4 5 6 7 8 9 10
3. Being urged to eat by someone else — 1 2 3 4 5 6 7 8 9 10
4. Feeling inadequate around others — 1 2 3 4 5 6 7 8 9 10

Emotional

5. Feeling bad, such as being anxious or depressed — 1 2 3 4 5 6 7 8 9 10
6. Feeling good, happy, or relaxed — 1 2 3 4 5 6 7 8 9 10
7. Feeling bored or having time on my hands — 1 2 3 4 5 6 7 8 9 10
8. Feeling stressed or excited — 1 2 3 4 5 6 7 8 9 10

Situational

9. Seeing an advertisement for food or eating — 1 2 3 4 5 6 7 8 9 10
10. Passing by a bakery, cookie shop, or other enticement to eat — 1 2 3 4 5 6 7 8 9 10
11. Being involved in a party, celebration, or special occasion — 1 2 3 4 5 6 7 8 9 10
12. Eating out — 1 2 3 4 5 6 7 8 9 10

Thinking

13. Making excuses to myself about why it's okay to eat — 1 2 3 4 5 6 7 8 9 10
14. Berating myself for being so fat or unable to control my eating — 1 2 3 4 5 6 7 8 9 10
15. Worrying about others, or about difficulties I am having — 1 2 3 4 5 6 7 8 9 10
16. Thinking about how things should or shouldn't be — 1 2 3 4 5 6 7 8 9 10

Physiological

17. Experiencing pain or physical discomfort — 1 2 3 4 5 6 7 8 9 10
18. Experiencing trembling, headache, or light-headedness associated with no eating or too much caffeine — 1 2 3 4 5 6 7 8 9 10
19. Experiencing fatigue or feeling overtired — 1 2 3 4 5 6 7 8 9 10
20. Experiencing hunger pangs or urges to eat, even though I've eaten recently — 1 2 3 4 5 6 7 8 9 10

Scoring

Total your scores for each area and enter them below. Then rank the scores by marking the highest score "1," next highest score "2," and so on. Focus on the highest ranked areas first, but any score above 24 is high and indicates that you need to work on that area.

(over)

Area	Total Score	Rank Order
Social (Items 1–4)	_____	_____
Emotional (Items 5–8)	_____	_____
Situational (Items 9–12)	_____	_____
Thinking (Items 13–16)	_____	_____
Physiological (Items 17–20)	_____	_____

What Your Score Means

Social　A high score on this factor means you are very susceptible to the influence of others. Work on better ways to communicate more assertively, handle conflict, and manage anger. Challenge your beliefs about the need to be polite and the obligations you feel you must fulfill.

Emotional　A high score here means you need to develop effective ways to cope with emotions. Work on developing skills in stress management, time management, and communication. Practicing positive self-talk can help you handle small daily upsets.

Situational　A high score here means you are especially susceptible to external influences. Try to avoid cues to eat and to respond differently to those you cannot avoid. Control your environment by changing the way you buy, store, cook, and serve food. Anticipate potential problems and have a plan for handling them.

Thinking　A high score here means that the way you think—how you talk to yourself, the beliefs you hold, your memories, and your expectations—have a powerful influence on your eating habits. Try to be less self-critical, less of a perfectionist, and more flexible in your ideas about the way things ought to be. Recognize when you're making excuses or rationalizations that allow you to eat.

Physiological　A high score here means that the way you eat, what you eat, or medications you are taking may be affecting your eating behavior. You may be eating to reduce physical arousal or deal with physical discomfort. Try eating three meals a day, supplemented with regular snacks if needed. Avoid too much caffeine. If any medication you're taking produces adverse physical reactions, switch to an alternative if possible. If your medications may be affecting your hormones, discuss possible alternatives with your physician.

From J. D. Nash. 1986. *Maximize Your Body Potential.* Shortened version. (Menlo Park, Calif.: Bull Publishing).

CHAPTER 11
Exercise for Health and Fitness

Multiple Choice

1. Exercise that achieves the target heart rate for an extended period of time is:
   a. very high intensity.
   b. isokinetic.
   c. aerobic.
   d. isometric.

2. The target heart rate is at least _____ percent of maximal heart rate.
   a. 35
   b. 55
   c. 75
   d. 95

3. The "natural high" that a person achieves as a result of vigorous physical activity may be the result of the release of:
   a. oxygen.
   b. endorphins.
   c. hypnotics.
   d. narcotics.

4. Maintaining strength is best achieved by:
   a. aerobic exercise.
   b. cycle training.
   c. resistance training.
   d. interval training.

5. Which of the following is NOT an element of health-related fitness?
   a. body composition
   b. strength
   c. endurance
   d. speed

6. Exercise intensity is measured by:
   a. a clock.
   b. pulse rate.
   c. check list.
   d. number of exercise bouts per week.

7. The least beneficial exercise for cardiorespiratory endurance is:
   a. jogging.
   b. cycling.
   c. rock climbing.
   d. swimming.

8. Cardiovascular fitness requires at least _____ bouts of exercise per week.
   a. two
   b. three
   c. four
   d. seven

9. The component of fitness that is most often neglected is:
   a. flexibility.
   b. duration.
   c. intensity.
   d. strength.

10. One way to help ensure consistency of exercise is to:
    a. keep a training journal.
    b. make goals consistent with national norms.
    c. increase your exercise volume by 10 percent or more per week.
    d. practice and play only one sport.

True or False

T F   1. A person can achieve a high level of cardiovascular fitness with two exercise bouts per week evenly spaced.

T F   2. The most crucial factor in attaining the training heart rate is the intensity of the workout.

T F   3. The fastest heart rate attainable before exhaustion is the training heart rate.

T F   4. Muscular force applied with movement is isometric exercise.

T F   5. Warm-up exercises will reduce the risk of injury but will not enhance performance.

T F   6. The best fluid replacement is cold water or diluted carbohydrate drinks.

T F   7. Exercise increases the efficiency of the body's metabolism.

T F   8. Exercise can help to protect women against osteoporosis.

T F   9. The old principle in physical training, *Use it or lose it,* no longer applies.

T F   10. An estimate of cardiovascular fitness can be obtained by checking your time in the 1.5-mile walk or run.

ANSWERS: Multiple Choice: 1. c; 2. b; 3. b; 4. c; 5. d; 6. b; 7. c; 8. b; 9. a; 10. a
True/False 1. F; 2. T; 3. F; 4. F; 5. F; 6. T; 7. T; 8. T; 9. F; 10. T

WELLNESS WORKSHEET 11.1

Do you need to improve your level of physical fitness?

Medical Clearance

In general, if you are under 35, have no physical complaints, and have had a medical checkup within the past two years, it is probably safe for you to begin an exercise program at your current level of physical activity and gradually increase it. To determine whether you need to consult your physician, read through the following list of statements and check any that are true for you.

_____ I am not feeling well.

_____ I have a specific health concern.

_____ I am over 20 percent above my desirable weight and much of the excess is body fat.

_____ I have been sedentary for a long time.

_____ I have a history of some type of cardiovascular disease.

_____ I can't walk more than two miles.

_____ I have one or more of the following symptoms after exertion:

    _____ Chest pain

    _____ Dizziness or faintness

    _____ Gastrointestinal upset

    _____ Difficulty breathing

    _____ Shortness of breath for more than 10 minutes after exertion

    _____ Lingering fatigue and difficulty in sleeping

_____ I am 35 or older and have a history of coronary heart disease risk factors:

    _____ Diabetes

    _____ Hypertension

    _____ High blood cholesterol levels

    _____ Cigarette smoking

    _____ A blood relative who had a heart attack before age 60

If you checked one or more of these statements, you should consult your physician before beginning any type of exercise program.

Assessing Cardiorespiratory Endurance: 1.5-Mile Run-Walk Test

(Don't attempt this test unless you have completed at least six weeks of some type of conditioning activity and, if indicated by the checklist above, have obtained medical clearance.) Before beginning this test, warm up with some walking, easy jogging, and stretching exercises.

1. Ask someone with a stopwatch, clock, or watch with a second hand to time you.

2. Take the test on a running track or course that is flat and provides measurements of up to 1.5 miles. Cover the distance as fast as possible, at a pace that is comfortable for you. You can run or walk the entire distance or use some combination of running and walking.

(over)

3. Note the time it takes you to complete the 1.5-mile distance.
   Your time: _____ : _____ (minutes:seconds)

4. Cool down by walking or jogging slowly for about 5 minutes.

5. Determine the rating for your score by consulting the table below. If you are unable to complete the entire 1.5 miles, consider yourself poor in CRE.

Standards for the 1.5 Mile Run-Walk (min:sec)

	High	Good	Fair	Poor
Males				
20–29	9:45	12:00	13:00	15:00
30–39	10:00	12:15	13:30	16:00
40–49	10:30	12:30	14:00	16:30
50–59	11:00	13:30	15:00	18:30
60+	11:15	14:30	16:30	19:00
Females				
20–29	11:00	13:15	14:15	16:15
30–39	11:15	13:30	14:45	17:15
40–49	11:45	13:45	15:15	17:45
50–59	12:15	14:45	16:15	19:45
60+	12:30	15:45	17:45	20:15

CRE Rating: _____

Source: I. Kusinitz and M. Fine. 1995. *Your Guide to Getting Fit*. 3rd ed. (Mountain View, Calif.: Mayfield).

CHAPTER 12
Cardiovascular Disease and Cancer

Multiple Choice

1. Smoking affects the cardiorespiratory system in which one of the following ways?
    a. It depresses the central nervous system.
    b. It increases the amount of oxygen available to the heart.
    c. It reduces levels of HDL in the bloodstream.
    d. It decreases blood thickness.

2. What total cholesterol level is suggested by your text as being too low?
    a. 240
    b. 210
    c. 170
    d. 140

3. Arteriosclerosis is:
    a. fatty buildup in the arteries.
    b. an aneurysm.
    c. hardening of the arteries.
    d. the same as atherosclerosis.

4. The factor that contributes least to risk of atherosclerosis is:
    a. age.
    b. hypertension.
    c. smoking.
    d. elevated cholesterol.

5. Which of the following systolic blood pressure readings would indicate the patient may have hypertension?
    a. 60
    b. 90
    c. 120
    d. 150

6. Mammography is recommended at least every one to two years for women over age:
    a. 20.
    b. 30.
    c. 40.
    d. 50.

7. Breast self-examination is recommended for all women over age:
    a. 20
    b. 30.
    c. 40.
    d. 50.

8. An imaging method in which sound waves are bounced off body structures to create an image on a television monitor is called:
   a. magnetic resonance imaging.
   b. ultrasonography.
   c. Papanicolaou test.
   d. CT test.

9. The most common form of cancer of the female reproductive system is:
   a. uterine cancer.
   b. ovarian cancer.
   c. vulvar cancer.
   d. cervical cancer.

10. The anti-carcinogen(s) found in broccoli and other members of the cruciferous family of vegetables is/are:
    a. emulsifiers.
    b. nitrates.
    c. antioxidants.
    d. sulforaphane.

True or False

T F   1. The type of fat that needs to be reduced most in the American diet is unsaturated fat.

T F   2. High blood pressure is considered a form of cardiovascular disease.

T F   3. Rates of CVD in the United States are higher for women than for men.

T F   4. Mexican-Americans and African Americans are more likely to suffer from cardiovascular disease than white Americans.

T F   5. Hypertension can lead to blindness.

T F   6. The terms malignant tumor and malignant neoplasm are synonymous with cancer.

T F   7. Sun exposure is a major cause of preventable cancer by damage to DNA in the cells.

T F   8. The best method for controlling prostate cancer is through hormone therapy.

T F   9. Sulforaphane is a potent carcinogen to which people are exposed if they consume a high fat diet.

T F 10. Two percent of all women are affected by breast cancer.

ANSWERS: Multiple Choice: 1. c; 2. d; 3. c; 4. a; 5. d; 6. c; 7. a; 8. b; 9. a; 10. d
True/False 1. F; 2. T; 3. F; 4. T; 5. T; 6. T; 7. T; 8. F; 9. F; 10. F

WELLNESS WORKSHEET 12.1

Are you at risk for cardiovascular disease?

Your chances of suffering an early heart attack or stroke depend on a variety of factors, many of which are under your control. To help identify your risk factors, circle the response for each risk category that best describes you.

1. Gender

    0 Female
    2 Male

2. Heredity

    0 Neither parent suffered a heart attack or stroke before age 60.
    3 One parent suffered a heart attack or stroke before age 60.
    7 Both parents suffered a heart attack or stroke before age 60.

3. Smoking

    0 Never smoked
    1 Quit more than 2 years ago
    2 Quit less than 2 years ago
    8 Smoke less than 1/2 pack per day
    13 Smoke more than 1/2 pack per day
    15 Smoke more than 1 pack per day

4. Environmental Tobacco Smoke

    0 Do not live or work with smokers
    2 Exposed to ETS at work
    3 Live with smoker
    4 Both live and work with smokers

5. Blood Pressure

    The average of the last three readings:

    0 130/80 or below
    1 131/81 to 140/85
    5 141/86 to 150/90
    9 151/91 to 170/100
    13 Above 170/100

6. Total Cholesterol

    The average of the last three readings:

    0 Lower than 190
    1 190 to 210
    2 Don't know
    3 211 to 240
    4 241 to 270
    5 271 to 300
    6 Over 300

(over)

7. HDL Cholesterol

The average of the last three readings:

0 Over 65 mg/dl
1 55 to 65
2 Don't know HDL
3 45 to 54
5 35 to 44
7 25 to 34
12 Lower than 25

8. Exercise

0 Aerobic exercise three times per week
1 Aerobic exercise once or twice per week
2 Occasional exercise less than once per week
7 Rarely exercise

9. Diabetes

0 No personal or family history
2 One parent with diabetes
6 Two parents with diabetes
9 Non-insulin-dependent diabetes (Type 2)
13 Insulin-dependent diabetes (Type 1)

10. Weight

0 Near ideal weight
1 Six pounds or less above ideal weight
3 Seven to 19 pounds above ideal weight
5 Twenty to 40 pounds above ideal weight
7 More than 40 pounds above ideal weight

11. Stress

0 Relaxed most of the time
1 Occasional stress and anger
2 Frequently stressed and angry
3 Usually stressed and angry

Scoring

Total your risk factor points. Refer to the list below to get an approximate rating of your risk of suffering an early heart attack or stroke.

Score	Estimated Risk
Less than 20	Low risk
20–29	Moderate risk
30–45	High risk
Over 45	Extremely high risk

Whatever your score, examine your responses carefully to identify your CVD risk factors. Consider planning a behavior change strategy to lower your risk by changing your lifestyle.

Name _____   Section _____   Date _____

WELLNESS WORKSHEET 12.2

Risk factors for cancer

Are you doing all you can to avoid cancer? You can directly influence some risk factors, such as diet and exposure to cigarette smoke, while others are beyond your control. The following statements relate to factors that can put you at increased risk for cancer. To identify your risk factors, check any statements that are true for you.

_____ I have a family history of cancer. Check any of the following family members who have had cancer; list the type(s).

    _____ Mother _____

    _____ Father _____

    _____ Sister _____

    _____ Brother _____

    _____ Paternal grandfather _____

    _____ Paternal grandmother _____

    _____ Maternal grandfather _____

    _____ Maternal grandmother _____

_____ I smoke cigarettes.

_____ I am constantly exposed to cigarette smoke at work or at home.

_____ I use smokeless tobacco.

_____ I live in a heavily polluted urban area.

_____ I work in one of the following industries:

    _____ Rubber   _____ Plastics

    _____ Paint and dye   _____ Cable

    _____ Petrochemical

_____ I am regularly exposed to one of the following substances:

    _____ Arsenic   _____ Asbestos

    _____ Benzene   _____ Benzidine

    _____ Coal combustion products   _____ Nickel compounds

    _____ Radiation   _____ Vinyl chloride

_____ My home, office, or school has high levels of radon gas.

_____ I have frequently gotten blistering, peeling sunburns.

_____ I am frequently exposed to sunlight and get a tan whenever possible.

_____ I have fair skin.

_____ I rarely use sunscreens.

(over)

_____ I am overweight or obese (I weigh more than 20% over my upper weight limit on a standard height-weight chart or have a measured body fat percentage above 25% [for males] or 30% [for females]).

_____ I am sedentary (I do not exercise at least three times per week).

_____ I eat a diet that is high in fat overall.

_____ I eat a diet that is low in fiber overall.

_____ My diet often includes the following:

    _____ Whole milk and milk products   _____ Beef, pork, poultry skin, egg yolks

    _____ Beer, wine, liquor   _____ Bacon, hot dogs, sausages, ham

    _____ Grilled or barbecued meats   _____ Moldy seeds, peanuts, or corn

_____ My diet seldom includes the following:

    _____ Cruciferous vegetables (cabbage, broccoli, cauliflower, brussels sprouts)

    _____ Yellow and orange fruits (apricots, cantaloupe, cherries, peaches, nectarines, mangoes, watermelon, persimmons, papayas)

    _____ Yellow and orange vegetables (carrots, yams, sweet potatoes, winter squash, pumpkin)

    _____ Dark-green leafy vegetables (broccoli, spinach, Swiss chard, kale, collard greens, sorrel)

    _____ Citrus fruits, tomatoes, strawberries, red peppers

    _____ Nuts and vegetable oils

    _____ Whole grains and dried beans (brown rice, kasha, bulgur, whole-grain breads, garbanzo beans, lentils, pinto beans)

For Women Only (Check statements that are true for you; ignore those that are not applicable.)

_____ I had early onset of first menstruation.

_____ My first pregnancy occurred late in life.

_____ I have never had a child.

_____ I had a child and did not breastfeed.

_____ I had prolonged high-dose estrogen treatment.

_____ I had late onset of menopause.

_____ I have had genital warts (exposure to HPV).

_____ I have genital herpes.

In addition to the factors mentioned here, early diagnosis is also important. Be sure you follow the guidelines for screening tests given in Table 12-3 in your textbook.

Your answers here can help you identify behaviors that you should change. Consider planning a behavior change program to alter one or more of your risky behaviors.

CHAPTER 13
Immunity and Infection

Multiple Choice

1. Any organism that causes disease is called a/an:
   a. allergen.
   b. pathogen.
   c. viral agent.
   d. parasite.

2. The release of histamines causes:
   a. infection.
   b. illness.
   c. contamination.
   d. inflammation.

3. The smallest pathogen, borderline between living and nonliving matter, is the:
   a. bacterium.
   b. protozoan.
   c. T-cell.
   d. virus.

4. Vaccines confer:
   a. attentuated organisms.
   b. toxoids.
   c. active immunity.
   d. passive immunity.

5. In most cases, antibiotics are useful against:
   a. bacteria.
   b. parasites.
   c. viruses.
   d. colds.

6. Which of the following statements about STDs is true?
   a. If you have syphilis or gonorrhea you will know it.
   b. STDs are preventable.
   c. STDs in the genitals cannot be transmitted to the mouth.
   d. You cannot have more than one STD at a time.

7. Which of the following STDs has been linked to increased risk of cervical cancer?
   a. herpes
   b. syphilis
   c. chlamydia
   d. genital warts

STUDY GUIDE

8. Epididymitis is an inflammation of the:
   a. urethra.
   b. testicles.
   c. nasal passages.
   d. rectum.

9. The patient who experiences repeatedly activated herpes infections is most likely to be treated with:
   a. antibody therapy.
   b. laser therapy.
   c. topical applications for pain relief.
   d. acyclovir.

10. Methods of protecting yourself against HIV will also protect you against:
    a. hepatitis A and B.
    b. hepatitis B and C.
    c. hepatitis C and A.
    d. hepatitis B only.

True or False

T F   1. Lymphocytes travel in both the bloodstream and the lymphatic system.

T F   2. The immune system "kicks in" only when you get sick.

T F   3. Acquired immunity is the ability of lymphocytes to "remember" previous infections.

T F   4. Allergic reactions occur when the immune system responds to a dangerous pathogen.

T F   5. Lyme disease can cause fetal damage.

T F   6. The most frequently prescribed drug for the treatment of syphilis is pentamidine.

T F   7. The customary treatment for pelvic inflammatory disease is penicillin.

T F   8. HIV is not spread through casual contact.

T F   9. All cases of AIDS, as defined by the Centers for Disease Control and Prevention, must be reported to public health authorities.

T F 10. Although it is expensive, there is a cure for herpes that includes treatment with zinc compounds, ointments, and ultrasound.

ANSWERS: Multiple Choice: 1. b; 2. d; 3. d; 4. c; 5. a; 6. b; 7. d; 8. b; 9. d; 10. b
True/False 1. T; 2. F; 3. T; 4. F; 5. T; 6. F; 7. T; 8. T; 9. T; 10. F

Name _____ Section _____ Date _____

WELLNESS WORKSHEET 13.1

Checklist for avoiding infection

The best thing you can do to prevent an infection is to limit your exposure to pathogens. The next best thing is to keep your immune system as strong as possible. Read through the following list of statements and check whether each is mostly true or mostly false for you.

True   False

Exposure to Pathogens

_____ _____ I receive drinking water from a clean supply.

_____ _____ The area in which I live has adequate sewage treatment.

_____ _____ I frequently wash my hands with soap and warm water.

_____ _____ I avoid close contact with people who are infectious with diseases transmitted via the respiratory route (e.g., influenza, chicken pox, and tuberculosis).

_____ _____ I do not use intravenous drugs.

When outdoors

_____ _____ When hiking or camping, I do not drink water from streams, rivers, or lakes without first purifying it.

_____ _____ I avoid exposure to insect bites.

_____ _____ When hiking in the woods or playing in a yard in an area where Lyme disease has been reported, I take appropriate precautions:

    _____ Cover as much of my body as possible with long pants and a long-sleeved shirt.

    _____ Tuck my shirt into my pants and my pants into my socks, shoes, or boots.

    _____ Wear light-colored, tightly woven fabrics.

    _____ Wear a hat.

    _____ Stay near the center of trails.

    _____ Check myself periodically for ticks.

    _____ Shower and shampoo after each outing.

    _____ Wash clothes and check equipment after each outing

    _____ Use an insect repellent containing DEET and a clothing spray containing the insecticide permethrin on my pants, shoes, and socks.

_____ _____ If I discover a tick attached to my skin, I remove it immediately in an appropriate

manner (fill in): _____

_____

_____

_____

(over)

STUDY GUIDE

True   False

In a sexual relationship

_____ _____ I am in a monogamous relationship with a mutually faithful, uninfected partner.

_____ _____ I use condoms with every act of intercourse.

_____ _____ I discuss STDs and prevention with new partners.

_____ _____ I avoid engaging in high-risk behaviors with any person who might carry the HIV virus.

In the kitchen

_____ _____ I wash my hands thoroughly with warm soapy water before and after handling food.

_____ _____ I don't let groceries sit in a warm car.

_____ _____ I avoid buying food in containers that leak, bulge, or are severely dented.

_____ _____ I use separate cutting boards for meat and for foods that will be eaten raw.

_____ _____ I thoroughly clean all equipment (cutting boards, counters, utensils) before and after use.

_____ _____ I wash fresh fruits and vegetables carefully to remove all dirt.

_____ _____ I cook all foods thoroughly, especially beef, poultry, fish, pork, and eggs.

_____ _____ I store foods below 40° F or above 140° F.

_____ _____ I do not leave cooked or refrigerated foods at room temperature for more than two hours.

_____ _____ I use only pasteurized milk.

_____ _____ I avoid coughing or sneezing over foods, even when I'm healthy.

_____ _____ I cover any cuts on my hands when cooking.

To Keep Your Immune System Healthy

_____ _____ I eat a balanced diet, following the guidelines presented in the Food Guide Pyramid and the Dietary Guidelines for Americans.

_____ _____ I maintain moderate weight.

_____ _____ I get eight hours of sleep per night.

_____ _____ I exercise regularly.

_____ _____ I have effective ways of coping with stress.

_____ _____ I get all recommended immunizations and booster shots (refer to Table 13-1 in your textbook).

False answers indicate areas where you could change your behavior to help avoid infectious diseases. Consider creating a behavior change strategy for any statement you checked false.

CHAPTER 14
The Challenge of Aging

Multiple Choice

1. The gradual decline in your ability to focus on objects close to you is called:
   a. presbyopia.
   b. osteoporosis.
   c. periodontitis.
   d. dendrites.

2. Which of the following statements about aging is true?
   a. Requirements for vitamins and minerals are lower for people over age 65.
   b. Glaucoma inevitably leads to blindness.
   c. The ability to hear high-pitched sounds increases with age.
   d. Alcohol and drug abuse are common problems among the elderly.

3. Glaucoma is elevated pressure in the:
   a. aorta.
   b. cerebral circulatory system.
   c. pulmonary artery.
   d. eye.

4. Which of the following is NOT associated with smoking?
   a. premature wrinkling
   b. premature balding
   c. glaucoma
   d. heart disease

5. Which of the following remains most stable in the aged?
   a. intelligence
   b. hearing
   c. eyesight
   d. flexibility

6. Which of the following is NOT a characteristic of brain death?
   a. unresponsivity
   b. incoherence
   c. flat EEG
   d. no movements of breathing

7. The testator of a will is the:
   a. attorney.
   b. person making the will.
   c. closest living relative.
   d. beneficiary of the will.

8. A hospice is:
   a. an institution where the dying are isolated from the rest of society.
   b. an institution that seeks to maximize quality of life for terminally ill patients.
   c. a hospital where people are kept alive with sophisticated equipment.
   d. a clinic where terminally ill patients go to test experimental treatments.

9. When someone dies without a will the state:
   a. distributes the property to the next of kin.
   b. appoints an administrator from the courts.
   c. puts the assets into the public coffers.
   d. pays the deceased's creditors before doing anything else.

10. Today, most people who die do so:
    a. with hospice involvement.
    b. at home.
    c. in a hospital or nursing home.
    d. under the direct care of a physician.

True or False

T F 1. A common physical consequence of aging is hearing loss.

T F 2. Behavior changes cannot extend the maximum human lifespan, which seems to be built into our genes.

T F 3. Alzheimer's disease is an incurable form of dementia.

T F 4. The average length of time we can expect to live is our lifespan.

T F 5. Males born in 1990 have a longer life expectancy than females born in the same year.

T F 6. Our attitudes toward death are formed in childhood and do not change considerably.

T F 7. It is ordinarily not possible to determine ahead of death how you want your body disposed.

T F 8. Acceptance is the final stage in Elisabeth Kübler-Ross' model of the psychological stages that a dying person experiences.

T F 9. Decisions about a will cannot be made until you are over 65.

T F 10. A person in a persistent vegetative state is responsive to stimuli.

ANSWERS: Multiple Choice: 1. a; 2. d; 3. d; 4. c; 5. a; 6. b; 7. b; 8. b; 9. b; 10. c
True/False 1. T; 2. T; 3. T; 4. F; 5. F; 6. F; 7. F; 8. T; 9. F; 10. F

Name _____   Section _____   Date _____

WELLNESS WORKSHEET 14.1

Are you prepared for aging?

Assess Your Current Behaviors

Are you doing everything you can now to enhance the quality of your life as you age? Read through the following list of statements and check the answer that best describes your current behavior.

Yes   No

____ ____ I exercise regularly.

____ ____ I eat wisely.

    ____ I eat meals high in complex carbohydrates (fresh fruits and vegetables, whole-grain cereals and breads, potatoes, brown rice, pasta)

    ____ I avoid saturated fats and get protein from fish and skinless poultry.

    ____ I use nonfat or low-fat dairy products.

    ____ I control caloric intake.

    ____ I limit the amount of sodium I consume.

____ ____ My weight is in the recommended range.

____ ____ I drink alcohol in moderation, if at all.

____ ____ I don't smoke or use smokeless tobacco.

____ ____ I recognize the stressors in my life and take appropriate steps to control and deal with stress.

____ ____ I perform appropriate self-examinations.

____ ____ I have regular physical examinations that include appropriate screening tests.

____ ____ I participate in activities that keep my mind sharp and active.

Thinking About Aging Have you thought seriously about the changes that aging can bring? To help you begin thinking now about your life as you grow older, answer the following questions.

1. What things come to mind when you think of an older person? Can you imagine those things applying to you? What do you think you will be like when you are 70 years old?

2. What do you most look forward to as you grow older?

(over)

STUDY GUIDE

3. What do you most fear as you grow older?

4. How long would you like to keep working? What would you like to do after you retire? What hobbies or volunteer opportunities would you pursue?

5. Have you considered the loss of income that retirement often brings? What can you do now to help meet your economic needs in the future?

6. Older people often find themselves alone more frequently (due to the death of a spouse and/ or close friends). Can you think of activities you enjoy doing alone?

7. If when you are older you are no longer able to care for yourself, what living and care arrangements would you prefer?

8. What would you do if your parents were no longer able to care for themselves?

9. List five positive and five negative things about aging.

CHAPTER 15
Environmental Health

Multiple Choice

1. In the future the population is likely to:
   a. increase least in developing countries.
   b. increase least in developed countries.
   c. decrease in developed countries and developing countries.
   d. decrease more in developing countries than developed countries.

2. The root of most environmental stress is:
   a. industrialization.
   b. population growth.
   c. urbanization.
   d. drought.

3. During the last century the highest priority in environmental health was controlling:
   a. infectious disease.
   b. air contamination.
   c. population growth.
   d. energy waste.

4. The increase in the concentrations of greenhouse gases is primarily the result of:
   a. the release of CFCs.
   b. energy use in the developed world.
   c. heavy metal contamination.
   d. deforestation.

5. Lead poisoning continues to be a serious problem particularly among children:
   a. who live in older buildings.
   b. had low birth weights.
   c. have not been vaccinated.
   d. have poor diets.

6. Which one of the following is a major source of acid rain pollutants?
   a. air conditioners.
   b. lead-based paints.
   c. synthetic building materials.
   d. coal-burning electric power plants.

7. The ozone layer protects the earth from excessive:
   a. radon exposure.
   b. nuclear radiation.
   c. ultraviolet radiation.
   d. chlorofluorocarbons.

8. A possible effect of exposure to excessive noise is:
   a. decibels.
   b. radiation.
   c. PCBs.
   d. tinnitus.

9. Faced with the vast array of confusing and complex ecological issues, people can accurately conclude all of the following EXCEPT:
   a. there isn't anything an individual can do.
   b. large corporations and manufacturers are primarily responsible.
   c. we can try to elect officials who have an environmental agenda.
   d. the little things individuals can do will make a difference.

10. A recent radiation concern related to certain soils, rocks, and building materials is:
   a. microwaves.
   b. asbestos.
   c. decibels.
   d. radon.

True or False

T F   1. We have reached a point in history when water is no longer a worldwide environmental concern.

T F   2. According to the World Health Organization, the majority of the world's people have an adequate water supply.

T F   3. Plastic waste makes up a larger proportion of waste than wood, glass, or food.

T F   4. It is estimated that each person in the United States suffers two to three episodes of food poisoning every year.

T F   5. Dust storms are a contributor to air pollution.

T F   6. The food distribution system in the United States is very safe and efficient.

T F   7. Many of the cases thought to be a 24-hour flu caused by a virus are actually episodes of food poisoning.

T F   8. Air pollution can cause illness and death.

T F   9. The thinning of the ozone layer of the atmosphere has thus far been confined to Antarctica.

T F   10. The problems associated with asbestos are minimal so long as it remains where it is applied and its protective coating is not disturbed.

ANSWERS: Multiple Choice: 1. b; 2. b; 3. a; 4. b; 5. a; 6. d; 7. c; 8. d; 9. a; 10. d
True/False 1. F; 2. F; 3. T; 4. T; 5. T; 6. T; 7. T; 8. T; 9. F; 10. T

_____ I recycle newspapers, glass, cans, and other materials.

_____ I have a compost pile or bin for my organic garbage or I take my organic garbage to a community composting center.

Reducing Chemical Pollution and Toxic Wastes

_____ When shopping, I read labels and try to buy the least toxic products available.

_____ I dispose of household hazardous wastes properly.

_____ If I am unsure of the proper way to dispose of something, I contact my local health department or environmental health office.

_____ Whenever possible, I buy organic produce or produce that is in season and has been grown locally.

Saving Water

_____ I take showers instead of baths.

_____ I take short showers and switch off the water when I'm not actively using it.

_____ I do not run the water while brushing my teeth, shaving, or hand-washing clothes or dishes.

_____ My sinks have aerators installed in them.

_____ My shower has a low-flow showerhead.

_____ I have a water displacement device in my toilet.

Preserving Wildlife and the Natural Environment

_____ I snip or rip plastic six-pack rings before discarding them.

_____ I don't buy products made from endangered species.

_____ When hiking or camping, I never leave anything behind.

Statements that you have not checked can help you identify behaviors that you can change to improve environmental health. Consider planning a behavior change program to alter one or more of your behaviors. To change some of the items listed, you may need the cooperation of your family and/or roommate(s). If there are environmental issues that are important to you, you can go beyond individual action by informing others, joining and volunteering your time to organizations working on environmental problems, and contacting your elected representatives.

WELLNESS WORKSHEET 15.1

Environmental health checklist

The following list of statements relates to your impact on the environment. Put a check next to the statements that are true for you.

Conserving Energy, Improving the Air

_____ I ride my bike, walk, use public transportation, or carpool in a fuel-efficient vehicle whenever possible.

_____ I keep my car tuned up and well maintained.

_____ I use only unleaded gas.

_____ My car tires are inflated at the proper pressure.

_____ I avoid jackrabbit starts and drive within the speed limit.

_____ I don't use my car's air conditioner when opening the window would suffice.

_____ My residence is well-insulated.

_____ Where possible, I use compact fluorescent bulbs instead of incandescent bulbs.

_____ I turn off lights and appliances when they are not in use.

_____ I avoid turning on heat or air conditioning whenever possible.

_____ I run the washing machine, dryer, and dishwasher only when they have full loads.

_____ I run the clothes dryer only as long as it takes my clothes to dry.

_____ I dry my hair with a towel rather than a hair dryer.

Saving the Ozone Layer

_____ I keep my car's air conditioner in good working order and have it serviced by a service station that recycles, rather than releases, CFCs.

_____ I check labels on aerosol cans and avoid those that contain CFCs.

_____ I avoid products containing methyl chloroform (1, 1, 1-trichloroethane).

_____ I don't have a halon fire extinguisher.

_____ I have an energy-efficient refrigerator, which I keep in good working order.

Reducing Garbage

_____ When shopping, I choose products with the least amount of packaging.

_____ I choose recycled and recyclable products.

_____ I avoid products packaged in plastic and unrecycled aluminum.

_____ I store food in glass jars and reusable plastic containers rather than using plastic wrap.

_____ I take my own bag along when I go shopping.

_____ Whenever possible, I use long-lasting or reusable products (such as refillable pens and rechargeable batteries).

(over)

STUDY GUIDE